"Hall and Flanagan's *Treatment of Childhood Disorders* represents a state-of-the-art engagement with evidence-based clinical child and adolescent psychology. It provides an extensive review of the related scientific psychopathology and treatment literature for each of the common disorders typically engaged in child psychopathology texts. This part of the work is done well enough to stand on its own as a useful survey of the field for clinicians and students in the mental health fields. Hall and Flanagan also address each area with thoughtful and informed analysis from both a developmental psychopathology and an integrative Christian perspective. The high-quality engagement with the influential literature in this specialty area is augmented by rich case examples that well illustrate the clinical issues and treatment approaches they cover. This will be an indispensable text for integrative Christian programs seeking to teach clinical child and adolescent psychology to graduate students. It also represents a valuable contribution for anyone in the broader field who seeks to culturally adapt evidenced-based clinical child and adolescent practice to Christian populations."

William L. Hathaway, dean and professor, the School of Psychology and Counseling at Regent University

---

Caring for the mental health of children and their families is complex and challenging —and meaningful. For Christian clinicians who work with childhood disorders, however, few resources exist to address such treatment from a research-based Christian integration perspective.

Treatment of Childhood Disorders fills this gap by combining biblical and theological understanding with current psychological literature on empirically supported treatments for children. Sarah E. Hall and Kelly S. Flanagan present an integrated approach based in developmental psychopathology that offers a dynamic, multifaceted framework from which to understand the processes that affect children's development.

In this unique textbook, Hall and Flanagan consider a variety of disorders commonly diagnosed in children and adolescents, including anxiety, depression, ADHD, and autism spectrum disorder. After discussing prevalence, risk and causal factors, patterns throughout development, and assessment, they focus on evidence-based practices that have been found to be effective in treating the disorders. Each chapter also features ideas for Christian integration in treatment and an extended case study that brings the content to life.

Sarah E. Hall (PhD, Pennsylvania State University) is associate professor of psychology, counseling, and family therapy at Wheaton College. With Kelly S. Flanagan she is the coeditor of *Christianity and Developmental Psychopathology*.

Kelly S. Flanagan (PhD, Pennsylvania State University) is clinical director of a pediatric development center in northwestern Illinois. She previously worked as associate professor of psychology and PsyD program director at Wheaton College.

Treatment *of* Childhood Disorders

Evidence-Based Practice in Christian Perspective

Sarah E. Hall & Kelly S. Flanagan

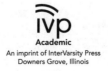

Academic

An imprint of InterVarsity Press
Downers Grove, Illinois

InterVarsity Press
P.O. Box 1400, Downers Grove, IL 60515-1426
ivpress.com
email@ivpress.com

InterVarsity Press® is the book-publishing division of InterVarsity Christian Fellowship/USA®, a movement of students and faculty active on campus at hundreds of universities, colleges, and schools of nursing in the United States of America, and a member movement of the International Fellowship of Evangelical Students. For information about local and regional activities, visit intervarsity.org.

While any stories in this book are true, some names and identifying information may have been changed to protect the privacy of individuals.

The publisher cannot verify the accuracy or functionality of website URLs used in this book beyond the date of publication.

Cover design and image composite: Autumn Short
Interior design: Daniel van Loon
Images: sketch backgrounds: © Ekateria Romanova / iStock / Getty Images
*   hands orange icon: © RobinOlimb / DigitalVision Vectors / Getty Images*

ISBN 978-0-8308-2868-5 (print)
ISBN 978-0-8308-2869-2 (digital)

Printed in the United States of America ♾

InterVarsity Press is committed to ecological stewardship and to the conservation of natural resources in all our operations. This book was printed using sustainably sourced paper.

Library of Congress Cataloging-in-Publication Data
A catalog record for this book is available from the Library of Congress.

P	27	26	25	24	23	22	21	20	19	18	17	16	15	14	13	12	11	10	9	8	7	6	5	4	3	2	1
Y	45	44	43	42	41	40	39	38	37	36	35	34	33	32	31	30	29	28	27	26	25	24	23	22	21		

To Jacob and Ian—SEH

To the brave children and families I work
with and learn from every day.
And to Caitlin, Quinn, and Aidan—you truly are gifts.—KSF

Contents

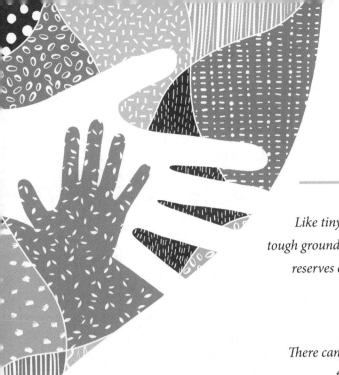

Introduction

*Like tiny seeds with potent power to push through
tough ground and become mighty trees, we hold innate
reserves of unimaginable strength. We are resilient.*

CATHERINE DEVRYE

*There can be no keener revelation of a society's soul
than the way in which it treats its children.*

NELSON MANDELA

OUR PURPOSE IN WRITING this book is to fill a need to integrate a thoughtful Christian perspective on child clinical psychology with the research about how to effectively treat psychological disorders in youth. As is widely recognized, children are not merely smaller versions of adults; their functioning and development are qualitatively different, as is the development and expression of psychopathology. The child clinical literature is well developed and addresses the unique characteristics of youth and the influences on them—and our collective knowledge of how and why certain symptoms manifest in some youth and not others is growing at a rapid rate as new studies build on previous work. However, the integrative literature has fallen behind. Many books and articles address clinical work with adults from a Christian perspective; however, much less has been written about clinical work with childhood disorders that is rooted in a biblical worldview, writing that should be foundational for Christian clinicians working with youth and their families. We are convinced of the value in combining all relevant sources of knowledge about psychopathology and treatment in youth. Therefore, in this volume we set out to fill what we see as a significant gap in the literature by integrating scientific child clinical research with a Christian perspective on children and childhood psychological disorders. Furthermore, we integrate these topics from the perspective of developmental psychopathology, which offers a dynamic, multifaceted framework from which to understand the pathways and processes that affect children's development, including the development of psychopathology, and thus identify the most effective approaches to treating disorders as informed by a variety of relevant perspectives.

To give our readers some personal background, we are both Christians who were trained in secular programs. We met as graduate students in child clinical psychology at Penn State, one in her first year and one in her last, and connected despite our cohort differences because we were two of the few Christians (that we were aware of) in the program. Our paths diverged as we continued in our training only to be connected again as faculty members at Wheaton College, an institution to which we were both drawn because of the emphasis on integrating our faith with scientifically based psychological theory, research, and practice. Though we taught in different programs (undergraduate and doctoral), we found common ground in our interest in combining our child clinical backgrounds and training in developmental psychopathology with a Christian perspective on disorders and treatment in childhood. These interests found their first major outlet in an edited book, *Christianity and Developmental Psychopathology: Foundations and Approaches,* published in 2014. When asked to coauthor a book that delved deeper into integration of a Christian viewpoint and specific child clinical research, for which the publishing company had been receiving requests, we chose to focus on evidence-based practice in the treatment of child and adolescent disorders to fill the void in the Christian psychological literature.

We hope and pray that the ideas we cover in this volume will be both empowering and challenging to current and future Christian clinicians who work with youth and families. Although the applications of these ideas will vary across clients—depending on their presenting problems, developmental stages, family situations, and religious and spiritual beliefs and practices—we recognize that we cannot separate our professional work from our theological understandings of the nature of human beings generally and children specifically. In the four parts of this book, we will cover the treatment of a variety of psychopathologies in youth. Part one provides two chapters of introductory material that is important for framing the disorder-specific parts of the book. The first chapter gives an overview of the field of developmental psychopathology and its implications for treatment, and introduces the concept of evidence-based practice in psychology (EBPP). The second chapter describes a Christian approach to treatment in general, taking into account best practices in the field in combination with biblical and theological principles. In part two, we review therapeutic approaches for internalizing disorders, in which the primary symptoms involve mood-related problems and their correlates; the three chapters in this part cover mood disorders, anxiety disorders, and posttraumatic stress disorder. In part three, we cover externalizing disorders, in two chapters on disruptive behavior disorders and attention-deficit/hyperactivity disorder. Finally, in part four, we discuss the treatment of autism spectrum disorder and eating disorders, which are other disorders that commonly affect youth. We also provide suggestions for approaching disorders with more theological complexity and less clear-cut treatment recommendations in a chapter that uses gender dysphoria as an illustration.

Within each disorder-specific chapter, we outline the diagnostic criteria, risk factors, developmental course, and assessment recommendations for the disorder(s). We then review the research on the most effective psychosocial interventions. Next, we explore integrative considerations in treatment that interweave psychologically based research and understandings of the disorder(s) with biblical and theological principles. Finally, we end each chapter with a case study that illustrates how risk factors, developmental considerations, and the application of empirically supported interventions might play out for individual youths and their families. We include these case studies in order to take the material from the theoretical to the practical, as our hope is that they will provide developing and practicing clinicians with examples of how the principles we have laid out might be applied in real-life clinical situations and of a variety of ways that integration may occur depending on client, family, clinician, and symptom variation. The case examples also highlight that no treatment is truly straightforward but rather requires individualization of evidence-based strategies. They are not meant to provide steps to follow but rather to illustrate some ways that a practicing integrationist might manage different issues that arise over the course of therapy and to inspire and encourage you as you integrate developmental psychopathology, evidence-based practice in psychology, and your Christian faith in your work with young clients.

Part One

Foundations

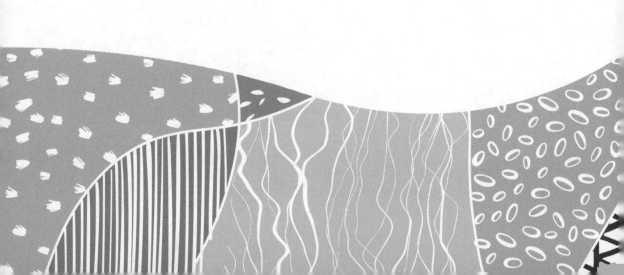

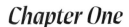

Chapter One

Developmental Psychopathology and Evidence-Based Practice

DEVELOPMENTAL PSYCHOPATHOLOGY

In 1984, *Child Development*, a prominent scientific journal, dedicated its first issue of the year to articles describing a burgeoning framework known as developmental psychopathology. This unique perspective combined the strengths of the previously largely separate fields of developmental psychology and clinical psychology in an effort to understand the complex dynamics that affect children's well-being (Sroufe & Rutter, 1984). In contrast to traditional, adult-oriented approaches to understanding psychopathology, developmental psychopathology focuses on individual pathways toward or away from disorder, taking into account the multitude of influences on the course of development from childhood through adulthood. Developmental psychopathologists recognize the value in studying youth who thrive throughout development, those who experience early hardship and subsequent or later disorder, children who survive highly adverse experiences yet bounce back, and individuals with seemingly low-risk early experiences but who develop psychopathology later in their lives. Prior to these initial writings in developmental psychopathology, clinicians and researchers generally only focused on the presentation of disorder at a given point in time in understanding psychopathology and treatment, missing the rich information that could be provided by a developmentally informed perspective that considers both normal and abnormal development. Since research based in a developmental psychopathology framework began in the 1970s, our understanding of the factors and processes that influence the course of development has increased exponentially. Still, much work remains to be done as we seek to understand how to treat and prevent psychopathology in youth in a manner thoughtfully informed by both research and clinical experience. In this chapter, we outline several key features of a developmental psychopathology–based approach to disorder and treatment and describe evidence-based practice in psychology.

NORMALCY AND ABNORMALITY

Though normal development and abnormal behavior have traditionally been studied separately, developmental psychopathology brings them together as developmental models are used to understand maladaptation over time. In other words, the study of normal development and the study of abnormal development inform one another (Hinshaw, 2017). On one hand, we cannot identify abnormalities unless we first understand the range of what is considered normal. We can only understand whether an older child's fears may be problematic if we understand the typical emotional experiences of similar-age youth. In order to identify toddlers whose delayed language development suggests that they are at risk for autism spectrum disorder (ASD), we need to know what communication skills are typical or normative at a given age. Indeed, the American Academy of Pediatrics recommends that all children be screened at eighteen- and twenty-four-month well-child visits for social and communication delays that may be signs of an ASD (Zwaigenbaum et al., 2015). On the other hand, research with youth who experience developmental abnormalities, including psychological disorders, contributes to our understanding of normal development. For example, studies of how maternal depression negatively affects infants' well-being gives us a better understanding of the dynamic, reciprocal interchanges between mother and baby that support the typical development of secure attachment, social communication, emotion regulation, stress reactivity, and even

cognitive abilities (Goodman & Brand, 2009). This perspective emphasizes continuities in development, even in the case of maladaptation, rather than the discontinuity between health and disorder traditionally highlighted in the study of psychopathology (Rutter & Garmezy, 1983). Therefore, a developmental psychopathology–based approach to treatment considers the literature on both normal and abnormal development.

Furthermore, psychopathology is conceptualized not as a disease state but as the result of development (Sameroff, 2014; Sroufe, 1997). Classic medical models understand psychological disorders as parallel to organic diseases, and traditional psychological approaches embrace some of their implicit assumptions. For example, the most commonly used diagnostic manuals contain categories of disorders with discrete names and symptom lists that rarely mention environmental factors. In contrast, developmental psychopathologists understand psychological disorders as the product of developmental progression that unfolds over time within a particular context. Furthermore, normal and abnormal development are not so much different processes as they are reflections of the same process as it is influenced by a variety of factors. Human behavior is understood to be an adaptation to the demands of the environment; some behaviors are healthy and others are problematic, but they all arise out of an individual's efforts to survive and thrive and navigate developmental tasks within a given context. For example, growing up with sensitive, authoritative parents, a child learns to express and manage anger by taking deep breaths and talking to a trusted adult as her parents teach her these techniques and model them in their own times of anger. In contrast, a child who grows up in an abusive household learns either to express her anger explosively and aggressively (as she imitates her parents) or not to express it in any way (since such expressions may call attention to herself and result in abuse), neither of which is the ideal manner for learning to manage strong emotions. Though these outcomes are dramatically different, the developmental processes therein—learning via modeling, regulating emotions in a way that promotes desired responses from others, and parenting as a significant contributor to children's behavior—are the same.

In addition, the boundaries between normal and abnormal behavior and development are often blurred (Cicchetti, 2006). Individuals are not best categorized as disordered or nondisordered; rather, states and behaviors at a given point are characterized as more or less adaptive, and individuals move between states of well-being and states of maladaptation depending on the interaction between the demands of the environment and their current development stage. A child with an anxiety disorder may display a high level of functioning at times, even in situations that are often anxiety provoking for her. An eating disorder may occur, remit, and recur as stressors ebb and flow across adolescence. Furthermore, youth at high risk for disorder may develop normally and healthily, whereas others who appear to be at low risk may unpredictably develop psychopathology. Rather than focus on end states of health or disorder, developmental psychopathologists argue that we must understand the pathway a given individual follows across development in order to best understand their outcomes and the factors that affect them.

DEVELOPMENTAL PATHWAYS

In a developmental model of disorder, psychopathology is considered an outcome of development, which suggests that we must understand how developmental processes unfold over time. In other words, individuals follow unique developmental pathways that lead them closer to or further from positive mental health outcomes (Sroufe, 1997). Common images of the variety of developmental pathways among children and even within an individual's lifespan include the numerous splitting and merging tracks at a train yard or a mature tree with branches reaching in many directions. The concept of developmental pathways necessitates understandings of both normal and abnormal development, as discussed previously. In order to identify progression toward problematic or abnormal outcomes, we must first know what constitutes normal or healthy development. In addition, a pathways-based approach suggests that there are many different courses from early to later development (Cicchetti & Rogosch, 1996; Sroufe, 1997). Two youth can experience similar early circumstances and deviate toward disparate outcomes, a pattern known as multifinality. For example, identical twins have a high concordance for schizophrenia occurrence due to the strong genetic underpinnings of the disorder; however, only about 50% of individuals with an identical twin with schizophrenia will develop symptoms (Gejman et al., 2010). This pattern, while highlighting the high heritability of the disorder, also suggests that differences in environmental exposures and experiences likely affect whether a high-risk genotype is ever expressed as schizophrenia. Similarly, siblings who grow up in the same home (i.e., sharing parents, economic resources, neighborhood variables, and schools) may diverge in mental health and other outcomes, particularly as they age. Alternately, the concept of equifinality explains that individuals with the same disorder may have followed different developmental pathways to arrive at the same end point. For instance, research on the etiology of anxiety suggests that it may develop as the result of a variety of genetic influences, endocrine dysregulation, temperamental predispositions, attachment and parenting patterns, and environmental conditioning (see chapter four).

The variety of developmental pathways that exist from early to later experiences and outcomes also highlights two competing ideas: development is both subject to change and constrained by prior development. On the one hand, there are many points in development when an individual's course may change. A child with a close relationship with her parents becomes distant and withdrawn following a period of bullying at school; an adolescent who lives in a poor, violent neighborhood seems increasingly likely to join a gang until an after-school job connects him with positive role models who help him consider a variety of choices. As we will discuss in more detail below, children are both vulnerable and resilient, and there are essentially an infinite number of pathways along which development can proceed as it is influenced by a wide variety of internal and external factors. However, development does not generally turn on a dime. Early developmental milestones and patterns set the stage for future behaviors and outcomes. Many classic developmental theorists describe this continuity (e.g., Erikson, 1950), and more recent

research supports it as well (e.g., Halligan et al., 2013; Neppl et al., 2010). This pattern of continuity is especially true for maladaptation; long periods of problematic behavior and negative environmental influences may deprive an individual of the opportunity to master developmentally appropriate tasks and gain the skills necessary to respond to the demands of their environment in an adaptive manner (Sroufe, 1997). For instance, a child who experiences ongoing abuse that disrupts her attachment to her parents may have trouble interacting appropriately with peers and teachers when she begins school, and as a result, she may miss out on crucial opportunities to build social skills and self-confidence in relationships with others; by adolescence, she is completely socially isolated and lacks both the social skills and support that teenagers typically rely on as they navigate the developmental challenges of this period.

RISK AND PROTECTIVE FACTORS

The course of an individual developmental pathway is not random or unpredictable; rather, it is affected by a multitude of influences within and around a child across development. These influences are known generally as risk and protective factors. A risk factor is any characteristic, influence, or experience that heightens the likelihood of a negative outcome. Risk factors can originate from many sources, including individual-level characteristics, the prenatal environment, families, peers, and the broader culture in which a child is embedded. In the disorder-focused chapters of this book, we explore a wide variety of risk factors, including certain genotypes, prenatal toxin exposure, dysfunctional family dynamics, and individual cognitive patterns. The goals of studying risk factors include both understanding the dynamics of how disorder develops and identifying who is at the highest risk for negative outcomes. To these ends, risk research is most useful for prevention and intervention when it identifies risk factors that are truly causal (rather than merely correlated with or markers of risk) as well as the mechanisms by which these factors raise the likelihood of maladaptation (Cicchetti, 2006; Grant et al., 2003).

Risk is both complex and dynamic. For many youth exposed to stressors, risk factors do not occur in isolation but alongside other risks (Sameroff et al., 1993; Sameroff, Seifer, Zax, & Barocas, 1987). Furthermore, risk has a cumulative effect, such that exposure to multiple risk factors exponentially increases the risk of a negative outcome, beyond what would be expected based on the individual effects of each risk factor by itself (Biederman et al., 1995; Sameroff et al., 1993; Sameroff, Seifer, Barocas, Zax, & Greenspan, 1987). Cumulative risk may negatively impact development by overwhelming a child's ability to cope with repeated and/or chronic stress (Evans et al., 2013; Evans & Kim, 2007). In addition, risk is generally nonspecific; particular variables raise an individual's risk of experiencing not only one but multiple disorders or negative outcomes (Atkinson et al., 2015). For example, maltreatment raises an individual's risk for a wide variety of mental health problems throughout childhood, adolescence, and adulthood (Jaffe, 2017). Similarly, disorders are not usually caused by a single risk factor but by exposure to variables that affect multiple developmental processes, often in interaction with one another. For example, posttraumatic stress disorder (PTSD) does

not automatically develop after exposure to a trauma; rather, whether PTSD develops is likely the result of a combination of biological, psychological, and interpersonal factors (see chapter five). Youth are at heightened risk for eating disorders when their exposure to a thin-body ideal in the media interacts with parental criticism of their weight to produce internalized body dissatisfaction (see chapter nine). Finally, risk factors are dynamic. When researchers operationalize a risk factor and consider individuals to be exposed or not exposed, they may oversimplify how risk is experienced differently by different individuals, depending on both the characteristics of the risk factor in question and how it interacts with other variables. For example, it is clear from decades of research that poverty has a deleterious effect on children's development. However, the experience of poverty is multifaceted and variable, and factors such as length of exposure (i.e., transient versus chronic poverty) and timing of exposure (i.e., early versus later childhood) may both affect youth differently and reflect the degree to which other risk factors (e.g., parental unemployment, housing instability, low levels of social support) are present (Kimberlin & Berrick, 2015).

However, risk factors are not deterministic; exposure to even a high level of a variable associated with negative outcomes does not guarantee them. Rather, risk factors interact with protective factors, influences linked with positive developmental outcomes (Luthar & Cicchetti, 2000). Protective factors can occur in all realms of influence on a child, including within the individual herself (e.g., good emotion regulation skills; Lengua, 2002), within the family (e.g., authoritative parenting; Fletcher et al., 2004), and in school or neighborhood contexts (e.g., sense of connection to school; Hawkins et al., 1999). These positive influences also impact risk exposure in different ways (Luthar, Cicchetti, & Becker, 2000). First, some factors are *promotive*, being linked with positive outcomes no matter the level of risk. For example, secure attachment in infancy predicts higher social competence and lower rates of emotional and behavioral problems later in childhood (Groh et al., 2014). Second, *protective-stabilizing factors* ameliorate the effects of risk on outcomes; inner-city adolescents who are exposed to violence do not experience increases in emotional distress when they report high levels of family support, in contrast to peers who feel less supported (Howard et al., 2010). Third, the presence of *protective-enhancing* factors leads to higher levels of competence in the presence of higher (versus lower) levels of stress. For example, among adolescent girls in Columbia, disclosure of thoughts and feelings to their mothers reduces feelings of hopelessness more in those who are exposed to violence than in those who are not (Kliewer et al., 2001). Fourth, *protective-reactive* factors ameliorate some but not all of the negative effects of risk exposure. For instance, parental aspirations for their children's education are correlated with adolescents' exam performance, but this link is weaker for youth from lower socioeconomic status (SES) backgrounds (Schoon et al., 2004). However, like risk factors, protective or promotive factors are probabilistic, linked statistically with a lower likelihood of negative outcomes but interacting with other variables to produce unique outcomes for any given youth. Also like with risk factors, research on protective factors is likely most impactful when it ex-

plores not only markers of protection but the mechanisms by which these factors promote positive outcomes; when mechanisms are identifiable, researchers and clinicians can incorporate them into interventions and prevention programs. For example, the Fast Track project was developed to promote positive outcomes in young children at high risk for academic and behavioral problems, including delinquency; a multifaceted intervention was designed to target emotional competence, social skills, self-control, reading abilities, and parenting skills through both school- and home-based treatment components. By targeting the mechanisms by which these youth were more likely than their peers to develop conduct problems, Fast Track has been found to be effective in reducing these negative outcomes even into early adulthood (Conduct Problems Prevention Research Group, 2011; Sorensen et al., 2016).

Some youth exhibit resilience, adapting well and displaying competence despite threats to healthy development (Masten, 2014; Masten & Coatsworth, 1998). Many youth who are born small or experience abuse or grow up in very impoverished families will not develop the negative outcomes for which these life experiences put them at heightened risk. These individuals display resilience due to the effect of protective factors that ameliorate the negative effects of risk. The definition of competence, commonly considered to be evidence of resilience, has varied widely in the literature (Masten & Coatsworth, 1995, 1998; Masten, 2014; Werner & Smith, 1992). Youth are generally considered competent when they adapt successfully to the demands of their environments; practically, competence may be operationalized as successfully navigating developmental tasks, including displaying socially acceptable behavior, succeeding in academics or work, forming healthy relationships, or having a subjective sense of success. Sometimes, competence is assumed in the absence of negative outcomes such as mental health problems or significant relationship failures (e.g., divorce), though the presence of positive indicators is more commonly emphasized. Furthermore, competence does not have to be continuously displayed throughout development for an individual to be considered resilient; rather, there are multiple pathways of resilience (Masten, 2014). Some resilient youth may appear to be essentially unaffected by risk, whereas others may experience either growth or a temporary decline in functioning following risk exposure after which functioning eventually improves. The interplay between risk and protective factors is dynamic, complex, and unique for individual youth; identifying such factors at a given point in time helps us predict who is likely to be more resilient but cannot definitively identify who will and will not overcome the effects of negative development experiences. However, understanding the various pathways from stress exposure to competence, in addition to the factors that promote healthy functioning and resilience, is crucial to designing effective prevention and intervention programs for youth at risk for psychopathology.

ROLE OF ENVIRONMENT AND CONTEXT

Broadly speaking, one of the most important sources of influence on a child's positive or negative development is the environment. Youth are embedded in multiple systems—family, school, neighborhood, peer group, religious community, broader culture, and particular point in history—which influence the child individually and through their interactions with one another (Bronfenbrenner, 1979). Developmental psychopathologists emphasize the role of the environment as both influencing behavior and providing a context within which development must be understood. The environment in which a child lives and functions provides a crucial set of influences on development. A review of the research on risk for psychopathology, such as the summary we provide near the beginning of each disorder-specific chapter of this volume, provides clear evidence that psychological disorders do not develop based solely on biological or genetic risk but as the result of both biological and environmental factors. For example, depression in youth appears to result from both genetic factors (e.g., a particular serotonin transporter promoter region genotype) and environmental factors (e.g., high stress exposure, family conflict), which likely combine to result in particular maladaptive patterns of individuals' functioning (e.g., cognitive distortions, rumination, emotional dysregulation; see chapter three for a review). Furthermore, the environment may play a more significant role than genetics in the development of psychopathology, especially in youth. The Rochester Longitudinal Study, which examined the effects of maternal schizophrenia and its correlates on children's outcomes from birth through age thirteen, found social and environmental predictors to have a bigger impact on children's development than mothers' diagnostic status. In other words, the genetic transmission of schizophrenia risk was less influential in children's behavioral, emotional, and cognitive outcomes than environmental variables such as parenting behaviors, family socioeconomic status, and stressful life experiences (Sameroff, Seifer, Zax, & Barocas, 1987; Sameroff et al., 1993). Recognizing the role of the environment in the development of psychopathology has important implications for prevention and intervention: "From a developmental psychopathology point of view, maladaptive behavior is caused by maladaptive environment; if we change those environments, we alter the behavior" (Lewis, 2014, p. 10).

However, the environment does not merely affect the individual in a one-way interaction; rather, the individual and the environment influence and change each other. This dynamic, two-way interaction is known as a transactional or transformational model of development (Lewis, 2014); a similar idea is found in the relational developmental systems paradigm (Overton, 2013). For example, a child may experience anxiety about starting school for the first time. In turn, manifestations of the child's anxiety actually change his environment (mainly in terms of the responses of other people). Perhaps sensitive parents spend extra time talking to the child to find out the specific causes of his worries about school; his teacher gives him the task of feeding the class hamster each day, which he looks forward to doing and which helps him view his presence at school as important; and a particularly empathic peer frequently seeks him out at recess so that he does not feel isolated. As these environmental responses occur, the child's anxiety decreases, and parents and teachers no longer need to make special efforts to reassure and comfort the child. The process of development is a series of back-and-forth interactions in which the youth and his environment are constantly

being affected by one another. Indeed, even as we recognize a child's context as a source of significant influences on her development, we cannot understand the nature of environmental influence without considering the characteristics of the individual (Hinshaw, 2017). Therefore, as we work to reduce the occurrence and negative effects of psychopathology in youth, we must consider how symptoms are created and perpetuated by the dynamic interaction between a child and her context. Throughout this volume, we discuss research elucidating the ways in which a child's individual characteristics interact with the environment in the determination of pathways and outcomes.

In addition, the environment provides a context within which we must view a child's development and behavior if we are to understand whether it is positive or problematic. We cannot know whether a child's running leaps are signs of developmentally appropriate activity or misbehavior if we do not know whether he is at recess or in math class. Spending a significant amount of time thinking about a difficult and stressful problem may lead to a creative invention when the target of the intense thought is a school project but could lead to depression when the focus is on the loss of a significant relationship. As youth age, they normatively gain the skills to make more nuanced adjustments to their own behavior based on the demands of a situation, but some youth may still exhibit behavior that is context inappropriate (whether due to psychopathology or other causes). Furthermore, exploring a child's environment allows for an understanding of how particular behaviors, even undesirable ones, are adaptive within their contexts. Developmental psychopathologists understand human behaviors to be attempts to adapt to the demands of the situation (Sroufe & Rutter, 1984; Sroufe, 1997). For example, biting another person can be a way for a young child to express strong anger and/or an attempt to make another person acquiesce to the child's wants (e.g., getting a toy back). Social withdrawal in depression can be understood as a way to reduce exposure to peer interactions that contribute to distressing thoughts and negative emotions. An adolescent with an eating disorder may restrict her food intake as a way of gaining a sense of control in a highly conflictual or emotionally overinvolved family. In all of these examples, intervening effectively with these clients and families necessitates an accurate understanding of the child's interaction with her environment and how the behavior serves an adaptive purpose for the youth.

Finally, all analysis of the adaptive or maladaptive nature of behavior must occur within the context of a child's age and developmental status (Cicchetti, 2006). An extended fit of crying when a child is not allowed to have his way might be clinically concerning in a fourteen-year-old but relatively normative in a two-year-old. The fears and anxieties that are common in youth change from early to later childhood (Muris et al., 2000). However, it is important to note that symptoms should not automatically be dismissed if they are common or developmentally normative; other aspects of the behavior, including its frequency and intensity and the impact on child and family functioning, need to be considered in determining whether and what type of intervention will be most beneficial. As we discuss throughout this volume,

symptoms and disorders may also present differently at various points throughout development; for example, in youth with bipolar disorder, the most salient depressive and manic symptoms change across development (Demeter et al., 2013; Freeman et al., 2011). Clinicians who work with youth must have a good working knowledge of normal development as well as how children's behavior may represent an attempt to adapt to the demands of the environment, remembering that the underlying developmental processes are the same whether the context promotes positive or problematic behavior.

EVIDENCE-BASED PRACTICE IN PSYCHOLOGY

The themes of developmental psychopathology are central to shaping a dynamic and complex view of youth and psychopathology, but they do not provide information about specifically how to most effectively treat disorders in childhood and adolescence. We find the most helpful framework for developing effective treatments for individual youth to be evidence-based practice in psychology (EBPP), which is "the integration of the best available research with clinical expertise in the context of [client] characteristics, culture, and preferences" (APA Presidential Task Force on Evidence-Based Practice, 2006, p. 273). Other authors have referred to the idea of utilizing therapist and client characteristics to inform the application of evidence-based treatment as "flexibility within fidelity" (Kendall et al., 2008). EBPP is generally considered the best approach to working effectively with clients across the lifespan in a variety of clinical tasks, including assessment, case formulation, and treatment. EBPP emphasizes three main sources of information and consideration in the treatment process: treatment research, clinical expertise, and client characteristics.

TREATMENT RESEARCH

There is an ever-growing body of literature examining the effectiveness of different treatment approaches for specific disorders in particular populations, including children and adolescents. Interventions that have been found by high-quality research to be effective psychological treatments are referred to as empirically supported treatments (ESTs; Chambless & Hollon, 1998) or evidence-based treatments (EBTs; Kazdin, 2008). Treatments are judged as empirically supported for specific disorders with specific populations. Research on ESTs should address two main issues: whether a treatment has been found to be efficacious in a highly controlled research setting and whether it is effective and useful in actual clinical settings (American Psychological Association, 2002; Chambless & Hollon, 1998). There are important differences between the studies that evaluate these two distinct but related questions, and both types of research are critical for understanding the clinical impact of an intervention.

Efficacy research aims to determine whether a particular intervention is effective in a research setting in which confounding variables and outside influences on client outcomes are as well controlled as possible. A number of practices characterize efficacy studies, including recruiting participants for the purpose of the study, conducting the intervention in a research setting, excluding individuals with comorbid or complex conditions, and utilizing appropriately trained researchers to administer the treatment over a fixed number of sessions (Weisz et al., 1995). In efficacy studies, the target intervention is generally compared to either another treatment or no intervention (with participants in such studies usually placed in a waitlist condition in which they will receive treatment at a later date in order to reduce ethical concerns). Randomized controlled trials (RCTs), in which participants are randomly assigned to one of the treatment groups, are commonly used to examine treatment efficacy. The main goal of this research design is to determine whether the treatment itself is the source of changes in symptoms; to this end, efficacy studies emphasize internal validity, aiming to establish the clearest cause-and-effect link possible between treatment and outcome by minimizing confounding factors. Based on efficacy research results, treatments are given one of four labels that summarize the strength of their evidence base (Chambless & Hollon, 1998; Silverman & Hinshaw, 2008). In order to be considered *well established* or *efficacious*, an intervention must be found to be either superior to a placebo or superior or equivalent to an established treatment in research conducted by two independent groups. In addition, this research must use a treatment manual, identify clear and consistent inclusion criteria, and assess participants' outcomes in a manner than is reliable and valid. The requirement of replication by more than one research group before a treatment is considered well established helps guard against bias or the limited usefulness of an intervention to a particular sample. *Probably efficacious* interventions are those which have been found by two studies to be more effective than a wait-list control or meet the well-established criteria based on research from only one research group. Psychosocial treatments are categorized as *possibly efficacious* if there is research evidence that supports the intervention but does not meet the criteria for a stronger rating, and treatments which have not yet been studied using sufficiently rigorous methodology are considered *experimental*. Efficacy is necessary but not sufficient to show that an intervention can reduce symptoms for clients in true clinical settings.

In contrast, studies of treatment effectiveness or clinical utility examine whether a particular treatment reduces target symptoms in a wider variety of clients being treated in "real life" clinical settings, including private practices, community mental health centers, hospitals, and schools. Effectiveness studies aim to maximize external validity, or the generalizability of findings, across a variety of clients as well as a variety of individual clinicians and clinical settings. To this end, these studies generally take place in clinical rather than research settings, use participants who have been referred for treatment for a presenting problem rather than recruited for the purpose of research (including participants with comorbid disorders or more complex clinical presentations), and employ clinicians to administer the intervention. Effectiveness studies are often conducted on interventions that have previously been found to be efficacious in order to determine their generalizability and feasibility within a wider range of clients and settings. For example, once a psychosocial treatment for social anxiety has been found to be efficacious in a research setting, it could be implemented within a classroom setting to see whether it is effective

as a school-based intervention. Not surprisingly, effectiveness studies generally produce much smaller effect sizes than efficacy research (Weisz et al., 1995). It is important to note that efficacy and effectiveness studies do not have to be completely separate; RCTs in which participants are randomly assigned to treatment conditions can be conducted in clinical settings and be administered by appropriately trained clinicians, increasing both internal and external validity (Chambless & Hollon, 1998).

CLINICAL EXPERTISE

EBPP values treatment research as an important component of treatment planning, but it does not consider a knowledge of ESTs to be sufficient for effective treatment (APA Presidential Task Force, 2006). Rather, clinicians must draw from treatment research in addition to their clinical expertise in order to develop and implement the intervention that is most likely to be effective for a given client. Clinical expertise is a clinician's ability to work effectively with clients that results from both formalized training and practical experience. Because people and problems are complex, standardized, systematic clinical trials cannot capture a full picture of the best practice in every therapy session. The ability to respond in the best manner possible to an individual client in a given moment is based not only on a strong empirical knowledge about disorders and interventions but also on an individual therapist's skill set. The complexity of effective clinical practice is captured in the common view that therapy is both an art and a science (e.g., Goodheart, 2006) that must draw from personal, subjective views and experiences as well as treatment research.

Clinical expertise can be manifested in a variety of clinical activities and skills and individual qualities (APA Presidential Task Force, 2006). Therapists with clinical expertise are skilled at assessing clients' symptoms and strengths and diagnosing accurately, conceptualizing cases thoughtfully, planning and implementing appropriate treatments that are likely to be helpful, and assessing treatment effectiveness and clients' well-being throughout the intervention and changing the course of treatment when necessary. They are aware of how client variables and contexts—such as age, culture, race, sexuality and gender, religious beliefs, and socioeconomic status—affect their experiences and values and tailor interventions appropriately. Expert therapists are interpersonally skilled, able to understand clients' verbal and nonverbal communication, express empathy, and build trust-based therapeutic alliances. In addition, such clinicians recognize their own abilities and limitations, displaying good self-awareness, understanding and limiting the effects of personal biases, and continuing to build clinical skills and knowledge through continuing education, training, reading, and consultation with other professionals. Finally, clinical expertise includes the ability to evaluate treatment and other clinical research critically.

CLIENT CHARACTERISTICS

Finally, evidence-based treatment approaches and clinical expertise are not applied in a vacuum; rather, they are used to help real people with unique needs, characteristics, and circumstances. Therefore, EBPP also involves taking these factors into account in the design and implementation of the most effective intervention possible (APA Presidential Task Force, 2006). Client characteristics that treatment providers may need to consider include age, developmental level, comorbid presenting problems, culture, race and ethnicity, socioeconomic status, gender and gender identity, sexual orientation, disability, family structure and dynamics, environmental context, stressors, personality, personal strengths, religious beliefs, values, and treatment preferences and expectations. Treatment research is seen as the starting point for selecting an intervention, but there is recognition that this research is conducted with a particular participant group which may range from very similar to very dissimilar to the client with whom a therapist is working. Furthermore, because there are many variables to consider, it is difficult to draw clear conclusions about the degree to which a client's characteristics are likely to impact the effectiveness of an empirically supported treatment. What differences are likely to interfere with the effectiveness of a treatment approach? How should a clinician utilize an intervention that was developed to treat depression in high socioeconomic status Asian female adolescents with no other diagnoses if her client is an eleven-year-old poor white male with comorbid anxiety? Is this intervention likely to be effective in spite of the differences between her client and the research population? In what ways might she adapt the intervention to better fit her client's characteristics, as she draws on her clinical expertise to make these decisions?

The importance of considering cultural influences on and variations between individuals in particular has received increasing attention in the clinical literature. Culture, which is defined as the practices, beliefs, and experiences shaped by one's membership in a particular group (Arnett & Jensen, 2019), is relevant for the clinical context for a number of reasons. Culture affects how psychological disorders and their causes are conceptualized, common symptoms or clinical presentations, whether and what type of treatment is sought, social stigma, and the dynamics of and assumptions about the relationship between client and clinician (Chen, Fu, & Leng, 2014; Comas-Díaz, 2006; Hall et al., 2016; Weisz et al., 1997). In addition, cultural variables need to be considered in applying or adapting empirically supported interventions with any particular youth and family. Sometimes interventions have been formally adapted and assessed with culturally, racially, and/or ethnically diverse youth (Huey & Polo, 2018; Murray et al., 2014). However, this work is very limited (Pina et al., 2019), and clinicians may need to modify a treatment after they engage in their own assessment of the client's cultural background and context. Culturally competent clinicians (1) work to be aware of their own views and biases, (2) empathically engage with clients from different cultural backgrounds in order to understand their worldviews, and (3) utilize culturally sensitive and appropriate interventions and clinical skills (Sue & Sue, 2013). Multicultural competence entails not only professional elements but also personal exploration. Though the task of working effectively and sensitively with culturally diverse youth and families is demanding, it is extremely important as we seek to serve all clients well in response to both ethical and theological principles. It is challenging to find specifically youth-oriented writings; however, many authors offer guiding principles for

working well with diverse adult clients (e.g., Ivey et al., 2011; La Roche et al., 2017; Sue & Sue, 2013; Suzuki et al., 2017).

The developmental psychopathology emphasis on context and the interaction between the individual and his environment similarly emphasizes the importance of considering client-level factors in assessment and treatment. McMahon and Frick (2005, 2007) present three areas that should be assessed when working with children with behavior problems; although their discussion focuses on disruptive behavior disorders, their recommendations are useful for clinicians working with any children within a developmental psychopathology framework. First, clinicians must assess the specific pattern and severity of symptoms a child is displaying as well as the level and type of impairment that results. For example, a child with autism spectrum disorder may have symptoms ranging from mild difficulties with social interactions and highly focused interests to profound difficulties with social communication and repetitive, self-injurious behavior. Assessing severity and impairment highlights the main targets of treatment, which will vary across children. Furthermore, on the far end of the spectrum, comprehensive assessment encourages clinicians to determine whether intervention is even necessary, which it may not be for a child who is displaying age-normative behavior that does not result in significant or lasting impairment. In addition, it may be helpful for clinicians and parents to assess the antecedents, consequences, and function of a particular symptom in order to understand the purpose it may serve for the child (Hanley, 2012). The most effective intervention for a child whose school refusal results in the regular one-on-one time with a parent that she craves is likely different from the client whose refusal to go to school allows him to avoid social interactions with peers that make him highly anxious. Second, children must be assessed for comorbid disorders. Comorbidity is common in children and adolescents (Merikangas et al., 2009), and children with two or more clinical conditions are likely to experience more severe symptoms and widespread impairment (Bauermeister et al., 2007; Schepman et al., 2014). In addition, the presence of comorbid disorders may change the treatment approach, particularly if one disorder is determined to underlie or exacerbate the symptoms of the other. Therefore, especially at the beginning of therapy, clinicians should utilize assessments, including interviews and questionnaires, that assess for a broad variety of symptom types. Once the presence or absence of particular symptom types has been established, the focus can shift to a more in-depth exploration of the presenting problems. Third, clinicians working within a developmental psychopathology framework should assess the risk or causal factors that have likely led to the child's current symptoms and level of functioning. A foundational assumption of developmental psychopathology is that a child cannot be understood apart from her context, which includes both past and present influences on development and functioning. In order to effectively treat oppositional defiant disorder in a young child, for example, it is critical to understand the family dynamics that may be inadvertently reinforcing problematic behavior as well as the stressors that may interfere with parents' abilities to respond sen-

sitively to their children (see chapter six). In many cases, these risk factors will become targets for intervention.

Finally, for Christian clinicians, the client's characteristics and preferences must inform how a biblical and theological framework is integrated into their work with individual youth and families (in addition, of course, to the characteristics, skills, preferences, training, and experience of the clinician with regard to integration in clinical practice). Some families, for whom their identification as Christians plays a significant role in all aspects of life, desire a treatment approach that explicitly integrates Christian faith with psychological principles, which can include discussion of spiritual issues, prayer, and the use of Scripture. Others families or youth view religion or spirituality as less important to them or even irrelevant for understanding psychological functioning, while still others hold worldviews that are in opposition to Christian beliefs (including atheism as well as other religious traditions). For these families, it would be inappropriate to impose the clinician's worldview in the therapeutic context. Indeed, respecting clients' rights to determine their own views and values is considered an important ethical principle (American Psychological Association, 2017). However, clinical work with youth and families of all faith backgrounds and worldviews can still be guided by a Christian therapist's general understandings of disorder, well-being, and how youth thrive. For example, the theologically informed views of children as gifts to be valued, individuals with full personhood, and active agents in their own and others' lives (Miller-McLemore, 2003) can be appropriately applied to enrich any treatment approach, whether religious elements are explicitly included or not (see this volume, chapter two). It is recommended that all clinicians ask youth and families about their religious or spiritual beliefs and practices, identifications, and/or communities as part of a thorough assessment of clients' worldviews and contexts (Josephson & Dell, 2004).

EXAMPLES OF EBPP APPLICATIONS

EBPP has gained attention even from researchers and practitioners who focus primarily on developing and testing ESTs. For example, there is increasing recognition that even though treatment manuals are an important element of most EBTs, the use of a manual does not eliminate the need for clinical judgment and flexibility. Clinicians can use their clinical expertise to flexibly apply manualized treatments while remaining faithful to the "main ingredients" of the intervention (Kendall et al., 2008). In order to accomplish this flexibility within fidelity, clinicians need to be careful to maintain the goals of each therapy session and to use techniques that are rooted in the theoretical basis of the treatment. Below we describe two examples of how the best application of empirically supported, manualized treatments for psychopathology in youth takes into account clinician and client factors.

Applied behavior analysis. Leaf and McEachin (2016) give some examples of the role of clinical judgment in applied behavior analysis (ABA), an evidence-based treatment for autism spectrum disorders (ASD; see chapter eight, this volume). They explain that the optimal application of the standardized elements of treatment during a particular session depends on both the individual characteristics of the child and those of the cli-

nician. A therapist needs to take into account the child's current state in order to maximize the likelihood that the child will respond to the operant conditioning principles designed to reduce symptoms and improve functioning. For example, a client may be more or less motivated to respond to the requests of the clinician, calm or upset, more or less cooperative and responsive to the therapist, or sick or hungry. In addition, the clinician must assess the function of the child's behavior in order to design the best behavior modification plan and apply it effectively during a given session. Clinician characteristics influence the application of the intervention as well; these characteristics can include the therapist's current mood and level of patience as well as her level of knowledge of behavioral therapy principles. Such factors then affect variables such as the language the therapist uses, how she addresses a particular behavior (e.g., the ways in which she prompts a child to behave appropriately or the rewards she uses to encourage positive behavior), and which presenting problems are prioritized at a given point. A less-experienced clinician working with a child who is tired and easily frustrated might focus on reinforcing a very simple positive behavior with a particularly desirable reward, whereas a clinician who feels encouraged and full of patience in a session with a child who is motivated and happy might target a more challenging or complex behavior. These authors compare the role of clinical judgment in therapy to the role of improvisation in cooking; the most-skilled cooks begin with a recipe, but they have learned from their previous experiences when to follow it closely and when to make changes that improve the meal in a particular way.

Coping Cat. The Coping Cat is a manualized, cognitive-behavioral treatment for anxiety in youth that is well supported in the treatment literature (Kendall et al., 2010). The intervention consists of several common elements of effective anxiety treatment, framing them with the acronym **FEAR** (**F**eeling Frightened, identifying and reducing the physiological signs of anxiety; **E**xpecting Bad Things to Happen, identifying and reducing cognitive distortions; **A**ttitudes and **A**ctions That Might Help, improving problem-solving skills; and **R**esults and **R**ewards, self-monitoring) in combination with exposure therapy (see chapter four, this volume). Despite the manualized nature of the Coping Cat program, the authors offer several suggestions for tailoring the intervention to meet individual clients' needs (Beidas et al., 2010; Kendall et al., 2008). In the "Feeling Frightened" module of treatment, therapists may explain relaxation differently to children of different ages, using a variety of concrete illustrations (e.g., muscle tension as "dry spaghetti" or diaphragmatic breathing as "blowing up a balloon") until one resonates with a particular youth. Clients and therapists can also try different progressive muscle relaxation scripts or guided imagery exercises to find the ones that work best for individual clients. Clinicians working with youth around not "Expecting Bad Things to Happen" might use characters that are of interest to a particular child as they complete thought bubbles with anxious and non-anxious self-talk. They might also help youth identify brief phrases that can serve as helpful self-talk in a variety of situations (e.g., "I can do it"), even creating visuals such as a keychain containing the phrase or a poster of a role model speaking the phrase. Identifying "Attitudes and Actions That Might Help" should be a collaborative process; rather than the therapist providing the client with a predetermined list of problem-solving ideas, the therapist and the youth can brainstorm possible solutions to a real-life problem that the child has identified as significant. Furthermore, a variety of techniques can be used to facilitate brainstorming, including the therapist and child competing to come up with more ideas, writing ideas on a dry erase board, or drawing pictures of or role-playing possible solutions. Exposure tasks and identifying "Results and Rewards" inherently need to be individualized to be effective in addressing a client's particular fears and anxieties. Examples can include the collaborative creation of a fear hierarchy, selection of rewards that are particularly motivating, discussion of the aspects of anxiety that are most distressing and likely to lead to avoidance, and customization of the scale used to rate anxiety during exposures (e.g., allowing the child to select or draw faces that communicate her experiences or using the emotion terms that the child prefers).

Other alterations help adapt the Coping Cat to be as effective as possible in light of a variety of client characteristics. Throughout the intervention, the content can be tailored to be developmentally sensitive for younger or older clients. For example, the therapist might use games or crafts to help younger children identify the symptoms of anxiety, whereas adolescents might be encouraged to keep a journal of therapeutic activities. Role-play and discussion targets should also be developmentally appropriate and relevant to the concerns of the individual client. Finally, clinicians should take into account comorbid conditions or difficulties that may necessitate changes in the application of the Coping Cat intervention. For youth with poor social skills, negative cognitions about social rejection may not be inaccurate, so clinicians may need to focus on helping these youth cope with stressful social situations rather than merely challenging what might be cognitive distortions for other clients. When working with youth with significant ADHD symptoms, clinicians may need to take frequent breaks during which they engage in fun, lively activities (such as doing jumping jacks) that build the therapeutic alliance while also increasing the likelihood that youth will be able to stay on task during other therapeutic discussions and activities. Clinicians working with youth with depression may help clients learn to identify and challenge not only anxious self-talk but also the cognitive distortions that may be related to depressive symptoms.

CONCLUSIONS

Clinicians working with youth and families are tasked with a challenging but meaningful undertaking, as they strive to understand the dynamic and complex interaction of factors that produce positive or negative changes in a child's mental health. Fortunately, the field of developmental psychopathology and the principles of evidence-based practice in psychology offer rich frameworks and tools for conceptualizing disorders and treatment. As we explore a variety of common disorders in youth throughout this volume, we integrate developmental psychopathology principles into our approach to understanding causal factors and effective interventions. We also present the current state of empirical evidence on the most effective treatments for these disorders, alongside which we encourage our readers to continually consider the individual youth, family, and clinician factors that shape the best application of evidence-based practice with any individual client.

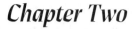

Chapter Two

A Christian Approach to Treating Children and Adolescents

WE BELIEVE THAT HUMANKIND has been blessed by God to be able to draw knowledge and understanding from a wide variety of sources, including both special revelation through the Bible and general revelation via creation and its study. For this reason, we take an integrative view of the relationship between psychology and Christianity (Jones, 2010). Though we suspect that most of our readers embrace the same approach, since Christian clinicians understand the interaction of science and faith in a wide variety of ways—including sometimes emphasizing one over the other in approaching treatment—we want to begin this chapter by clearly laying out our assumptions and understandings. We will start with a definition of our view: "Integration of Christianity and psychology . . . is our living out . . . of the lordship of Christ over all of existence by our giving his special revelation—God's true Word—its appropriate place of authority in determining our funda-

mental beliefs and practices toward all of reality and toward our academic subject matter in particular" (Jones, 2010, p. 102). Integrationists believe that the best way to understand people and their functioning—including psychopathology and treatment—is by integrating all the knowledge we can access from all reliable sources. Scripture is, of course, the foremost and most trustworthy source of information; it provides "everything necessary to a full life in Christ" (Jones, 2010, p. 110) as well as information about many patterns of human experience and striving within the bigger picture of God's redemptive story. However, we believe that Scripture is not intended to be our only source of information about every aspect of creation and humanity; for example, the Bible is not an anatomy textbook, a cookbook, a symptom checklist, or a truck mechanic's manual. Truth is revealed not only in Scripture but also through human beings' thoughtful, discerning engagement with each other and the world around them, which occurs formally in vocational and academic study and informally in our everyday personal and professional relationships and experiences. As other authors have noted, in a perfect (sinless) world, all sources of truth would be integrated in seamless harmony and connection with one another (Entwistle, 2015; Jones, 2010); as integrationists, then, we strive to bring back together that which has been separated following the fall. Therefore, high-quality psychological theory and research offer a rich source of information for those who wish to understand patterns of human biological, cognitive, emotional, and behavioral functioning, development, and well-being. At the same time, as Christian integrationists who take the authority of Scripture seriously, we recognize that our biblical and theological knowledge provides an important framework for the ways in which we understand and apply psychological ideas. In this chapter, we discuss some of the implications of Christian understandings of the nature of human beings, suffering, healing, and children on how we think about and approach treatment.

CHRISTIANITY AND PSYCHOLOGICAL TREATMENT

An integrative approach to Christianity and clinical applications of psychology emphasizes biblically and theologically based understandings of human beings as the context in which we understand scientific theory and research about disorder and treatment. Therefore, we will draw from a variety of Christian sources as we outline some of the understandings that we see as crucial to integrate with psychologically based knowledge. We use the framework of many integrative

writers (e.g., Entwistle, 2015; McMinn & Campbell, 2007) that a Christian worldview is grounded in the themes of creation, fall, and redemption to discuss human nature, suffering, and healing, respectively. We then contend specifically with how theological understandings of children shape the application of these ideas to a therapeutic context.

THEOLOGY OF CREATION AND HUMAN NATURE

The Bible opens with an account of God as creator of all things, including human beings, who are given a special place in his creation as bearers of his image (Genesis 1:26). The image of God is an inherent part of personhood that is universally present in all people, including Christians as well as nonbelievers, and imbues each person with dignity and worth (Erickson, 2013). The presence of the *imago Dei* in human beings has been interpreted as having three main manifestations (Erickson, 2013; McMinn & Campbell, 2007). First, the *imago Dei* can be understood as having functional implications, in that people are meant to be God's representatives in the management and stewardship of the rest of the created order. Second, substantive or structural views emphasize the presence of certain aspects of the nature of God in humans, since we are created in his image. As image bearers, humans have the capacity to reflect many aspects of God's nature, including nobility, creativity, justice, mercy, emotionality, and the capacity for moral and rational thought (Entwistle, 2015; McMinn & Campbell, 2007). Third, God's image manifests itself in people in their relational nature, a reflection of God's relational character. We will focus on the implications of this final view and its emphasis on relationality for psychological treatment.

The three-in-one God of the Bible is understood as inherently relational; therefore, people created in his image are also imbued with relational capacities and drives. Some theologians have even posited that the image of God is not manifest fully in individuals but rather within our relationships with other people (Barth, 1945/2009; Grenz, 2000). In any case, it is clear that we are created in the image of a relational God whose purpose for us is to be in right relationship with him and with other people (John 1:12; Romans 5:10-11; Ephesians 4). The best model of relationality we have is in Jesus, whose image bearing is not tainted by sin. Jesus' life sets examples for us in terms of his relationship with God and his relationship with people (Erickson, 2013). First, Jesus' relationship with God is perfect. He is one with the Father, whom he glorifies (John 17). Jesus also obeys the Father perfectly, submitting his own will to that of his Father (Matthew 26:39; John 4:34). Second, Jesus displays deep compassion for human beings and their needs and suffering (Matthew 9:36; Mark 10:21; Luke 7:13). In his ministry on earth, he spends a great deal of time teaching, shepherding, and healing people. Jesus does not hesitate to engage with people who are sick, unclean, or outcast by society (Matthew 9:20-22; Luke 19:1-10; John 4:7-26). God's intention for the people he created in his image is to live in authentic, compassionate relationships with other people and in perfect, obedient fellowship with him.

The importance of supportive, healthy relationships and their impact on development are frequently emphasized by psychological theories and research. For example, in the psychological literature, there is consistent evidence of the importance of high-quality

relationships with other people in promoting mental health and well-being (Ozbay et al., 2007), which may occur at least partially through the impact of social support on how our brains process potential threats (Maresh et al., 2013). Furthermore, common factors research suggests that the client-therapist relationship or alliance is a significant determinant of the effectiveness of treatment (Laska et al., 2014). As people who have been universally imbued with God-given relationality, our drive to connect deeply with others is an inherent part of our nature. Our clients and their families will experience pain and grief when their relationships with other people are difficult, damaged, or absent, and recognizing the importance of healthy relationships for well-being should play a role in shaping the goals of therapy. Furthermore, to be effective clinicians, we must draw on our relational nature to build therapeutic relationships with clients that form a foundation for treatment that produces change. We have the privilege of connecting deeply with both youth and their families, mourning their suffering and celebrating their victories and growth alongside them, particularly when they also belong to the body of Christ (1 Corinthians 12:26). One of the challenges unique to clinical work with youth is the necessity of being able to build relationships not only with our young clients but also with their parents and other caregivers, stretching our relational skills as we connect with individuals across the lifespan. Further, while it is a privilege for any clinician to be allowed into a client's life, it is a particularly special opportunity to be allowed into the lives and hurts of children, who are more vulnerable members of society, and our relationship-building work with parents forms an important foundation in their ability to entrust their children's suffering and hope for change to us.

THEOLOGY OF THE FALL AND SUFFERING

Of course, the manifestation of the *imago Dei* in people was disrupted by the entry of sin into the world through the disobedience of the first man and woman (Genesis 3; Luther, 1545/1958). The effects of sin are far-reaching and impact both the created world broadly and human beings specifically; in Genesis 3, the Lord explains that, as a direct result of sin, people will experience physical pain, relational disharmony, difficult work, and ultimately death. We want to be careful to note that the theological concept of sin is generally understood to include both sin as a state and sin as an act (Augustine, 398/1986; McMinn & Campbell, 2007). McRay and colleagues (2016) describe the DSM as "not a catalog of sin but a catalog of the state and consequences of sin" (p. 103). In other words, our fallen nature and world might be considered causal at the root level for all human problems, including psychological disorders. Indeed, it has been argued that the risk factors that we consider to cause psychopathology at biological (e.g., neurotransmitter abnormalities) or other levels (e.g., cognitive distortions) are only imperfect and problematic because of the entry of sin into the world at the time of the fall (McMinn, 2004; McRay et al., 2016).

With regard to areas of functioning of particular interest to clinicians, the fallen state of the world affects our biological, behavioral, emotional, cognitive, and social functioning (McMinn, 2004; McRay et al., 2016). Because of sin, our genes mutate, our neurotransmitter and hormone levels are too low or too high,

our brains form and function imperfectly, and our bodies respond to stress ineffectively. Because of sin, we behave in ways that are maladaptive, selfish, impulsive, and harmful to ourselves and others. Because of sin, our emotions become twisted, reflecting our desire to see our own purposes thrive rather than God's, and we are easily overwhelmed by dysregulated feelings and their expression. Because of sin, we think about ourselves, others, and the world in ways that are inaccurate, unhelpful, and self-focused. Because of sin, we accidently and purposefully hurt other people through our words and actions. Psychological symptoms—along with everything that is imperfect and painful in the world and in human experience—exist as a result of the presence of sin.

Beyond the general effects of the sinful condition, individual acts of sin can affect psychopathology, though some cautions are in order as we begin this discussion. First, we note that there is not a clear, consistent correlation between individual sin and psychological well-being. People who live clearly sinful, God-dishonoring lives may not exhibit a single symptom of psychopathology as categorized by our diagnostic system, whereas individuals with mental illness may be extremely faithful in their Christian walk. In the book of Job, friends suggest that Job's sufferings are the result of unconfessed sin, a belief that is debunked in God's response to Job, supporting the idea that suffering—including psychological suffering—may happen to righteous individuals (Webb, 2012). Jesus himself addresses the misconception that disability is the result of sin, explaining that one man's blindness was caused not by his sin or the sin of his parents but that "this happened so that the works of God might be displayed in him" (John 9:3). Second, it is important to recognize that different people have different predispositions to areas of difficulty or weakness. Johnson (1987) discusses the difference between the biblical concepts of sin and weakness, particularly as they pertain to psychological disorder. Sin is active disobedience to God's perfect commands for us, it is displeasing to him, and we will be judged or held responsible for our sins. In contrast, weakness is imperfection or inadequacy that we passively receive and for which we are not judged by God; rather, human weakness can glorify God and testify to his power (2 Corinthians 12:9). This distinction is important as we understand the differences among people that may predispose them to certain psychological illnesses. We know from psychological research, as we will review throughout this book, that psychopathology results from a variety of genetic and environmental influences. From a Christian perspective, the predisposition that results from such influences outside of the individual's control might best be understood as weaknesses. One child has genetic and temperamental predispositions toward anxiety; one adolescent is at higher risk for alcohol abuse due to his biological makeup. In these cases, we view the predisposition toward a disorder as the result of weakness, not in the sense of moral failure but in the sense of innate susceptibility. This susceptibility may interact with individual sin, as we will discuss, but it is not sinful in itself. Finally, we must approach the process of discerning the effects of individual sin on disorder with humility, as it may be difficult to look into another person's life and easily distinguish sin versus weakness or action re-

sulting from free will versus strong predispositions. It may be particularly tempting to let our own biases color our views of the role of sin in psychopathology; for example, a clinician to whom self-control comes naturally may find it difficult to empathize with a client whose poor impulse control she sees as a failure to display self-control rather than an underlying predisposition toward impulsivity. Further, we cannot presume to have the wisdom or insight to know God's will or make these distinctions. God is patient to meet us where we are; may we do the same for our clients and their families.

With these ideas in mind, we do consider that an individual's sins as well as the sins of others at individual and larger societal levels may affect the occurrence and course of psychological disorders (McRay et al., 2016). For example, an adolescent with conduct disorder may have opportunities to choose whether to join a group of peers who are setting out to steal alcohol from a store, which would generally be categorized as a sinful behavior. The idea of weakness or predisposition does not excuse us from action; we have free will and agency to make choices that move us toward or away from God as well as mental health. With youth, it is important to note that the ability to make healthy and/or godly choices—particularly in the face of susceptibility to emotional or behavioral problems—is significantly impacted by both developmental stage and environmental influences. Younger children are likely to have more difficulty making healthy or right choices in such situations, and youth surrounded by powerful environmental influences may have more trouble resisting them. For these reasons, youth who struggle with predispositions toward psychopathology are in particular need of sensitive, informed adult support, particularly as their brains are maturing, they are developing self-regulation, and they are learning to make right choices in times of temptation or when the influence of their weakness is particularly strong.

Of course, adults frequently fail youth, both in individual interactions and at the level of societal structures. These two areas represent additional ways in which sin can affect psychopathology. First, mental health can be negatively affected by the specific sins of others. Examples include the adolescent who develops PTSD following sexual assault, the youth who becomes depressed and suicidal as the result of bullying by peers, and the child whose externalizing behavior develops as an adaptation to his parents' severe marital conflict. In these cases, addressing the sin that has contributed to the youth's symptoms is extremely important; depending on the setting and the individual's worldviews, the behavior may or may not be labeled as "sin" but should be seen as problematic either way. Second, sin that occurs at an institutional, structural, or societal level may also impact psychopathology in youth. For example, the idealization of thinness as beautiful in Western societies—and the related devaluing of a variety of body types as acceptable—is thought to have contributed to the incidence of eating disorders in adolescents and young adults (Derenne & Beresin, 2006). There is growing popular concern that the pressure from parents and teachers to achieve at high levels in every area of life has contributed to significant increases in anxiety, depression, and suicidality in adolescents (Schrobsdorff, 2016). Such undue pressure on children and adoles-

cents is a reflection of societal-level sin. Furthermore, due to their lack of power relative to adults, youth are particularly vulnerable to the effects of others' sin at both the individual and the structural/societal levels; the implication of this vulnerability is that adults have a special responsibility to address this sin and its effects (Jensen, 2005).

THEOLOGY OF REDEMPTION AND HEALING

Fortunately, the story of humanity does not end with the fall; God does not leave us to drown in our sin. Jesus' life, death, and resurrection offer redemption, reconciliation to God, freedom from the bondage of sin, and eternal life through faith (John 3:16). "Every aspect of creation is to be redeemed and restored" (Entwistle, 2015, p. 80) as God "reconcile[s] to himself all things" through Jesus' death (Colossians 1:20). This promise signifies that all the realms of human functioning that have been tainted by sin—biological, behavioral, emotional, cognitive, and relational—have the potential to be purified, redeemed, and restored to the form and function that God originally intended for them. Therefore, alongside the hope of healing and freedom from sin and death available to us through Jesus' death and resurrection is hope for healing from pain and suffering that result from ailments and illnesses, including psychological disorders. God cares about people who are hurting, suffering, and vulnerable (Deuteronomy 10:18; 2 Corinthians 1:3-5); as the Great Physician, he can heal any disease or disorder. As we have previously discussed, Jesus' ministry involved many healing encounters with the sick and hurting. Furthermore, as clinicians created in the image of a healing God, we can understand ourselves as agents of his healing power over suffering and disease (while simultaneously recognizing that only God provides the ultimate healing and delivery from sin and death that was bought by Jesus' blood). Sometimes, healing occurs suddenly and miraculously; other times it is a more gradual process that occurs through care facilitated by other support systems, professionals, and technological advances, including psychotropic medications or empirically supported psychosocial treatments. Whatever form healing takes, we should recognize it as an outpouring of God's kindness and redemption. Jesus came to live, die, and rise not just that we might merely live but that we might live abundant, full lives filled with joy (John 10:10; Romans 5:21). Sometimes, that joy and abundance may not take the form we expect; while we might hope and pray for God to remove our sufferings and symptoms, Scripture is consistently clear that God is constantly at work, including through our trials and problems (Romans 8:28). Indeed, some of the work that God does in our hearts, lives, and character is made possible only by the experience of suffering (Romans 5:3-5; James 1:2-4). The deep desperation of depression may provide an adolescent with the opportunity to trust in God's goodness and provision in a way that she would not have been able to in the midst of joy and hope. The challenging task of parenting a child with severe autism might provide a father with the opportunity to develop truly self-sacrificial, Christlike actions and attitudes that he would not have been spurred to without the occurrence of his child's disorder. The concept of posttraumatic growth (Tedeschi & Calhoun, 1995) high-

lights the role of suffering in the reevaluation of one's beliefs and priorities that can lead to a richer sense of self, purpose, and relationships following a traumatic experience. God's work in the world and in individuals' lives occurs not merely in spite or in relief of psychological symptoms but in the midst of them.

In addition, we recognize that though God's redemptive work has already begun, it has not yet been completed and will not be finished until the consummation of God's rule, the reestablishment of his authority, and the creation of the new heaven and the new earth (Entwistle, 2015; McMinn & Campbell, 2007). We will continue to suffer and be imperfect until Christ comes again, establishing his full reign and completely and finally eliminating the effects of sin (Romans 8:18-21; 2 Peter 3:13; Revelation 21). Even though Jesus has conquered sin and death, we continue to live in a fallen world and struggle against the sinful nature and the effects of individual and corporate sin (Entwistle, 2015). Therefore, illness, disorder, and imperfection still exist. Children and adults still experience depression, anxiety, ADHD, and other symptoms that cause distress and impair functioning. Indeed, the research we will review throughout this volume suggests that while psychological interventions effectively treat disorders for many youth, some will continue to struggle with their symptoms throughout the course of life. However, the promise of the new heaven and the new earth in which we are fully healed, restored, comforted, and made anew offers unique hope for youth and families whose struggles with psychopathology are persistent and resistant to treatment.

THEOLOGY OF CHILDHOOD

Though all children are people, all people are not children. Theological writing and thought that focus mainly on adults help us think about and understand youth, but they are not sufficient. Working with youth and their families is a unique calling that must be informed by theological understandings of children specifically in addition to a broader theology of human nature, suffering, and healing. In this section, we will use Miller-McLemore's (2003) three themes—that children should be (1) valued as gifts, (2) respected as full persons, and (3) viewed as agents—to structure our discussion of theological views of children (see Flanagan & Hall, 2014, for further discussion of these themes and their application to clinical work with youth).

Children as gifts. First, we must recognize that children are blessings and gifts, to families specifically and to the community more broadly. Scripture communicates this idea in a variety of ways. Throughout the Old Testament, children are described as a reward and a sign of God's blessing (Deuteronomy 7:12-14; Psalm 127:3-5). Furthermore, they are the fulfillment of God's consistent promises to the patriarchs to make his people into a great nation (Genesis 15:4-5; Genesis 22:15-18). In the New Testament, Jesus interacts with children in a way that displays their significance. He explicitly welcomes children and commands others to do the same (Mark 9:33-37); he lays hands on them and heals them (Mark 5:39-42; Matthew 17:14-18). Finally, God chose for his Son to enter the world as a newborn, the ultimate gift to a fallen world.

We will discuss two main implications of the gift nature of children for those who work with them. First, we should recognize that children do not ultimately belong to us but to their heavenly Father. As parents and other significant adults, we act as the direct agents of God's love, grace, instruction, and discipline to children. Throughout Scripture, parents are commanded to teach their children about God and his commands (Deuteronomy 6:6-9; Ephesians 6:4), to discipline their children in order to shape their character (Proverbs 22:15; Hebrews 12:7-10), and to delight in their righteousness (Proverbs 23:24-25). The process of parenting a child from birth to adulthood has been compared to the process of discipling a believer from a new faith commitment to a mature spiritual life (Balswick & Balswick, 2014). From a Christian perspective, the goal of parenting is to support children's healthy development toward godly life and character as an expression of the duty that comes with the reception of this particular gift (Miller-McLemore, 2003). It is clear that parental choices and behaviors have a lasting impact on children's well-being and even the well-being of their future descendants (Exodus 20:4-6; Deuteronomy 4:40; 2 Timothy 1:5).

Furthermore, the care of children is not entrusted to parents in isolation but, ideally, with the support of the larger community. Stonehouse (1998) points out that Moses' iconic instructions to parents to teach their children constantly about God in Deuteronomy 6 are given to the nation of Israel as a whole community. Parents have special responsibility for the care and support of their children, but God's design for families is for their efforts to be aided and sustained by the broader body of Christ as other adults support parents in their efforts, play direct instructive and supportive roles with youth (e.g., Sunday school teachers, youth leaders, mentors), and pray for youth and families. Clinicians are included in the broader community of care for youth who suffer from psychopathology. Children in general are a vulnerable population, due to their weakness relative to adults and the power structure of society, and some children face circumstances or conditions (e.g., poverty, displacement, abuse, physical or mental illness) that enhance their vulnerability to negative outcomes (Jensen, 2005). God's care for the vulnerable is evident, from commands to Israel to leave some of the harvest from their fields and vineyards for immigrants, widows, and orphans (Deuteronomy 24:19-22) to God's role as their helper and sustainer (Psalm 10:14; 68:5; 146:9) to the characterization of "pure and faultless religion" as including care for the orphan and the widow (James 1:27). Because of the continuity of mental health problems throughout development for some individuals, youth who suffer from persistent psychopathology might also be characterized as particularly vulnerable. If we recognize that children are gifts whom God has entrusted to our care, we must also recognize that caring for them well means providing special, truly helpful care for those who are suffering or at high risk. For orphans, this care may entail community members stepping into the roles of family members to meet practical and emotional needs; for children with a psychological diagnosis, this care involves support and intervention from adults involved in their lives, including clinicians. We believe that for clinicians, providing the best possible care for this segment of the population must include drawing from the great resource of treatment research.

Second, we recognize that children are gifts in our acknowledgment that the acts of interacting with and caring for them affect our own spiritual development and well-being. Children can teach us how to better worship God. Psalm 8:2 states, in praise of God, "Through the praise of children and infants you have established a stronghold against your enemies, to silence the foe and the avenger." John Calvin, in his commentary on Psalms (1847–1850), understands this verse to reflect the capacity of even the preverbal newborn child to praise the Lord. He refers to the fact that infants are created with the ability to suckle for nourishment from birth as evidence of God's good provision for his people. This goodness is so powerful and overwhelming that it can defeat all those who stand in opposition to God's purposes. So, when we look at children, we ought first and foremost to see God's hand in their design— the creativity, power, care, and goodness embodied by the Maker who forms us in the womb (Psalm 139:13-14). In addition, in Matthew 18, Jesus sets children as an example for his followers about how they should think about greatness. In their humility, openness, and trust, children set an example for older believers about how to receive the kingdom of God. From watching, caring for, and engaging with children, we learn about our own proper stance before the Lord. The "lowly position" of children is a gift in its instructional value. Finally, if we recognize children as gifts from the Lord, we might better understand our interactions with them to ultimately be opportunities to worship God. God is glorified when we delight in our children, when we instruct them in his Word, and when we care for them in a manner that shapes their lives and character in godly ways that contribute to the advancement of God's kingdom.

Children as persons. The view of children as gifts must be balanced by an understanding that children are also fully human individuals who should be viewed and respected as such. At times, adults are tempted to emphasize the ways in which children are "lesser" than adults—in stature, strength, knowledge, skill level, reasoning ability, emotional self-control, power, or life experience—and to allow such comparisons to characterize their view of children. The result is a condescension in which children may come to be viewed as not yet fully human, and their views, experiences, and characteristics may be easily dismissed. However, a biblical view of children is founded on the recognition that though they are still developing, youth are as fully human as adults who are both created in the image of God and affected by sin.

Like adults, children are imbued with the *imago Dei* from the beginning of life (Towner, 2008). Although the full expression of God's image in them may still be developing (e.g., creativity, justice, rationality), even the young child possesses this image and the resulting worth and value. Furthermore, youth whose behavior, emotions, thoughts, or overall functioning are affected by psychological disorder are still image bearers through whom we might see their Creator. Combined with the understanding of children as gifts, their possession of God's image highlights the importance of treating them with kindness, respect, and dignity. Such theological understandings provide even stronger underpinnings to the professional ethical commitment clinicians have to "respect the dignity and worth of all people" (American Psychological Association, 2017, p. 4).

Theologians who write about children vary in their views of how sin is expressed, as well as the degree to which individuals are accountable for sin, in early childhood, but they generally agree that as fully human persons, children are affected by sin (Jensen, 2005). Returning to the view of sin as both state and act, we recognize that both manifestations affect youth. As a result of our fallen state, children's bodies, including neurotransmitter and hormone levels, sometimes function in ways that do not promote optimal physical and mental health. Children experience overwhelming and dysregulated emotions, they think in ways that are distorted by sin, and sin provides the background for the formation of relationships with others, which fall short of God's design for perfect unity among believers. (Note: developmental immaturity in areas such as language, cognition, emotional development, and social skills do not necessarily represent the effects of sin but rather human limitation. The apparently "selfish" actions of a young child who does not yet possess theory of mind—the ability to take another person's perspective into consideration—are probably better understood as reflective of children being developmentally incapable of true selflessness than as acts of a sinful nature.) However, like adults, children do sin in active and specific ways. It may be easy to perceive external sins of commission in younger children (e.g., hitting, biting, willfully disobeying adult comments), but as youth age, their sins may become more "adultlike" in their complexity and their ability to disguise them (e.g., lying, cheating, displaying relational aggression, harboring internal hatred and anger toward others). In any case, recognizing that youth are fully human means acknowledging their sinful nature and the role of sinful choices in their lives and addressing the effects of sin when appropriate. As with adult clients, decisions about the degree to which sin is explicitly addressed in a therapeutic context are complex and need to include consideration of the client's worldview, the difficulty of separating the effects of the sinful nature/weakness from the sin as act, and the effect that a discussion of sin is likely to have on the client's well-being. Because of the importance of developmental considerations, clinicians working with youth should be especially cautious about introducing the idea of individual sins' role in mental illness and treatment in order to avoid placing an undue sense of blame or responsibility on a young client, who is likely to have trouble understanding the complexity of the factors that affect psychological well-being, which may interfere with the treatment and recovery process.

Another aspect to our humanity is the interconnection of the various aspects of our functioning and development, including physical, cognitive, social, emotional, and spiritual. For youth, promoting psychological well-being may be especially significant because of its role in the process of healthy development, including spiritual development. Stonehouse (1998) discusses children's mastery of Erikson's (1985) developmental tasks as forming the foundation for the development of their faith and relationship with God. For example, infants who develop a sense of trust in their caregivers are better prepared to rely on God as trustworthy and consistent than those who view the world with mistrust because of early experience with unreliable or unresponsive parents. Older children who master a sense of industry, the ability to work productively and cooperatively, have the skills and sense of purpose that may help them see themselves as productive members of the body of Christ. Many experiences, including psychopathology and its correlates, can interfere with the mastery of these developmental tasks. The young child with high levels of anxiety may experience the world as frightening, unsafe, and unpredictable, making it difficult for her to trust others, including God. The older child whose disruptive behavior disorder symptoms make it difficult to engage cooperatively with others may develop a sense of inferiority rather than industry, coming to view himself as isolated from others in the church whose behavior is viewed as more productive and appropriate. In both of these examples, the amelioration of symptoms is likely to help children master the developmental tasks they are faced with as they age and, as a result, to have a stronger foundation for spiritual growth. Treating childhood psychopathology, therefore, can be understood as having both psychological and spiritual implications.

Children as agents. Emphasizing the links between the *imago Dei* and the idea of agency, Erickson (2013) notes that "because all are in the image of God, nothing should be done that would encroach upon another's legitimate exercise of dominion" (p. 473). If we understand children as fully human, we must also recognize that they have been imbued by their Creator with the capacity to impact their environments and that they are worthy of the dignity of being allowed to direct their own lives in appropriate ways. The manifestation of agency changes with age, of course, but it is a relevant topic from the first moments of life. Research on newborns indicates that when given the opportunity and freedom, they will, within one to two hours of birth, actively seek out the mother's breast and begin nursing (Widstrom et al., 1987). Young babies are even understood to regulate their sensory intake through simple actions such as turning away or expressing distress when they are overwhelmed or overstimulated (Kopp, 1989); one of the functions of the relatively large amount of time newborns spend asleep is understood to be helping their immature nervous systems manage the barrage of sensory information in the world (Brazelton, 2013). These behaviors are best understood as reflexes rather than purposeful, planful actions; however, they still reflect the God-given agency that allows us from birth to express our needs and impact our environments in ways that promote our own well-being.

As children develop, their expression of agency changes and becomes more purposeful. Toddlers, who are beginning to have a sense of themselves as unique from others and are able to move around much more freely than they could as infants, are navigating a newfound sense of independence. These children often express their agency in any way they can, which can result in disruptive behaviors; parents or caregivers familiar with the concept of the "terrible twos" (or threes, or fours) recognize that the young child's developing expressions of agency may clash with adults' desires for the child's behavior or environment to be shaped in specific ways. As adults who interact with young children, our task is often to structure their environments and interactions in a way that promotes appropriate agency even as we do not allow them to have agency in every area of life. For example, a child may be allowed to

wear her favorite swimsuit inside the house but not outside during the winter; even if the parent would prefer that she wear more "appropriate" clothes in the house, she can express her own desires and preferences in a way that is not potentially harmful (as going outside in a swimsuit when the temperature is below freezing would be). A Sunday school teacher might allow each child to choose whether to have pretzels or graham crackers for a snack; the teacher sets some boundaries (e.g., snack is served at a specific time, children must sit at the table while they eat, they cannot have cookies for snack, they are only permitted two servings) but allows children to have appropriate choices. It is important to recognize that respecting children's agency means offering them more ways to express and apply it in developmentally appropriate ways as they age. The toddler whose parents would not allow her to wear a swimsuit outside in February might become an adolescent who, aware that it is a cold day, refuses to wear a coat while waiting for the bus. Since she is older, her parents might allow her to exercise her agency in choosing her clothing and to learn from the consequences of her behavior (e.g., she feels cold and decides to wear a coat on the next cold day) while still setting limits when appropriate (e.g., she can choose her friends, but her parents need to meet the friend's parents before she is permitted to go over to her house). Miller-McLemore (2003) argues that youth whose parents are overly controlling and who are not allowed some freedom of choice as they grow become adolescents and adults who have not developed the skills to make good decisions on their own, such as when they are faced with peer pressure to drink alcohol or use drugs. She notes that "children need instead a gradual transfer of power that involves receiving responsibility for progressively greater choices within a range appropriate to their age and situation" (p. 143). Allowing children to express their agency in developmentally appropriate ways not only recognizes this theologically significant element of personhood, it also promotes positive development and the adaptive implementation of power, choice, and agency as they grow into adolescents and adults.

The concept of agency has important implications for understanding psychopathology and treatment. Youth who feel little control in their own lives—little opportunity to express their agency—are at higher risk for developing a variety of psychological symptoms; in contrast, youth with an internal locus of control are more likely to be resilient and have positive outcomes following adverse experiences (Culpin et al., 2015; Weems et al., 2003; Sullivan et al., 2017; Zhang et al., 2014). Furthermore, we must take children's agency into account as we approach treatment in a manner that truly embraces our theological understandings of youth. If we understand youth to have God-given agency, then our approach to intervention should make room for the child's or adolescent's self-direction and voice in the process. Of course, respecting a child's agency does not mean allowing her to have complete freedom of choice in whether to seek treatment, what form it should take, or other decisions in the treatment process. Rather, parallel to our discussion of respecting agency in parenting more generally, this space must be developmentally appropriate and tailored to an individual child's needs and abilities. For a young child with a disruptive behavior dis-

order, facilitating his agency may take the form of having him participate in the selection of rewards he will receive for positive behaviors in a behavior management plan as well as giving him the opportunity to talk with the therapist about his experience of anger and its causes (even as his clinician and parents make decisions about the behaviors targeted for change). An older child with depression should play an active role in talking with the clinician and her parents about how her symptoms affect her functioning, what she would like to change through therapy, and how she might apply the techniques she is learning in therapy to different situations in her life (even as her parents and therapist also identify therapeutic goals and support her in the application of therapeutic techniques). Facilitating the exercise of agency for an adolescent with ADHD may include allowing him to decide whether to take his medication on days he does not have school (even as he is expected to take his medication on school days), what methods for organization and planning would be most acceptable and effective for him, and the self-advocacy steps he feels most comfortable with at school. The American Academy of Pediatrics recommends that practitioners solicit assent from youth to whom they prescribe medications for ADHD, allowing the child or adolescent to have an opportunity to express her agreement with or objection to this element of treatment despite not needing to provide true legal consent (Koshy & Sisti, 2015). Particularly for youth who are likely to experience prolonged or recurrent symptoms into adulthood, bringing them into the treatment process as active agents better prepares them to take over the decision-making roles in their own treatment that shift from parents (as youth) to oneself (as older adolescents and adults). Finally, the empowerment of allowing youth to appropriately exercise their agency in the treatment process can be an element of healing and improvement in and of itself. Empowering youth in this manner can help counteract the sense of helplessness and powerlessness that youth, particularly those affected by psychopathology, may experience. We will talk in future chapters of this volume about the potential impact of recognizing and making room for children's agency in the treatment process for specific disorders.

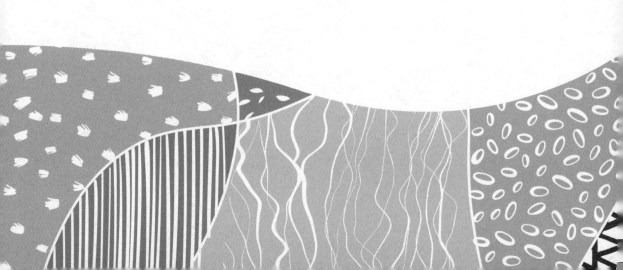

Part Two

Internalizing
Disorders

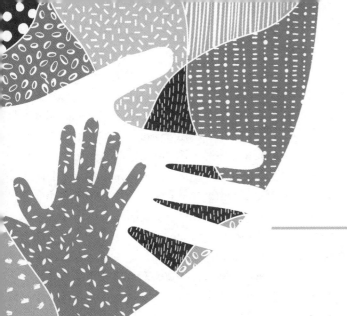

Chapter Three

Depression and Bipolar Disorders

DEPRESSION

AS ONE OF THE MORE frequently diagnosed psychological disorders, depression is sometimes referred to as the "common cold of psychopathology" (McRay, Yarhouse, & Butman, 2016, p. 199). Depressive disorders are characterized by sadness or irritability as well as accompanying cognitive and behavioral symptoms. Two depressive disorders, differing in length and severity of symptoms, are commonly seen in children. Youth with *major depressive disorder* experience persistent depressed or irritable mood and/or diminished pleasure in enjoyable activities for at least two weeks (American Psychiatric Association, 2013). They may also display a variety of other symptoms, including appetite and/or weight changes (or a lack of expected weight gain), changes in sleep, psychomotor agitation or retardation, fatigue or loss of energy, extreme feelings of worthlessness or guilt, difficulty thinking or concentrating, and thoughts of death or suicidality. At least five symptoms must be present for a diagnosis of major depression. *Persistent depressive disorder*, or *dysthymia*, requires fewer symptoms with a longer duration for diagnosis. Youth with dysthymia display depressed or irritable mood, along with at least two other symptoms, for at least one year.

At any given point in time, around 2-3% of children and 3-6% of adolescents meet the criteria for major depression; by age eighteen, nearly 13% of youth will have experienced a depressive episode (Bitsko et al., 2018; Costello et al., 2006; Ghandour et al., 2019; Perou et al., 2013). The rate of depression in American youth has remained fairly stable since the 1960s; the apparent rise in the rate of depression over time according to some sources appears to be due to methodological and reporting differences across studies rather than actual changes (Costello et al., 2006). In childhood, boys and girls experience depression at similar rates, but starting around age thirteen, the rate of depression in females rises significantly, reaching a rate that is double the rate for males by the end of adolescence (Galambos et al., 2004; Twenge & Nolen-Hoeksema, 2002). In light of research exploring a variety of potential explanatory factors for this difference in gender rates beginning in adolescence, Hilt and Nolen-Hoeksema (2006) propose an interactional model in which genetic, neurobiological, cognitive, and relational differences combine with puberty-related changes to produce higher symptom levels in girls.

Comorbidity between depression and other disorders is common. In one clinic-referred sample, 74% of youth with depression met the criteria for a comorbid disorder (Hammen et al., 1999). Anxiety disorders and disruptive behavior disorders are the most common comorbidities among depressed youth (Hammen et al., 1999). One-quarter to one-half of youth with depression also meet the criteria for an anxiety disorder, a link thought to be best explained by common biological underpinnings of the two types of disorders (Axelson & Birmaher, 2001). When depression and anxiety are comorbid, it is more common for the anxiety disorder to appear first (Essau, 2003), and the presence of anxiety is associated with more severe depression (McCauley et al., 1993). The influence of shared genetic factors on depression and anxiety increases with age, suggesting that environmental factors may play a stronger role in this comorbidity in childhood, whereas genetic factors play a larger role in adolescence (Waszczuk et al., 2014). Rates of comorbidity between depression and disruptive behavior disorders vary widely, with some studies finding that more than half of youth

with depression also meet the criteria for conduct disorder or oppositional defiant disorder (Fleming & Offord, 1990; Nottelmann & Jensen, 1995). The research is mixed as to the temporal order in which the disorders appear, with some studies finding that conduct problems precede depression and others showing that depression appears first (Rohde, 2009). In addition, depression may co-occur with substance use (Armstrong & Costello, 2002) and eating disorders (Hughes et al., 2013) in adolescence. Finally, depression in youth is commonly preceded by academic difficulties, including poor attendance or poor performance at school (Hammen et al., 1999). Difficulties with concentration and attention that begin before the onset of a full depressive episode may explain these school problems; alternatively, academic struggles, which may reflect learning difficulties, may lead to frustration and hopelessness that in turn raise the risk for depression (Mufson et al., 2004). Finally, youth with depression are more likely than depressed adults to develop later bipolar disorder (Kovacs, 1996).

RISK/CAUSAL FACTORS

Biological factors. Twin and sibling studies of depression in adolescents and adults suggest that depression is moderately heritable, with genetic factors generally contributing more strongly than environmental factors to depressive symptoms (Chen, Li, et al., 2014; Lau & Eley, 2006; Sullivan et al., 2000). Though studies implicating specific genes or gene groups in depression risk have had inconsistent results, the most promising evidence has begun to link a particular genotype of the 5-HTTLPR, or serotonin transporter promoter region, with a heightened risk for depression; however, this genetic risk is generally only expressed in the presence of environmental risk, such as stressful life events, peer victimization, and poor parenting, supporting a diathesis-stress model of disorder (Banny et al., 2013; Hayden et al., 2009; Koss et al., 2018; Little et al., 2015). Youth with a particular genotype may show an increased sensitivity to their environments and, therefore, to environmental and social triggers for depression (Brouillard et al., 2018; Way & Taylor, 2010). Further highlighting the complexity of understanding causal factors, the 5-HTTLPR genotype interacts with both environmental factors and other genetic factors, such as genes linked to brain-derived neurotrophic factor (BDNF), in the prediction of depressive symptoms (Cicchetti & Rogosch, 2014; Wang, Tian, & Zhang, 2020).

A variety of structural and functional abnormalities are seen in neuroanatomical studies of youth with depression, including abnormalities in and among structures within the corticolimbic region of the brain, including the prefrontal cortex (PFC), orbitofrontal cortex (OFC), anterior cingulate cortex (ACC), and amygdala, which are involved with emotional processing and regulation (Hulvershorn et al., 2011). In addition, certain patterns of chemical abnormalities appear to characterize depression, including elevated cortisol levels and dysregulation within the hypothalamic-pituitary-adrenal (HPA) axis of the endocrine system (Guerry & Hastings, 2011; Lopez-Duran et al., 2009), which are thought to be shaped by exposure to environmental stressors (Heim et al., 2008).

Psychological factors.

Cognitive patterns. There is significant theoretical and empirical work linking particular

styles and patterns of thinking with depression across the lifespan. For example, youth who describe themselves in more negative than positive terms experience higher levels of depressive symptoms (Alloy, Black, et al., 2012; Timbremont & Braet, 2004). One of the factors linked to higher rates of depression in adolescent girls and women involves gender differences in rumination, or the tendency to dwell on problems, negative experiences, and/or negative emotions (Butler & Nolen-Hoeksema, 1994; Morrow & Nolen-Hoeksema, 1990). Indeed, across childhood and adolescence, girls show higher levels of rumination than boys, which in turn predict depressive symptoms as well as increases in symptoms over time (Broderick & Korteland, 2002; Hankin, 2008; Moore et al., 2013). In young adults, rumination interferes with cognitive and behavioral patterns that promote mental health and positive mood, including positive thinking, hopefulness, engaging in enjoyable activities, and effective problem solving (Abela et al., 2002; Lyubomirsky & Nolen-Hoeksema, 1993, 1995). Interestingly, rumination may also increase depression risk via its impact on other environmental factors; for example, rumination predicts increases in peer victimization over time, suggesting that cognitive factors may affect youths' interactions with others in a way that further increases their risk for depression, a phenomenon known as interpersonal stress generation (McLaughlin & Nolen-Hoeksema, 2012).

Individuals with depression often show particular explanatory patterns in how they understand causes of events, known as attributional style. Explanations for events can be internal (caused by my characteristics/actions) or external (caused by influences outside myself), stable (unchanging over time) or unstable (fleeting or situationally bound), and global (applying to many situations or domains) or specific (true only of events related to the one in question). For example, if an adolescent receives a poor grade on a test at school, there are a variety of explanations she could offer herself for this event, including that she did not study enough (internal, unstable, specific), the exam was too hard (external, unstable, specific), the teacher dislikes her (external, stable, specific), or she is stupid (internal, stable, global). Across childhood and adulthood, individuals with depression tend to make internal, stable, and global attributions for negative events but explain positive events as having external, unstable, and specific causes (Gladstone & Kaslow, 1995; Hankin et al., 2018). Blaming oneself for negative events, and failing to recognize one's role in positive events, contributes to negative emotions and maladaptive behaviors, such as social withdrawal (Zimmer-Gembeck et al., 2016), which in turn reinforce this explanatory style. In the example given above, the adolescent who believes she is stupid is likely to feel sad or angry and to not put forth any effort to improve her performance, whereas the teen who believes she failed the test because she did not study enough might be frustrated but is likely to change her study habits in order to try to do better on the next exam. It is important to note that there are developmental changes in the links between explanatory style and outcomes. In middle childhood, explanatory style does not predict depression; however, by late childhood, youth who display a more pessimistic explanatory style (i.e., blaming themselves for and perceiving negative events as

their fault while attributing positive events to external and fleeting causes) are more likely to develop depressive symptoms (Nolen-Hoeksema et al., 1992). This difference suggests that environmental variables, rather than still-developing psychological factors, are more influential in mental health at a younger age.

It is important to note that there are complex interactions among causal factors, including between cognitive and other risk factors for depression. For example, heritability studies suggest a significant link between genetic factors and rumination (Moore et al., 2013). In addition, depressive symptoms predict changes over time in attributional style, suggesting a bidirectional relationship between these variables (Gibb et al., 2006). Finally, it appears that attributional style does not increase hopelessness in individuals who are not experiencing significant negative life events or other stressors (as they do not have negative experiences to attribute to their own stable characteristics), meaning that attributional style interacts with environmental risk in a diathesis-stress fashion to produce depressive symptoms (Hayden et al., 2009; Rueger & Malecki, 2011).

Emotion regulation and coping. Difficulty regulating emotions effectively has been linked with internalizing symptoms broadly (Alink et al., 2009; Kim & Cicchetti, 2010) and depressive symptoms specifically (Cole et al., 1996; Hughes et al., 2011). There are a number of aspects of emotion regulation that have been linked to depression risk. First, adolescents who experience more intense and frequently changing emotions, which may be challenging to regulate, have higher levels of depressive symptoms (Silk et al.,

2003; Turpyn et al., 2015). Indeed, youth with higher levels of depressive symptoms are more emotionally out of control and more likely to experience negative emotions that interfere with adaptive behavior (Hughes et al., 2011; Neumann et al., 2010). Poor emotional self-awareness also predicts depressive symptoms (Hughes et al., 2011). Second, certain regulatory patterns appear to be associated with depressive symptoms. Youth who have higher levels of depressive symptoms tend to utilize fewer emotion regulation strategies when they experience negative emotions; use effective and adaptive emotion regulation strategies less frequently; use maladaptive strategies such as internalization (i.e., direct emotions at themselves), avoidance, disengagement, and rumination when they are upset; and view their emotion regulation attempts, as well as their mothers' attempts to help them regulate emotions, as less effective than their peers (Flett et al., 2012; Garber et al., 1995; Hughes et al., 2011; Neumann et al., 2010; Silk et al., 2003). In contrast, adolescents who utilize effective and adaptive strategies for managing negative emotions, such as engaging in distracting activities and seeking support, experience lower symptom levels (Flett et al., 2012; Moore et al., 2013).

As with other risk factors, emotion regulation interacts with other influences on a child's functioning and development. For example, girls who do not regulate sadness well have higher levels of depressive symptoms, but only when their parents are not highly accepting and warm (Feng et al., 2009). In addition, executive function deficits, such as poor working memory and cognitive flexibility, may impede some youths' coping ef-

forts and increase their risk for depression (Evans et al., 2016). Executive functioning supports skills such as cognitive flexibility, problem solving, and planning ahead, which appear to be important components of identifying and implementing effective strategies for coping with negative experiences and emotions. Temperament-based characteristics of positive and negative emotionality (the tendency to experience positive and negative emotions, respectively), which are likely to affect emotion regulation and coping abilities, have also been linked to depression risk (Compas et al., 2004; Van Beveren et al., 2019). Indeed, difficulties with emotion regulation may be the mechanism through which other risk factors, such as temperament and interpersonal stressors or traumas, increase a youth's risk for depression (Chang et al., 2018; Fussner et al., 2018; Yap et al., 2007, 2010). For example, when parents express strong negative emotions and critical comments toward their children, adolescents may experience significant sadness and anger without the regulatory support of their parents, which may be especially likely to happen for youth who are temperamentally prone to readily experiencing negative emotions. These youth may ruminate on these emotions and their parents' words and actions toward them rather than distracting themselves or seeking others' support, cognitive and regulatory strategies which create further emotional and behavioral consequences that raise the risk for depression.

Environmental factors.

Stressors. There is a significant body of literature linking stressors with an increased risk for depression in children and adolescence (Cole et al., 2006; Ge et al., 1994; Nishikawa et al., 2018; Nolen-Hoeksema et al., 1992; Rudolph et al., 2009). Life events which are identified as disappointing may put youth at particular risk for ongoing depression (Goodyer et al., 1997). Research on the effect of poverty or socioeconomic status on depression in youth is mixed (Costello et al., 1996; Eamon, 2002; Twenge & Nolen-Hoeksema, 2002). Studies that have found a positive association between poverty and depression risk point to mechanisms such as violence and disengagement in the neighborhood, a lack of engagement in academic and extracurricular activities, maternal depression, and physical punishment (Eamon, 2002).

Stress exposure appears to interact with cognitive and behavioral patterns in the prediction of depressive symptoms (Robinson et al., 1995). For example, adolescents who experience more interpersonal stressors have more depressive symptoms but only when they also display certain cognitive patterns, such as low self-worth and a negative attributional style (Carter & Garber, 2011). In addition, peer victimization shows a strong link with depressive symptoms, which may be mediated by maladaptive coping responses as well as a negative attributional style (Gibb et al., 2012; Hawker & Boulton, 2000; Troop-Gordon et al., 2015). Stress also affects explanatory style, with children who report more negative life events becoming more pessimistic in their explanatory style over time (Nolen-Hoeksema et al., 1992). Finally, the symptoms of and behaviors associated with depression may actually increase the occurrence of interpersonal stressors in girls, rather than stress simply acting to increase symptoms, supporting a transactional model of depression (Rudolph et al., 2009). Therefore,

it is important to assess not only the stressors present in a client's life or history but also their impact on behavioral and cognitive patterns and functioning.

Family dynamics. Clinical samples of depressed youth commonly report a number of family stressors, including parental divorce, low levels of parental marital satisfaction, high levels of parental stress, low levels of parental support, and frequent marital and parent-child conflict (Eamon, 2002; Hammen et al., 1999). For example, adolescents whose parents divorce experience greater increases in depressive symptoms than their peers with nondivorced parents, a link that is explained by stressful life events, which often increase following disruptive family events such as divorce (Ge et al., 2006).

The dynamics within families have also been linked with depression risk (Goodyer et al., 1997: Liu & Merritt, 2018; Wang, Tian, Guo, & Huebner, 2020). High levels of parental criticism and negativity are associated with higher levels of depressive symptoms, a link that may be mediated by youths' emotional reactivity (Turpyn et al., 2015; Yap et al., 2010). Similarly, parents who are more aggressive and less approving and affectionate toward their children have adolescents who develop higher levels of depressive symptoms over time (Schwartz et al., 2012, 2014). Adolescents also experience more depressive symptoms and greater increases in symptoms over time when their parents are highly psychologically controlling (El-Sheikh et al., 2010; Kouros & Garber, 2014). Interestingly, one study found controlling parenting to predict depressive symptoms only in girls who displayed low levels of positive emotions, suggesting an interaction between parent and child characteristics in the development of depression (Feng et al., 2009). Lower levels of support and cohesion within families have also been linked with higher levels of depressive symptoms in youth (Flett et al., 2012; Kouros & Garber, 2014; Sheeber et al., 1997; White, Shelton, & Elgar, 2014). Certain parental characteristics, such as maternal depression, increase the likelihood of negative parenting behavior that promotes children's depression (Kuckertz et al., 2018; Wolford et al., 2019). Furthermore, family dynamics can affect response to treatment. Adolescents who experience higher levels of parent-child conflict show less improvement in response to both cognitive-behavioral and psychopharmacologic treatment (Feeny et al., 2009). There may even be a genetic element underlying the link between parent-child conflict and depression in youth; the same parental genetic predisposition that increases youths' biological vulnerability to depression may make parents themselves more likely to interact in conflictual ways with youth (Samek et al., 2018).

It is important to note that family factors interact with one another and with other risk and protective factors in the development of disorder. For example, warm and supportive parenting can attenuate the negative effects of stressors or adolescents' attributional style on depressive symptoms (Ge et al., 1994; Rueger & Malecki, 2011), but low levels of positive parenting can enhance the impact of other stressors on adolescents' depression risk (Oppenheimer et al., 2018). In addition, one study found adolescents' mood lability to predict later negative parent-child interactions but not the reverse (e.g., negative interactions predicting symptoms; Maciejewski et al., 2014), suggesting that youths' symptoms can affect family functioning and highlighting the dynamic interactions that affect psychopathology in youth. Finally, as discussed earlier, it is clear that genetic and biological risks interact with environmental stressors to shape an individual's path toward or away from disorder. Such interactions can help us understand why some children who experience high levels of family conflict or stress, for example, develop depression, whereas others do not; they can also help us understand how to better promote resilience or intervene to change the course of a disorder.

Developmental Course

Like other disorders, depression may manifest differently depending on the age and developmental level of the individual. Differences in presentation may be due to developmental abilities that change over time (e.g., cognitive abilities, language abilities, self-awareness, abstract thought, future orientation) or differences in the causal factors that are linked to depression at different stages (Weiss & Garber, 2003). Previous DSM criteria for depressive disorders have been widely criticized for being developmentally insensitive and difficult to use to accurately diagnose these disorders among youth (Essau & Ollendick, 2009), and DSM-5 criteria remain little changed. However, a number of developmentally oriented researchers have studied how depression may present differently across childhood and adolescence. Some writings talk about a very early form of depression that can appear in eighteen- to twenty-four-month-olds and may present as sustained social withdrawal and avoidance (Guedeney, 2007). As this very early depression is understood as the manifestation of particular parent-child dynamics that result from factors such as maternal depression (Luby, 2009), interventions focus on changing these interactions and are unique to this age group (e.g., Jung et al., 2007). In preschoolers with depression (roughly ages three to five), symptoms commonly reflect DSM criteria; for example, sadness or irritability and anhedonia are common symptoms (Luby et al., 2003, 2006). However, many young children will not meet DSM diagnostic criteria if they are applied strictly and may be underdiagnosed when clinicians rely on them exclusively. One study found that a modified set of criteria may better capture depression at this age; these criteria are based largely on the DSM criteria for adults but include alterations such as symptoms that may be less persistent (e.g., depressed mood "for a portion of the day for several days" rather than "most of the day, nearly every day"), feelings of worthlessness or guilt that may appear through play rather than explicit verbal statements, and suicidal or self-harming themes in play rather than explicit suicidal thoughts or behaviors (Luby et al., 2002). Some depressed preschoolers may also exhibit significant disruptive behavior (Luby et al., 2006). Children who experience depression in preschool are at heightened risk for depression and other disorders later in childhood and adolescence (Gaffrey et al., 2018; Luby et al., 2014).

There is some similarity between childhood and adolescent depression, such as in episode duration and severity and in rates of recurrence (Birmaher et al., 2004). However, some changes occur with development. As childhood progresses, parents of depressed youth generally report decreases in crying but increases in sad mood and feelings of worthlessness (Achenbach, 1991a). Youth with depression self-report an increase in negative mood as they enter adolescence (Achenbach, 1991b); indeed, sadness is the most common and severe symptom of depression in adolescents and is more likely to characterize the disorder than anhedonia (Rohde et al., 2009). In depressed girls uniquely, sad mood continues to worsen across adolescence, and withdrawal, concentration difficulties, insomnia, low energy, and weight gain or loss are common symptoms during the teen years (Achenbach et al., 1991; Rohde et al., 2009). Symptoms such as hopelessness and guilt also appear more frequently in adolescents than in children, likely due to the development of more advanced and future-oriented cognitive abilities (Weiss & Garber, 2003). In contrast with adults with depression, adolescents are more likely to have appetite and/or weight changes, difficulty sleeping, and loss of energy and less likely to experience anhedonia or difficulty concentrating (Rice et al., 2019). Adolescents with depression are more likely than their healthy peers to drop out of high school and to be unemployed in adulthood (Clayborne et al., 2019).

ASSESSMENT

Assessment of youth depressive symptoms most commonly includes both diagnostic interviews and questionnaires and should elicit information from multiple sources, including youth, parents, and teachers (Essau & Ollendick, 2009; Rudolph & Lambert, 2007). Interviews can be unstructured or structured; an example of the latter is the Schedule for Affective Disorders and Schizophrenia in

School-Age Children (K-SADS; Kaufman et al., 1997), which assesses children and adolescents' symptomatology through separate parent and child interviews. Perhaps the most commonly used self-report rating scales are the Beck Depression Inventory (BDI; Beck & Steer, 1993), designed for use with adults but suitable for adolescents; the Children's Depression Inventory (CDI; Kovacs, 1992), an adaptation of the BDI for children as young as age seven; and the second editions of the Reynolds Child Depression Scale (RCDS-2; Reynolds, 2010) and Reynolds Adolescent Depression Scale (RADS-2; Reynolds, 2002), which are scored based on both age and gender norms. The depression subscales from broadband symptom measures such as the Child Behavior Checklist (CBCL; Achenbach, 1991a) and its related forms can also be used and allow for the concurrent assessment of other types of comorbid symptoms. Essau and Ollendick (2009) argue for the use of dimensional rather than categorical assessment tools for depression in youth. Categorical assessments, commonly including structured interviews, aim to determine whether each symptom is present or absent and whether the total number of symptoms meets the cutoff criteria in the DSM. In contrast, dimensional assessments such as the CBCL allow for the measurement of constellations of symptoms along continua and facilitate data-based comparison to same age and gender peers.

It is important to remember during the assessment process that the presentation of depression changes across childhood and adolescence (Rudolph & Lambert, 2007). Therefore, a developmentally sensitive approach necessitates awareness of the way in which the client's age may affect observed or reported symptomatology; this awareness is important to ensure that youth who do not fit the largely adult-based symptom descriptions in the DSM-5 are not underdiagnosed. Furthermore, childhood and particularly adolescence may be periods of more normative mood fluctuations and difficulties learning to regulate emotions than adulthood. Clinicians need to understand what is developmentally typical in order to judge whether mood-related symptoms represent passing stages or true, clinically significant aberrations. Clinicians must also consider whether the child's current functioning is a change from past functioning.

Thorough assessment should include evaluation for comorbid disorders, particularly anxiety disorders (Rudolph & Lambert, 2007). Clinicians should be cautious about the use of certain rating scales in this process, as many questionnaires do not distinguish well between depressive and anxious symptoms (Joiner et al., 1996). However, some instruments, such as the Positive and Negative Affect Scale for Children (PANAS-C: Laurent et al., 1999) have been found to differentiate between depression and anxiety (Lonigan et al., 2003), as both are characterized by negative emotions, but depression is more likely to involve the absence of positive emotions. Well-designed, thorough clinical interviews with children and parents can assist in this process as well. Finally, in addition to evaluating depressive symptoms, a thorough assessment should include specific information about social functioning, stressful events, and family history (Klein et al., 2005) in order to inform treatment planning from a developmental psychopathology framework.

TREATMENT

A significant amount of research has explored the effectiveness of a variety of treatments for childhood and adolescent depression. While research on the effectiveness of antidepressants for children and adolescents is much more limited than that with adults, selective serotonin reuptake inhibitors (SSRIs), which increase available serotonin by blocking its reuptake (Stark et al., 2006), appear to be the most effective psychopharmacological treatment (see Emslie, 2012, for a brief review). In general, a combination of medication and a psychosocial treatment, such as cognitive-behavioral therapy (CBT) plus an SSRI, is more effective than either treatment alone (TADS, 2004; Kennard et al., 2014; Vitiello et al., 2006); however, medication may be a particularly crucial component of treatment for severe depression, with some studies finding that combination therapy has no added effectiveness (Curry et al., 2006; Goodyer et al., 2007). Among psychosocial interventions, CBT and behavioral interventions have been found to be the most effective treatments for children, though they are still considered only possibly efficacious. For adolescents, CBT and interpersonal therapy (IPT) have strong research support, and various forms of both types of interventions are considered well established or probably efficacious (Weersing et al., 2017). Each intervention is discussed in detail below. (Note: Because the complete intervention programs that are utilized to treat depression in youth rarely contain behaviorally focused interventions without accompanying cognitive components, the descriptions of the behavioral components of CBT capture the essence of behavioral interventions, which are not discussed separately. An example of a more purely behavioral intervention and its supporting research can be found in Stark et al., 1987.)

Cognitive-behavioral therapy (CBT).

Treatment for Adolescents with Depression Study (TADS). TADS is a randomized clinical trial comparing the effectiveness of an SSRI, CBT, a combination of CBT and an SSRI, and a placebo on depression in adolescents (TADS, 2000). The TADS CBT intervention utilizes the traditional CBT foci on changing cognitive processes and enhancing social and behavioral skills. The program emphasizes the importance of a strong therapeutic alliance between the client and the therapist that is supported by parental involvement. Individual and parent sessions occur over a twelve-week "acute" treatment phase that is followed by three to six weeks of continuation and skill consolidation and then more infrequent booster sessions focused on relapse prevention (TADS, 2005).

TADS CBT begins with psychoeducation about the nature of depression from a CBT model (i.e., that thoughts, feelings, and behaviors affect one another and can create negative as well as positive spirals) in addition to individualized goal setting for treatment. Goals should be concrete, achievable, and mutually agreed upon by the client, parents, and therapist. Adolescents are introduced to the "Emotions Thermometer" as a way to monitor the types and intensity of their emotional experiences as well as triggers, thoughts, and behavioral responses. Using this information, clients and clinicians begin to identify patterns in the adolescent's experience of depression, including situations and cognitions that negatively affect mood. The early sessions of TADS CBT also aim to establish a therapeutic alliance between the client and the clinician. Throughout all stages of TADS CBT, homework and questionnaire-based symptom monitoring are used to promote and track improvement.

As the acute phase of TADS CBT progresses, the focus of therapy shifts to identifying and utilizing strategies to change the maladaptive cognitive and behavioral patterns that underlie depressive symptoms. Behaviorally focused interventions aim to increase behavioral activation, or the use of changes in behavior to activate changes in thoughts and moods. The links among emotions, thoughts, and behaviors are reviewed, and the value of changing behaviors in order to impact thoughts and emotions is discussed. Adolescents are then encouraged to create a list of activities they enjoy (or previously enjoyed) and to select some activities in which to purposefully engage in the coming week. Emphasis is placed on selecting activities that are social, give the client a sense of success, are realistic (e.g., inviting two friends over for dinner rather than making a meal for one's entire class), and are adaptive and not potentially dangerous to oneself or others. Through a discussion of how many enjoyable activities the client has engaged in over the last several days, a concrete goal that represents an increase in these activities is set, and adolescents track their engagement in pleasant activities each day. In addition, therapists work to help clients develop problem-solving skills in order to promote the ability to cope with stressors and challenges and decrease the likelihood that problematic experiences will worsen depressive symptoms. Clinicians and clients discuss the steps of problem solving using the mnemonic RIBEYE (**R**elax

or calm down, **I**dentify the problem, **B**rainstorm possible solutions, **E**valuate possible solutions, say **Y**es to the best solution, and be **E**ncouraged by oneself and others) and then apply these steps to specific problems a client is facing. Finally, to link behavioral and cognitive skills, therapists explain that it is important to identify whether a situation can be changed (i.e., sometimes problem solving and other direct methods may be the best approach, and sometimes they may not be) and that changing our behaviors may not always lead to immediate changes in our thought processes, which can be targeted in other ways.

Cognitive interventions include identifying and challenging cognitive distortions. These distortions may include (often automatic) problematic, inaccurate, and/or unhelpful beliefs that contribute to symptoms of depression. In addition, cognitive work aims to identify clients' attributional style (e.g., internal/external, stable/unstable, global/specific) and the ways in which this pattern may contribute to self-blame or failure to recognize one's positive abilities. Therapists may use hypothetical scenarios as well as material from the client's at-home mood monitoring to guide the client to identify patterns of cognitive distortions or maladaptive attributions. Once adolescents are able to identify their automatic cognitions, they are taught to examine the validity of their thoughts using techniques such as Socratic questioning ("How else might someone see that situation?"), looking for contradictory evidence ("What is the evidence in support of that thought? What is the evidence against it?"), role-playing (having the therapist model self-questioning and generating alternative thoughts), and reverse role-playing (having the therapist embody the adolescents' cognitive distortions while the client offers alternative thoughts to counteract them). For some clients, it may be helpful either to make a list of alternative thoughts to use when "talking back" to their cognitive distortions or to depersonalize the discussion, talking about situations and beliefs that might apply to other adolescents and pretending to coach other individuals to listen to alternative thoughts.

After behavioral and cognitive interventions have been applied, the focus of treatment shifts to skill development in the areas of social interaction and affect regulation. Clinicians use role-playing to model and promote the development of social skills, including conversation skills, assertiveness in social interactions, effective communication, listening skills, and the process of compromising. Adolescents' emotion regulation abilities are promoted by instruction and practice in the areas of emotion identification, identification of emotion-evoking triggers, emotion regulation techniques, and relaxation (including guided imagery, deep breathing, and progressive muscle relaxation). During skill building, family members become a more active part of treatment, with some sessions involving both the parents and the adolescent in order to promote the application of social and emotion regulation skills to interactions within the family.

Finally, the acute stage of treatment ends with a review of individual goals, principles and skills learned in treatment, and progress. The focus of treatment then shifts to a maintenance-oriented relapse prevention stage, with more infrequent sessions that involve a review of previously learned skills and their application to new situations as well as discussion of how to distinguish between a "slip" (brief symptom reappearance) and true relapse. TADS has been found to be effective in reducing depressive symptoms and suicidality in adolescents (TADS, 2009).

ACTION program. The ACTION program is a manualized, cognitive-behavioral group intervention aimed at nine- to thirteen-year-old girls with depression (though the program can be adapted for use with boys; Stark et al., 2010). The program embraces developmental psychopathology assumptions, including an understanding of depression as the outcome of a non-normative developmental pathway in which the effects of a variety of individual risk factors result in disorder, with an emphasis on the effect of risk on girls' emotion regulation skills. The ACTION program consists of child and parent components and has three main goals for clients: (1) to learn and apply coping skills, (2) to identify and effectively solve problems, and (3) to recognize and change cognitive distortions. The child component of the intervention is administered mainly in small groups in a school setting, with each girl also meeting individually with the therapist twice. The parent component also consists of small group meetings, which the client participates in with her parents every other week.

The ACTION program has six core therapeutic components that are the focus of the child intervention, with the parent program promoting skills that support these components. First, clients are provided with affective education, which includes information about depression and the links among thoughts, feelings, and behaviors. Clients are taught to be more aware of their emotional experiences by paying attention to emotion signals in the "three Bs": **B**ody (physiological signs), **B**rain (thoughts), and **B**ehavior. Second, an individual meeting between the client and the therapist focuses on goal setting for treatment as well as linking the group treatment components to the client's goals. Goals are then shared with the group (with the client's permission), and monitoring of progress as well as brainstorming about how group members can help each individual work toward her goals occurs throughout the intervention. Third, the girls are taught coping skills to manage negative moods and cope with difficult situations they cannot change. Emphasis is placed on techniques such as engaging in enjoyable activities, practicing relaxing activities, seeking others' company and support, and being active. Clients are encouraged to keep a "catch the positive diary" (CPD) in which they record positive events and activities in their lives in order to help them find and focus on their positive rather than negative experiences. The CPD also helps girls see the constructive impact of using coping skills on their moods and behaviors. Fourth, therapists work with clients to help them develop problem-solving skills to address situations that can be changed rather than merely coped with. In the ACTION program, the "five Ps" of problem solving are described as **P**roblem (identify the problem), **P**urpose (identify the goal or desired outcome), **P**lans (brainstorm potential solutions), **P**redict and pick (evaluate consequences of identified solutions and pick the best one), and **P**at on the back (evaluate the outcome of the solution). Fifth, group members are reminded of the links among thoughts, feelings, and behaviors and learn to identify and change their distorted cognitions through cognitive restructuring. They are taught that there are many possible interpretations of our thoughts about a given situation and that they can choose which thoughts to believe are true. Clients then learn to recognize negative thoughts and be "thought detectives," testing their thoughts against reality, and identifying alternative cognitions that are more positive and accurate. One helpful, developmentally appropriate framework for externalizing and concretizing the problem of cognitive distortions is to describe them as coming from the "Muck Monster," who gets youth stuck in negative thoughts, and teaching girls to "talk back to the Muck Monster" as they identify and speak alternative thoughts. The Muck Monster can even be represented by an empty chair, in which the therapist can sit when she is representing a client's negative thoughts and toward which clients direct their restructured thoughts. Finally, therapists help clients create a self-map in order to foster a more positive sense of self. Self-maps are visual representations of a client's strengths. Clients themselves—in addition to group members, parents, teachers, and therapists—contribute to the list of strengths that are represented by bubbles on the self-map, which can be significantly influential in broadening a client's sense of herself and helping her recognize her positive qualities.

While clients are working in their small groups to develop self-awareness, coping skills, cognitive restructuring abilities, and problem-solving skills, parents are learning techniques for supporting their children and promoting the use of these skills in the home. Parents work with therapists to develop positive strategies for managing their children's behavior, to learn and model problem-solving skills within the family context, to listen empathically and resolve conflict effectively, and to change any of their own behaviors that support their children's core depressive beliefs (e.g., words or actions that might support a client's view that she is not loved).

Research has shown the ACTION program to be an effective treatment for depression in preadolescent girls, with improvement apparent both immediately following treatment and at a one-year follow-up (Stark et al., 2010). More specifically, the child component, with or without the parent component, leads to a decrease in depressive symptoms and a more positive view of oneself and the future, whereas the parent component of the intervention has been found to improve family cohesiveness and communication.

Interpersonal psychotherapy for depressed adolescents (IPT-A). Interpersonal therapy (IPT; Weissman et al., 2000) was developed as a treatment for depression in adults and has been successfully adapted for use with adolescents, an approach known as interpersonal therapy for depressed adolescents (IPT-A; Mufson et al., 2004). IPT is based in psychodynamic and attachment theories and emphasizes that individuals with depression are in relationships with others that influence the onset of and recovery from the disorder. IPT-A targets the developmentally specific social and relational problems experienced by adolescents with depression, particularly in family relationships, in a twelve- to sixteen-week treatment format. IPT-A takes a developmental psychopathology perspective on depression in adolescents, understanding the negative impact of relational difficulties on developmental tasks as well as the impact of depressive symptoms on interpersonal interactions (Gunlick & Mufson, 2009). The goals of IPT-A include the reduction of both interpersonal problems and overall symptoms of depression.

IPT-A is divided into three phases (Mufson et al., 2004). The *initial phase* involves the assessment of symptoms and associated interpersonal problems, psychoeducation, and goal identification. Treatment begins with a thorough assessment of current symptoms and functioning as well as family, symptom, and psychosocial history. Information is provided by both the adolescent and her parents. During this phase, the suitability of IPT-A as a treatment for a particular youth is also assessed, with a focus on identifying the adolescent's ability to form an open and trusting relationship with the clinician, the mutual recognition of the presence and significance of interpersonal problems, and the family's ability and willingness to support treatment. Following assessment, psychoeducation begins. The IPT-A clinician aims to help the adolescent and her family understand the nature of depression and its impact, including the time-limited and treatable nature of the disorder. Therapists then assign the client a "sick role," in which the negative impact of symptoms is recognized as not being the adolescent's fault but despite which the adolescent should try to function as well as possible in her daily life and roles. The "sick role" is meant to provide a balance between the pressure on the adolescent to overcome the effects of her symptoms on a day-to-day basis and the expectation that she will not be able to function at all in the midst of a depressive episode.

The focus of IPT-A then shifts to the identification of the interpersonal problems the adolescent is facing and goal setting relating to these difficulties. Therapists utilize a tool called the interpersonal inventory to visually map the client's relationships. The template for the interpersonal inventory consists of an *x*, representing the client, surrounded by a series of concentric circles, or "closeness circles." The client is asked to write the names of the people she feels closest to in the smallest circle, with larger circles populated with the names of people with whom the client has relationships of decreasing closeness. This relational map is then used as a prompt for a discussion of the adolescent's significant relationships, including the dynamics of these relationships and how they have been affected by the depressive symptoms. This discussion continues and deepens across subsequent treatment sessions. The therapist may also encourage the adolescent to explore recent major life events in order to better understand how such stressors have contributed to the development of depression and interpersonal problems. As the adolescent's significant relationships and interpersonal difficulties are explored, possible goals for the remainder of treatment may begin to emerge. IPT-A therapists are encouraged to focus on goals in the areas of (1) grief over the death of a loved one, (2) conflicts in relationships with family and friends, (3) relationally oriented role transitions (e.g., beginning puberty, adding family members), and/or (4) social skills deficits. These areas of relational difficulty are common among adolescents and well suited for IPT-A's focused and short-term format. Clinicians and adolescents work together to identify specific, realistic goals for treatment by exploring which relational problems are of the highest priority to resolve and are likely to be malleable. Goals, as well as other logistic details of treatment, are laid out in a verbal treatment contract between the therapist and the client (and optimally, with the support of the parents), marking the end of the initial treatment phase.

The middle phase of treatment focuses on the development of skills for addressing the interpersonal problems identified in the initial phase. This phase of IPT-A is less manualized than aspects of this and other treatments due to the need to tailor skill building to the unique interpersonal difficulties faced by each client. However, there are some techniques and approaches that are commonly utilized. A general recommendation is for the clinician to be aware of the dynamics of the therapeutic relationship and bring to the client's awareness any interactions within this relationship that reflect the types of problems the client is having in other relationships. One specific therapeutic technique is *encouragement of affect*, in which the therapist aims to help the client understand and manage her emotions so as to improve tolerance of negative emotions as well as awareness of how emotions affect interpersonal interactions. To achieve this goal, IPT-A clinicians often work with clients to create "depression circles," visual representations of the cyclical links among stressful life events, the client's emotions, symptoms of depression, and relational difficulties. Depression circles highlight the self-perpetuating nature of depressive symptoms and offer an opportunity to identify ways to break the negative cycle. A second therapeutic technique that is often useful in IPT-A is *communication analysis*, in which the client and therapist analyze specific interactions the client has had with others in order to understand the impact of communication techniques on relationships and help the client communicate more effectively. Common patterns of ineffective communication include ambiguous and unclear messages, incorrect assumptions that are communicated to others, "the silent treatment," and hostile communication (Weissman et al., 2000). Using communication analysis, clients and therapists work to identify these patterns and replace them with more effective communication techniques, including communicating messages directly and clearly and using empathy to understand the other person's feelings and perspectives on the interaction. Third, as cognitive distortions often interfere with depressed adolescents' abilities to make good decisions, IPT-A therapists may use *decision analysis* to walk a client through problem-solving steps when he needs to make a decision related to an area of interpersonal difficulty. Clients and therapists (1) identify the problem or situation, (2) identify the client's main goal, (3) create a list of possible options, (4) evaluate the options and the consequences, (5) select an option, (6) implement the decision, and (7) evaluate the outcome and return to step four if necessary. In this process, clinicians should be aware that adolescents may struggle to identify a wide range of possible options as well as to implement the best option when they are embedded in a situation; therefore, work with teenage clients may focus on these challenges throughout the decision analysis. Fourth, *role-playing* can be a helpful technique for exploring a client's emotions and behaviors and practicing new skills. As some adolescents will be self-con-

scious about acting out situations in the therapy room, the clinician may need to begin with a simple role-play task, making it as fun as possible or even framing it as if the client and the therapist were putting on a play together. Role-play in IPT-A can be used to practice more effective communication skills, combat social anxiety, build self-confidence, test out an option selected during decision analysis, and identify potential obstacles to applying new skills in a real-life context. Finally, to a more limited degree, clinicians may use direct techniques such as modeling skills and strategies, advising clients in their behavioral choices, and providing education and information (Weissman et al., 2000).

The termination phase of IPT-A revolves around the review of previously learned skills, promoting continued improvement, and preventing relapse. There are seven termination tasks in IPT-A (Mufson et al., 2004). First, the clinician should help the client express her emotions about the end of therapy and communicate that negative emotions are common. If possible, the therapist can also link the client's emotions around termination to the interpersonal experiences and difficulties that have been the focus of therapy. Second, the therapist reviews the signs and symptoms of depression, as well as the specific effects depression has had on the client, in order to prepare the adolescent to recognize them in case of recurrence. Third, the positive changes that have occurred during therapy are reviewed to help the client see his areas of competency as well as his active role in his own improvement. Fourth, the client and the therapist should review the interpersonal stressors that the client has faced, which may involve a review of the goals of treatment. Following the discussion of interpersonal strategies, the fifth termination task involves encouraging the client to recognize the interpersonal strategies she has developed in therapy for interacting and communicating well with others during difficult interpersonal interactions. Discussion of specific situations in which the client successfully used—or could have used—these strategies can be helpful in encouraging the client to use them again in the future, which is the focus of the sixth termination task. To promote continued use of adaptive interpersonal strategies, clients and clinicians brainstorm relational stressors or difficulties that the client is likely to face in the future and link acquired strategies to these situations. Seventh, if the reason for termination is not the completion of all therapeutic goals (e.g., therapy is ending because of a change in the therapist's or client's situation), therapists should assess the need for further treatment. This evaluation might include a discussion of identified problem areas, treatment goals, the degree of progress that has been made, and the benefits and challenges of continuing treatment. For all clients, regardless of termination reason, less frequent booster or maintenance sessions that occur for a period of time following termination (e.g., biweekly sessions for three months, monthly sessions for one year) can help maintain gains and prevent relapse.

IPT-A is considered a well-established individual treatment for depression in adolescence. A number of studies have shown that IPT-A leads to a reduction in symptoms and distress and an improvement in functioning immediately after therapy and at a one-year follow-up (see Gunlick & Mufson, 2009, for a review).

INTEGRATIVE APPROACH TO TREATMENT

CBT. Cognitive-behavioral interventions emphasize the links among thoughts, feelings, and behaviors, a concept which is supported by Scripture (Elliott, 2006). For example, we see the potential impact of our emotions on our behavior and cognitions when we are told, "See what this godly sorrow has produced in you: what earnestness, what eagerness to clear yourselves, what indignation, what alarm, what longing, what concern, what readiness to see justice done" (2 Corinthians 7:11) and when Moses follows the presentation of the Ten Commandments with the instruction to his listeners, "God has come to test you, so that the fear of God will be with you to keep you from sinning" (Exodus 20:20). We are given examples, particularly in the gospel of Mark, of how Jesus' view (thoughts) of sin and injustice provokes anger and subsequent action (Mark 3:5; 10:13-16; 11:15-16). Jesus also gives verbal instruction linking a change in thinking with a change in emotion (John 21:23-24), and true repentance and submission to God (behavior) is sometimes portrayed as involving an emotional component (James 4:9). Therefore, the idea that our emotions, cognitions, and behaviors affect one another is consistent with biblical portrayals of human nature.

Furthermore, we can utilize biblical and theological principles to create a uniquely Christian approach to CBT interventions for depression in youth. Behaviorally focused components of intervention include helping clients learn to monitor and increase their engagement in enjoyable activities as well as to develop problem-solving skills. From a behavioral standpoint, it is important to note that youth with depression often feel hopeless and helpless. They may have essentially lost the sense that they have any agency to change their experiences or contribute to improvements in their symptoms; rather, they often feel at the mercy of their circumstances and their disorder. However, recognizing that these youth, like all others, do have God-given agency (Miller-McLemore, 2003), we might approach behavioral interventions with the theological goal of helping them regain this recognition in their own lives. Although changing emotions and cognitions can feel abstract and challenging when one is in the middle of a depressive episode, counting and increasing pleasurable activities is often a much more concrete and achievable task. (This is one reason behavioral interventions are often implemented before the cognitive components of CBT.) Because this task is usually fairly easily and enjoyably achieved by youth in treatment, it can contribute to increasing not only positive emotions, which God expresses toward us and wants us to experience (Zephaniah 3:17; Galatians 5:22-23), but also a client's sense of agency in her own life. Similarly, teaching children and adolescents problem-solving skills and helping them to implement them during difficult situations can help them shift from a sense of helplessness (e.g., "I always get into trouble at school") to more adaptive responses and behaviors that contribute to a positive view of their own agency (e.g., "I was able to try a new solution, and it had a positive outcome!"). The potential for, and importance of, improvement in a client's sense of agency and its role in improving symptoms of depression also highlights the balanced role of parents and clinicians; these adults help, teach, and

support but do not become intrusive or over-involved in the tasks that youth need to be doing themselves, such as choosing enjoyable activities to engage in more or selecting the best solution to a problem.

Cognitive interventions focus on identifying and challenging cognitive distortions. In order to call a particular thought pattern a distortion, we must first understand the truth by which we are judging the accuracy of the cognition and according to which we are testing it. Some truths are more individual and experientially based, with evidence for or against them stemming from personal circumstances. For example, youth with depression often struggle with the thoughts that other people do not like them or that they are stupid. Although it is possible that these facts are true for a given individual, for the vast majority of youth, these thoughts are inaccurate and, therefore, are considered distortions (e.g., thinking that "no one likes me" after the dissolution of one friendship or that "I am stupid" following poor performance in a single class). In these cases, the client and the CBT clinician are likely to engage in a search for evidence in the client's life that supports or refutes these beliefs (e.g., "Who are some people in your life who you still have relationships with? What is the evidence that these individuals like you?" or "How has your present and past performance in other classes been? What is the evidence across a variety of academic and other pursuits that your intelligence is low?"). In other cases, the negative thought patterns that permeate depression may revolve around greater issues of truth that go beyond one's life circumstances. For example, the beliefs that "no one likes me" or "I am stupid" are likely distortions in and of themselves, but they have an impact on emotions and behaviors because they have a deeper level of meaning. One individual could believe that she is disliked by others and have no emotional reaction, while another displays this belief and becomes extremely sad and hopeless and withdraws socially as a result. The difference in these reactions is in the meaning that is ascribed to the belief. If the therapist and the client dig more deeply into the thoughts of the second individual, they are likely to uncover beliefs such as "being disliked means that I am an unlikable person" and "my sense of value comes from being likable and/or liked by others." These deeper distortions deal with broader issues of truth that are not unique to an individual's circumstances. As Christians, we share an understanding of certain universal truths based on our Scriptures and theology, and these truths can be utilized to counter these deeper cognitive distortions that may truly underlie the emotional and behavioral symptoms of depression. Scripture can be a particularly useful tool for challenging distorted beliefs with Christian clients (Pearce, 2016; Tan, 1987; Walker, Ahmed, Milevsky, Quagliana, & Bagasra, 2013; Walker et al., 2014). The client who believes that her sense of value comes from human perceptions of her might spend time memorizing and meditating on verses that speak about God as the source of human value (e.g., Genesis 1:27; Zephaniah 3:17; Luke 12:24; Galatians 2:20; 1 John 3:1) so that she can use these Scriptures as self-statements to counter her cognitive distortions. An adolescent who feels an overwhelming sense of guilt might be directed to find comfort in Scriptures that speak about God's forgiveness and love (e.g., Matthew 26:26-28; John 3:16;

Romans 8:37-39; Ephesians 2:4-7; Colossians 2:13-14). We might think about the ACTION program technique of teaching clients to "talk back to the Muck Monster" as a developmentally appropriate representation of the use of Scripture to counter the lies that we believe that can come from the devil or have their source in evil roots (John 8:44). One note of caution: we should be careful not to communicate to clients that a "good Christian" will be able to read and learn more Scripture and quickly experience symptom improvement as a result, a message that may induce more guilt and negative feelings by simplistically reducing the solution to depression or other disorders to the performance of spiritual practices. Rather, we should emphasize the use of Scripture as a tool to speak truth as one component of treatment.

The self-mapping component of the ACTION program represents a specific focus on the development of a more positive sense of self in clients, which is another cognitive intervention. During this process, the therapist solicits feedback from other people who can speak to the client's strengths, a contribution that can make a significant difference in whether the client truly believes that she has positive qualities (rather than just being encouraged by the clinician to identify these in herself). The role of this external feedback highlights for those of us who interact with and care for youth the importance of not only valuing children as gifts but also communicating our valuing to them. While we have previously discussed the importance of encouraging youth not to find their meaning in others' opinions, we also recognize that Scripture exhorts us to love one another through our words and our behaviors (John

13:34-35; Ephesians 4:29), and the expression of this love and care may be particularly significant for youth who struggle with the depressive symptoms of sadness, hopelessness, self-blame, and negative self-concept. Therefore, as parents, teachers, mentors, and clinicians, we might view it as a theological duty to communicate to the youth we live and work with that they are worthy, loved, and valuable, in our eyes and in the Lord's.

Finally, intervention components that target emotions, such as emotion regulation skill building, also affect the links among behaviors, thoughts, and feelings. We see a wide variety of examples of emotional expressions throughout the Bible, ranging from those that are condemned in the text to those that are portrayed as "right" or help the author connect with God, as well as emotions displayed by Jesus himself. Therefore, it is not the experience or expression of particular feelings that are inherently good or bad from a theological perspective; rather, it is the thoughts an emotion reflects as well as the effect it has on our behavior that influence our understanding of its nature and desirability (Elliott, 2006). Furthermore, there are a number of biblical examples of commands related to self-control or self-regulation as well as to methods of changing our emotions (e.g., Proverbs 25:28; Philippians 4:6; see Hall, 2014, for a more complete discussion of emotion regulation in Scripture and theology). Therefore, in the process of helping clients become more skillful emotion regulators, we should seek to understand the prompts and dynamics of each emotional experience in order to determine how it is best regulated (reduced versus enhanced, changed via cognitive versus behavioral components) or whether it should

be fully experienced and expressed as a means for contributing to development, including one's relationship with God. In specific consideration of depression, we see many examples in the Psalms of the expression of sorrow and pain to the Lord (Psalm 22:1-2; 77:1-2; 102:1-11; 119:28; 120:1). Yet, many of these Psalms begin with the expression of sorrow but move into praise for God and recognition of his goodness and faithfulness, often even culminating in expressions of faith and joy. God hears our cries and welcomes our genuine expressions of grief and sadness, but he does not desire for us to stay in a state of distress. The acts of crying out to God in our sorrow and also reminding ourselves of his goodness and faithfulness to his people, as displayed through the fulfillment of his promises, are methods for managing and addressing the strong negative emotions that often occur within depression. In addition, we can be comforted and encouraged by the reminder that God has purposes and plans that are much greater than merely our happiness; through our trials and difficulties, which may include periods of deep sadness, God is at work in us, refining us and growing us in ways that are uniquely facilitated by the challenges we experience (Romans 5:3-5; James 1:2-4).

IPT-A. The IPT-A focus on the centrality of relationships to well-being, and their vulnerability during times of difficulty and stress, is consistent with a Christian theological and biblical view of our interactions with others. Bonhoeffer (1954) states, "The physical presence of other Christians is a source of incomparable joy and strength to the believer" (p. 19). Intentionally including the youngest members of the body of Christ in our community is of special importance to many theologians who write about children (e.g., Mercer, 2005). We are created by a relational three-in-one God to be in helping and supporting relationships with other people (Genesis 2:18-24). Beginning shortly after the fall, however, discord, shame, blame, and even violence are introduced into relationships (Genesis 3–4). We see the continued effects of sin and its nature on brokenness in relationships throughout Scripture and Christian history as well as in our daily lives. For this reason, biblical writers such as Paul devote a good deal of time and space to instructions for living in right relationships with family and friends (e.g., Romans 13–14; 1 Corinthians 5–7, 12; Ephesians 4–6), and Scripture portrays healthy interactions with others as an important component of godly life. During his time on earth, Jesus devoted significant time and energy to developing and nurturing his relationships with his disciples, who played an important role in supporting him and his ministry (despite their many failings and denials). Due to both the importance and the difficulty of maintaining healthy relationships, treatment for depression that targets relational dynamics is supported on a theoretical level by the value Christians place on relationships.

Theologians' views of children's sinfulness vary widely, with some writers advocating a balanced approach that views children as both victims and agents of sin (Jensen, 2005). Such a view recognizes that children may not evidence a sinful nature in the same way and with the same level of personal responsibility as adults; in addition, the effect of sin on children may be primarily through the sinful actions of others, such as in cases of abuse and other forms of violence. On the other hand, as fully human persons, children are affected by original sin and possess a sinful or fleshly nature. We should not, therefore, view them as entirely innocent, holy, or incapable of sinning (as anyone who has parented small children would likely agree); children can sin and even contribute to violence against others. This balanced view of children's sin natures parallels the IPT-A idea of assigning the client a "sick role." The adolescent (and her family members) should recognize that her symptoms will impact her functioning and not see her as being at fault for impairment in relationships, schoolwork, and self-care; however, her depression is not viewed as an "excuse" to purposefully neglect the areas over which she can still exert some control or to not make her best attempt (limited though it may be) to function as well as possible in the different arenas of her life. Just as this balanced view of sin in childhood promotes both care for children in their vulnerability and responses to them that aim to improve and shape their behavior toward right living, so also the idea of the sick role helps family members (and the client herself) to show the client grace during a depressive episode but maintain the expectation that she has still has agency to work toward her own improvement and function as well as she can in a given situation.

Similar to our discussion of integration within CBT approaches, the skill-building or behaviorally focused components of IPT-A—including improving self-understanding, communication skills, and problem-solving skills—have the potential to improve a client's sense of his own agency in the midst of a disorder that can make this recognition especially challenging. Working with youth to support the development of these skills helps them to gain confidence in their abilities to navigate difficult relationships and interactions rather than feeling helpless to change them. The emphasis on communication skills in IPT-A is particularly important in helping adolescents develop the ability to create and maintain the healthy relationships that theology and Scripture portray as central to human purpose and well-being.

BIPOLAR DISORDERS

Bipolar disorders are diagnosed in the presence of manic or hypomanic episodes and their frequently accompanying depressive episodes (American Psychiatric Association, 2013). The criteria for a depressive episode in bipolar disorders are identical to that in depressive disorders. Manic episodes, in contrast, are characterized by the presence of unusually elevated, expansive, or irritable mood and an increase in goal-directed activity or energy for at least one week. Individuals must also display three additional symptoms (four if their mood is irritable rather than euphoric), including grandiosity or an inflated sense of self-esteem, a decreased need for sleep, talkativeness or pressured speech, flight of ideas or racing thoughts, distractibility, an increase in goal-directed activity or psychomotor agitation, and an increase in risky behaviors. The symptoms must be severe enough to cause impairment or necessitate hospitalization or be accompanied by psychotic features. Some individuals may experience hypomanic rather than full manic episodes. Hypomanic episodes involve the same symptom criteria as manic episodes, but symptoms only need to last for four days for diagnosis, and significant impairment, psychotic features, or the po-

tential for harm to self or others is not present. The DSM-5 identifies three bipolar disorders that are distinguished by episode type. Bipolar I disorder consists of at least one manic episode (and may include depressive or hypomanic episodes). Individuals with bipolar II disorder have experienced at least one major depressive and one hypomanic episode. Finally, a child or adolescent can be diagnosed with cyclothymic disorder if he experiences periods of subclinical depressive and manic symptoms over the course of a year without ever meeting the full criteria for a depressive, manic, or hypomanic episode.

The diagnosis of bipolar disorder in children and adolescents has risen drastically since the mid-1990s, from .025% of youth in 1994 to 1% in 2003 (Moreno et al., 2007), with this increase continuing and resulting in more recent prevalence estimates at 1-3% of youth (Birmaher, 2013). Mental health professionals disagree about whether the increase in diagnoses is due to a better understanding of the presentation of the disorder in youth (and, therefore, accurate diagnosis of youth who would not have been identified previously) or an inaccurate overapplication of the diagnosis (Parens & Johnston, 2010). Further complicating diagnosis, comorbidity is the norm rather than the exception in child and adolescent bipolar disorder. Up to 75% of youth with bipolar disorder also have a disruptive behavior disorder (DBD; Findling et al., 2001). Bipolar disorder is also very commonly comorbid with attention-deficit/hyperactivity disorder (ADHD) in youth, with estimates ranging from 32-98% (Biederman et al., 1996; Moreno et al., 2007; Wozniak et al., 1995. Youth with bipolar disorder also have a heightened risk for substance use and anxiety disorders and obsessive-compulsive disorder (Goldstein et al., 2013; Harpold et al., 2005; Lewinsohn et al., 1995; Masi et al., 2018).

RISK/CAUSAL FACTORS

Biological factors. Bipolar disorders are strongly influenced by genetic factors. It is not unusual for youth with bipolar disorders to have a parent with a depressive or bipolar disorder (Findling et al., 2001). Indeed, children who have a parent with bipolar disorder have a five-fold risk of developing the disorder themselves compared to youth with two healthy parents (Youngstrom et al., 2005). Data from twin and adoption studies point to heritability estimates of at least 80% (Mick & Faraone, 2009; Smoller & Finn, 2003; Youngstrom & Algorta, 2014), suggesting that the link between bipolar symptoms in parents and children has a significant genetic component and is not due merely to environmental factors.

There are a number of biological processes that have been linked with bipolar disorder symptoms. There is evidence of dysfunction in emotional processing in youth with bipolar disorders, including increased amygdala activity and decreased activity in the dorsolateral prefrontal and ventromedial prefrontal cortices, which help regulate emotional responses, as well as abnormalities in the connectivity between these regions (Garrett et al., 2012; Ladouceur et al., 2011; Pavuluri, West, Hill, Jindal, & Sweeney, 2009; Singh et al., 2015; Weathers et al., 2018). These findings suggest that increased neurobiological sensitivity to emotional information and decreases in regulatory abilities may underlie the strong emotion responses and dysregulation, including mood shifts, that characterize bipolar

disorder (Strakowski et al., 2012). In addition, it is thought that individuals with bipolar disorder may have dysregulation within their behavioral activation systems (BAS), which regulate approach behaviors and goal-driven activity, as heightened BAS activity is associated with manic and hypomanic episodes, while low BAS activity occurs during depressive episodes (Alloy et al., 2008, 2012; Gruber et al., 2013; Youngstrom & Algorta, 2014). Finally, a number of structural brain abnormalities, including reduced volume in the amygdala and regions of the hippocampus, are associated with bipolar disorder in youth (Blumberg et al., 2005; Tannous et al., 2018; Youngstrom & Algorta, 2014).

Environmental factors. Family dynamics have been found to impact functioning and recovery in individuals with bipolar disorder. One such aspect of family functioning is the level of expressed emotion (EE) present in families. High EE is often operationalized as the number of critical comments, the amount of emotional involvement, and/or the level of hostility observed in family interactions (Miklowitz et al., 2009). In one sample of young adults with bipolar disorder, almost half had families who were high in EE (Butzlaff & Hooley, 1998; Miklowitz et al., 1988). Adults with bipolar disorders whose family members express higher levels of EE are more likely to relapse (Priebe et al., 1989). There is limited research exploring EE in the families of younger bipolar clients, but high EE does appear to predict higher levels of symptoms, particularly depressive symptoms, in children and adolescents (Miklowitz et al., 2006; Rosenbaum Asarnow et al., 2001). High EE has also been linked to lower levels of family cohesion and flexibility among families with a bipolar adolescent (Miklowitz et al., 2009; Sullivan & Miklowitz, 2010). It is likely that the relationship between EE and bipolar symptoms is bidirectional; critical and hostile interactions increase symptomatology and decrease response to treatment, while a family member's active symptoms may also contribute to negative family interactions. In addition, there is some question as to whether high EE may be a manifestation of mood disorder symptoms in family members, suggesting that the link between EE and symptoms might be both environmentally and biologically understood (Miklowitz et al., 2006).

Other aspects of family-related stress may affect the occurrence and course of bipolar disorder. Adolescents with bipolar disorder who report higher levels of interpersonal stressors (with family members, peers, or romantic partners) show less improvement over time in their manic and depressive symptoms, with the effects being particularly strong for older adolescents and females (Kim et al., 2007). High levels of family stressors and conflict have also been linked to higher levels of suicidal ideation in adolescents with bipolar disorder (Goldstein et al., 2009). In addition, parental psychopathology, in the presence of poor parental coping skills, predicts increased symptom severity in youth with bipolar disorders, a link that may be explained environmentally by both parental modeling of emotional dysregulation and decreased parental support (Peters et al., 2015). Finally, physical or sexual abuse in childhood is linked with an earlier age of onset, more time in manic or depressive episodes, faster cycling, and more comorbidity with other disorders in adults with bipolar disorder (Post et al., 2001).

Interactional processes. From a developmental psychopathology perspective, it is important to understand the interplay between biological and environmental influences in the development of bipolar disorder in children and adolescents, recognizing that these risk factors do not exist in isolation. For one, environmental experiences may impact biological processes and trigger manic or depressive episodes. Furthermore, a kindling or sensitization model of bipolar disorder, which posits that the progression of the disorder changes neurological functioning such that each successive mood episode is more easily triggered by environmental factors, has some empirical support (Post, 2007). On the other hand, genetic factors and biologically based tendencies, such as the experience of intense emotions without well-developed regulatory skills, influence environmental variables, straining interpersonal relationships and potentially increasing family conflict and stress (Youngstrom & Algorta, 2014). However, the processes by which these factors interact to influence the onset and course of an individual client's disorder is unique, highlighting the importance of assessing individual risk and protective factors and taking these into consideration in treatment implementation.

DEVELOPMENTAL COURSE

The influence of developmental factors and stages on the presentation and course of bipolar disorder is less clear than for some other disorders in youth. However, there is some work that informs developmentally oriented understandings. During manic episodes in particular, bipolar disorder in youth looks fairly similar to its adult counterpart (Findling et al., 2001). However, it is important to note that there may be significant differences between certain aspects of the presentation of bipolar disorder in adults and that in children and adolescents. For example, youth with bipolar disorder are more likely to experience ultrarapid or ultradian cycling (as frequently as more than once per day), little to no interepisode recovery (e.g., a chronic course), minicycles that occur between full manic or depressive episodes, mixed episodes, irritability rather than euphoric mood, and explosive angry/violent outbursts or "rages" (Biederman et al., 1996; Findling et al., 2001; Geller et al., 1998, 2002; Wozniak et al., 1995). However, in the DSM-5, children who display outbursts of rage may be more accurately diagnosed with disruptive mood dysregulation disorder (American Psychiatric Association, 2013).

Rapid cycling and mixed episodes, common occurrences in pediatric bipolar disorder, do not appear to change in frequency across development (Demeter et al., 2013). However, some symptom changes do occur with age. Among bipolar youth, certain manic symptoms—such as motor activity, irritability, and aggression—decrease with age, while most depressive symptoms—including sadness, anhedonia, fatigue, low self-esteem, and suicidality—increase into adolescence (Demeter et al., 2013). Such changes are thought to reflect normative developmental changes in self-regulation as well as cognitive ability. Parental report indicates that hypersexuality and impulsive spending during manic episodes increase in adolescence (Freeman et al., 2011).

When youth present with bipolar disorder, it generally begins early in life; for example, one study of clinically referred children found that over two-thirds of youth with a bipolar diagnosis had symptoms that began before age six, though it is important to note that, due to the chronic nature of the disorder, parents may have trouble pinpointing when symptoms began (Wozniak et al., 1995). However, adolescence appears to be the peak period of onset for bipolar disorders (Merikangas et al., 2012). While prospective continuity studies are few, there appears to be a high level of continuity between bipolar disorder in youth and later mood problems (Youngstrom & Algorta, 2014). One study found that 40% of youth with a bipolar disorder experienced a manic episode between the ages of eighteen and twenty (Geller et al., 2008). However, given the significant decrease in the occurrence of the disorder from the early to the later twenties, it has been proposed that there may be a "developmentally limited form" of bipolar disorder that occurs in youth who then grow out of their affective symptoms as the result of brain maturation (Cicero et al., 2009). Therefore, given the difference in presentation between childhood and adult bipolar disorder, we must be cautious in making predictions about individual outcomes, as we do not yet understand how to best distinguish developmentally limited from persistent forms of the disorder. Rather, symptoms should be assessed, diagnosed, and treated as they occur at a given time with as much developmental sensitivity as possible, focusing on their developmental appropriateness as well as the impairment and distress they cause in determining whether they are presently problematic.

ASSESSMENT

Because of the controversies around the accurate diagnosis of bipolar disorder in youth, careful assessment is especially crucial in possible cases of this disorder. Youngstrom and colleagues (2005) offer four main guidelines for assessment of bipolar disorders in children and adolescents. First, given the genetic links and biological underpinnings of the disorder, a family history should be taken to determine whether bipolar disorder is present in any family members. It is important to note that the presence of familial bipolar disorder is more informative than its absence (the former suggests heightened risk whereas the latter does not rule it out). Second, given the potential for misdiagnosis based on symptom overlap or confusion with other disorders, clinicians should thoroughly assess the "handle symptoms" that are unique to bipolar disorder. For example, certain symptoms of bipolar disorder and ADHD—such as distractibility, impulsivity, high energy, and talkativeness—may be mistaken for one another. However, there are a number of symptoms that appear to be unique to mania, including grandiosity, decreased need for sleep, elevated mood, and racing thoughts (Geller et al., 1998). Therefore, thorough assessment of manic symptoms is important for distinguishing between the two disorders. Third, though the pattern of mood cycling may look different in youth than adults, clear cycling may occur for many clients, and unusually intense or frequent mood swings are often present. Therefore, assessment should focus on mood *changes*, whether they are truly episodic according to the DSM definition, that are generally central to the disorder. Fourth, assessment should ideally take

place over an extended timeframe, continuing through the process of treatment. The evaluation of a child's symptoms at a given point in time only provides information about the presence or absence of a current episode, whereas the diagnosis of a bipolar disorder will be enhanced by information about episodes over time (including recurrence and length of individual episodes). In addition, assessment should cover not only current symptoms but past functioning in order to establish a baseline by which to evaluate whether current and present symptoms truly represent a change in mood and/or functioning.

It is tricky to identify a single assessment tool that provides sufficient data to inform a bipolar disorder diagnosis in youth. Some youth-oriented structured interviews do not take into account developmental variation in symptoms, while others do not assess manic symptoms (Youngstrom et al., 2005). Interviews that elicit developmentally sensitive information about mania and depression from multiple reporters (child/adolescent, parents, teachers) are certainly crucial to the diagnostic process; if a suitable structured interview cannot be located, it may be helpful to combine information gathered from an interview with questionnaire data. Two surveys that have been found to be helpful in reliably identifying manic symptoms in youth, and distinguishing mania from other potentially confounding symptoms, are the General Behavior Inventory (GBI; Depue et al., 1989) and its parent-report adaptation (Youngstrom et al., 2001) as well as the parent-report adaptation of the Young Mania Rating Scale (P-YMRS; Gracious et al., 2002).

Finally, due to the high level of comorbidity with other disorders seen in bipolar youth, good assessment must include screening for other disorders, especially ADHD, disruptive behavior disorders, anxiety disorders, and substance use. Improvement in a client's symptoms and functioning will likely be limited by other disorders that are left untreated, though it may be important to address bipolar symptoms first, even if other disorders are present, due to its significantly impairing nature (Kowatch et al., 2005).

Treatment

Effective treatment of bipolar disorders in youth most commonly involves medication. Similar to psychopharmacological treatment in adults, lithium, anticonvulsants, and second generation (atypical) antipsychotic medications have been found to be effective in treating bipolar disorders in children and adolescents, with a limited number of comparative studies suggesting that antipsychotic drugs are more effective than the others (Geller et al., 2012; Goldstein et al., 2012). The addition of an antidepressant may be necessary to most effectively reduce depressive symptoms (Atkin et al., 2017). The use of these drugs is very common: up to 90% of youth receiving outpatient treatment for bipolar disorder are prescribed medication (Moreno et al., 2007). Some researchers and clinicians have expressed concern that, given the drastic increase in diagnoses, medications for bipolar disorder are being overprescribed to youth (Parens & Johnston, 2010). Therefore, providers must recognize the role not only of medication in the treatment of bipolar disorder but also of thorough, accurate assessment in determining whether the disorder is truly present. Following an empirically informed assessment but before beginning

other therapies, young clients with bipolar disorder should be referred to a prescriber for an evaluation of the need for medication. Finally, response rates to treatment vary widely across studies, suggesting that individual differences between clients and families may moderate the effects of treatment (Vitiello, 2013) and highlighting the importance of a developmental psychopathology–informed view of bipolar disorder as the outcome of the interaction of risk and protective factors.

Psychosocial interventions are also commonly an important component of treating bipolar disorder in youth, with empirical support for these treatment approaches increasing rapidly. Family psychoeducation plus skill building is considered a well-established treatment (Fristad, 2016), dialectical behavior therapy is categorized as probably efficacious (Goldstein, Fersch-Podrat, et al., 2015), and cognitive-behavioral therapy is possibly efficacious (Fristad & MacPherson, 2014). Each of these therapeutic approaches is described below.

Family psychoeducation plus skill building. Family-based interventions for bipolar disorders recognize the role of environmental factors in the development and exacerbation of symptoms in youth. They serve to target these risks, which are not likely to be ameliorated by medication and may have an especially powerful effect on youth, who are generally strongly embedded in their family environments. One such approach, family-focused therapy for adolescents (FFT-A; Miklowitz et al., 2004; Miklowitz, Mullen, & Chang, 2008), aims to reduce the effect of family stressors by (1) changing family interactions to decrease expressed emotion and (2) helping clients develop tools for managing these stressors effectively. FFT-A is an adaptation of an adult intervention that addresses bipolar disorder as it presents and is uniquely shaped by developmental considerations in adolescence. The intervention is administered in twenty-one sessions over nine months, with meeting frequency decreasing as treatment progresses, and consists of three phases: psychoeducation, communication enhancement training, and problem-solving skills training.

The psychoeducation phase focuses on helping clients and families understand bipolar disorder and its treatment. Initial sessions begin building the therapeutic alliance and identifying each family member's view of the main problems and goals for treatment. Subsequent sessions revolve around education about the symptoms of bipolar disorder in adolescence as well as how biological and environmental risk and protective factors interact in the development of the disorder. Adolescents and parents begin to (separately) track the client's daily moods and sleep/wake cycles as well as events associated with significant mood changes. The goal of utilizing mood charts early in therapy is to help families understand that mood changes are not entirely unpredictable but can be linked to sleep/wake patterns and environmental events. In addition, the recognition of these individual patterns allows for discussions about how to prevent future episodes as well as to manage difficult moods and minimize their impact on functioning. Parents and siblings are encouraged to view themselves as allies who can both understand the impact of varying states (e.g., stable, manic, depressed) on the adolescent's functioning and well-being and help reduce risk and promote pro-

tective factors, such as regular sleep patterns and positive family interactions.

In the communication enhancement phase, family members are taught skills for effective communication, including (1) giving positive feedback, (2) listening actively, (3) using positive strategies for asking family members to change their behavior, and (4) giving negative feedback constructively. Ineffective communication is viewed as an expression of the family's distress around the adolescent's disorder, so improved communication skills may both strengthen the family's ability to cope with the client's mood changes and reduce the impact of negative family dynamics on the adolescent. The clinician teaches about and models each skill for family members, who then use role-playing to practice the skills with one another. Work focuses initially on the first two skills, which tend to promote positive feelings among family members, and moves to the last two more conflictual skills as treatment progresses. The adolescent adaptation of this phase is much less formal than the adult version, to reduce the potential for resistance, and uses real-life situations whenever possible (e.g., a family comes into a session experiencing conflict around chores). In addition, family members are asked to record their use of each skill outside of the therapy setting in order to promote generalization of communication skills to the home environment.

Finally, the problem-solving skills phase focuses on giving clients the tools to effectively address problems and difficulties they may face, a task that many youth with bipolar disorder find challenging. Families learn the steps of problem solving—identify the problem, generate possible solutions, evaluate these solutions, and select and implement the best option—which is seen as a collaborative process in which parents and adolescents work together to generate and select solutions. Problems can include conflicts within the family, and these conflicts can be reduced by both improvements in clients' and parents' problem-solving skills and the identification of behavior management strategies that parents can use to shape adolescents' behavior. Common topics discussed during the problem-solving stage include increasing compliance with medication, improving sleep habits and consistency, completing schoolwork and improving behavior at school, and decreasing conflicts within the family. In addition, parents and siblings are encouraged to apply problem-solving skills to situations within their own lives that affect their well-being and ability to interact well with the client.

Following the completion of the three phases of FFT-A, quarterly maintenance sessions involve a review of information and skills presented in previous sessions in order to maintain gains and reduce the risk of relapse. Though research has generally utilized small samples, when combined with medication, FFT-A effectively reduces the symptoms of bipolar disorder in adolescents (Miklowitz et al., 2004, 2014) and increases positive family interactions (Simoneau et al., 1999). The intervention has a particularly marked effect on youth from families high in expressed emotion (Miklowitz et al., 2009). Multifamily psychoeducational psychotherapy (MF-PEP; Fristad, Gavazzi, & Mackinaw-Koons, 2003; Fristad et al., 2009), a group intervention with very similar educational and skill-building components as FFT-A, has been found to decrease young adolescents' mood disorder symptoms as well

as to increase positive family interactions, parents' support for clients, and treatment utilization (Fristad, Goldberg-Arnold, & Gavazzi, 2003; Fristad et al., 2009). MF-PEP is particularly effective for youth with poorer functioning and higher levels of stress and trauma (MacPherson et al., 2014).

Dialectical behavior therapy (DBT). Dialectical behavior therapy (DBT) was originally designed as a treatment for adults with borderline personality disorder (Linehan, 1993). Since its initial implementation, it has been adapted for use with adolescents with a variety of emotional and behavioral difficulties, including suicidality and bipolar disorder (Miller et al., 2006; Rathus & Miller, 2015). DBT for adolescents with bipolar disorder includes individual and family sessions over the course of one year (Miklowitz & Goldstein, 2010). During the first six months of treatment, considered the acute treatment phase, clients meet weekly with the therapist; sessions are biweekly during the next three to four months (the continuation phase) and monthly during the final two to three months of treatment. Over the course of the intervention, the clinician (referred to as the "skills trainer") provides psychoeducation about the disorder and works with the client and her family to develop five sets of skills that underlie improvements in emotional and behavioral regulation (Miklowitz & Goldstein, 2010; Rathus & Miller, 2015).

The goal of the *mindfulness* module is to help adolescents learn to be fully present with their current emotions and experiences without judging or trying to change them. Mindfulness skills can help reduce impulsivity, increase positive and decrease negative emotions, support good decision making, and improve attentional focus. Clients learn about the roles of the Emotional Mind (state of being overwhelmed by emotions), the Reasonable Mind (thinking logically and non-emotionally about a situation), and the Wise Mind (the ability to combine emotional and rational input to make the best choices and cope well with stressors). Clients learn how to be mindfully present and practice this skill through a variety of in-session and homework exercises, including mindfully listening to music, smelling a candle, or unwrapping a piece of chocolate. Next, clients learn *distress tolerance*, or the ability to tolerate negative emotions and challenging situations. Two types of distress tolerance skills are taught. Crisis survival skills help adolescents manage negative emotions in the moment so that they do not lead to maladaptive, impulsive outcomes (such as substance use or self-harm). Crisis survival skills include distraction (e.g., doing a puzzle), self-soothing (e.g., stretching, listening to calming music), praying, practicing relaxation, exercising, improving self-talk (cognitive restructuring), and listing the pros and cons of engaging in an impulsive behavior. Though they are important for reducing risky behavior in moments of intense emotion, these skills do not move the client toward a more long-term solution. Rather, management of distress in healthy ways that promote long-term growth focuses on reality acceptance skills, the ability to accept pain and difficulty as parts of life so that adolescents can move on from dwelling on how to reduce their suffering or how it is unfair (which often serves to worsen negative emotions).

During the third module, clients are taught to *walk the middle path*. Walking the middle path involves accepting a dialectical view, that opposing ideas can both be true and that there is more than one way to solve a problem; this module brings together the skills of accepting one's experiences (including negative emotions) while also working to improve emotion management and problem solving. To develop this skill, clinicians help clients identify situations in which opposing ideas are both true (e.g., "My friend can be kind and mean") and practice looking at the same situation from multiple perspectives (e.g., why a client might want her sister to share her clothes but why the sister may not want to do so). The focus of parent sessions during this module is on understanding and resolving dialectical dilemmas that often occur in families, including the balance between permissiveness and strictness, considering an adolescent's problem behavior as both undesirable and developmentally normative, and "holding on while letting go" (fostering appropriate dependence and independence). The fourth module emphasizes *emotion regulation skills* in order to help youth with bipolar disorder learn to manage their strong emotions in developmentally appropriate ways. Clients learn about emotions and the purposes of emotion regulation and then are taught specific emotion regulation skills using the acronym ABC PLEASE. Adolescents explore how to **A**ccumulate positive experiences (increasing their engagement in activities they enjoy), **B**uild mastery (planning activities and setting goals that will increase their sense of mastery and control), and **C**ope ahead (visualizing an upcoming difficult experience and planning and rehearsing the coping skills that will be used). Then the focus turns to taking care of the body in ways that support healthy emotional functioning, including treating **P**hysical i**L**lness,

Eating a healthy diet, **A**voiding mood-altering drugs, improving **S**leep, and **E**xercising.

The final module focuses on interpersonal effectiveness skills to help clients form and maintain healthy, supportive relationships, with which youth with bipolar disorder often struggle. Three skill sets are covered. Adolescents learn how to increase positive interactions and reduce conflict in relationships using the GIVE skills (be **G**entle, act **I**nterested, **V**alidate others, and use an **E**asy manner), to assert oneself effectively and appropriately using the DEAR MAN skills (**De**scribe the situation, **E**xpress your feelings using "I" statements, **A**ssert what you do or do not want, **R**einforce the other person by explaining the benefits of your request, be **M**indful and focused on what you want, **A**ppear confident, and be willing to **N**egotiate), and to maintain self-respect in relationships using FAST skills (be **F**air to yourself and the other person, don't over-**A**pologize, **S**tick to your values, and be **T**ruthful). Throughout all modules, worksheets, exercises, and homework assignments are used to facilitate practice and refinement of skills. DBT has been found to reduce depressive symptoms, decrease suicidality and self-injurious behavior, and improve emotion regulation in adolescents with bipolar disorder (Goldstein, Axelson, et al., 2007; Goldstein, Fersch-Podrat, et al., 2015).

Cognitive-behavioral therapy (CBT). CBT-based interventions may be more appropriate for children with bipolar disorder than family psychoeducation and skill-building interventions. One CBT approach, child- and family-focused cognitive-behavioral therapy (CFF-CBT; Pavuluri et al., 2004; West & Pavuluri, 2009), is based on the FFT-A model with adaptations to make it developmentally appropriate for younger children. CFF-CBT is based on the understanding that bipolar disorders in children result from the interaction of biological factors, particularly neurologically based difficulties with emotion reactivity and regulation, and environmental stressors in children's home and school settings to produce a unique symptom presentation in childhood. In addition, the intervention utilizes behavioral and cognitive techniques that help both children and parents manage bipolar symptoms, rather than intervening mainly with the client and including adjunctive parental support and education. It is important to note that the program is designed for use with children who have been stabilized on medication before beginning the psychosocial intervention.

CFF-CBT contains seven treatment components, represented by the acronym RAINBOW. *Routine* emphasizes the importance of keeping a predictable, consistent, and simple schedule and routine for children with bipolar disorder. Routines can help reduce reactivity in youth, conflict within families, and changes in the sleep-wake cycle that can trigger episodes. *Affect Regulation* skills are taught to families, beginning with the importance of monitoring clients' mood states in order to guide the responses of family members, who are taught strategies for managing strong emotions in the client. Psychoeducation about the symptoms of bipolar disorder is also provided to help families better understand the clients' mood-related symptoms. *I Can Do It!* is a component of treatment in which clients and family members learn how to promote a positive self-image in the child, particularly during depressive episodes; clients practice creating positive self-statements, while family members are encouraged to give clients feedback about their positive characteristics. Parents are also taught to use limit setting and positive reinforcement to shape children's behaviors in a calm manner (as opposed to yelling and punishing). In *No Negative Thoughts and Live in the "Now,"* the role of cognitive distortions in promoting negative emotions and family conflict is discussed. Clients and family members learn to examine their thoughts in order to identify and challenge distortions. In addition, in order to combat the feeling of being overwhelmed that youth with bipolar disorder and their families may face, participants learn mindfulness-informed self-statements (e.g., "Crossing one bridge at a time") that help them focus on the present rather than dwelling on the past or being discouraged by the prospect of future difficulties. In the fifth treatment component, clients learn how to *Be a Good Friend*, while parents learn to develop a *Balanced Lifestyle*. Youth with bipolar disorder may have a variety of social skills deficits but significantly benefit from meaningful friendships; therefore, therapists use instruction and role-playing to help clients develop social skills, and parents are encouraged to facilitate their children's peer relationships through activities such as playdates and sleepovers. In addition, in order to combat the weariness that adults caring for a child with bipolar disorder may experience, therapists work with parents to help them identify ways to balance engaging in enjoyable and renewing activities with their need to care for others. *Oh, How Can We Solve the Problem?* focuses on the development of problem-solving skills when

clients are in a calm state, with an emphasis on parents and children working together and viewing one another as allies. Finally, in *Ways to Get Support*, the therapist works with the parents and children to identify sources of help, support, and acceptance. The therapist and the client create a "support tree," a visual representation of supportive individuals identified by the child who could help her in challenging situations. In addition, the teacher is given information about the child's diagnosis and treatment in order to help her understand how to support the child in the school context.

When used in combination with medication, CFF-CBT has been found to reduce manic and depressive symptoms in children between the ages of seven and thirteen, though there is some mixed research as to whether the intervention produces more robust or lasting changes in one type of symptoms or with clients with particular characteristics (Weinstein et al., 2015; West, Jacobs, et al., 2009; West et al., 2014).

INTEGRATIVE APPROACH TO TREATMENT

Medication. Recognizing children's full humanity includes recognizing that they possess the same multifaceted complexity as adults, with their personhood consisting of biological, emotional, psychological, social, and spiritual elements. Perhaps even more significantly for children than for adults, from a developmental psychopathology framework, we must consider the influence of a wide variety of risk and protective factors on each of these aspects of functioning and how their interplay results in a child's current state of adaptation or maladaptation, well-being or disorder. For youth with bipolar disorder, biological influences seem to play an especially influential role in the development of symptoms. Unfortunately, we may sometimes be tempted to view children's behavior reductionistically, viewing undesirable behavior as something that results from a child's poor self-control or family factors that can be relatively easily changed, such as disciplinary techniques. Indeed, Rondeau (2003) expresses concern about the disconnection between the church's lip service about caring for children and the degree to which youth who display the symptoms of bipolar disorder—including anger, aggression, moodiness, and/or risky sexual behavior—may be rejected by the body of Christ. She emphasizes the importance of supporting rather than rejecting these youth and their families, given the challenges of the disorder and the importance of caring for those among us who are suffering (1 Corinthians 12:26-27). If we are too quick to take a simplistic view of children's problem behavior, including symptoms of bipolar disorder, as something that is explained by individual sin and should be addressed by emphasizing repentance and a purposeful change in behavior, we underestimate the role of complex causal factors and may dismiss the need for psychological treatment. However, in recognition of the full humanity of youth and the complexity of factors that lead to behavior at a given point in development, we need to acknowledge the role of uncontrollable biological factors that can contribute to tendencies and behaviors that we view as unacceptable for "good Christians." Rather, we should seek to care for these youth and their families by seeking to better understand their symptoms in light of their biological, psychological, and spiritual elements as legitimate aspects of being fully

human. Therefore, given the research on effective treatment, one element of supporting youth with bipolar disorder and their families should involve encouraging them to seek treatment, which may include medication, given the role of biological factors in the development of the disorder. This encouragement might also involve expressing understanding, supporting, and purposefully including these families within the full activities of the church community.

Psychosocial approaches. Each of the effective approaches to treating bipolar disorder in youth recognizes the importance of involving all family members in the process of symptom treatment; neither work with the client alone nor work with parents alone will suffice. Such an approach recognizes the balance of the theological ideas that children are both gifts and agents (Miller-McLemore, 2003). Viewing children and adolescents as gifts, for whom we are called to provide care and nurturing, highlights the role of parents in examining their own lives and actions and investing in new knowledge and skills that can help us improve communication, reduce hostility and criticism, manage family members' difficult emotions, and more effectively solve problems and disputes within the family. We cannot claim that our youth are precious gifts if we are not willing to do the work required to learn about their unique challenges and characteristics and to care for them well, which may be especially difficult and complex in families with a child or adolescent with bipolar disorder. As a complement to this view, we also understand youth to have agency in their own lives. The implication of this idea for family therapy is that family members cannot by themselves effect change in the lives of an older child or adolescent; the client also plays a role in taking responsibility for his behavior and being an agent of change in his own life. In turn, the parents of these youth must work to make the appropriate changes in their own lives while also supporting the client's growth and allowing him the necessary freedom to develop and implement new skills (and sometimes even granting him the right to choose not to make changes at the current time, recognizing that enacting one's agency may sometimes involve a lack of action or change that cannot be forced by others).

The idea of the multigenerational effects of sin also helps us understand the importance of involving family members in the treatment of disorders in youth (Lastoria, 1990). We are warned repeatedly in Scripture that sin has a negative effect on many subsequent generations (Exodus 20:5; Psalm 37:18; Jeremiah 32:18). Though we must be cautious about trying to identify the specific manifestations of intergenerational sin in every family situation, it is clear that parents' negative behaviors and choices have an effect on their children and that mitigating the role of these factors on children is crucial. In a family-focused approach to treating bipolar disorder, we recognize that each family member plays a role in the dysfunctional and maladaptive interactions and individual symptoms that have developed; therefore, the involvement of multiple family members in treatment is necessary to reduce symptoms and problems. Furthermore, we understand that individuals' choices and behaviors can have a strong positive ripple effect through subsequent generations (Genesis 22:17-18; Exodus 20:6), offering hope that the investment of time and energy

that families make to improve their skills and interactions can not only reduce the negative effects on younger generations but even promote ongoing positive interactions and health through new cycles of care, warmth, effective communication, and support.

Finally, there can be spiritual significance to the improvement of communication skills that are taught in family skill building, DBT, and CBT interventions for bipolar disorder. The influence of speech on others and on one's own well-being is a common theme throughout the Bible (Proverbs 13:3; Matthew 12:33-37). One message involves supporting others and displaying our care for them through our words (Proverbs 16:24; Ephesians 4:29), a skill supported by work on how to give positive feedback to others. Other messages revolve around the communication of critical or negative messages. There are times when such interactions are harmful to the person receiving them, and we are instructed to refrain from negative communication in these situations (Ephesians 5:4; James 3:6-12). At other times, however, we are called to speak critically for the good of others, which may include confrontation about sin or wrong behavior (Matthew 18:15; James 5:19-20). In these instances, especially within a family where there is a proneness to sensitivity or strong emotional reactions, it is important to communicate critical feedback in constructive and effective ways, another skill that is emphasized in these interventions. The communication and support skills that are learned in a family-focused intervention have the potential to be useful for both improving a family member's symptoms and helping individuals to speak in ways that build up the body of Christ at large.

DISRUPTIVE MOOD DYSREGULATION DISORDER

Disruptive mood dysregulation disorder (DMDD) was included as a new disorder in DSM-5 to help differentiate between clinically significant mood lability and behavioral dysregulation and true childhood bipolar disorder (American Psychiatric Association, 2013). Beginning in the 1990s, understandings of the presentation of bipolar disorder in childhood underwent significant change, with many clinicians categorizing nonepisodic irritability or emotional lability in youth as bipolar disorder, despite the DSM description of the disorder as consisting of discrete manic or depressive episodes, regardless of age (Parens & Johnston, 2010; Roy et al., 2014). However, increasing recognition of the clinical significance and impairment of emotional and behavioral outbursts, sometimes known clinically as "rages," led to the development of DMDD as a more appropriate categorization for some youth. Indeed, with the introduction of DMDD in DSM-5, there was a decrease in diagnoses of mood disorder not otherwise specified (NOS), which is a catchall category that can be used to diagnose youth with atypical mood disorder symptoms (Le et al., 2020). DMDD is characterized by recurrent, extreme verbal and/or physical outbursts of temper that are developmentally inappropriate and occur at least three times per week. Even between outbursts, children with DMDD are consistently irritable or angry. DMDD is diagnosed in children ages six to eighteen who display the first symptoms of the disorder by age ten, and the symptoms must be present for at least twelve months to meet diagnostic criteria. As a newer diagnosis, there is little research on DMDD and its cor-

relates, but it is estimated to occur in 2-5% of youth and present most commonly in children, with some continuity through childhood but decreasing prevalence throughout adolescence (American Psychiatric Association, 2013; Dougherty et al., 2016). Studies of children with bipolar disorder and ADHD, which share some symptoms with DMDD, can inform current treatment planning (Roy et al., 2014; Tourian et al., 2015), and work examining treatment efficacy has begun (Linke et al., 2020); however, more research is needed to establish an understanding of the developmental course, risk factors, and effective treatments that are specific to DMDD.

CASE STUDY

Pertinent history. Kelsey is a fourteen-year-old African American teenager who resides with her father, Jasen Williams, and paternal grandmother and legal guardian, Camella Williams. Kelsey is in regular education in the ninth grade at Wonder High School and receives average grades. Before beginning therapy, Kelsey was admitted into a children's hospital inpatient psychiatry unit (IPU) due to suicidal ideation. She told a classmate she had thought about killing herself by jumping from a window. She also attempted to stab herself in the chest with a butter knife four days prior to her admission, though she did this in front of her father who stopped her. At the time of admission, Kelsey said she was feeling sad and lonely and that she had felt that way for the past few years. She said she frequently cried and felt worthless.

No previous psychiatric history was reported for Kelsey. Her sister and maternal grandmother have a history of mood disorders effectively treated with psychopharmacological interventions. Kelsey's mother lives in Louisiana, and Kelsey visits her for two weeks every summer. Kelsey and her father have lived with her paternal grandmother since age nine when her parents divorced after years of "intense battles." She describes a generally good relationship with her father and grandmother but says she misses her mother sometimes. She understands that her young mother experiences addictions to alcohol and drugs and that she has more opportunities living with her father. Kelsey reports feeling "safe" with her father. Kelsey has never experimented with drugs or alcohol and does not have a desire to do so because of her mother's difficulties.

Kelsey has a scar on her face due to a burn that occurred when she was an infant. She said she has experienced a high level of verbal and physical victimization from her peers at school and in the neighborhood regarding her scar. Kelsey's best friend provided support in middle school; however, this friend attends a different high school. Kelsey currently has a few peers she sits with at lunch, but she could not identify any close, intimate friendships. She states that she does not have hope that things will change for her in the future. Her church is a safe place for her from these peers, though she continues to display withdrawn behavior at church and feels lonely there. Her faith is important to her, and she notes that praying, journaling, and singing worship songs in her bedroom help her cope when she gets "really low."

According to hospital staff, Kelsey verbalized her feelings well and was able to identify stressors. She enjoyed writing in her journal about her feelings. She was compliant and cooperative with staff. However, she also appeared inattentive and easily distractible regarding topics that were emotionally difficult for her (family, school, suicidal ideation). She interacted well with her peers and quickly built friendships with the other teenage girls. After six days, Kelsey was discharged from the hospital with the diagnosis of persistent depressive disorder, moderate severity, early onset, with pure dysthymic syndrome. The family was given the recommendation for Kelsey to participate in weekly individual outpatient therapy and for her family to participate in family therapy.

Course of treatment.

Individual therapy sessions. In order to assess the severity of her depressive symptoms, Kelsey completes the Children's Depression Inventory (CDI-2) in the first session. Her responses to this measure and her suicidal ideation are monitored throughout treatment. At the first session, her total score is Elevated, and her responses result in Very Elevated scores on the Interpersonal Problems and Negative Self-esteem scales; that is, Kelsey experiences low self-esteem and self-dislike as well as hopelessness, perceived problems interacting with her peers, and feelings of being lonely and unimportant. Kelsey identifies difficulties with peer relationships as a major stressor. Kelsey is quiet during this initial session. In order to build rapport, the clinician and Kelsey listen to Kelsey's favorite music, including Christian songs, and Kelsey explains why she likes it. They look up the lyrics to several of the songs, and the clinician notices a theme of feeling lost, disillusioned, and desperate but awaiting God's love and comfort. Kelsey cries when this observation is made but has difficulty explaining why it bothers her.

In the second individual session, Kelsey's identified primary stressor is discussed. As requested by the clinicians, Kelsey brings her yearbook from last year, and they spend a large part of the session going through the yearbook. The clinician gains insight into Kelsey's school context and is able to ask questions about different peers in order to better understand Kelsey's experiences. Kelsey notes that during the school day she becomes sadder and more withdrawn as the day progresses. She has felt this way for most of middle and high school. She also says she often worries about being victimized and that she constantly has to "watch her back." She often does not want to go to school. Kelsey agrees to complete a homework activity consisting of monitoring both her mood and enjoyable activities she engages in with ratings of how much joy they bring her.

In the third session, Kelsey's mood monitoring and pleasant events charts, which she completed on four of the seven days, are reviewed. Kelsey and the clinician graph the information from the charts together, and Kelsey is asked what she observes in her charts. She quietly reflects on these data, and after a period of silence, makes a few observations: her mood is not always sad/low, she feels the worst at school when she chooses to be alone (e.g., going to the library for lunch to eat by herself), whereas the activities that result in the most elevated mood are creative tasks or helping someone else. The clinician reviews pleasant event scheduling, and together they identify a list of activities that bring Kelsey joy. They also discuss her coping strategies and whether her prominent strategies are indeed helpful (e.g., withdrawal and avoidance, rumination to try to "think of

ways to correct everything that [she] did wrong"). Kelsey asks if they can pray together, and the clinician suggests they open and close each session in prayer. They decide together that Kelsey will engage in contemplative silence as a way to facilitate self-awareness and acceptance of her sadness, to provide a space in which her mind can quiet down, and to allow God to speak to her during prayer. The homework activity for this week is for Kelsey to practice daily contemplative silence and to engage in pleasant event scheduling.

During the fourth session, Kelsey is introduced to the specific cognitive interventions of identifying and challenging cognitive distortions. Kelsey's distorted, unhelpful beliefs that contribute to her symptoms of depression indicate self-blame, worthlessness, and her belief that nothing will ever go right for her. Further, Kelsey often attributes anything good that happens to external, unstable, and specific causes, whereas she articulates well her internal, stable, and global attributions for the difficulties that occur in her life. Kelsey agrees to keep a thought record and attempt to challenge these thoughts.

In the fifth session, Kelsey presents with flat affect and withdrawal. She describes a recent experience in which she overheard some girls talking about her at school. She tried to talk to her grandmother about the situation but felt like she got the message to "get over it." Kelsey reports thinking again that dying might be easier than living. She is able to identify reasons she wants to live, though she doubts whether her hopes for the future will be attained. Kelsey has been ruminating on the experience at school and has found it difficult to let go (as reflected in her thought log). The clinician reflects on what a difficult experience this must have been, particularly given her history of feeling unwanted by peers, and Kelsey's recent attempts to be engaged at school. The clinician also discusses the harm that rumination can have on us; in other words, what we devote ourselves to will have the deepest effect on our innermost being. The clinician has brought a sketchpad for Kelsey to use. She has not depicted her thoughts or feelings through drawing before, although she loves to draw, but she is willing to try. They both take time to draw Proverbs 4:20-25 and discuss how Kelsey can guard her heart and keep her gaze before her. Kelsey's commitment to pleasant event scheduling is discussed and she notes that she is trying hard to engage in the activities that bring her joy. She also notices again the connection between activities and her mood with the charts she is keeping about half of the time.

In the sixth individual session, Kelsey brings her sketchpad to show her depiction of several meaningful verses for her, including Romans 5:1-5, which is discussed frequently at her church and by her family. Kelsey feels there is truth she can have hope, even during suffering. God is working in her life, but she finds it difficult to sense that hope and wonders if her faith is weak because she questions why she has to go through this suffering. The therapist normalizes this questioning and encourages Kelsey to cognitively challenge this belief about her faith. In discussing the character she is developing, Kelsey is unable to identify many positive qualities about herself and states that she cannot feel confident in new situations due to fear that someone will make a negative comment about her appearance. A mindfulness exercise in which she writes down the words that come

to mind when she thinks of herself, and then writes them repeatedly until they are just words, results in the following list: dull, ugly, uninteresting, weak, unimportant, and unworthy. Kelsey and the clinician then review her meaningful verses and what is important to her in her true identity in Christ. She lists: worthy, loved, welcomed, and welcoming. They also go back to the list of events that bring Kelsey joy (from session three) and discuss how joy represents her heart and the gifts God has given her, which are reflected in her list (honest, creative, aesthetic, compassionate, loving, objective, patient, welcoming, vulnerable). Kelsey continues to complete her thought record and is asked to reflect on these deeper truths about herself to counter the beliefs that underlie her cognitive distortions.

During the next session, the clinician brings a white rock for Kelsey. They open the session with prayer following the reading of Revelation 2:17 ("Whoever has ears, let them hear what the Spirit says to the churches. To the one who is victorious, I will give some of the hidden manna. I will also give that person a white stone with a new name written on it, known only to the one who receives it."), followed by contemplative silence. They discuss all the names she has been given by her peers and the expectations placed on her by her family. She can see these names are hurtful and untrue in many ways. They agree Kelsey will listen over the next few weeks through contemplative prayer and journaling to hear the name God has given to her, with the white rock being a promise of God's view of her. Kelsey also shows a drawing she did of God as her shelter (Deuteronomy 33:12).

Knowing that the eighth session would focus on problem solving, Kelsey had visually depicted verses read at church the past week (Psalm 66:17-20). In session, she talks about God being her guiding light and setting the right path before her, if she only walks with her eyes open and listens to him. The clinician suggests she reflect on Isaiah 30:15 ("By waiting and by calm you shall be saved, in quiet and in trust shall be your strength" [NABRE]), which Kelsey, after quiet contemplation, imagines herself on the side of a lake with God's light coming across the water and shining on her. They then place behind her in this visualization exercise two interpersonal problems that are currently contributing to her sadness, including how to deal with a particularly mean peer and frequent conflict she has been experiencing with her grandmother. Kelsey is led through a problem-solving activity in which she identifies possible strategies to deal with these problems, including effective communication and responses to this peer and her grandmother. Kelsey's comfort with asserting herself and expressing her feelings and needs is discussed. Kelsey and the therapist decide that a family therapy session will be scheduled in which Kelsey will try out these solutions with her grandmother in the supportive space of the therapy room.

In the ninth session, Kelsey and the clinician continue to work on problem solving with regard to her peer relationships and the negative interactions she experiences with certain peers. They identify several strategies for developing and strengthening relationships with other peers and review the negative effects of withdrawal and avoidance on Kelsey's depression. Because Kelsey feels helpless in the face of these problems but "desperately wants to be strong" as emphasized by

her family, they discuss what it means to be "strong." Kelsey says it is difficult to acknowledge her own strength because she often recognizes her weakness and loss of what to do to maintain hope in the future. The therapist helps Kelsey challenge the belief that strength means never fearing or doubting, replacing it with the thought that acknowledging our own weakness and vulnerability can be part of strength. They then review the ways Kelsey has demonstrated strength during treatment. Through this discussion, Kelsey also identifies trust in God and reliance on his promise and refuge as part of her strength. Another family session is scheduled to discuss this topic.

Sessions ten to fourteen reflect the emphases of the termination phase within treatments for mood disorders. Kelsey has recognized the benefits of the skills she has learned in therapy and consistently practices them throughout the week. Her motivation to improve her well-being and her commitment to her family relationships are assets to treatment. Her CDI score has decreased slightly by session six but is within the Average range for the total score and the High Average range for the two scales that were initially Very Elevated. Though little has changed in the way some peers treat her at school, she feels good about standing up for herself, focusing on her own interests, and developing friendships with two peers she relates to easily. Kelsey has begun to sing in her church choir and soon after was asked to sing some solos, which improved her self-esteem. She has also become involved in her school's chorus and photography club and started to volunteer in the special education classroom at her school, using her love of music and art to connect with the children. In this final phase of treatment, the clinician meets with Mr. Williams to review the signs and symptoms of Kelsey's depression so he can support her and determine whether she needs psychotherapy in the future.

Family therapy sessions. Four family sessions are held with Kelsey, Mr. Williams, and his mother, Mrs. Williams. The focus of these sessions is on facilitating discussion about Kelsey's feelings and identifying appropriate interventions. Her grandmother and aunt indicate surprise about Kelsey's depressed mood and interactions with her peers. They note their perceptions of Kelsey's high self-esteem, strength, and motivation to succeed at whatever she puts her mind to. They state that Kelsey has always been teased by her peers, the neighborhood kids, and family members but that "she can handle it." They do not report any depressive symptoms for Kelsey. Kelsey says she did not feel comfortable telling her family about her feelings because they would tell her to "be strong" and "get over it." Her grandmother and father agree that being able to overcome obstacles is a trait they want to instill in Kelsey. The benefits of open communication between Kelsey and her family are discussed. Also, the difficulty of experiencing victimization as an adolescent without support from any friends or family is discussed.

In the second family therapy session, psychoeducation about depression is presented. The clinician explains that Kelsey has good social skills, but over time her interactions with peers have left her feeling unsure of herself, withdrawing and isolating herself, and demonstrating poor assertiveness skills. After Kelsey is provided the

opportunity to discuss these links with her caregivers, the clinician reviews Kelsey's task of engaging in pleasant activities and the need for support from her family. The need for Kelsey to be permitted to choose the activities that bring her joy is discussed. Kelsey presents the list she has developed and solicits feedback from her family about these ideas and any others they have. The clinician facilitates discussion about the positive qualities the family sees in Kelsey as represented in her interests. The family provides positive feedback to Kelsey, which is meaningful to her.

The third family therapy session focuses on the way the family members show love to and recognize love from each other. Emphasis is placed on the need for openness and non-judgment as they discuss this topic because it is based on subjective experiences which are all valid. They depict these displays of love either in words or pictures on a large sheet of paper with each of their names represented. The target of this session is to allow open communication about Kelsey's experience of her father as absent and her grandmother as un-accepting and insensitive as well as to better understand their experience of Kelsey. The family's experience of Kelsey as dismissive and remote is apparent, and the clinician relates it to her depressive symptoms and the developmental transition between a parent-child to a parent-adolescent relationship. Through this activity, each family member comments on their surprise and sadness about how information and experiences can be misunderstood or even missed completely. The clinician facilitates discussion regarding how they can better show and recognize love for each other.

In the fourth family therapy session, ways to communicate effectively in the midst of conflict are reviewed. Kelsey and her grandmother develop several ways they can calm down during conflicts in order to present their own perspectives and listen to others' perspectives. The need to respect each other's points of view even if they disagree is reviewed. Kelsey then discusses her shame for not feeling strong enough for her family. She discusses what it means to her to be strong and asks whether that fits her grandmother's view of strength. Kelsey's father and grandmother hear her pain and agree with Kelsey's explanation. However, her grandmother also discusses her fear that Kelsey's weakness (depression) is a sign that Kelsey's faith is weak and that it will prevent her from being a woman who can handle challenges in life. The different ways Kelsey demonstrates strength are again reviewed, and ways that Kelsey's father and grandmother can support her and continue to facilitate her strength when she feels weak are explored.

Additional considerations from a developmental psychopathology framework. Kelsey's father consults with her physician about the utility of psychotropic medication given the chronic course of Kelsey's depression. After discussing the benefits and Mr. Williams's concern regarding medication, they decide medication would be started should psychotherapy not decrease her depressive symptoms. It is also recommended that Kelsey's father meet with school staff to discuss the bullying Kelsey has experienced and determine whether there are strategies to support Kelsey and prevent further bullying. In response, the school provides counseling support to Kelsey and aligns her class schedule the following

quarter with the schedules of a few peers who are nice to Kelsey. Kelsey is moved that her father took this step to support her and feels more at ease about her upcoming course schedule. Kelsey also participates in group therapy activities at school designed to allow for expressing her feelings, connecting with other students, and learning social problem-solving strategies. She seems to enjoy the activities and wants to develop a friendship with one of the other students in the group. Kelsey's counselor reports that she interacted well with her peers and demonstrated good social skills, frequently helping her peers engage in effective problem solving. Finally, Kelsey and her father decide she would visit her mother over spring break as well as during the summer, which gives Kelsey something to look forward to and helps with her feelings of missing her mother. Future booster sessions will include check-ins about Kelsey's use of the skills she found effective and provide the opportunity to discuss her feelings about her family relationships and whether she feels supported and loved.

Conclusion

Youth with depression or bipolar disorder struggle with affective and mood-related symptoms that are often accompanied by cognitive, behavioral, and physical correlates and may present differently across development. While both depression and bipolar disorder appear to have significant biological underpinnings, environmental and family factors also play a role in their development, emphasizing the need for multifaceted treatment approaches. Fortunately, research has identified a number of effective interventions for these youth, with SSRIs, CBT, and IPT-A being useful treatments for depression, and second generation antipsychotic medications, family-focused therapy, and CBT showing promise as effective methods for improving symptoms. Finally, it is recommended that Christian cli-nicians consider biblical and theological ideas that support youths' agency and full personhood and serve as resources for work that aims to improve their cognitive, behavioral, and interpersonal skills.

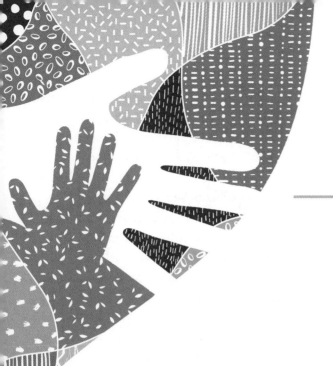

Chapter Four

Anxiety Disorders

ANXIETY, FEAR, AND WORRY are a normal part of the human experience; the prevalence of references to these emotions in Scripture speaks to this reality. Often recognized by their common physiological signs (e.g., racing heart, shallow breathing, shakiness, sweatiness, lightheadedness, stomach discomfort), these emotions are often accompanied by certain cognitive and behavioral reactions that signal a threat to one's well-being. Anxiety and fear reflect the activation of the sympathetic nervous system's fight-or-flight response, which prepares us to protect ourselves from potential harm (Comer & Comer, 2018). When an actual threat is present, this physical process and its accompanying thoughts and actions can help us keep ourselves safe and promote well-being; for example, fear or anxiety can prepare you to slam on the brakes when a deer jumps out in front of your car or prompt you to study for a final exam. However, when fear or worry is excessive, creates distress, and/or interferes

with functioning, it reflects a distortion in the helpful nature of these emotions and may signal the presence of an anxiety disorder.

The DSM-5 recognizes seven specific anxiety disorders that can be diagnosed in children, adolescents, or adults (American Psychiatric Association, 2013). *Separation anxiety disorder* in youth is characterized by excessive anxiety about separation from a parent or other attachment figure that is developmentally inappropriate and lasts for at least four weeks, including three of the following: distress about anticipated separations, excessive worry about loss of or harm to an attachment figure, excessive worry about adverse events that could result in separation (such as being kidnapped), difficulty going to places such as school because of separation fears, fear of being alone or without one's attachment figures, difficulty sleeping away from home or far from attachment figures, nightmares about separation, and somatic symptoms such as headaches upon actual or anticipated separation. *Selective mutism* is the refusal to speak in one or more social situations in which this behavior is expected (despite the ability to speak in other situations and the lack of a communication disorder), lasting for at least one month and negatively affecting educational, occupational, or social functioning. Most commonly, selective mutism manifests in the school setting and is associated with significant social anxiety in settings outside the home; it may not become apparent until it leads to school avoidance. *Specific phobias* are disproportionate fears of particular objects or situations, such as dogs, spiders, heights, water, flying, or needles that last for at least six months. Encountering the feared object or situation, which is often avoided, leads to immediate anxiety. Individuals with specific phobia will often express significant fear around multiple stimuli or situations, and these phobias lead to significant distress or impairment. Youth with *social anxiety disorder* experience significant and persistent anxiety about embarrassing oneself in social situations that involve being evaluated by others, such as meeting new people or giving a speech. (Children who are anxious only when they interact with adults are not considered to have social anxiety disorder.) This fear is out of proportion to the situation and may result in avoidance of the anxiety-provoking social situations. *Panic disorder* consists of recurrent, unexpected panic attacks, periods of intense but time-limited fear that can include racing heart, sweating, shaking, shortness of breath, choking sensations, chest pain, nausea, dizziness, numbness, feelings of derealization, fear of losing control, and fear of dying. Panic attacks result in worry about subsequent attacks and their effects and

lead to maladaptive behavior changes. Individuals with *agoraphobia* experience significant fear about situations in which escaping or seeking help in the event of panic-like or embarrassing symptoms might be difficult, such as using public transportation, being in open or enclosed spaces, being in a crowd, or being away from home by oneself. This fear is out of proportion to the actual threat of the situation, may result in avoidance, is distressing or impairing, and is persistent. Finally, *generalized anxiety disorder* (GAD) involves excessive, persistent, and uncontrollable worry and anxiety about a number of topics and situations. Individuals experience symptoms such as restlessness, fatigue, difficulty concentrating, irritability, muscle tension, and difficulty sleeping. (Only one of these symptoms is needed for diagnosis in children, whereas adolescents and adults are required to exhibit at least three.) For GAD to be diagnosed, the anxiety must be distressing or impairing.

Overall, between 3% and 5% of youth are estimated to have an anxiety disorder (Bitsko et al., 2018), but rates vary depending on the specific disorder (American Psychiatric Association, 2013). Selective mutism appears to be the rarest of the anxiety disorders and is generally only seen in young children. In children, panic disorder, agoraphobia, and GAD are rare, with social anxiety disorder (7%) and specific phobia (5%) being the most common. Separation anxiety is more common in children than adolescents. From least to most common, the anxiety disorders that occur in adolescence are GAD (0.9%), separation anxiety (1.6%), agoraphobia (1.7%), panic disorder (2-3%), social anxiety disorder (7%), and specific phobia (16%). Anxiety disorders are more common in females than males (American Psychiatric Association, 2013). Some research has found that girls experience higher levels of anxiety than boys as early as the toddler years, while other work suggests that these differences do not emerge until adolescence (Carter et al., 2010). Finally, anxiety disorders are commonly comorbid with one another as well as with depression, somatic symptom disorders, substance use, attention-deficit hyperactivity disorder, and disruptive behavior disorders (Angold et al., 1999; Biederman et al., 2007; Essau, 2003; Verduin & Kendall, 2003). The overlap among anxiety disorders and between anxiety and depression appears to be the result of both genetic and environmental factors, with the relative role of genetic factors increasing from childhood and adolescence (Waszczuk et al., 2014).

Risk/Causal Factors

Biological factors. There are significant links between parental and child anxiety disorders (Lawrence et al., 2019; Turner et al., 1987); however, these links could reflect either genetic or environmental influences on children's anxiety. Twin studies suggest that genetics play a stronger role than environment in the development of anxiety disorders; however, genetic influences decrease across childhood relative to environmental influences (Bartels et al., 2007). For example, heritability estimates, or the proportion of variance in anxiety symptoms explained by genetics, are 39-64% at age four but drop to 22-43% by age nine (Eley, Bolton, et al., 2003; Hallett et al., 2009). Some studies have specifically implicated one genotype of the serotonin transporter gene (5-HTT) in the development of anxiety; however, findings have been in-

consistent (Murray et al., 2009). Further research suggests that these apparent inconsistencies might be explained by the need to also take environmental factors into account. Indeed, there appears to be an interaction between the presence of the 5-HTT allele and environmental factors. Youth with the 5-HTT allele are only at heightened risk for anxiety when they are also exposed to environmental risk, such as low social support, life stress, or prenatal maternal anxiety (Fox et al., 2005; Petersen et al., 2012; Tiemeier et al., 2012).

Genetic factors generally convey risk via neurobiological factors. Youth with anxiety disorders have higher levels of cortisol, a hormone that is released by the endocrine system in response to threat, both when they are stressed and when they are not (Brand et al., 2011; Higa-McMillan et al., 2014). There are also differences in when cortisol levels rise and fall throughout the day in anxious youth as compared to their peers, suggesting a dysregulation within the hypothalamic-pituitary-adrenal (HPA) axis of the endocrine system (Dierckx et al., 2012). Prolonged elevated cortisol exposure, especially early in development, is neurotoxic (Lupien et al., 2009). The brains of youth with anxiety disorders may also differ in important ways from those of their peers. Youth with GAD have larger amygdalas than non-anxious youth (De Bellis et al., 2000). The amygdala is also more active in anxious individuals during exposure to fear-provoking stimuli, suggesting that anxiety disorders may be linked with high biologically based sensitivity to danger or threat in one's environment (Craske et al., 2009; Davis et al., 2019; Nitschke et al., 2009; Pérez-Edgar et al., 2007). The activity and connectivity of the prefrontal cortex (PFC), which is thought to regulate the responsivity of the amygdala to threat, has also been found to differ between anxious and non-anxious individuals (Jalbrzikowski et al., 2017; Monk et al., 2006, 2008). In addition, a heightened neural response to mistakes is linked with anxiety disorder risk (Meyer, Carlton, et al., 2018; Meyer, Nelson, et al., 2018). Finally, research with adults has found other neuroanatomical patterns associated with anxiety, such as increased activity in the bed nucleus of the stria terminalis (BNST) and the insular cortex and dysfunction within the anterior cingulate cortex, though less is known about these patterns in childhood and adolescent anxiety (see Higa-McMillan et al., 2014, for a summary). It is also important to remember that biological variables interact with other risk factors. For example, experiencing more stressors predicts lower levels of connectivity between the amygdala and other parts of the brain, which is in turn linked to more anxiety symptoms (Pagliaccio et al., 2015).

Psychological factors.

Attachment. Attachment is the emotional bond between two individuals, most commonly studied between children and their parents (Ainsworth, 1979). Children who are characterized as securely attached find a sense of security and comfort in being with their parents; they seek their parents out for reassurance but are able to explore their environments based on the sense of safety their parents provide. Children who are insecurely attached do not see their parents as secure bases from which they can explore; instead, they may cling to parents, not be distressed when they leave the room, be inconsolable following a separation, and/or push their parents away when they try to comfort them. Insecure

attachment is thought to result from suboptimal parenting behaviors, including inconsistency, insensitivity, and unresponsiveness to children's needs. Youth who are insecurely attached to their parents show higher levels of anxiety across development (Bosquet & Egeland, 2006; Brumariu et al., 2012; Colonnesi et al., 2011). Because these children's relationships with their parents do not provide a sense of safety and predictability, they do not receive the support they need to develop a view of others as caring and responsive or the world as safe (Bowlby, 1989). These views, or internal working models, then guide children's interactions and behaviors, which are likely to reflect fear and anxiety. As with all risk factors, however, attachment status varies, even within youth with anxiety; anxious youth may be securely attached to their parents, so it is important for clinicians to assess the relationship quality of any given client rather than assuming that anxiety is caused by parental unresponsiveness or inconsistency.

Attachment security interacts with other factors in the prediction of anxiety. For example, one study linking insecure attachment in infancy with heightened risk for the development of anxiety symptoms in adolescence found this relation to be mediated by adolescents' views of their peers (Bosquet & Egeland, 2006). This pattern supports the role of internal working models; children who develop a sense that their parents and the world are unsafe and unpredictable may view their peer relationships in the same way, leading to fearfulness in social interactions. The link between attachment security and anxiety in children and adolescents has also been found to be at least partially mediated by problems with emotion regulation (Bender, Sømhovd, et al., 2015; Brumariu et al., 2012). In other words, children who display lower attachment security are more likely to have difficulties regulating their emotions, which in turn predicts anxiety. Parents play an important role in regulating young children's emotions (Sroufe, 1995) and helping children to manage their own emotions, and insecure attachment may reflect a lack of parental availability and support for these important developmental tasks. Indeed, insecure attachment is associated with certain parenting behaviors, including negativity and high levels of control, which in turn can heighten children's anxiety (Hudson et al., 2011; van Brakel et al., 2006). Finally, children who are insecurely attached are also more likely to have certain temperamental characteristics that also predispose them to anxiety (Hudson et al., 2011; van Brakel et al., 2006).

Temperament. Temperament is an individual's characteristic pattern of reacting to the environment and regulating those reactions (Rothbart & Bates, 2006). Temperamental characteristics are thought to be innate and to form the core of personality. Different theorists and researchers have focused on different aspects of temperament, but one temperamental trait that has received significant attention in anxiety research is behavioral inhibition, which is described as non-normative shyness and fearfulness in new situations (Hirshfeld-Becker et al., 2004). Behavioral inhibition can be operationalized in terms of either external behavior (e.g., the frequency with which children speak to peers and adults, expressions of distress) or physiological signs (e.g., heart rate, blood pressure, cortisol level; Kagan et al., 1988). Throughout childhood, behavioral inhibition has been linked to

higher levels of concurrent and later anxiety, with some studies pointing to particularly strong links with social anxiety (Broeren et al., 2013; Hudson et al., 2011; Kerns et al., 2011; Muris et al., 2011; Sandstrom et al., 2020; Schwartz, Snidman, & Kagan, 1999). Temperamental characteristics may play a role in whether children's anxiety persists across development (Bufferd et al., 2018), particularly in combination with other variables, such as stressor exposure (Mumper et al., 2020). In addition, children who are naturally more reactive to potentially threatening situations—and subsequently have difficulty managing their strong emotions—may be more prone to experiencing anxiety that is overwhelming, distressing, and/or interfering. Indeed, behavioral inhibition is linked with children's less effective regulation of emotions (Feng et al., 2008; Penela et al., 2015).

Emotion regulation. As noted, youth with anxiety disorders have trouble regulating emotions effectively (Esbjørn et al., 2012; Hambour et al., 2018; Schneider et al., 2018). These difficulties manifest themselves in a number of ways. Youth with anxiety disorders endorse fewer attempts to regulate negative emotions (Suveg & Zeman, 2004), and the use of fewer emotion regulation strategies is linked with higher levels of anxiety symptoms (Lougheed & Hollenstein, 2012). When they do attempt to regulate their emotions, children with an anxiety disorder use fewer effective strategies, such as reappraisal and problem solving, than non-anxious youth. Instead, they are more likely to identify and use maladaptive emotion regulation strategies, such as avoidance and suppression (Carthy et al., 2010; Folk et al., 2014; Keil et al., 2017; Mathews et al., 2014; Suveg et al., 2008). In addition, adolescents who do not see themselves as knowing how to effectively regulate negative emotions have higher levels of anxiety (Neumann et al, 2010). Similarly, children with anxiety disorders believe that their attempts to regulate negative emotions, particularly anxiety, will fail (Carthy et al., 2010; Mathews et al., 2014; Suveg & Zeman, 2004). Older children and adolescents who see themselves as having less control over their emotions and emotion-evoking experiences have higher levels of anxiety (Weems et al., 2003).

Youth with higher levels of anxiety may experience emotions differently than their peers. For example, youth with anxiety disorders experience more frequent and intense negative emotions, particularly worry and anger, than their non-anxious peers (Carthy et al., 2010; Suveg & Zeman, 2004). They also experience more physiological signs of anxiety when exposed to a stressor (Tan et al., 2012; Nelemans et al., 2017). Higher levels of anxiety symptoms are also associated with heightened emotional reactivity and lower levels of positive emotions (Lonigan et al., 2003). In addition, children and adolescents who experience more symptoms of anxiety than their peers have poorer emotional awareness and more difficulty identifying their emotions (Brumariu et al., 2012; Mathews et al., 2014; Schneider et al., 2018; Suveg & Zeman, 2004).

From a dynamic developmental psychopathology perspective, it is important to note that the relationship between emotion regulation and anxiety is complex and affected by other factors. While the relationship between emotion regulation difficulties is likely bidirectional, there is some evidence that poor emotion regulation contributes to the development of anxiety. For example, children who

display difficulties regulating their emotions in early childhood have a higher risk of later elevated anxiety (Bosquet & Egeland, 2006). In addition, difficulties with emotion regulation predict increases in anxiety symptoms over time (McLaughlin et al., 2011). Finally, the link between difficulties with emotion regulation and symptoms of anxiety may be affected by other variables, such as attachment (as discussed earlier). This link may also be affected by gender; indeed, the relation between emotion regulation and anxiety is stronger for girls, who experience higher levels of each (Bender et al., 2012). Paradoxically, it may be girls' greater awareness of their emotions and attention to emotional experiences that enhances the emotional consequences of stressful situations and interactions.

Cognitive patterns. Cognitive models of anxiety in youth are newer than adult models, but they outline the ways in which information processing might differ in anxious versus non-anxious youth (Daleiden & Vasey, 1997; Hadwin et al., 2006). There are several stages of information processing, and the first two, encoding and interpretation, have received the most empirical attention in relation to childhood anxiety. First, anxious youth show certain patterns in the information they select to attend to and encode in memory. Specifically, these youth display threat-related attentional biases, paying more attention to information that indicates a threat in the environment than they pay to nonthreatening stimuli (Bar-Haim et al., 2007; Vasey et al., 1996). Second, perhaps because of bias in the encoding process, anxious youth interpret information in their environments as more threatening than non-anxious youth. Children with anxiety disorders are more likely than their peers to view ambiguous situations as threatening (Barrett, Rapee, Dadds, & Ryan, 1996; Cannon & Weems, 2010; Higa & Daleidan, 2008). In turn, these interpretations increase the likelihood of their choosing an avoidant response to the situation (Barrett, Rapee, Dadds, & Ryan, 1996). Interestingly, anxiety predicts increases over time in the tendency to view ambiguous situations as threatening, rather than the other way around, suggesting that being anxious may change youth's perceptions of their environments (Creswell & O'Connor, 2011).

Certain patterns of thinking, which may be categorized as interpretations, are also associated with anxiety in children and adolescents. Children who display higher levels of particular types of cognitive distortions have higher levels of anxiety symptoms (Brumariu et al., 2012). The specific cognitive patterns that have been linked to anxiety include catastrophizing (anticipating the worst possible outcome of a situation), overgeneralization (applying the outcome of one experience to all other similar experiences), personalizing (blaming oneself for negative events), and selective abstraction (paying more attention to the negative than the positive aspects of a situation; Leitenberg et al., 1986). Similarly, more frequent negative self-statements (e.g., "I am going to make a fool of myself"), as well as a higher ratio of negative to positive self-statements, predicts anxiety severity in children with anxiety disorders (Treadwell & Kendall, 1996). It is important to note that cognitive patterns do not develop in a vacuum; children may develop a tendency to talk to themselves in negative ways as the result of environmental influences. For example, children's anxious self-talk is pre-

dicted by mothers' anxious self-talk (Wei et al., 2014). This link suggests that thought patterns might best be changed by targeting both the child's internal information processing and family interactions.

Environmental factors.

Parenting. In addition to internal factors, family dynamics and parenting behaviors affect youths' anxiety symptoms. (However, it is important to note that while a number of parenting variables have been linked to anxiety disorders in youth, they only account for a small percent of the variance in children's anxiety; McLeod et al., 2007). First, familial warmth and support may affect childhood anxiety. Mothers of anxious children express less warmth and praise than mothers of non-anxious children, and low levels of social support, acceptance, and validation within families are linked with higher levels of social anxiety in youth (Festa & Ginsburg, 2011; Moore et al., 2004). In addition, youth with higher levels of anxiety are more likely than their peers to experience harsh discipline, high levels of negative parental emotions, criticism, and parental rejection; furthermore, parental verbal aggression (e.g., anger, belligerence, cruelty, argumentativeness) predicts increases in adolescents' anxiety symptoms over time (Hummel & Gross, 2001; Rodriguez, 2003; Schwartz et al., 2012). Youth whose interactions with their families are primarily negative rather than positive may experience even their family environments as threatening, leading to increases in fear and anxiety, in contrast to healthy youth, for whom families are safe havens that support development.

Second, parents who are controlling or overly protective of youth are more likely to have children who struggle with anxiety. Parents of anxious children grant them less psychological autonomy (i.e., encouraging the child's independence and respecting the child's unique views) than parents of non-anxious children (Moore et al., 2004; Siqueland et al., 1996). Similarly, high levels of parental psychological control are linked with higher levels of anxiety in children and adolescents (Festa & Ginsburg, 2011; Luebbe & Bell, 2014). The relationship between psychological control and anxiety appears to be mediated by children's perceived control (Nanda et al., 2012). In other words, children whose parents are highly controlling of their behavior view themselves as having less control over events in their lives, which in turn leads to increased anxiety. In addition, parental overprotectiveness is linked with children's anxiety symptoms (Pereira et al., 2014). For example, when toddlers exhibit high levels of distress during a new situation and their mothers act protectively (e.g., moving or turning the child away from the anxiety-eliciting object or situation), children's fearfulness decreases less than when their mothers do not protect them from the situation (Buss & Kiel, 2011). This finding suggests that exposure is important for decreasing anxiety, even in young children, and overprotective parents can interfere with this process. Furthermore, anxious parents are more likely to exhibit overprotectiveness, indicating that they may transmit risk to their children in multiple ways, including via not only parenting practices but also genetic factors (Orgilés et al., 2018).

Finally, the dynamics of emotion socialization differ between families with and without an anxious child. Emotion socialization is the process by which families com-municate information, explicitly and implicitly, about the acceptability and regulation of various emotions (Eisenberg et al., 1998). This socialization process, in turn, affects youths' views of emotion and their psychological well-being. For example, during discussions about emotion, parents of youth with anxiety disorders engage in less discussion of the causes and consequences of emotions and display more negative and less positive emotion than parents of non-anxious youth (Suveg et al., 2008). In addition, compared to families with non-anxious youth, parents of anxious children are less supportive when their children experience negative emotions, a factor that may impact anxiety through its effect on children's emotion regulation abilities (Hurrell et al., 2015). Furthermore, when children with anxiety disorders and their parents problem solve about how the child should respond in a challenging situation, the children are more likely to endorse avoidant behavior as a solution than they were prior to the family discussion, suggesting that family dynamics may reinforce avoidance in anxious children (Barrett, Rapee, Dadds, & Ryan, 1996). Family dynamics related to emotion socialization are one mechanism that may explain the link between parental anxiety and children's anxiety (Kerns et al., 2011; Pereira et al., 2014). For example, parental social anxiety disorder predicts toddlers' anxious and avoidant behavior in potentially frightening situations, including exposure to a stranger and the presence of a remote-controlled robot (Aktar et al., 2014). Such new experiences are considered "social referencing situations" because young children will generally look to their parents in order to know how to feel and behave. This finding suggests that socially anxious parents communicate (even nonverbally) to their children that these situations are threatening, warranting anxiety and best being addressed through avoidance. Indeed, parental anxiety predicts youths' bias toward viewing their environment as threatening, which in turns predicts youth anxiety (Affrunti & Ginsburg, 2012). For example, when anxious mothers read a picture book with their preschool-aged children about starting school, they are more likely than non-anxious mothers to tell the story in a way that portrays it as less positive and more threatening (Murray, Pella, et al., 2014). This narrative, in turn, predicts higher levels of later child anxiety. Other research has specifically explored the cognitive patterns linking parental and youth anxiety. As mentioned earlier, mothers' anxious self-talk predicts youths' anxious self-talk (Wei et al., 2014), and mothers' beliefs about anxiety (e.g., worrying can help me avoid problems, worrying is dangerous) are correlated with children's beliefs about anxiety (Lønfeldt et al., 2017). Interestingly, maternal catastrophizing has been linked to children's anxiety, even in non-anxious mothers (Moore et al., 2004). This pattern suggests that anxious children's cognitive patterns may actually impact their parents' way of thinking, indicating that influences between youth anxiety and parenting behaviors may be bidirectional (Ahmadzadeh et al., 2019).

Conditioning. Fear and anxiety can be learned, or conditioned, by one's experiences and interactions with the environment. One type of environmental learning involves our observations of others, a phenomenon known as social or vicarious learning (Bandura, 1977). Children may learn anxious and avoidant be-

haviors by observing others performing or modeling them. For example, a child attending his first street fair may see his mother's anxious reaction to the crowd and hear her make comments such as, "I need to get out of here. I can't breathe with so many people around." The idea of crowds as a threatening or anxiety-provoking stimulus has been modeled for the child, who is likely to imitate his mother's words and actions as he develops his own response to the situation (see the discussion of social referencing above). Indeed, this pattern helps explain the nongenetic links between parental and child anxiety.

In addition, children's direct experiential encounters with their environments can shape their behaviors and reactions, including anxiety, which can develop or be maintained through classical and operant conditioning. In classical conditioning, a conditioned stimulus becomes associated with an unconditioned stimulus that naturally elicits a particular response, such that the conditioned stimulus comes to elicit the same response (Comer & Comer, 2018). In the case of anxiety, this usually involves learning to associate a nonthreatening (or minimally threatening) stimulus with significant threat or danger and, therefore, reacting with extreme anxiety. For example, consider a child with a specific phobia of bees that developed following a bee sting. The sting caused the child considerable distress and pain, and she now associates bees with stings, leading to the anxious anticipation of distress and injury whenever she sees or thinks about bees or going to a place where bees may be present (e.g., a park). Classical conditioning can play a role in the development of other anxiety disorders as well, such as when separation from parents, social interactions, or being in public or crowded places comes to be associated with danger or threat and reacted to with fear and anxiety. Experimental studies consistently show that classical conditioning can create an anxious association in youth, and there is some evidence that youth with anxiety disorders may be particularly predisposed to develop and maintain these associations (Craske et al., 2008; Lau et al., 2008; Liberman et al., 2006).

In operant conditioning, behaviors are learned through their consequences; actions that are reinforced (rewarded) are likely to recur, whereas those that are punished are not (Comer & Comer, 2018). Reinforcement and punishment can be implemented purposefully by other people or occur without intentionality, as the result of environmental circumstances or others' responses. Like other behaviors, anxiety and its associated behaviors increase in frequency when they are reinforced and decrease when they are punished or not rewarded (Fisak & Grills-Taquechel, 2007). For example, an adolescent who experiences social anxiety may skip class on the day she is scheduled to give a presentation. By missing class, she avoids having to present, and her anxiety is reduced. Because her avoidance has been reinforced, she begins to skip classes that require public performances or even significant social interactions. Without intervention, her anxiety, as well as her avoidant behavior, will likely continue. A similar pattern may ensue with a child who experiences anxiety when she starts preschool, screaming and crying and clinging to her parents due to separation fears as well as anxiety about interacting with her peers. If her parents decide that this experience is too distressing for everyone and pull her out of preschool after three days, her anxiety and anxious behaviors have been reinforced and are even more likely to persist when she encounters another situation that requires separation and/or social interaction. However, if she continues to attend preschool, her anxiety will not be reinforced, and eventually it will decrease (especially if other aspects of attending preschool are enjoyable for her).

From a developmental psychopathology perspective, it is important to emphasize a multifaceted approach to understanding behavior. While a conditioning model helps us to understand an important influence on the development of anxiety, it is not the only piece of the puzzle. The child who experiences significant anxiety upon beginning preschool may benefit from continuing to attend, so that her anxiety is not reinforced, but she may also need additional support and understanding. Perhaps she is fearful for some reason that her parents will not come back to get her (a cognitive distortion), so she would be comforted by being able to wear her father's watch while she is at preschool. Perhaps she has a behaviorally inhibited temperament and is overwhelmed by the number of children who are present when she is dropped off; in this case, she might benefit from being brought to preschool early enough that she is among the first few children to arrive. Furthermore, if her anxiety is due in part to bullying by peers, these negative interactions need to be appropriately addressed by parents and school staff. The complex and dynamic nature of environmental influences on anxiety highlights the importance of thorough assessment for each case.

Interactional model. In order to illustrate some of the many interactions among risk factors for anxiety, let us consider a fictional child. She is born to two parents who experience high levels of anxiety, predisposing her to genetic and neurobiological patterns that make her more prone to experiencing anxiety. She also displays high levels of behavioral inhibition and strong negative emotions as a young child, which are challenging for her to regulate. She learns through her experiences that she cannot manage her anxiety well, and without the necessary warmth and support from her parents to be able to tolerate her negative feelings, stops trying to manage them and starts avoiding anxiety-provoking situations. Her parents, due to their own anxiety, perceive these situations as threatening, and become overprotective and psychologically controlling in order to reduce their daughter's clear distress in new situations. They may even explicitly communicate to her that it is better to avoid a difficult situation than to experience anxiety. The child sees her parents' reactions to the situation and to her behavior, and her interpretation of the situation as dangerous is confirmed and likely to occur again the next time she faces a new situation. In addition, her parents' overprotectiveness prevents her from experiencing anxiety-provoking situations, which (1) removes the role of desensitization to her anxiety through exposure, and (2) prevents her from practicing strategies for regulating her anxiety. Her avoidance of new situations is reinforced by temporary decreases in her anxiety, and the cycle of avoidance that has been started by her parents' behavior is further perpetuated by her own experiences. The end result is a child who is fearful and anxious as the result of the dynamic interaction of biological, psychological, and environmental factors.

DEVELOPMENTAL COURSE

There is moderate stability in anxiety across childhood and adolescence (Bosquet & Egeland, 2006); however, there are also significant developmental variations in common anxiety symptoms and their expression. Between the ages of one and three, general anxiety increases (though more for girls than for boys), whereas separation anxiety and fearfulness of new situations normatively decrease (Carter et al., 2010). Indeed, most toddlers do not experience significant separation anxiety, and among young children who do, only a small percentage (less than 7%) continue to display separation anxiety into early elementary school (Battaglia et al., 2016). Fear and anxiety are common in young children and normatively decrease in both amount and intensity (Gullone, 2000). Fears about specific objects and situations—such as dogs, the dark, being alone, and doctors—are common and developmentally normative in young children; indeed, 75% of four-year-olds report experiencing fears, worries, or scary dreams (Gullone, 2000; Muris et al., 2000). Fears and scary dreams decrease with age, while worries increase from early to late childhood (Muris et al., 2000).

Older children most commonly report worrying about illness and injury, supernatural phenomenon, and school performance (Gullone, 2000). The content of youths' worries also varies by gender and socioeconomic status, highlighting the importance of considering demographic variables when evaluating the context for children's anxiety. Some research has found that animal fears and anxiety about death and harm to self or others are among children's top worries across childhood (Muris et al., 2000). Among children with clinically significant anxiety, separation anxiety and some specific phobias (e.g., of animals and blood) generally first emerge in childhood (Becker et al., 2007; Kessler et al., 2005). As childhood progresses, different types of anxiety show different developmental patterns (Broeren et al., 2013). In general, social anxiety decreases, and separation anxiety is fairly stable (i.e., consistently low, moderate, or high for a particular child). However, an interesting pattern emerges for generalized anxiety and specific phobias. For most children, these types of anxiety are moderate but stable, whereas for a smaller group of youngsters, these anxieties are low to moderate in early childhood, increase and peak around age eight, and decrease again in late childhood. This increasing-decreasing trajectory is considered non-normative and may reflect clinically significant levels of anxiety that peak in midchildhood for reasons that are unclear.

Adolescents most commonly endorse anxiety about economic and political issues (Gullone, 2000), though normative levels of anxiety vary across adolescence. In studies of adolescents as a group, anxiety symptoms generally decrease from early to middle adolescence and then increase between middle and late adolescence (Costello et al., 2003; Van Oort et al., 2009). These changes may represent differences in the developmental tasks and experiences across the adolescent years. For example, early adolescence generally marks the start of puberty as well as the transition from elementary to middle school, changes which are commonly anxiety provoking. Midadolescence may be characterized by fewer significant changes as well as increases in independence that are experienced as positive, whereas older adolescents are commonly experiencing more psychological individuation from their parents as well as higher levels of adult expectations. When researchers seek to elucidate different pathways of anxiety (through an individual-differences approach), three anxiety-symptom trajectories emerge among adolescents. Most adolescents experience low levels of anxiety across the teen years, whereas smaller groups of youth experience some elevated anxiety that peaks in midadolescence and then declines (Legerstee et al., 2013). In boys, the third trajectory involves anxiety that begins high but then decreases across adolescence, whereas the third group of girls experiences anxiety that increases from mid- to late adolescence. The risk of developing an anxiety disorder is elevated for the girls who experience increasing anxiety across adolescence and the boys who experience trajectories of anxiety that peaked in early or midadolescence.

Finally, the behavioral manifestations of fear and anxiety change across development. For example, young children with separation anxiety disorder often display school refusal and anxiety upon actual separation but a lack of cognitive symptoms (e.g., fear of loss of attachment figure or events that would lead to separation), whereas older children express more cognitively based worries about specific threats or anticipated separations. Children with phobias may display their anxiety in different ways, such as crying, freezing, throwing tantrums, or clinging to adults when they encounter a feared stimulus or situation (American Psychiatric Association, 2013). Other disorders are more rarely seen in young children. For example, social phobia is most likely to emerge in late childhood or adolescence, with a median age of onset of thirteen

(American Psychiatric Association, 2013; Beesdo et al., 2007; Kessler et al., 2005). The occurrence of panic disorder increases through adolescence, agoraphobia peaks in late adolescence and early adulthood (American Psychiatric Association, 2013), and most individuals do not experience GAD, panic disorder, or agoraphobia until late adolescence or adulthood (de Graaf et al., 2003; Kessler et al., 2005). While GAD tends to have an adult onset, many individuals with the disorder report having experienced anxiety since childhood or adolescence, and an earlier age of onset is associated with higher levels of comorbidity and impairment (American Psychiatric Association, 2013). These developmental changes may explain the fairly low homotypic continuity of anxiety disorders throughout childhood and adolescence, as only a small number of youth meet the criteria for the same disorder at two or more points in time (Beesdo et al., 2009). However, many children continue to display anxiety symptoms over time, even though the form of their anxiety may change or they may meet the criteria for multiple anxiety disorders. It is likely that changing environmental factors interact with the biologically based emotional dysregulation displayed by children with anxiety disorders to change the form of anxious symptoms across development. Based on this conceptualization, one approach advocates focusing on core features of dysregulated anxiety rather than the various behavioral symptoms that characterize distinct anxiety disorders (Weems, 2008).

ASSESSMENT

As with all disorders, developmental sensitivity in the assessment of anxiety disorders is paramount. It is particularly important with these disorders, however, given the normative nature of many fears and worries across development and the changing form of anxiety as youth age. Therefore, assessment must incorporate the evaluation of not only the content and frequency of a child's worries but also the degree to which they lead to distress, impairment, and/or the avoidance of tasks and experiences due to anxiety (Silverman & Ollendick, 2005). Huberty (2012) recommends that assessment of anxiety include several specific components, such as: gathering developmental and family history; interviewing the child, parents, and teachers about cognitive, behavioral, and physiological symptoms; using developmentally appropriate questions when interviewing youth; using a structured interview to differentially diagnose among anxiety disorders; observing children's speech, behavior, and social interactions in a clinical or school setting; and utilizing both broad-based and symptom-specific questionnaire measures of symptoms. Broad-based measures that assess a wide variety of symptoms include the Behavior Assessment System for Children, Third Edition (BASC-3; Reynolds & Kamphaus, 2015) and the Child Behavior Checklist (CBCL; Achenbach, 1991a). Such instruments are useful as screening tools for identifying areas for further evaluation as well as potential comorbidities. Commonly used symptom-specific self-report measures of anxiety in youth include the Revised Children's Manifest Anxiety Scale, Second Edition (RCMAS-2; Reynolds & Richmond, 2008); the Multidimensional Anxiety Scale for Children (MASC; March, 1997); and the Screen for Child Anxiety Related Emotional Disorders (SCARED; Birmaher et al., 1999).

Each of these questionnaires has both parent and child forms. The Anxiety Disorder Interview Schedule for DSM-IV—Child Version (ADIS-C; Silverman & Alfano, 1996a, 1996b) is a structured interview that has forms for use with both children and parents and assesses the symptoms of the various anxiety disorders as well as depressive and externalizing disorders. Given the significant changes that occur in anxiety and its common targets across childhood, it is particularly important to utilize assessment tools that have been designed for use with and normed on child or adolescent populations (Silverman & Ollendick, 2005). Finally, there is often significant disagreement between child and parent reports of children's anxiety, with children generally becoming more reliable reports as they age (Affrunti & Woodruff-Borden, 2015; Becker et al., 2016; Silverman & Ollendick, 2005). Therefore, best practice in anxiety assessment generally involves gathering information from both youth and their parents.

TREATMENT

Both psychopharmacological and psychosocial treatments have been found to be effective for reducing anxiety symptoms in youth. The medications most commonly used to treat anxiety are antidepressants (including selective serotonin reuptake inhibitors [SSRIs], tricyclics [TCAs], norepinephrine serotonin reuptake inhibitors [NSRIs], and monoamine oxidase inhibitors [MAOIs]) and anti-anxiety medications. SSRIs have received the most empirical support as effective medications for the treatment of childhood anxiety, though the type of medication that is most effective depends on the specific anxiety disorder (Compton et al., 2007; Fonagy et al.,

2015; Huberty, 2012; Ipser et al., 2009). Benzodiazepines, anti-anxiety medications commonly used in adults, have not been found to be effective for anxious youth. Studies comparing psychopharmological and psychosocial treatments and their combination are limited and have had mixed findings. Some evidence suggests that SSRIs are more effective than cognitive-behavioral therapy (CBT) in treating childhood anxiety, whereas some suggests that there is no difference in outcomes between the two; however, research that compares monotherapy with a combination of medication and psychotherapy points to a combination of these interventions as being superior to either implemented individually (Calati et al., 2011; Gonzalez et al., 2015; Segool & Carlson, 2008; Piacentini et al., 2014; Taylor et al., 2018; Walkup et al., 2008). One challenge in using medications are the significant side effects some youth experience, leading some researchers and clinicians to recommend psychosocial treatments, alone or in conjunction with medication (Leckman, 2013; Segool & Carlson, 2008).

CBT and behavioral treatments involving modeling and exposure are considered well-established psychosocial interventions for the treatment of anxiety in children and adolescents (Comer et al., 2019; Higa-McMillan et al., 2016). A wide variety of other approaches have good empirical support; these include family psychoeducation, relaxation training, assertiveness training, attention control, cultural storytelling, hypnosis, and stress inoculation. Although there are a variety of effective treatment packages that have been developed for the treatment of anxiety disorders in youth, they share a number of common elements, including psychoeducation and emotion education, coping skills and problem-solving skill training, cognitive restructuring, exposure, and relapse prevention (Mallott & Beidel, 2014; Seligman et al., 2014). Each of these elements, as well as some specific examples of full treatment programs with high levels of empirical support, is discussed below.

Common treatment elements.

Psychoeducation and emotion education. Psychoeducation often comprises the first phase of treatment and focuses on helping clients and families understand basic information about anxiety disorders and their treatment (Seligman et al., 2014). Parental components of psychoeducation may include information about anxiety disorders themselves as well as the distinction between what does work in the treatment of anxiety (e.g., practicing skills and facing fears) in contrast with what does not help an anxious child (e.g., telling a child to "not be afraid" or "just relax" or merely talking about their fears; Chorpita, 2007). An early emphasis in the child-focused portion of many treatment approaches is on helping youth understand the labels for, physiological signs of, and facial expressions linked with various emotions, especially anxiety. Therapists might act out different emotions with clients or create a "feelings dictionary" or "feelings collage" using drawings or pictures cut out from magazines to illustrate various emotions (Kendall et al., 2002; Kendall & Hedke, 2006). Once youth understand how people experience emotions generally, the focus may shift to their personal experiences of anxiety, including how it feels and what triggers it. Some approaches use a "feelings thermometer" as a concrete way to illustrate that the same emotion can be experienced at different levels of intensity; youth may use this

thermometer to rate how anxiety provoking different stimuli or situations are on a scale of one to ten (Kendall & Hedke, 2006). Therapists encourage youth to use this information about their own anxiety signs and triggers to raise their awareness of whether they are anxious at a given moment, which is the first step in implementing strategies for reducing anxiety. In addition, helping the child to be able to place her anxiety around a particular stimulus or situation on this hierarchy informs the exposure component of therapy.

In addition to learning about the physiological signs of anxiety, youth are taught that anxiety has cognitive and behavioral components (Chorpita, 2007). The cognitive patterns associated with anxiety are explored further in the cognitive restructuring component of therapy. It can be useful, however, to link the child's experience of anxiety with their behavioral reactions (e.g., clinging to a parent, avoidance of the situation). It is also important to make youth aware that everyone experiences anxiety and that it is the way our body and mind make us aware of danger, acting as a sort of alarm (Chorpita, 2007). Therefore, anxiety is neither inherently good nor inherently bad. It can be good or helpful when it alerts us to an actual danger that we need to address, but it can be problematic when it is overwhelming, impairing, or out of proportion to the actual danger, as is often the case with anxiety disorders. Disordered or problematic anxiety might be described to youth as a "false alarm." This framework sets the stage for future treatment components that involve the use of relaxation (to turn off the false alarm), problem-solving skills (to address situations that may actually be problematic or dangerous), cognitive restructuring

(to examine the thoughts that may errone-
ously lead a child to believe that a false alarm
signals actual danger), and exposure (to help
reduce the occurrence of false alarms).

Coping and problem-solving skill training.
Some youth with anxiety disorders struggle
to cope with and make decisions in anxiety-
provoking situations. Therefore, treatment
often includes the use of relaxation and other
coping skills to help youth manage their
anxiety in real-life situations (Mallott &
Beidel, 2014). The distinction between
emotion-focused and problem-focused
coping is helpful here (Lazarus, 1999). When
an individual experiences a negative emotion,
such as anxiety, there are two general ways
that the negative emotion can be managed.
On one hand, sometimes the most effective
way to address the emotion is to take an action
to change the situation (problem-focused
coping). For example, if an adolescent is
anxious because she has a physics test to-
morrow, the most adaptive way to manage her
anxiety is to study or otherwise prepare for
the test. On the other hand, there are some
situations that cannot be easily changed, in
which case a focus on regulating the emotion
itself (emotion-focused coping) is the most
beneficial approach. For instance, a child who
is fearful of riding in cars will be best served
by finding techniques for managing his
anxiety before and during car travel rather
than trying to change the situation or avoid
car rides altogether. It is important to remember that in some situations, the best
course of action is a combination of approaches. Interventions for anxious children
provide tools for both problem-focused
coping, in the form of problem-solving
training, and emotion-focused coping, in the
form of relaxation training.

Because relaxation (i.e., a state of low
arousal) is the opposite of fear or anxiety (i.e.,
states of high arousal), effectively creating a
sense of relaxation inherently reduces the
physiological experience of anxiety. There are
two common types of relaxation training that
are taught in the treatment of anxiety in youth.
First, youth may learn to use deep or diaphragmatic breathing to slow their breathing
(which often becomes faster and shallower
when people are anxious) and reduce their
physiological arousal. The child is instructed
to get in a comfortable position and close her
eyes, and at the therapist's prompting, to take
a deep, slow breath. The therapist might count
to four slowly as the client breathes in and
then count again as she releases the breath.
Youth often find it helpful to think about
filling their stomach or the bottom of their
lungs with air first, which then fills their lungs
up to the top as the breath progresses, with
breathing out following the reverse pattern.
The deep breath is repeated several times. Visualization can also be used to promote deep
breathing. For example, younger children
might be instructed to put their hands on
their stomachs and think about blowing up a
balloon or to imagine smelling roses and then
blowing out candles as they breath in and out
(Eisen & Schaefer, 2005; Kendall & Hedke,
2006). The therapist might instruct older
children to visualize themselves going to a relaxing place, such as the beach, where they
then take deep breaths. This relaxation technique is very useful because it can be done in
almost any setting and can be hard to observe
by others, making it fairly discreet.

Second, progressive muscle relaxation (PMR;
Wolpe, 1990) involves tensing and relaxing each
muscle group in the body in sequence. PMR

takes fifteen to thirty minutes as the therapist instructs the child to (1) tense a specific muscle, (2) hold the tension for five to ten seconds while focusing on the physical sensation of tension, (3) relax the muscle, and (4) focus on the feeling of relaxation and how it contrasts with tension (Huberty, 2012). Therapists often begin with the feet and work their way up the body to the neck and face. The final stage of PMR may involve tensing and relaxing all the muscle groups in the body. PMR helps youth to release physical tension following the muscle exhaustion of forced tension as well as to learn the difference between feeling tense and feeling relaxed. With younger children, concrete descriptions of tension versus relaxation (e.g., dry versus wet spaghetti) can be useful. Once youth are trained in PMR, they can go through the exercise on their own, either by coaching themselves or through the use of audio materials, such as a recording by the therapist. One useful resource that includes a variety of audio versions of all three relaxation techniques is *I Can Relax! A Relaxation CD for Children* (Child Anxiety Network, 2007). Mindfulness training, which aims to increase awareness of bodily sensations through simple activities (such as mindful breathing and eating), is commonly used with adults and gaining support as effective for reducing anxiety in youth (Borquist-Conlon et al., 2019; Semple, Reid, & Miller, 2005).

In problem-solving training, youth learn the skills for identifying and selecting effective solutions to problems they encounter (Seligman et al., 2014; Ugueto et al., 2014). Anxiety-provoking situations are generally the target for problem solving in this population, as difficulty navigating potential solutions to problems, in addition to deficits in identifying when there is a problem that can be solved, often contribute to fear and worry. In this component of intervention, therapists and clients work through the steps of effective problem solving. First, the problem needs to be defined. Clinicians should help youth identify a specific, concrete problem that can potentially be solved by the youth's actions. Second, the child and the therapist work together to generate as many potential solutions as possible. As anxious children may tend to generate solutions that involve avoidance or escape, the clinician should include these in the list of ideas but also encourage the child to generate more adaptive (but realistic) solutions. Third, the strengths and weaknesses, or positive and negative consequences, of each solution are discussed. The therapist should support the client in identifying both short- and long-term outcomes that are likely to occur, which may help the client to better see the downsides of avoidant behavior. Fourth, based on the consequences identified and the likelihood of success in solving the problem, the best solution is chosen. If there are many potential solutions to choose from, it may be helpful to rank the solutions from most to least desirable in order to identify the best ones. The therapist should allow the child to identify and select the best solution, even if the therapist disagrees with the choice. Finally, the child implements the chosen solution (usually as a homework assignment), and the child and the therapist subsequently evaluate its effectiveness and consequences. If the solution did not produce the desired outcome, a different solution is selected (perhaps based on the rankings made in step four), and the new solution is implemented and evaluated. It is important for therapists to encourage anxious clients that (1) there is no correct or perfect solution to a problem, and (2) the experience of problem solving should be viewed as a learning process, as the first solution may not always work, and it is acceptable to need to try a different one (Ugueto et al., 2014). Problem-solving skills might first be applied to a low-stress or low-anxiety situation, with work progressing to their application in high-anxiety situations (Kendall & Hedtke, 2006). For example, a child who experiences mild worries about the dark might be encouraged to identify possible solutions to this problem first (e.g., turn on a night-light at bedtime, put a lock on her closet door to keep the monsters from getting out, go into her parents' bedroom when she wakes up during the night) and evaluate them based on likely outcomes. After successfully implementing the steps of problem solving to change this situation, the child may be better prepared to apply them in a situation that provokes more anxiety and avoidance behavior.

Cognitive restructuring. Cognitive restructuring comprises a significant component of a CBT approach to treating anxiety disorders. During this element of treatment, youth learn to identify unhelpful or inaccurate thoughts (cognitive distortions) by testing them against reality and to replace them with more realistic and adaptive self-statements (Seligman et al., 2014). In order to begin to identify cognitive patterns, a child might be encouraged to think about what she was saying to herself during a time when she was anxious (Kendall et al., 2002). The child and the therapist then work together to ask whether those thoughts are accurate or inaccurate, helpful or unhelpful. With support, the youth is likely to be able to recognize dis-

torted thoughts during in-session discussion (even though this task may be challenging while she is highly anxious). One approach outlines common "thinking traps," or patterns of cognitive distortions, such as overestimating the probability of negative outcomes, walking with blinders (focusing only on the negative aspects/possible outcomes of a situation), the repetitor (believing that because something went wrong once, it will always go wrong), the catastrophizer (expecting the worst in every situation), the avoider (believing situations will be scary without being willing to experience them), the fortune teller (jumping to conclusions without having all the facts), the should (believing that there are certain ways one should always be/feel/perform), and the perfectionist (setting expectations for oneself that are too high; Chorpita, 2007; Kendall et al., 2002; Kendall & Hedke, 2006). Thought diaries, in which clients record their emotional, cognitive, and behavioral reactions to different situations throughout the week, are a common homework assignment used to support the identification of cognitive patterns.

Once a child has practiced identifying cognitive distortions, and she and the therapist have a good sense of the client's common patterns of thinking when she is anxious, work to challenge negative thought patterns begins. Therapists may begin this transition by helping youth see the negative consequences of falling into the thinking traps, or cognitive distortions, previously identified (Chorpita, 2007). Clinicians then work with youth to help them test the accuracy of their thought patterns. This process is often approached in an almost scientific manner, with therapists supporting youth as they ask questions about their thoughts, such as "What is the proof?" "Are there any facts that will back this up?" "Is there any evidence that this won't happen?" or "How likely is it that this will really happen?" (Chorpita, 2007). For example, an anxious child might be convinced that he is going to throw up at school and humiliate himself in front of his classmates, prompting him to refuse to go to school. The therapist might help the client examine the probability that this will happen. If he has thrown up at school one day out of six years of attendance (roughly 1,080 days of school), based on previous experience, there is a .09% likelihood that he will throw up on a given school day, and he has had 1,079 days at school when he did not throw up. The thought that he will "humiliate himself" in front of his classmates could also be challenged, as the child is asked to think about times that any of his classmates have been hurt or ill at school and his peers were sympathetic and supportive. The client and the clinician then work to identify alternative thoughts that might be more accurate or helpful. In the example just discussed, the child who is sure he will throw up at school might think to himself instead, "The odds of that happening are very low. And if I did get sick at school, it wouldn't be the end of the world; other kids have gotten sick at school and then come back and still had friends there." The therapist may play a more active role in challenging cognitive distortions and modeling restructured thoughts at the beginning of this component of therapy, with independence and responsibility for these tasks shifting to the youth himself as he builds skills. Decreasing negative self-talk appears to be the most important target of cognitive restructuring in reducing symptoms, though this change in thinking is also sup-

ported by skills development (Treadwell & Kendall, 1996).

Exposure. Anxious youth often avoid anxiety-provoking situations as a coping mechanism (Barrett, Rapee, Dadds, & Ryan, 1996); however, this avoidance is generally distressing and/or impairing and, so, is considered maladaptive. Therefore, helping youth to be able to tolerate anxiety-provoking situations through exposure therapy can be very helpful in overcoming symptoms, particularly in youth with GAD, social anxiety disorder, specific phobia, and separation anxiety disorder (Kendall et al., 2005; Seligman et al., 2014). Exposure to anxiety triggers helps youth develop skills to manage and cope with anxiety in addition to teaching them that anxiety (and the perceived threat) are not as dangerous and intolerable as they have believed (Huberty, 2012). This aspect of treatment is generally approached systematically and gradually, beginning with exposure to stimuli that create low levels of anxiety, which allows the youth to develop skills for managing and tolerating anxiety. Once skills are built at lower levels of exposure, the therapist may expose the child to situations or objects that produce moderate or higher levels of anxiety and support the child as he applies his previously learned skills to these more challenging situations. Exposure often begins with the client imagining the feared stimuli and shifts to in vivo exposure as skills are built and mastered (Huberty, 2012). Exposure is most helpful when the client is fearful about specific objects, situations, or tasks, such as in the case of specific phobias or social anxiety disorder. Systematic desensitization uses the principles of classical conditioning to help a client uncouple the object or situation with a sense of threat and relearn to associate it with relaxation and positive emotions (or at least the absence of anxiety). Flooding, which is sometimes used with adults and involves intensive, nongraduated exposure to the most highly feared stimulus, is not generally recommended for use with youth (Ollendick et al., 2004).

In order to implement systematic exposure and desensitization, the client and the clinician work together to create a fear hierarchy (Huberty, 2012; Kendall et al., 2005). They often start by identifying a stimulus that provokes little to no anxiety. For example, if the child has a fear of spiders, the first step on the hierarchy might be thinking about a picture of a friendly cartoon spider that is not experienced as threatening. The therapist and the client then identify fear-related stimuli that evoke increasing amounts of anxiety. A SUDS (subjective units of distress) rating scale from either one to ten or one to one hundred can be used to help the child assign a numeric value to the anxiety she associates with each stimulus. Following the imaginal task, the spider-phobic child's fear hierarchy might include looking at a picture of a spider, watching a video of a cartoon spider, watching a video of a live spider, having a spider in a glass cage across the room, standing next to the spider cage, taking the lid off the spider cage, watching the therapist take the spider out of the cage, petting the spider, and, finally, holding the spider in her hand. Fear hierarchies typically have eight to twelve steps that can be adjusted or expanded on during the exposure process (Huberty, 2012). The child should be exposed to the lowest (least threatening) remaining step of the hierarchy while she utilizes relaxation or other previously

learned techniques for coping with anxiety until her anxiety level has significantly decreased. The client and the therapist then work their way up the hierarchy at whatever pace is necessary until the child can tolerate exposure to the most highly anxiety-provoking stimulus on the hierarchy, either through the active use of coping techniques or because she has become desensitized to the object or situation via gradual exposure. With training and support from the therapist, parents can also help implement exposure hierarchies out of the session when appropriate; for example, a child with separation anxiety might benefit from time at home that increases in distance from the parent, beginning with playing in another room and working her way up to being left with a babysitter while the parent goes out (Kendall et al., 2005). Finally, it is important to be developmentally sensitive when implementing exposure tasks; the child's developmental level may affect the complexity of explanation given for the tasks, the child's ability to identify feared objects or situations as well as to provide accurate SUDS ratings, the child's ability to regulate strong emotions during exposure, and the degree of family involvement in the task (Kendall et al., 2005).

Relapse prevention. Finally, because it is not uncommon for anxiety symptoms to recur (Keller et al., 1992), the final sessions of anxiety treatment often focus on consolidating the skills that have been previously learned with the goal of relapse prevention (Seligman et al., 2014). Maintenance and relapse prevention involve several components (Chorpita, 2007). First, basic information about anxiety should be reviewed with the client and linked with her experiences in treatment. Second, the therapist should explore whether the child understands that improvement in her symptoms is due to learning and practicing the skills learned in treatment; if not, this link should be made explicit and the child encouraged by her role in the process of improvement. A client's belief in her ability to manage her anxiety is a predictor of treatment effectiveness (Kendall et al., 2016). Both the child and her parents should be praised for their hard work during treatment. Third, the role of continued exposure in maintaining treatment gains should be discussed and the child encouraged to think about how she will continue to challenge herself to face potentially anxiety-provoking situations. Fourth, the difference between a "lapse" and a "relapse" should be discussed. Lapses are small steps backward that are normal and do not constitute an emergency or need to panic. Lapses are especially common during times of stress or transition. Relapses, on the other hand, represent significant deterioration in functioning and anxiety-management skills that are difficult to overcome without assistance. The goal in identifying lapses and using the skills learned in therapy to overcome them is to avoid a full relapse. Finally, the child's progress and skill gains, in addition to the importance of continued exposure, should be reviewed with the parents as well. Following (or during the course of) relapse prevention, sessions may be tapered to a reduced frequency until treatment is ended altogether, with tapering occurring either more rapidly (for children who appear to be maintaining treatment gains) or more slowly (for those who need more support to maintain their progress).

Specific treatment approaches.

Coping Cat. Perhaps the best-known manualized treatment for anxiety disorders in youth is the Coping Cat program for children (Kendall & Hedtke, 2006), with an adolescent adaptation known as the C.A.T. Project (Kendall et al., 2002). (The term "Coping Cat program" will be used henceforth to describe techniques used in both the child and adolescent versions of the intervention.) The goal of the Coping Cat program, which is a CBT approach suitable for youth with comorbid disorders, is the reduction of the physical, cognitive, and behavioral symptoms of anxiety (Kendall et al., 2017). Treatment is conducted over the course of sixteen weekly individual sessions with the child and includes two parent sessions (though parents may choose to be more involved in goal setting, supporting the child's use of CBT skills, and/or building their own anxiety-management techniques). The first half of the intervention is considered the educational phase; the second half focuses on skill application.

The first phase of the Coping Cat program revolves around the mnemonic FEAR, which represents four steps to addressing anxiety and is represented by questions used to guide the client and help her remember the steps. The "Feeling Frightened?" step includes education about the physical symptoms of anxiety as well as relaxation techniques for reducing them. Modeling and role-playing are used to allow children to view and practice emotional awareness and relaxation strategies in a non-threatening setting. Parents are provided with the same information that their children are given, with youth teaching their parents relaxation skills. In "Expecting Bad Things to Happen?" the role of thought patterns in anxiety is explored. Children are taught to identify and then challenge cognitive distortions that contribute to their fear and worry.

In order to help children with the potentially abstract task of identifying patterns of self-talk, clients begin by filling in the thought bubbles of cartoon characters in various situations. Modeling and role-playing are also heavily utilized in this step, which emphasizes reducing negative thoughts rather than increasing positive self-talk. The third step, "Attitudes and Actions That Might Help," involves a focus on problem-solving skills as a way to increase the client's self-confidence. The client and the therapist work together to implement the steps of effective problem solving—identify the problem, generate possible solutions, evaluate these solutions, select the best solution, and make a plan to implement it. The therapist begins by modeling these steps, inviting the child to join in and eventually supporting the child as she follows them more independently. Finally, in the "Results and Rewards" step, clients learn to self-monitor their thoughts and behaviors and the impact these have on their anxiety. Children also work with the therapist to identify ways they can reward themselves when they effectively implement cognitive or behavioral anxiety-reduction techniques, such as with material prizes, fun activities, or social rewards.

The second phase of the Coping Cat program is more behavioral and focuses on systematic, hierarchical exposure to anxiety-provoking situations in which the client practices applying the skills that have been learned in the FEAR plan. Exposure can be imaginal or in vivo and progresses to situations that are increasingly anxiety provoking as the child tolerates and masters her anxiety in less intense situations. The therapist monitors the child's anxiety levels throughout the exposure and supports the child as she ap-

plies relaxation and self-talk skills. In addition, the child creates a "manual" (e.g., video, booklet) that instructs others about how to manage anxiety. This task serves multiple purposes, including consolidating and reinforcing skills, improving the child's self-esteem and self-efficacy, and allowing the therapist to monitor the child's understanding of the skills learned in treatment. The parent session generally takes place at the beginning of the phase in order to facilitate parental understanding of the purpose and process of exposure. The Coping Cat has been found in several randomized clinical trials to be effective in reducing anxiety disorder symptoms both immediately following the intervention and at a one-year follow-up (Kendall, 1994; Kendall et al., 1997).

FRIENDS program. The FRIENDS program (Barrett, 2000, 2004a, 2004b) is a CBT-based family intervention for childhood anxiety that began as an adaptation of the individually focused Coping Cat program complemented by a family component (Barrett, Dadds, & Rapee, 1996). The program consists of ten weekly sessions and two booster sessions and includes both child and parent components that are usually administered in group settings (Shortt, Barrett, & Fox, 2001). The child component includes the usual elements of a CBT intervention for anxiety, including emotional education, coping and problem-solving skills, relaxation, identification of cognitive distortions, cognitive restructuring, and relapse prevention. The treatment protocol also includes helping children to focus on positive experiences, emotions, and thoughts as well as to identify role models and sources of support in their lives. The FRIENDS acronym outlines these elements as follows: *Feelings, Remember to Relax, I can do it! I can try my best!, Explore solutions and coping step plans, Now reward yourself! You have done your best!, Don't forget to practice!,* and *Smile! Stay calm and talk to your support networks.* The FRIENDS acronym also represents the wide applicability of the concept of friendship, including (1) thinking about their bodies as friends that warn them of potential danger, (2) being their own friends by rewarding themselves for using anxiety-management skills, and (3) making and talking to their friends when they are anxious in order to benefit from social support (Shortt et al., 2001).

The family or parent component of the FRIENDS program is designed to complement the youth component in several ways (Barrett, Dadds, & Rapee, 1996; Shortt et al., 2001). First, parents are taught behavioral methods to reward the child's adaptive behavior and use of anxiety-management strategies. For example, parents might praise a child with social anxiety for introducing herself to a new peer at church rather than avoiding the interaction. Ignoring, or not reinforcing, anxious and maladaptive behaviors can help extinguish them; a child's constant expression of worry that her brother's tardiness in coming home from school is due to a terrible accident might not be acknowledged by the parent, who instead encourages the child to use the anxiety-management strategies she has learned. Second, parents are taught strategies for managing their own anxiety and other strong emotions. These strategies include relaxation as well as cognitive restructuring. Third, parents learn to use effective communication and problem-solving skills to work as a parental team to manage child and family difficulties. This el-ement includes training in conflict reduction and management skills, a discussion of the importance of setting aside time to listen empathically to one another each day, and the encouragement to schedule problem-solving sessions in which the family meets together each week to discuss and problem solve around child and family challenges. The group format also allows for the development of a support network among parents. The FRIENDS program has been found to be effective in reducing anxiety symptoms in youth (Barrett, Dadds, & Rapee, 1996; Shortt et al. 2001). The inclusion of a family-based component in CBT may be especially important for younger children and for girls.

Social Effectiveness Therapy for Children and Adolescents (SET-C). Social Effectiveness Therapy for Children and Adolescents (SET-C; Beidel & Roberson-Nay, 2005; Beidel et al., 2000) was designed as a treatment for social anxiety in youth ages eight to twelve that is modeled after adult treatments for social difficulties. The goals of SET-C include reducing anxiety symptoms, improving social skills, and increasing social involvement. SET-C consists of four components, which focus mainly on individual and group work with clients themselves. First, a brief psychoeducational component includes information for both children and parents about social anxiety and its treatment. Second, social skills training occurs in a group format. Youth are taught social skills such as introducing yourself to a new person, beginning and maintaining conversations, actively listening to others, joining a group, being assertive, and talking on the phone. Training includes instruction by the therapist followed by modeling, practice, and constructive feedback and praise from other group members. Nonverbal skills (e.g., eye contact, tone of voice) are also addressed as needed. Homework is assigned in order to encourage clients to practice these skills outside of therapy. Third, a peer generalization component allows children to practice the social skills they have learned in a more naturalistic situation. Immediately following each social skills session, a small group of children (including some from the therapy group and some recruited peers) participates in an unstructured group activity, such as bowling, a pizza party, or going to a museum. The activity always involves a meal or snack, and the recruited peers are instructed not to allow any of the children to isolate themselves or withdraw from social engagement. Finally, individual exposure sessions facilitate approach behaviors and desensitization to situations that the youth personally identifies as anxiety provoking. Youth participate in these situations—such as giving a speech, eating in front of others, asking an adult for help, or taking a difficult test in front of others—until their anxiety during the experience has been essentially eliminated, which takes an average of sixty minutes. SET-C takes place over the course of thirteen weeks, including one psychoeducational introductory session and sessions focusing on social skills training, peer generalization, and exposure. Notably, this intervention is purely behavioral; it does not include an explicit cognitive restructuring component, based on research suggesting that it is not necessary for symptom improvement in this population (Beidel & Roberson-Nay, 2005). SET-C has been found to reduce the symptoms of social anxiety in youth, with gains maintained over three- and five-year follow-ups (Beidel et al., 2000; Beidel, Turner, et al., 2005; Beidel et al., 2006).

INTEGRATIVE APPROACH TO TREATMENT

Psychoeducation and emotion education.

Anxiety and fear are mentioned frequently throughout the Old and New Testaments. One implication of this pattern is the recognition that anxiety is an inherent part of the human experience. In Scripture, worry and fear are discussed in a variety of different contexts, which may help us to understand that these emotions do not have a single cause or inherent acceptability. Some passages discuss fear and anxiety as emotions that we should not experience as Christians (e.g., Psalm 27:1-3; Matthew 6:25-34; Philippians 4:6; 1 John 4:18); these passages generally focus on worry that reflects a lack of trust in God and his provision. Other Scriptures portray fear positively (e.g., Exodus 20:20; Deuteronomy 10:12-13; Philippians 2:12; 1 Peter 1:17); in these cases, this fear is awe and respect that is rightly directed toward God. Therefore, the Bible portrays fear and anxiety differently depending on their targets and causes, which indicates we need to approach our interpretation of anxiety cautiously and thoughtfully. That which is the result of the belief that people are more powerful than God or that he cannot protect or provide for us is fear which we should strive to banish. On the other hand, the fear of God is encouraged and reflects more biblically based thinking about his power and greatness. These ideas are consistent with a clinical view that anxiety cannot be assessed merely by its presence or absence but that functional effects (e.g., how does anxiety affect behavior?) and context (e.g., is the anxiety proportional to the actual threat?) must be taken into account. Furthermore, the fact that fear can be viewed by Christians as either positive or negative is consistent with a CBT emphasis on the connections among thoughts, behaviors, and emotions (Elliott, 2006). Fear in Scripture is differentiated by the thoughts that underlie it (worry about people and harm to ourselves versus fear of God).

In addition, these different types of fear may be linked with different behaviors. The fear of harm that we are instructed to avoid can enslave us, leading us to undesirable behaviors such as apathy, complaining, and even drunkenness to dull the pain (Bonhoeffer, 2012). On the other hand, it has been argued that the fear of God is a necessary underpinning for right relationships with God as well as other people, as it guides our obedience to commandments about serving him and treating others in right ways (Fout, 2015). For Christian families, a discussion of the portrayal of fear and anxiety in the Bible will be important, given its prominence and varied meaning. Furthermore, families, youth, and clinicians might explore what children's anxiety reflects about their image of God as well as how a broader or different understanding of God and his nature might shape their experience of the world as safe versus threatening (Olson et al., 2013).

Coping and problem-solving training. Some mentions of anxiety and fear in Scripture, particularly fear that is undesirable or caused by thoughts that do not reflect trust in God, also include instructions for managing it. Resources for managing anxiety include comfort from God himself, kind words from others, seeking God's kingdom first, praying to God about our needs, and casting our anxiety on him (Psalm 94:19; Proverbs 12:25; Matthew 6:33-34; Philippians 4:6; 1 Peter 5:7). Lifting up our burdens and worries

to God, and receiving his comfort, can be important components of managing anxiety for Christians. For example, a client might begin to practice regular prayer that is focused on these tasks (Walker, Doverspike, et al. 2013). Spiritual elements can also be integrated into relaxation training. One study found that spiritual meditation leads to greater decreases in anxiety than secular meditation among healthy young adults (Wachholtz & Pargament, 2005). During spiritual meditation, participants were instructed to focus on a spiritual phrase (e.g., "God is love," "God is peace") during daily twenty-minute meditation periods. Particularly with older youth, the process of focusing on certain qualities of God and his power and goodness may help induce relaxation and be a component of decreasing anxiety.

It is worth taking the time to explore families' views of the meaning and implications of these anxiety-management strategies. Because of their instructional nature and relatively frequent occurrence, some families view passages such as Philippians 4:6-7 ("Do not be anxious about anything, but in every situation, by prayer and petition, with thanksgiving, present your requests to God. And the peace of God, which transcends all understanding, will guard your hearts and your minds in Christ Jesus") as a cure-all for anxiety, including clinically significant anxiety. In other words, if a Christian experiences anxiety, she needs only to pray to God, and she will receive his peace, and her anxiety will dissipate. If her anxiety persists, this is an indication that her faith is weak or that she is not performing "good Christian tasks" (e.g., reading her Bible, praying) frequently or wholeheartedly enough. Such messages can be very hurtful toward individuals, who may then start to question their faith or experience guilt because of their inability to improve their anxiety through spiritual practices. Youth may be particularly vulnerable to the negative effects of these implicit or explicit messages if they come from influential adults, including parents and church leaders. It may be helpful to communicate to families that the causes of anxiety are multifaceted and generally require interventions with multiple components targeting these varying causes. Although Scripture is often a helpful tool in promoting relaxation as well as cognitive restructuring (discussed in the next section), youth with anxiety disorders may be so strongly predisposed to fear and worry through biological and temperamental vulnerabilities that these must be addressed as well. Even secular approaches (Chorpita, 2007) note the importance of helping parents understand the difference between helpful and unhelpful messages (such as those that promote simplistic solutions) in the treatment of significant anxiety.

Problem-solving training is a component of many CBT interventions, and with anxious youth, its focus is on helping them develop the skills to more confidently and effectively approach rather than avoid problems and anxiety-provoking situations. From a theological perspective, working with children to develop these skills is a part of respecting them as full persons with developing cognitive and planning abilities that support their growth. One important component of these skills involves the ability to assess consequences and long-term outcomes. As Christians, we see the importance of such abilities in Scriptures that emphasize

eternal over earthly or temporal outcomes, such as 2 Corinthians 4:17-18 ("For our light and momentary troubles are achieving for us an eternal glory that far outweighs them all. So we fix our eyes not on what is seen, but on what is unseen, since what is seen is temporary, but what is unseen is eternal") and 1 Peter 1:6-7 ("In all this you greatly rejoice, though now for a little while you may have had to suffer grief in all kinds of trials. These have come so that the proven genuineness of your faith—of greater worth than gold, which perishes even though refined by fire—may result in praise, glory and honor when Jesus Christ is revealed"). Teaching youth to generate and evaluate possible plans of action in difficult situations encourages them to think beyond what feels good in the moment to how their choices will impact themselves and others in a broader way. Because of their tendency to avoid anxiety-provoking situations, anxious children may need extra help and support in this process. However, respecting the child's personhood and agency may also entail allowing him to choose and implement a solution that will fail. As many treatment approaches emphasize, part of the learning process involves making and evaluating mistakes and poor decisions; from a theological perspective, allowing a youth to fail—not overstepping the therapist's role as a guide—also supports his God-given agency. Of course, as adults charged with the care for the youth over whom God has given us influence, we do not merely leave them in the midst of their failures; rather, we support them in processing their choices, their consequences, and their effectiveness, the final step in the problem-solving process.

Cognitive restructuring. Cognitive restructuring is predicated on the idea that cognitive errors can be identified and compared to truth or reality. As in the treatment of other disorders, Scripture is helpful in identifying the realities against which worries and thoughts about threat can be tested (Tan, 2007; Walker, Ahmed, et al., 2013). A child whose separation anxiety revolves around discomfort of being separated from her mother might find truth and comfort in passages that emphasize God's constant presence with us, such as Joshua 1:9 ("Have I not commanded you? Be strong and courageous. Do not be afraid; do not be discouraged, for the LORD your God will be with you wherever you go") and Psalm 139:7-10 ("Where can I go from your Spirit? Where can I flee from your presence? If I go up to the heavens, you are there; if I make my bed in the depths, you are there. If I rise on the wings of the dawn, if I settle on the far side of the sea, even there your hand will guide me, your right hand will hold me fast"). An adolescent with GAD who displays catastrophic thinking, constantly worrying that something bad will happen to her or her loved ones, might counter those thoughts with Psalm 32:7 ("You are my hiding place; you will protect me from trouble and surround me with songs of deliverance") or Romans 8:28 ("And we know that in all things God works for the good of those who love him, who have been called according to his purpose"). Of course, a rich understanding of passages such as these, in light of the experiences of Christians throughout history, suggests that they do not indicate that God will keep every one of his followers physically safe at all times. Rather, they speak of God's protection over our souls and our eternal well-being, including the shaping of our character and faith, which further suggests that threats to our physical health and safety are of relatively little significance in the grand scheme of eternity. For this reason, clinicians and families might be wise to limit the use of such passages to challenge distorted cognitions to older children and adolescents who can understand the nuances of their meaning. Otherwise, children who take them more literally may actually experience worsening anxiety, as well as doubt in the veracity of God's Word, if they or others experience any harm. However, used in a developmentally sensitive manner, Scripture that is incorporated in cognitive restructuring has the potential to both reduce anxiety and increase a client's sense of safety and being grounded in God and his truth.

Exposure. Exposure is clearly a critical element in the treatment of anxiety. Given that the experience of exposure may be difficult and unpleasant (for both the client and her parents), it can be important to remind ourselves that caring for youth and treating them as the gifts they are does not always entail facilitating positive emotions. The process of disciplining and shaping our children to have the character that we—and, more importantly, God—desire may be painful and difficult (Hebrews 12:7). For youth with anxiety disorders, exposure to the object(s) of their fear and the reduction of avoidance are important processes in shaping their character and their mental health. We see throughout Scripture, particularly in the New Testament, the idea that though this world is not our home, we are to be fully engaged with it (John 17:14-16). We have great biblical models of individuals who were called to face difficult, anxiety-provoking situations, and whose courage God used for his purposes. Some of these examples include Gideon fighting the Midianites with only three hundred soldiers (Judges 7), Esther approaching the king to share the truth that would save the Jewish people from destruction (Esther 5), Stephen preaching the gospel to the religious leaders who would stone him to death (Acts 7), and Jesus facing his crucifixion and separation from his Father (Matthew 26–27). Some youth may find it helpful to explore the passages in which biblical heroes willingly enter into even life-threatening situations as a model of those who choose not to avoid but to follow what God desires for them.

However, in the process of exposure (including discussion about others who have chosen approach rather than avoidance), we must be sensitive to children's feelings, words, developmental levels, levels of understanding, and readiness to face a highly feared stimulus or situation. The effectiveness of exposure and adults' role in facilitating it for children's own health and development does not mean that we "force" them to face their fears. Rather, we encourage, explain, and support until children are willing participants (knowing that for some youth, willingness may never equal eagerness). By being careful to support rather than force in the process of exposure, we are better able to hear children's needs and desires and to respect their agency as individuals with a will and a voice. Indeed, the effectiveness of exposure in reducing fear can help youth gain a sense of mastery over formerly anxiety-provoking stimuli and situations, and this sense will be enhanced for youth who have an ownership role in the process of exposure. Furthermore, the way we approach this element of intervention has implications for children's spiritual development and well-

being. When we encourage appropriate self-determination and agency for youth in areas that are especially significant for them (such as allowing a child with an anxiety disorder to be involved in choosing how to face his fears), they are likely to develop a sense of efficacy and agency that carries over into other areas of their lives, including their relationship with God and their spiritual practices.

Relapse prevention. Fully human youth, like fully human adults, fail sometimes. Even when we have been freed from the sinful nature, we may still sometimes act like we are slaves to it (Romans 7:21-23). Those who have overcome their struggles with anxiety will still sometimes feel anxious and resort to the avoidant and maladaptive behaviors they used to perform regularly. For these reasons, it is important to recognize that we all fail sometimes and to encourage youth who have completed treatment for anxiety that failure and setbacks are normal. As many approaches discuss, recognizing the difference between a lapse (temporary setback) and a relapse (full-blown recurrence) is helpful in reminding these youth that failure and setbacks do not mean that all progress has been lost. Trials and challenges can support the development of skills and character (Romans 5:3-4; James 1:2-4). It is also important to recognize the role of supportive adults in preventing relapse in anxious youth. One study found adolescents' level of anxiety to be related to their perceptions of the supportiveness of their religious communities; youth who reported that people in their congregations were more supportive and helpful during times of trouble and less critical and conflictual had lower levels of anxiety (Desrosiers & Miller, 2008). Finally, in the concluding stages of therapy, children and adolescents are learning to apply acquired skills in new situations more independently, without the level of support they have been receiving from the therapist throughout weekly treatment. It is crucial to acknowledge and help a child recognize her own agency in order for her to develop autonomy in this process. If a child sees herself as completely dependent on adults to put her coping and other skills into action when she encounters a challenging situation, discouragement and relapse into significant anxiety are more likely. If she views herself as capable of approaching and mastering new situations (i.e., having agency and self-efficacy), in contrast, the transition out of therapy will be smoother and more successful. Furthermore, it is much easier to encourage a child to leave therapy embracing this view if she has been an active agent throughout the process of therapy, including implementing coping techniques and problem-solving skills, practicing cognitive restructuring, and having a voice in the exposure process.

CASE STUDY

Pertinent history. Marcos Perez is a seven-year-old Latino boy in the second grade at a private Catholic school. His parents Sonia and Martín Perez describe him as a nervous child who has been bothered by small things since the age of two. He tends to worry about various topics, such as the weather, illness, and social situations. Marcos worries about things he cannot control as well as the future (what might happen); for example, he worries that his neighbors may not get home safely. He frequently makes physical complaints and worries about physical pain (e.g., if he gets hurt, he may think he has broken his toe or his

back). He has specific fears that he worries about when in particular situations (e.g., the dark, thunderstorms, flipping over in a car). He worries about other children when they are upset and worries about whether his peers like him. Marcos is indecisive, often worrying about hurting others' feelings when making decisions. He frequently asks questions and talks about whatever worries he has, and at times he cannot sleep because he is thinking about the targets of his anxiety. He also appears tense and restless when worried and seeks to avoid situations that bother him (e.g., watching Disney movies in which a character dies). Marcos is described by his parents as "perfectionistic, sensitive, and dramatic"; for instance, he will not attempt tasks if he thinks he will make a mistake, sleeps with a stuffed animal that he "treats like a person," and cries during commercials about children or animals.

Marcos also becomes irritable when worried. He reportedly does not frequently tantrum but will sit and pout for long periods. According to his parents, Marcos "has to be talked out of a bad mood." At school, Marcos reports feeling embarrassed when he is called on, as he thinks other children stare at him. If something is difficult for him or if he cannot immediately do it correctly, he sits under his chair and cries. Marcos frequently gets frustrated with his schoolwork and runs out of the classroom. His mother receives weekly phone calls or texts from his school about Marcos's refusal to do his work; his teachers say he "shuts down" and refuses to talk. Recently, Marcos hid a homework assignment in his closet because he could not understand how to do it; however, he cried about and confessed this behavior, saying that he was worried about making mistakes. In addition,

Marcos tends to focus on the negative. He often makes negative self-statements (e.g., "I'm just dumb," "I'm a terrible person," "Nobody likes me"). Marcos has a couple of friends at school who help him when he becomes upset, but he does not hang out with any peers outside of school. Marcos's anxiety has persisted since beginning full-day kindergarten, occurs at home and school, and is associated with physical symptoms, problems with completing his work, and his developing negative attitude toward school. Marcos currently meets criteria for generalized anxiety disorder.

Marcos is the only child of Sonia and Martín Perez. Mr. and Mrs. Perez describe Marcos as "talkative, loving, and sensitive"; one of his strengths is being quick to help others when asked or when he sees a need. Mrs. Perez describes her relationship with Marcos as strong with open communication, though she notes that it can be frustrating to her to watch Marcos struggle. Mrs. Perez describes her husband as hardworking and loving, often showing affection toward Marcos; however, he is not home much due to his two jobs. Mr. Perez expresses his desire to support his wife in parenting Marcos and his worry that she often seems stressed and overly anxious about Marcos. The family attends Catholic mass weekly, and Marcos attends a religious education class (Confraternity of Christian Doctrine, or CCD) after the mass. They describe spirituality as important to them, frequently praying together and talking about God. They would like the therapist to "have God present" in therapy with Marcos as they believe God can heal Marcos. They are also worried that he will not be able to take First Communion because it requires him to stand up in front of others in church. They

have a large extended-family network, though Marcos's cousins are all much older than he is. They are open to mental health treatment and want to do "what it takes" to help Marcos, though Mr. Perez will not be available for sessions due to his work schedule.

Individual therapy is recommended for Marcos with a focus on helping Marcos gain skills for coping with his worries. Evidence-based interventions will help Marcos understand and recognize his anxiety, understand how his worries affect his behavior, challenge his anxious thoughts, and use effective coping strategies. It is also recommended to Marcos's parents that they actively participate in therapy each week and with parent consultation sessions in order to better understand his difficulties and how they manifest in his behaviors, remove any reinforcement of his anxiety, and promote his use of coping strategies outside of therapy.

Course of treatment.

Individual therapy sessions. Marcos's mother reports that he is hesitant about beginning therapy. At first, Marcos presents as quiet, nervous, and reticent to talk to the therapist in the waiting room (e.g., wringing his hands, looking to his mother for support, and glancing shyly at the therapist). The therapist normalizes his feelings about meeting a new, unfamiliar adult and helps him transition into the therapy room by first playing a game that includes his mother with the understanding that she will leave the room after the game. After the game, Marcos becomes talkative and easily engages in conversation with the therapist during a second game to build rapport. Marcos and the therapist ask one another questions and share responses in the context of a tower-building game. Marcos is willing to identify strong emotions he wants help coping with and recent instances at school and home in which he felt angry or scared and cried. Marcos often laughs nervously, but he listens attentively and is compliant with all activities.

By the end of the session, Marcos appears comfortable with the therapist. Marcos identifies his goal for therapy as learning what to do when he feels angry, scared, or worried. He says he wants to use drawing and playing games to learn about feelings and regulation strategies. Together, the therapist, Marcos, and his mother identify the following treatment goals: (1) Marcos will learn to express his feelings verbally rather than "shutting down"; (2) Marcos will develop the ability to self-regulate when he becomes emotionally overwhelmed; (3) Marcos will develop frustration tolerance if he cannot easily solve a problem at school; (4) Marcos will learn and implement coping strategies to help him cope with his worries (e.g., making mistakes, the dark, thunderstorms, social fears); and (5) Mr. and Mrs. Perez will implement parenting strategies that support Marcos's coping with anxiety and that communicate confidence in his abilities.

In the second session, Marcos again presents as nervous in the waiting room but also expresses positive affect and eagerness to begin the session. The therapist first meets with Marcos and his mother to provide psychoeducation about anxiety and the treatment plan. Marcos and the therapist then meet individually and work on emotion recognition exercises to identify different feelings. They first read a children's book about emotions while applying the content to Marcos's own experiences. They then engage in an art ac-

tivity in which Marcos selects four emotions to depict on paper-bag puppets. He displays some rigidity in wanting to make his art project come out exactly how he wants and begins to shut down with mistakes, but he responds well to the therapist's support and continues to engage in the activity. The therapist reinforces the idea that mistakes are okay and can help us learn. Marcos describes each emotion and the physical sensations in his body that accompany each emotion. Regarding worry or nervousness, Marcos identifies feeling a rapid heartbeat, sweating, and experiencing muscle tension. Marcos has difficulty identifying situations that make him feel specific emotions, though he tells the therapist that he has "very strong" emotions and that he is "overemotional." The therapist emphasizes that his emotions are not bad, and some people naturally feel very strong emotions. He and the therapist discuss how emotions vary in intensity and change throughout the day (i.e., they pass and do not last). Marcos becomes more open and engaged with the therapist throughout the session, although he reports that it is "not very much fun" to talk about all of his feelings. His mood improves when he plays a short card game with the therapist at the end of the session. The therapist assigns Marcos and his mother the homework of writing down any situation in which Marcos feels one of the four emotions and placing it in the emotion puppet bag over the next week.

Marcos brings his homework to the next session. With his mother's help, he was able to identify at least two times during the week that he felt each emotion, which was more than expected! The therapist explains the reward system for homework completion that will be used in therapy, and Marcos expresses his excitement. Marcos is willing to discuss his feelings, the situations in which he experiences these feelings at home and school, and how he typically responds. He demonstrates a desire to learn skills that will help him to feel in control and to have a better day at school. However, he needs processing time to respond to questions. He also seems more comfortable discussing anger and sadness than anxiety and has difficulty describing physiological and behavioral responses to distressing situations. The therapist provides psychoeducation regarding the similarities of physiological arousal between fear and anger and explains that the same coping strategies they will learn for worries can also be used to reduce anger. The therapist models imagining two situations in which she feels nervous and describes her somatic experience using a feeling thermometer. Marcos begins to open up about things that upset him. He reports an elevated level of anxiety regarding being away from his family (e.g., being upstairs when his mother is downstairs in the home, sleeping at a friend's house) and fear of certain things (e.g., the dark, bridges, riding in a car and being next to a semi-truck since he saw a crash a year ago). Marcos notes he used to have lots of nightmares and sometimes is scared because "he sees things in the dark." He describes staying away from things that upset him (e.g., movies in which the main character is separated from a parent) and trying to do everything exactly right. Marcos states that he gets frustrated when he makes a mistake, feels sick to his stomach with a rapid heart rate, and wants to cry, hide, or rip up the paper. The therapist writes each of these situations on an index card, and they begin to

categorize them as "small, medium, or huge" worries. For homework, Marcos is asked to write about two times he experiences anxiety during the week and record his physiological responses to those experiences.

The therapist reviews the session with Mrs. Perez and explains Marcos's homework of monitoring his emotions and physiological responses related to these emotional experiences to build self-awareness. He and his mother express willingness to engage in monitoring of emotions over the next week. Mrs. Perez appears apprehensive when the therapist describes that Marcos will earn points for each homework assignment that he can use to redeem various prizes at the clinic. The therapist reflects her apparent apprehension, and Mrs. Perez admits that they do not use rewards in their home because it feels like bribing. The therapist explains how difficult it is for children (and adults!) to face their anxiety and that it is important to help Marcos remain motivated toward working on the difficult tasks that will be part of therapy and also to acknowledge the hard work he does.

In the fourth session, the therapist and Marcos discuss difficult situations in which Marcos became upset on his first day back to school from the winter break. Marcos sits quietly while his mother describes his difficulty returning to school but answers questions readily when asked. Through role-play, Marcos is able to identify his feelings of anxiety and worry as well as his negative thoughts ("I am different than the other kids," "Am I going to make it through the day?"). His tendency to avoid what he does not think he is good at is discussed. Marcos responds well to the use of a color-coded gauge for emotions that shows differing levels of the intensity of his emotions. The therapist introduces the metaphor of Marcos as a "brave knight" who utilizes different strategies to remain calm to be able to make decisions. Each of the strategies is part of the knight's armor. Large butcher paper is used to outline Marcos's body, which the therapist explains they will "dress with protective armor." They first focus on breathing to help his body feel calmer, which is the chest plate that will calm his heart. The therapist teaches "star breathing" while incorporating a breath prayer, "The peace of God will guard my heart" (from Philippians 4:6-8). Using a visual of a star, they breathe in while saying in their mind, "The peace of God . . . ," hold their breath, and breathe out, " . . . will guard my heart" five times for each point of a star. The therapist also leads Marcos through a developmentally appropriate progressive muscle relaxation exercise. Marcos enjoys both exercises and reports feeling calmer after them. He seems surprised about the possibility that if he implements a calming strategy prior to the intensity of his emotions becoming elevated (crying, hiding, yelling), then outbursts could potentially be prevented. Marcos then teaches his mother the relaxation strategies. Marcos is assigned the practice of breathing at home with his mother's support. If he practices breathing at school, he is to tell his mother so he can get extra points for practicing.

The next session again focuses on relaxation strategies, as Marcos reports enjoying them and wants to learn more strategies. The therapist invites Mrs. Perez into the session so she can hear about the use of meditation and so the therapist can answer any questions she has. The therapist explains that meditation is a time to listen and rest in the peace offered by God, describing contemplative prayer and the use of a mantra to increase their focus and attention on God within them. It is suggested that Marcos repeat the verse "The Lord is with me; I will not be afraid" (Psalm 118:6) during this silent period. Mrs. Perez expresses some reticence about meditation, as she has heard it is un-Christian. The therapist explains that contemplative Christian prayer has been a part of Christian practices and the Catholic Church for centuries. Information is provided regarding endorsement of contemplative prayer from bishops of the Catholic Church and the pope as a way to draw near to God. The idea is discussed that all methods of prayer that are inspired by Christ can lead to him through the power of the Holy Spirit. Mrs. Perez is encouraged to talk to her priest about the practice and her concerns and to continue dialogue with the therapist. In the practice, Marcos and his mother are instructed to be still and silent with their eyes softly closed instead of squeezing their eyes shut. Marcos says he feels weird sitting on the sofa and doing this in front of his mother and the therapist; thus, yoga mats are provided for Marcos and his mother to rest with their heads on their arms. Given his age, they start with four minutes of meditation in this therapy session with the aim of practicing for five to seven minutes at a time at home when there are no distractions. Marcos is first instructed to be aware of his breathing (air entering and leaving his body, his belly rising and falling like a balloon inflating and deflating) while settling into contemplative prayer. The breath is to lead him into stillness of his mind and body with no other purpose than to be still while in God's presence (Psalm 46:10). During this period, Marcos will repeat the verse "The Lord is with me; I will not be afraid." The therapist explains that he will likely have many thoughts that enter his mind that could be distracting, particularly the worries he experiences. Marcos enjoys this practice, and he and his mother identify bedtime as a time to practice at home in order to calm his mind before sleeping. The therapist and Marcos then meet to review a situation in which Marcos was upset over the past week. He did not know how to complete a writing assignment and then made a mistake completing a math worksheet. He crumpled the worksheet and hid under his desk, crying. He had difficulty calming down until he was allowed to talk to his mother on the phone. Marcos identifies that his mother helps him calm down through two messages: "It's okay," and "You will get through this." He and the therapist reflect on the similarities to the verse he just meditated on and how important the mantra is to him. The therapist then facilitates role-playing this situation while having Marcos identify his ongoing feelings (nervous about the assignment, angry about his mistake) and arousal level. They then role-play again with Marcos incorporating breathing prior to becoming so aroused that he wanted to hide.

Marcos is eager to begin the next session and immediately tells the therapist about his practice of meditation and how excited he is that a friend is coming over to his house the next day. The therapist praises Marcos for his practice and for inviting a friend over to his house. The therapist then explains the focus of this session, which is to introduce monitoring our thoughts and linking different thoughts to different feelings and responses. The therapist introduces two new pieces of

armor (Ephesians 6:10-18). The first, a sword, he has already learned—to identify and communicate his feelings to others ("use your words"), which helps him feel more knowledgeable and in control of the big feelings. The next piece of armor is a helmet that protects Marcos through positive self-talk. They first read a children's book about an anxious main character, and Marcos practices identifying the character's negative self-talk and replacing it with positive self-talk. They then talk about a situation over the past week in which Marcos became anxious at school when the teacher yelled at the class for being too rowdy, and Marcos hid under a beanbag chair in the back of the room. The therapist has Marcos draw comic strips to assist him in identifying his thoughts in anxiety-provoking situations. In the first comic strip he describes what happened. He has difficulty accepting that his behavior does not have to be perfect at school and seems to fixate on his "bad days." He expresses worry that his parents will be angry with him if he gets upset. In his second comic strip, Marcos is able to identify his negative self-talk ("I'm a bad kid") and replace it with a positive statement ("I care about my behavior. I'm trying the best I can"), which results in feelings of calmness and engagement in the classroom. His homework is to continue practicing breathing and meditation and to also monitor his feelings and thoughts. Mrs. Perez joins the session, and Marcos teaches his mother this cognitive strategy. Mrs. Perez is able to talk with Marcos about his fear of getting in trouble at home, and they decide that negative consequences happen only at school, whereas her role is to help him learn how to deal with his big feelings. She says it seems helpful when Marcos is able to call her from school, and the therapist indicates that she will work with the school to see if they will regularly permit this support. In the session, Marcos is able to identify his feelings and accept calming strategies to do with his mother over the phone (breathing, identifying his feelings or "using his words," practicing positive self-talk).

In the subsequent session, the therapist focuses on teaching Marcos to use cognitive-behavioral strategies to "talk back" to his worries. They begin by reviewing the thoughts that Marcos identified over the past week. He and the therapist create a story and draw comic strips to illustrate how "anxious thoughts" make the story characters more worried whereas "coping thoughts" make them feel better. They illustrate how thoughts can influence the outcome of a situation (i.e., either cause people to become more worried and avoid situations or to become less worried and face the feared situation). They add a new piece of armor to his coping strategies, a belt of truth that is buckled around his waist so he can find the truthful thoughts. They identify how worry can trick Marcos with "thinking monsters" that cause him to worry more (e.g., "Mr. Perfect," who sets very high goals for him all the time; "Mind Reader Gremlin," or assuming other people's thoughts and feelings; "MagMin Monster," who focuses on the negative and minimizes the positive; "Conclusion Jumper," who thinks the worst will happen; "Labelpus," who puts negative labels on everyone). Specifically, they discuss how perfectionism causes Marcos to worry more and feel worse. The therapist shares examples of when she has paid attention to the perfectionist monster, and Marcos predicts the outcome of these stories (i.e., that the therapist worried

more and performed worse). He independently identifies the therapist's negative thinking. Marcos identifies that perfectionism seems helpful at first and seems to offer a way to make him feel better because it prevents mistakes. However, he recognizes that it ultimately causes problems for him.

In the next session, Marcos and the therapist continue to focus on identifying Marcos's unhelpful thoughts, especially those that arise during difficult academic tasks, by first reviewing his thought monitoring over the past week with his mother in the room. Marcos's mother reports that he frequently "shuts down" during schoolwork if he does not understand the task immediately. Marcos describes how he views the characteristics of the perfectionist monster ("Mr. Perfect"); he is able to identify that perfectionistic thoughts occur to him frequently and that they make him worry and cause him to avoid difficult school material. The therapist reflects his increased awareness and insight into his own thinking patterns. The therapist helps to link his avoidant (shut-down) behavior with these anxious thoughts so Mrs. Perez can more accurately understand his behavior in light of the underlying feelings and thoughts. While engaging in a difficult logic puzzle, Marcos and the therapist identify the thoughts that the "should monster" and the "perfectionist monster" are telling him (i.e., "I should know this already!" "I shouldn't make any mistakes," "It's not okay to have to cross something out"). They record these thoughts on strips of paper and identify ways to "talk back" to these worries, which they write on the flip side of the paper. They then practice a more difficult activity for Marcos—writing a response to an open-ended question on the room's whiteboard. Marcos successfully practices talking back to his worry thoughts with the support of the therapist.

Marcos has shown an increased willingness to approach his worries and situations that are more difficult for him, but before they move on to explicit exposure tasks, the therapist uses this session to reinforce his problem solving and use of coping strategies. The therapist first explains that his protective armor is not complete without a shield of faith that he can use to get through difficult situations. They discuss the belief that God will protect him and help him. A "stop and think" strategy is presented in which Marcos is encouraged to pause, engage in problem solving, and then implement a coping strategy or try a solution to the situation. During their discussion of "highs" and "lows" from the week, Marcos describes his nervousness about standardized testing at school this upcoming week, and his desire to not do the language arts testing in particular, as that subject is more difficult for him. The therapist engages in reflective listening and supportive processing of Marcos's emotions. They then discuss the power of "stop and think" to problem solve the situation. Marcos identifies that he could ask his teacher if he could do the testing in another location or in a quiet area of the classroom to increase his comfort, he could engage in breathing and positive self-talk, and he could gather information about the testing (i.e., ask his teacher what it is used for). The therapist and Marcos discuss how his pieces of armor could be used in different situations, including breathing, positive self-talk (a "mantra"), labeling his feelings ("use your words"), and using cognitive challenging. They make and decorate a paper fortune teller with the coping strategies.

Marcos then teaches his mother the different coping strategies through playing the fortune teller with her. His mother reports that his anxiety was not apparent through the week, and they experienced low stress as a family due to not having school for the week because of winter weather. He was nervous returning to school after the snow days, but he was able to use his coping strategies. Marcos responded positively to praise for his use of these strategies. Marcos is given an assignment to complete a worksheet to identify connections between thoughts-feelings-behaviors and engagement in problem solving.

In the next stage of therapy, the focus is on exposure to his worries and fears. The therapist, Marcos, and his mother first review his homework and situations in which Marcos became worried (forgetting his lunch at home, a thunderstorm) and his use of coping strategies in these situations. His mother reports that Marcos did not display any behavior problems at school during the past week. Marcos expresses pride and excitement about this achievement and about his ability to use breathing and cognitive challenging during a thunderstorm and to problem solve when he forgot his lunch. This discussion leads into the therapist's presentation of exposure tasks. Marcos and the therapist discuss the meaning of bravery as stepping into situations even when we feel scared or nervous. The therapist focuses on the importance of confronting fears and the negative effects of avoidance strategies. The therapist describes a situation that made her feel anxious in the past week and invites Marcos to "tag along" and predict the somatic experiences of her anxiety and how she got through the experience of anxiety. They discuss the physical manifestations of anxiety, how anxiety "peaks" and then "falls" quickly, and how anxiety grows through avoidance but subsides through confronting the situation. Marcos recognizes that when he faces a fear his "worry gets smaller," whereas when he avoids a fear his "worry gets bigger." He describes situations in which his worry got bigger when he avoided a fear (e.g., fear of heights on a family vacation) and got smaller when he faced a fear (e.g., asking his teacher for help on an assignment). The therapist asks Marcos which of his worries he would like to focus on first. Then Marcos works on creating a "fear ladder" (i.e., a hierarchy of anxiety-producing situations), which the therapist explains will be linked to a reward system. They discuss the use of prayer prior to each exposure task so Marcos feels ready to go where God will be with him so he is safe and strong.

At the beginning of the next session, the therapist meets with Marcos and his mother together to discuss exposure tasks and the need for his parents to coach him through these tasks through use of coping strategies rather than enabling avoidance or taking over tasks for him to make him feel better. Mrs. Perez reports that Marcos is making significant improvements in his emotion regulation skills. She describes how Marcos became upset at soccer practice and started shutting down but was able to identify his emotions and rejoin the practice. He later voluntarily discussed his feelings with his mother. Marcos expresses he avoids some soccer skill practice at soccer because the skills are challenging for him. They use this scenario to discuss the value of doing difficult things, because facing difficult things increases his strength. Marcos and the therapist review psychoeducation about avoidance and the importance of confronting his fears,

specifically how worries "grow" if you avoid them but "shrink" if you face them. Together they create a reward system for using his coping skills and not avoiding "brave steps." They plan the first exposure task to be conducted in a therapy session and then play a challenging but fun board game together at the end of the session with modeling of positive self-talk and perseverance when things are not easy. The therapist also reinforces Marcos and his mother's teamwork. Throughout Marcos spontaneously catches himself making negative self-statements.

The first exposure task Marcos chooses for his hierarchy is to watch scenes from Disney movies he has always wanted to watch but avoids because he knows a parent dies in them. The therapist and Marcos first talk about what he may feel and think while watching the movie clips. They then look at images from the movies found online while Marcos engages in relaxation exercises. He then watches the actual scenes; by the end of the second movie clip, Marcos states with surprise that he does not feel anxious and the experience was not as bad as he expected. The therapist reinforces how avoidance can make our fears bigger.

The next session focuses on preparing for the first out-of-session exposure (being tardy to school). Marcos presents as anxious at the thought of having to be late to school but practices using his coping skills with the therapist during imaginal exposure. They also discuss coping strategies Marcos could utilize for his anxiety (e.g., identifying his feelings, positive thinking on the way to school, asking for help from his teacher) and incorporate these strategies into a story they write about being late. Marcos is very engaged and enjoys writing the story. He tells the therapist he wants to write other stories to "help other kids be brave." Marcos and his mother agree the exposure will occur before the next session and Marcos will not know when it will happen (but he is aware it will be happening once over the next week). Mrs. Perez will help remind Marcos of his coping skills while the exposure is happening. Marcos and his mother will report the outcome of this exposure to the therapist. The next session will focus on reviewing this task through role-play and identifying the anxiety Marcos experienced during the exposure and his use of coping strategies.

Marcos presents for the next session with excitement, running up to the therapist in the waiting room to report that he completed his exposure homework and that it went well. He states he felt anxious at home when getting ready for school knowing he would be late. He engaged in relaxation and breath prayer and challenged the thinking traps he experienced (e.g., that it was "the end of the world" if he was late). He identifies it was "not as big of a deal" as he had originally feared. Marcos and the therapist then prepare for his homework for the next session, which is to forget his homework folder for school one day next week when he has papers to return to school. He presents with more anticipatory anxiety with this task but identifies the armor he will use in the moment. The therapist assures Marcos that his teacher will be notified and asked if she can remind him to use his coping skills if needed.

At the next session, Marcos describes how he felt sick to his stomach while his teacher was collecting the class's homework folders that he did not have. He used a mantra and engaged in breathing, and noticed that his

high level of anxiety peaked and then "just went away" after the teacher organized them into groups for an activity. He expressed greater motivation to continue his brave steps based on his successes. Marcos and the therapist prepare for his next exposure task, which is to purposely make mistakes on a spelling test at school. They role-play the situation, practice using Marcos's coping skills, challenge his anxious cognitions, and create a plan to continue to prepare himself for the exposure. Marcos presents with substantial anticipatory anxiety while talking about this exposure and says he is "the smartest kid in the class" and is afraid other students will view him as "stupid" if he makes a mistake. Marcos and the therapist acknowledge these thoughts as thinking traps and challenge them. He agrees to continue to work with his mother to prepare for the exposure on Friday.

When the therapist greets Marcos and his mother in the waiting room the next week, Marcos displays anxious behavior (eyes averted, head down, fidgeting, picking at his hands). His mother asks to meet with the therapist about a recent meltdown at school. Mrs. Perez describes how Marcos defied his teacher's requests (not wanting to return to the classroom after recess) and was disrespectful toward his teacher (e.g., "This is stupid"). The therapist utilizes drawing comic strip boxes on the whiteboard to examine Marcos's thoughts, feelings, and behaviors because he has difficulty talking about this incident. Marcos depicts how he felt nervous because his teacher told them about an upcoming practice for First Communion and "made a big deal about it." Marcos is nervous about being in front of others and in front of the priest and having their attention be on him. He admits that although he has participated in education for his First Communion, he does not know what actually will happen at the ceremony. He responds positively to discussion about the benefit of practice to help him understand it and is willing to identify and challenge his thoughts. They discuss Marcos's motivation to receive his First Communion with a focus on the sacrament signifying his love for Jesus Christ. He also expresses surprise that he is not getting in trouble with the therapist for his behavior at school and that the expectation is that he learn from these experiences rather than get through anxious situations with no difficulty at all. They add practice for First Communion to his exposure hierarchy, and Mrs. Perez agrees to contact Marcos's teacher and the parish priest to find a time to meet in the church to walk Marcos through the practice on his own first before he practices with his class. With Marcos in an improved mood, they discuss his successful completion of his most recent exposure task. They then prepare Marcos for the next task, to go to a friend's house that he has never been to before, with imaginal exposure and role-playing. Mrs. Perez had reached out to a peer Marcos wants to play with and asked if the parent would be able to have Marcos over while she ran some errands. Identifying something for Mrs. Perez to do would also help her get through the time period that Marcos would be at his friend's house by providing a distraction from her own worry about him. They plan for him to complete this task prior to the next session.

For the next session, the therapist meets Marcos and his mother at the local public library, where Marcos will practice going to the bathroom on his own. They first engage in relaxation exercises to help Marcos feel calm prior to the task. Next he walks away from his mother down an adjacent book aisle and back to experience being apart from her in public. Marcos wants to practice this several times until he feels comfortable with it and his anxiety level has decreased (from a seven out of ten to a zero out of ten, with ten being the highest). He is then to walk toward the bathroom and back to his mother as the next step, but he walks to the bathroom and proceeds into it. Marcos is proud of himself and asks if they can play hide-and-seek in the library before they go. Mrs. Perez expressed some anxiety but was able to engage in coping strategies herself when Marcos went to the bathroom. She lets Marcos know that she believed he could do it and how proud she was of him. They then enjoy a game of quiet hide-and-seek among the book aisles.

Given Marcos's successful exposures during the last couple of sessions, the therapist introduces the idea of "graduation" from therapy to Marcos and his mother. With Mrs. Perez, the therapist reviews Marcos's progress over the past several months. Mrs. Perez expresses concern that Marcos will need a "long time" to anticipate and prepare for saying goodbye to the therapist and that he may get worse again. The therapist normalizes how clients can sometimes re-experience symptoms during the process of termination and reinforces the knowledge and skills they now have to manage his feelings. Mrs. Perez expresses that she would like to have the option of contacting the therapist for continued treatment for Marcos if he ever struggles in the future. The therapist then discusses termination with Marcos. Together they begin a "timeline project" to review everything Marcos has learned in therapy. Marcos begins the timeline project by creating an "emotionomitor" (a large thermometer that represents his level of emotion). He and the therapist identify different situations he has experienced over the past few months and discuss the intensity of his emotion during each event and how he got through it. The therapist reinforces his bravery in facing his worries and situations that make him nervous. At first, Marcos is reticent to discuss his feelings about ending therapy. He tells the therapist that he would "definitely not feel happy." The therapist encourages Marcos to express all of his emotions (e.g., sadness, anger, worry) about saying goodbye to the therapist. They discuss how Marcos would like to celebrate his "graduation" and identify having balloons, an ice cream sundae bar, and a Silly String war during the final session. Marcos attends his last session with a story he wrote about a boy who overcomes anxiety with the help of God, his parents, and a "nice friend" (who resembles the therapist).

Parent and family therapy sessions. At all of the individual sessions, the therapist meets with Mrs. Perez at the beginning of the session to check in about Marcos's functioning over the last week, and then again at the end of the session so Marcos can explain the session content to his mother and homework assignments can be reviewed. However, there are also important parent and family sessions held over the course of therapy. At the intake, Mr. and Mrs. Perez express the belief that God can heal their son. The therapist explores this belief, and Mrs. Perez admits she feels frustrated that anxiety is so prevalent in their family despite their expressed faith. They discuss how God will and does help them, but they need to be willing to do things differently.

Mrs. Perez in particular can overtly communicate her trust in God's protection and guidance to model this for her son (in prayer, during daily interactions) rather than reinforcing his avoidance of situations that cause distress. Both Mr. and Mrs. Perez are also asked to monitor their communications about anxiety. Throughout therapy, the therapist gently points out their anxious messages that suggest Marcos should be nervous in certain situations or may not be able to handle the situation. The therapist also is mindful about modeling for Mrs. Perez how to encourage Marcos's confidence that he can handle difficult situations instead of undermining his confidence.

During the exposure stage of therapy, the therapist meets with Mr. and Mrs. Perez to encourage their support for Marcos to identify and communicate about his emotions throughout the exposures, particularly regarding First Communion. Mrs. Perez is receptive to hearing his experiences and is able to identify her own embarrassment and worry that Marcos will suffer a major setback as a result of this experience and will not be able to "handle things when he's older." The therapist helps Mrs. Perez process her experience and affirms her desire for the best for Marcos's future. The therapist also helps Mrs. Perez identify the progress Marcos has made in the past couple of months (e.g., the ability to identify and express his emotions, the courage to face things that are difficult for him). Additionally, the therapist discusses with Mr. and Mrs. Perez all of Marcos's "protective factors" (e.g., his close relationship with his parents, his parents' motivation and insight to obtain treatment for him, Marcos's intelligence and ability to communicate with supportive adults, his social skills, and his sense of humor). Mrs. Perez and the therapist discuss different ways Mrs. Perez can validate Marcos's experience and communicate confidence in his ability to handle difficult situations.

In an individual session, Marcos relates to the therapist that he experienced a "low" when he heard his parents fighting. He describes how he goes to his bedroom to cuddle with a stuffed animal when he hears his parents fighting. Marcos is able to label his emotions about his parents' fighting, and identify questions he has (e.g., Are they going to get a divorce? What will happen next? Why can't they figure out how to get along? Why can't they be nice to each other? Is it something I did?). A family session is scheduled to talk about Marcos's experiences. The therapist reinforces open communication, affect expression, active reflection, and physical touch (hugs, rubbing his back, cuddling) to increase Marcos's sense of security. Marcos expresses feeling awkward asking his parents questions regarding their fighting, but he is interested in their answers. He and his parents hug and Marcos smiles after the discussion. His parents let the therapist know they had been stressed about money over the past few months, and this session was a "wake up" for them to realize that their stress was affecting Marcos.

After the sixth session, a parent session is held with Mrs. Perez to prepare for a problem-solving meeting at Marcos's school (see below). The therapist and Mrs. Perez identify the topics Mrs. Perez would like to review at the meeting. She reports that Marcos's teacher and the principal interpret his shutting down as noncompliance and subsequently punish him. She would like the therapist to educate the team working with Marcos about his anxiety. They discuss ways Mrs. Perez can advocate for environmental supports for Marcos's development of regulation skills, since he still needs those external reminders and redirection. Mrs. Perez reports she also has difficulty regulating her emotions when he calls her upset from school, which she and the therapist process.

Additional considerations from a developmental psychopathology framework. It is recommended that Marcos's parents continue to promote his engagement in extracurricular activities despite his desire to avoid them. They acknowledge that once he engages in the activity, he is able to participate and enjoy it. These activities provide supervised social interactions with his peers, physical activity, and a sense of confidence and self-efficacy. His interaction with friends outside of school for playdates is also encouraged. Mrs. Perez reports her desire and willingness to continue to promote his social interactions, though it took the therapist's weekly check-ins with her to ensure she obtained contact information of classmates he could invite over.

Though Marcos would benefit from counseling within the school setting to help him deal with worries and fears that occur during the school day and develop a greater level of self-mastery in a supportive environment, counseling is not available at his school. Thus, the therapist first connects with Marcos's teacher in a phone call to explain the nature of Marcos's anxiety, to help her be aware of physical symptoms of anxiety and frustration, and to encourage her to provide support to him when she notices his anxiety. Marcos's daily expressed worry ("What if I have a bad day at school?") is described, as is his excitement about receiving praise at school and his desire to continue getting praise for positive behavior. Marcos has some somatic symptoms related to his anxious feelings, which when expressed by Marcos to adults can be a "cue" or "warning" that he may be feeling anxious or overwhelmed and may need some time to calm himself. The therapist presents the coping strategies he is learning in therapy that can easily be implemented at school.

A few weeks after the phone call, Marcos's teacher asks Mrs. Perez for a problem-solving meeting at school to address Marcos's refusal behaviors. Mrs. Perez asks the therapist to attend the meeting as she does not believe school staff understand Marcos's anxiety but rather think he is "a bad kid." The therapist seeks a collaborative relationship with school staff during the meeting, serving as a consultant to the school but also contributing to problem solving. The therapist provides perspective about Marcos's underlying anxiety, low self-esteem, and deficits in self-regulation that require support from adults as he cannot self-soothe or choose to utilize coping strat-

egies once he is already aroused. This perspective is important as the team had outlined a behavior plan with one target for Marcos to follow adult orders. He would be given strikes when he does not comply. Together, the team develops a positive reinforcement system rather than the "strike" system used in his classroom. He will earn points for asking for help when he needs it, for using coping strategies when upset, and for complying with directions. Marcos's teacher identifies a way for Marcos to communicate when he is feeling frustrated or nervous (e.g., a hand signal) in order to prevent shut-down behavior and refusal to work, as well as the use of a visual on his desk to remind him of the coping strategies he has been learning. A designated area is identified in the classroom for Marcos to use to calm down when upset and be able to think about the situation. This meeting and then follow-up phone calls during the course of therapy set the stage for collaboration with Marcos's teacher for the exposure tasks.

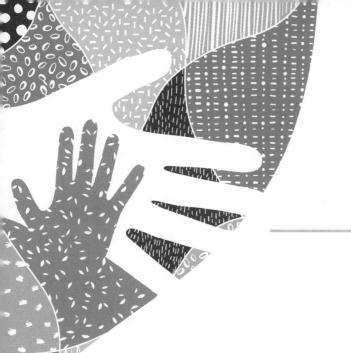

Chapter Five

Posttraumatic Stress Disorder

MANY YOUTH experience traumas such as abuse, assault, accidents, community violence, natural disasters, and political conflict. Some of these children and adolescents will recover quickly or show few symptoms following trauma exposure. Other youth, however, will develop a trauma- or stressor-related disorder, such as *posttraumatic stress disorder* (PTSD) or *acute stress disorder* (ASD). The DSM-5 (American Psychiatric Association, 2013) presents different diagnostic criteria for individuals above age six and those six years old and under. For anyone, regardless of age, a diagnosis of PTSD necessitates exposure to "actual or threatened death, serious injury, or sexual violence," which can result from directly experiencing, witnessing, learning about, and/or being exposed repeatedly to negative details about a traumatic event (American Psychiatric Association, 2013, p. 271). For older children, adolescents, and adults, exposure must also be accompanied by symptoms in four categories.

First, *intrusive symptoms* involve recurrent and distressing memories or dreams, dissociative periods when the individual re-experiences the event ("flashbacks"), and intense distress or physiological reactions to reminders of the trauma. Second, individuals with PTSD *avoid* internal (e.g., memories) and external (e.g., places) situations and stimuli that remind them of the traumatic events. Third, significant *cognitive and mood* symptoms occur; these may include dissociative amnesia, cognitive distortions, self-blame for the traumatic event, strong negative emotions, difficulty experiencing positive emotions, diminished interest or pleasure (anhedonia), and feeling detached from others. Fourth, individuals experience increases in *arousal and reactivity*, such as disproportionally angry outbursts, self-destructive behavior, hypervigilance, an exaggerated startle response, difficulty concentrating, and trouble sleeping. Children ages six and younger are diagnosed with PTSD according to similar criteria with some developmentally appropriate changes. First, young children with PTSD experience intrusive symptoms, though these may be expressed either in memories/dreams/flashbacks or through play themes. Second, avoidance and cognitive changes are grouped together. To be diagnosed with PTSD, children must display avoidance, increased negative emotions, decreased positive emotions, anhedonia, and/or social withdrawal. Third, young children display increases in arousal and reactivity; these symptoms may manifest in ways that are largely similar to older individuals but can also appear as extreme temper tantrums. At any age, symptoms must last for at least one month and be significantly distressing and/or impairing for diagnosis. (Individuals who experience symptoms with a shorter duration—three days to one month—receive a diagnosis of ASD.) Most individuals display symptoms within three months of trauma exposure, but the onset of the disorder may be delayed until six months or longer after the trauma (American Psychiatric Association, 2013).

Rates of PTSD in youth are difficult to determine, as figures vary drastically across studies (from less than 2% to 35% or higher) depending on the population surveyed, the trauma type, and the length of time since the trauma exposure (Cohen et al., 2010; Taylor & Weems, 2009; Wang et al., 2013). The DSM-5 criteria for PTSD, which differ somewhat from their DSM-IV predecessors, may result in higher diagnostic rates for both children and adolescents (Modrowski et al., 2017; Wolmer et al., 2015). Findings on the relation between gender and PTSD in youth are mixed. Some studies have found that girls experience PTSD at higher rates than boys following trauma exposure (Cénat & Derivois, 2015; Kessler et al., 2012; Marthoenis et al., 2019; Nordanger et al., 2013; Udwin, Boyle, Yule, Bolton, & O'Ryan, 2000). However, other studies have found no gender differences in rates of PTSD in preschoolers, children, or adolescents (Contractor et al., 2013; Scheeringa & Zeanah, 2008; Taylor & Weems, 2009). When gender differences exist, they appear to be due to the higher rate of sexual assault for girls as well as the development of an external locus of control and stronger biological reactions to a stressor (see Nader & Fletcher, 2014, for a review).

Among youth with PTSD, psychiatric comorbidity is common. One study found that 40% of youth who had experienced a trauma met the criteria for a comorbid diagnosis of a disruptive behavior, mood, or anxiety disorder (Copeland et al., 2007). Furthermore, youth with high levels of other types of symptoms, such as depression and anxiety, have higher levels of PTSD symptoms as well (Taylor & Weems, 2009; Udwin et al., 2000). Comorbidity may vary by age. For example, in a sample of preschoolers in New Orleans who developed PTSD following Hurricane Katrina, nearly 90% of them had a comorbid diagnosis, most frequently oppositional defiant disorder or separation anxiety disorder (Scheeringa & Zeanah, 2008). In adolescents, PTSD commonly co-occurs with substance use disorders, which appear to begin with or after the onset of trauma symptoms (Evans et al., 2007; Giaconia et al., 2000; Lipschitz et al., 2003). In some settings and cultures, PTSD may be accompanied by somatic symptoms such as stomachaches, headaches, shortness of breath, and dizziness (Zhang, Zhang, Zhu, Du, & Zhang, 2015; Zhang, Zhu, Du, & Zhang, 2015).

RISK/CAUSAL FACTORS

Though many youth are exposed to traumatic or potentially traumatic events, only a small number develop clinical levels of trauma symptoms (Adams et al., 2014; Copeland et al., 2007; Nordanger et al., 2013). Therefore, while trauma exposure is a risk factor for PTSD that is inherent in the definition of the disorder, other individual and environmental factors affect a child's vulnerability to experiencing clinically significant problems following a traumatic event.

Biological factors.

Genetic factors. Heritability studies in adults suggest that 30-40% of the variability in PTSD symptoms following trauma exposure is due to genetics (Stein et al., 2002; True et al., 1993). One specific genetic finding involves a gene region known as FKBP5, which is involved in the regulation of the glucocorticoid receptor (GR), to which cortisol binds in the body. Among adults who experienced childhood abuse, the allele (version) of FKBP5 present in their genome predicted the severity of their trauma symptoms in adulthood (Binder et al., 2008). This finding suggests that certain individuals have a genetic vulnerability to a more severe reaction to trauma. The serotonin transporter gene region HTTLPR-5, which has been implicated in risk for multiple disorders, also interacts with trauma exposure in the prediction of PTSD symptoms (Gressier et al., 2013; Xie et al., 2009). Of individuals who experienced trauma as children, those with a certain genotype within this region are more likely to develop PTSD at some point in their lives.

Stress reactivity. The human body and brain are equipped with the ability to respond fairly effectively to environmental stressors. The body's stress response system involves several brain regions (including the hippocampus, the prefrontal cortex, and the amygdala) as well as multiple nervous and endocrine circuits (including the hypothalamic-pituitary-adrenocortical [HPA] axis, the sympathetic nervous system, and the parasympathetic nervous system; Bremner, 2006; Del Giudice et al., 2011). The systems work optimally when stressors are manageable and/or temporary as they adjust to address the stressor and return to a resting state when the stressor abates (Hulme, 2011). However, when stressors are intense, frequent, or chronic, or when the individual's stress management abilities are limited (such as in young children), they may overwhelm the body's ability to respond in healthy ways and to return quickly or fully to a normal level of functioning. Indeed, exposure to trauma in childhood alters the functioning of the stress response systems in the body, notably the HPA axis (Gillespie et al., 2009; Heim et al., 2008). This overwhelming of the body's stress management systems is thought to underlie the symptoms of trauma disorders (De Bellis, 2001).

Much of the neurobiological research on PTSD has focused on dysregulation within the HPA axis. Under normal conditions, when humans are stressed, the HPA axis stimulates the temporary release of glucocorticoids, such as cortisol, which help the body respond to the threat and recover once it is over (McEwen, 2002). However, severe or prolonged stress can cause abnormalities in cortisol. Generally, findings about cortisol levels in youth who have experienced trauma are inconsistent, sometimes indicating that trauma leads to higher cortisol levels and sometimes associating it with lower levels

(De Bellis, 2001). These inconsistencies may be due to variability in cortisol levels—and their reaction to trauma—across development and throughout the day (De Bellis, 2001; Gunnar & Vazquez, 2001). They may also suggest that trauma does not affect overall cortisol levels per se but rather changes stress reactivity, as reflected by cortisol secretion. This idea is supported by research that has found that traumatized youth may have cortisol levels that change more drastically throughout the day than their peers (Weems & Carrión, 2008). One more consistent finding is that PTSD is associated with lower than normal levels of cortisol in the morning in traumatized youth (Goenjian et al., 2003; Keeshin et al., 2013; Pfefferbaum et al., 2015). Both heightened cortisol—reflecting increased reactivity to stress—and abnormally low levels of cortisol—reflecting a dampening in the body's ability to adapt to stressors— may be problematic. It is important to note that HPA axis dysregulation resulting from childhood trauma has been found to persist into adulthood (Gunnar & Vazquez, 2001; Hulme, 2011), underscoring the importance of early and effective treatment.

It is clear that though PTSD, by definition, has an environmental trigger (trauma), underlying genetic and/or biological vulnerabilities interact with environmental and psychological variables and are important for understanding an individual's response to a traumatic event. Even psychologically focused treatments affect biological stress reactivity. For example, amygdalar responses are linked to degree of improvement in trauma-focused cognitive-behavioral therapy (TF-CBT), with adolescents who show less improvement displaying amygdala activation to threatening and nonthreatening stimuli, whereas adolescents whose symptoms improve more show amygdala activation only in response to threatening stimuli (Cisler et al., 2015).

Neurological abnormalities. Certain patterns of brain structure and functional abnormalities are associated with PTSD. Some studies suggest that certain neuroanatomical patterns, particularly those in brain regions involved in the body's stress response, may increase vulnerability to trauma disorders. Among maltreated youth, those with PTSD have smaller left amygdalae, right hippocampi, and ventral medial prefrontal cortices (vmPFC) than those without the disorder (Morey et al., 2016). One possible explanation is that these patterns may enhance fear reactivity. Alternatively, stress exposure may also alter the developing brain. For example, older adolescents with PTSD have larger right amygdalae than their nontraumatized peers, but this difference does not exist earlier in development (Weems et al., 2015). Early trauma is also associated with a decrease in white matter in certain parts of the corpus callosum, which connects the left and right hemispheres of the brain; this reduction in volume is hypothesized to reflect an overstimulation of the developmentally normative pruning process by severe stress, possibly via high levels of stress hormones (Daniels et al., 2013; Rinne-Albers et al., 2013). Finally, youth with PTSD display patterns of brain activity that indicate increased reactivity to negative stimuli (e.g., distressing images, angry or frightened facial expressions), particularly in the amygdala (Keding & Herringa, 2015; McLaughlin et al., 2014; van den Bulk et al., 2016). Such findings suggest that trauma may sensitize the brain to potentially threatening stimuli, leading to symptoms such as strong anger and anxiety, hypervigilance, an exaggerated startle response, avoidance, and cognitive distortions.

Psychological factors.

Emotion regulation. Children with PTSD have more trouble regulating their emotions than children without a trauma disorder (Bender, Pons et al., 2015; Bennett et al., 2015; Espil et al., 2016; Feldman et al., 2013; Khamis, 2015; Powers et al., 2020). There appears to be a dynamic interaction between trauma exposure and the ability to regulate one's emotional experiences. On the one hand, some studies suggest that children who have more trouble regulating their affect are at higher risk for PTSD and other negative outcomes following trauma (Chaplo et al., 2015; Mohammad et al., 2015; Sundermann & DePrince, 2015). When these youth experience a trauma that creates strong negative emotions, they may not be well equipped to cope with those feelings in adaptive ways, which may in turn result in trauma symptoms. For example, youth who experience overwhelming anxiety around stimuli and situations that remind them of the trauma and who are not able to manage that anxiety will likely avoid those reminders; they may also experience hypervigilance and difficulty sleeping. In contrast, better emotion regulation skills help protect youth against the development of posttraumatic stress symptoms following trauma exposure (Levey et al., 2016; Punamäki et al., 2015).

On the other hand, trauma exposure itself appears to affect emotion regulation skills (Kim & Cicchetti, 2010; Maughan & Cicchetti, 2002; Shields & Cicchetti, 1998). From a developmental psychopathology perspective, we must consider a child's context in order to understand the development of a particular behavior or symptom and how it represents an adaptation to the environment. When youth are traumatized, they shift from processing information in a learning orientation to engaging with their environments with a survival orientation (Ford, 2009; Greene et al., 2014). In survival mode, the goals of emotion regulation are threat perception and self-protection rather than healthy engagement with the environment. These goals are extremely useful and may, in fact, be lifesaving; the maltreated young child who learns to suppress her own fear and anger expressions may be less likely to attract the attention of an abuser in a given moment. However, when these strategies are used in nonthreatening situations, such as at school or in peer interactions, they are maladaptive, interfering with development, learning, and/or relationships. Constant suppression of emotions may lead to an inability to engage fully with the environment or to accurately read and understand others' emotional expressions. Indeed, poor emotion regulation appears to be one mechanism by which trauma exposure leads to PTSD symptomatology (Alink et al., 2009; Bennett et al., 2016). Furthermore, improvements in emotion regulation abilities over the course of cognitive-behavioral treatment for PTSD predict decreases in symptoms both at the end of treatment and at a six-month follow-up (Sharma-Patel & Brown, 2016; Thornback & Muller, 2015). Therefore, consideration of emotion regulation may both help identify the youth who are at heightened risk for a trauma disorder following stressor exposure and be an important consideration in treating a child's full constellation of symptoms and impairments.

Cognitive patterns. Youth who experience a trauma may have a variety of cognitive responses and develop more or less adaptive and accurate ways of thinking about themselves, their experiences, and the world. Youth who consistently exhibit negative patterns of thinking are at higher risk for the development of a trauma disorder. For example, among adolescents who survived a major earthquake, the degree to which their core beliefs about themselves, others, and the world were challenged by the trauma predicted PTSD symptoms (Zhou et al., 2015). Negative thoughts about the world (e.g., "The world is a dangerous place") and about oneself (e.g., "I am a coward") are associated with worse PTSD symptoms in traumatized youth (Kaur & Kearney, 2015; Liu & Chen, 2015; Nixon et al., 2010; Palosaari, Punamäki, Peltonen, Diab, & Qouta, 2016; Ross & Kearney, 2015). Youth also have more severe PTSD symptoms when they display higher levels of negative appraisals (e.g., "Bad things always happen," "I will never be able to have normal feelings again") and lower levels of positive appraisals (e.g., "Getting over the event will make/has made me better at coping") about the traumatic event (Hitchcock et al., 2015; Meiser-Stedman et al., 2009).

Specific types of cognitive distortions have also been linked to risk for a trauma disorder. One such pattern is self-blame (e.g., "The event happened because of the sort of person that I am," "Somebody else would not have gotten into this situation"; Foa et al., 1999). Following a variety of types of trauma, youth who endorse higher levels of self-blaming or guilt-ridden thinking are more likely to develop PTSD (Klasen et al., 2015; Moscardino, Scrimin, Capello, & Altoè, 2014; Ross & Kearney, 2015).

Some traumatized youth exhibit the cognitive pattern of overgeneralization, applying negative beliefs stemming from their traumatic experiences to a wide variety of other situations (e.g., coming to believe that "everyone is out to hurt me" after being assaulted by a single individual). These youth have higher levels of internalizing and externalizing symptoms, even following treatment for a trauma disorder (Ready et al., 2015). Another type of cognitive distortion is emotional reasoning, or basing conclusions about a situation on one's emotions (e.g., "I feel afraid; therefore, this situation must be dangerous"). Traumatized youth who exhibit higher levels of emotional reasoning have more severe PTSD symptoms shortly after trauma exposure (but not a few months later; Verduijn et al., 2015). Finally, some youth may show patterns of religious or spiritual cognitions that make them more susceptible to trauma symptoms. For example, Muslim youth in Indonesia who agreed more strongly with the belief that honoring their God (Allah) will prevent bad things from happening in the future actually had more severe trauma symptoms following a tsunami (Dawson et al., 2014). This finding has some interesting possible explanations. Youth who endorse this belief may also believe (perhaps implicitly) that it was their own lack of faith or honoring behavior that caused the past trauma. Alternatively, youth who have more severe symptoms may find hope and a sense of control in the belief that their religious faith/action can help prevent future disasters.

While it is clear that there is a correlation between certain negative cognitive patterns and PTSD, one might wonder about the direction of causation. In other words, do distorted cognitions following a trauma lead to more severe trauma symptoms, or does PTSD lead to erroneous ways of thinking? Studies of therapeutic change suggest that it is the former. During the course of treatment for trauma, reductions in cognitive distortions predict reductions in trauma symptoms but not the other way around (Kleim et al., 2013; McLean et al., 2015; Smith et al., 2007). This finding highlights the role of cognitive patterns as a true risk factor for psychopathology following trauma exposure as well as their potential importance as a target of intervention.

Finally, as with all intertwined risk and protective factors, thought patterns do not occur in isolation but rather interact with other child characteristics, such as social support. One study of war-affected children found that negative posttraumatic cognitions mediate the effect of peer difficulties on trauma symptoms, such that being unpopular with one's peers leads to more cognitive distortions following trauma exposure, which in turn predicts higher levels of PTSD symptoms (Palosaari et al., 2016). In contrast, youth who have higher levels of social support following a trauma exhibit fewer negative cognitions and more adaptive or healthy cognitions, which in turn predict lower levels of trauma symptoms (Hitchcock et al., 2015). However, to illustrate the complexity of the relationship among these factors, some apparent social support can actually enhance symptoms. For example, peer-victimized adolescents are at a higher risk for PTSD when they co-ruminate, interacting with friends in a manner that focuses extensively on negative information and events (Guarneri-White et al., 2015).

Environmental factors.

Trauma type and exposure intensity. The experience of trauma varies widely among youth,

and the types of traumas and intensity of exposure impacts risk for PTSD. The types of traumas that youth with PTSD most commonly report are exposure to violence (in person or through the media, within and outside of their families) and separation/loss within their families, though youth report a wide variety of traumatic experiences (Taylor & Weems, 2009). Traumas that are interpersonal in origin carry a particularly high risk for PTSD (Deeba & Rapee, 2015; McLaughlin et al., 2013); 30-50% of individuals who are the victims of violence (e.g., physical abuse, sexual assault) or witness interpersonal violence (e.g., domestic violence, military conflict) develop the disorder at some point in their lives (De Bellis, 2001). Trauma that occurs from the purposeful actions of other people may be especially disruptive to a child's sense of well-being and security and her view of others and the world as safe. Furthermore, interpersonal traumas such as maltreatment may be likely to be associated with other risk factors for PTSD, such as lack of social support, parental psychopathology, and additional traumatic experiences (De Bellis, 2001). In addition, exposure to multiple traumatic experiences increases the risk for a trauma disorder, whether the traumas are unique or repetitions of the same type of event (Adams et al., 2014; de Albuquerque & de Albuquerque Williams, 2015; Enlow et al., 2013; Hicks et al., 2020; McLaughlin et al., 2013). It is thought that early stressor exposure actually "sensitizes" a developing child to the negative effects of subsequent traumas, increasing the risk of a trauma disorder following exposure to multiple traumas (Shao et al., 2015; Smid et al., 2012).

Regardless of trauma type, youth who have higher levels of proximity or exposure to a trauma are more likely to develop PTSD symptoms (Trickey et al., 2012), a phenomenon known as the "dose effect" (Furr et al., 2010; Ying et al., 2014). More intensive exposure to specific threat-related aspects of a traumatic experience is associated with a heightened risk for a trauma disorder; such exposure can include experiences such as being in a boating accident as a poor swimmer, seeing blood at the site of a trauma, staying in the path of a hurricane rather than evacuating, being at the site of a terrorist attack, or being trapped or seeing someone else injured during an earthquake (Marthoenis et al., 2019; Nordanger et al., 2013; Scheeringa & Zeanah, 2008; Udwin et al., 2000; Ying et al., 2014). In addition, experiencing physical injury or witnessing death is linked to PTSD risk, as is losing a loved one in a traumatic incident (Nordanger et al., 2013; Udwin et al., 2000; Wei et al., 2013; Wolmer et al., 2015). Finally, a higher level of exposure to the details of the event following its occurrence—such as through information discussed by family members or media exposure—also represents heightened risk for trauma symptoms (Busso et al., 2014; Wolmer et al., 2015; Yeung et al., 2018). Being exposed to these types of situations and experiences during a trauma may increase the sense of personal threat that results from the trauma and underlies PTSD symptoms. It is important for clinicians to assess not only trauma type but also a child's exposure level and subjective experience.

It is important to note that intensity of exposure may interact with other risk factors. For example, individuals who are able to evacuate ahead of a hurricane may be of higher socioeconomic status (SES) than those who do not have the means to travel, and SES itself may impact risk for PTSD (Trickey et al., 2012). Indeed, trauma exposure explains the link between low SES and heightened risk for PTSD (Enlow et al., 2013). In addition, exposure does not occur in isolation from internal variables; for example, media exposure interacts with physiological reactivity in the prediction of trauma symptoms, such that adolescents with lower levels of reactivity only have a heightened risk of PTSD when they are exposed to large amounts of media coverage of a terrorist attack (Busso et al., 2014).

Social support. Family and friends are an important source of help, comfort, and support for all youth but perhaps especially those who have experienced a trauma. Indeed, there are significant links between supportive relationships and reduced risk for PTSD in trauma-exposed youth (Trickey et al., 2012; Udwin et al., 2000; Xu & Yuan, 2014). Social support can come from a variety of sources. Youth who feel more connected to and supported by their peers, classmates, and teachers are less likely to develop PTSD following a trauma (Banks & Weems, 2014; La Greca, Silverman, Lai, & Jaccard, 2010; Leshem, Haj-Yahia, & Guterman, 2016; Morley & Kohrt, 2013; Moscardino et al., 2014; Vernberg, La Greca, Silverman, & Prinstein, 1996). Support from one's family also appears to be important in reducing PTSD risk following traumas such as natural disasters or violence exposure (Banks & Weems, 2014; Guerra et al., 2018; Ozer & Weinstein, 2004; Xu & Yuan, 2014). Some specific aspects of family support, such as social engagement and open emotional communication, have been found to predict lower levels of trauma symptoms (Halevi et al., 2016; Leshem et al., 2016; Otto et al., 2007; Vernberg et al., 1996). Other aspects of family functioning and relationships which may affect social support have been linked with a heightened risk for trauma disorders even from very early in development. Youth who were insecurely attached to their mothers as infants are at higher risk for developing PTSD following risk exposure later in development (Enlow et al., 2014). These youth may lack the sense of a secure base and ability to use their parents as a source of comfort that securely attached youth possess, making them both more reactive to trauma and less able to solicit appropriate support from others. Parents who struggle with their own psychological disorders, including depression and PTSD, appear to be less able to support their trauma-exposed children, who are at a higher risk for PTSD (Kiliç et al., 2003; Landolt et al., 2005; Levendosky et al., 2013; Meiser-Stedman et al., 2006; Smith, Perrin, et al., 2001). Furthermore, the relation between parental psychopathology and child PTSD symptoms appears to be reciprocal (Neill et al., 2018).

The influence of social support must be understood in its complexity and relationship with other variables. For example, trauma exposure and relational dynamics are not independent. Youth from families with poorer functioning have a higher risk of exposure to certain traumas, such as community violence (Gorman-Smith et al., 2004), representing the phenomenon that risk factors often aggregate for particular individuals. In addition, the links between social support and trauma may actually be reciprocal, as higher levels of trauma symptoms have been found to predict difficulties in relationships (Butcher et al., 2015), and youth who experience more cascading negative life events resulting from a trauma (e.g., losing one's home following a

hurricane) experience lower levels of social support over time (La Greca et al., 2010). Therefore, increasing children's resilience is not merely a matter of increasing the availability of support but may also entail working with youth to be able to engage with others in socially skilled ways that allow them to access that support. Similarly, the relation between family functioning and children's symptoms may be bidirectional; that is, poor family functioning may increase trauma-exposed youths' symptomatology, but having a child with significant trauma symptoms may also interfere with healthy family dynamics. Indeed, children's trauma symptoms predict the level of stress parents report around interactions with their children (Salloum et al., 2015). Furthermore, some studies have not found parenting variables to predict children's symptom severity following a trauma (Kiliç et al., 2003; Scheeringa et al., 2015), suggesting perhaps that it is not merely family functioning on its own but rather how family dynamics interact with other variables (e.g., other sources of support, parental mental health, the child's personality) that shapes a child's response to a trauma.

Interactive risk factors. Trauma, especially early trauma, has such a significant impact on children's development and functioning that there is a subfield within psychiatry dedicated to exploring its effects. Developmental traumatology (De Bellis, 2001) understands early trauma as having the potential to overwhelm a child's ability to manage stressors, a capacity that is affected by the interaction of genetic, biological, and environmental factors. For example, consider two young children who survive a serious school bus accident. One child, a girl, is severely injured in the crash, and the friend she was sitting next to on the bus is killed. She is a child who is already more biologically prone to be sensitive to stress, and the accident enhances her body's stress reactivity and HPA axis dysregulation. She becomes irritable and anxious and is unable to manage the anxiety she feels when she thinks about the event. She also has trouble sleeping at night due to her heightened physiological arousal and recurrent nightmares about the accident. She withdraws socially and does not appear to enjoy interacting with her peers or her family members. She also refuses to get in any motor vehicles. Her mother, who was also on the bus as a chaperone, is experiencing her own trauma symptoms, including flashbacks and constant worry that one of her children will die suddenly. The girl's mother is unable to discuss the events with her daughter without getting overwhelmingly anxious and panicked, leaving her unable to help her daughter manage her strong negative emotions and facilitating her avoidance of reminders of the event. The little girl throws a tantrum every morning before school, and her emotionally and physically exhausted mother eventually allows her to stay home every day rather than fighting with her hysterical child. The little girl loses the contact she had with supportive peers and teachers at school, and her trauma symptoms continue to worsen.

In contrast, a second child, a boy, is also on the bus but is not injured and does not witness any serious injuries or fatalities. He is a child who is normally calm, emotionally well regulated, and not highly reactive to stress. His parents, who were not at the scene of the accident and do not have depressive or trauma symptoms, are able to be sensitive to his needs and emotions following the accident. The boy expresses some fearfulness about riding the bus again, but his parents are able to convince him that he will be safe getting on the bus again, and after a few days of riding it to and from school without incident, his anxiety disappears. The little boy is able to talk openly with his parents when he feels anxious or thinks about the accident, and they are supportive, validating his concerns but not allowing him to avoid reminders of the trauma. His play with toy vehicles often involves accidents, but he does not get emotionally overwhelmed during these times, and after several weeks, the accident themes in his play decrease. He never develops significant trauma symptoms, and his long-term functioning is not impacted by the accident. These two children, surviving the same traumatic experience, have very divergent outcomes due to the interaction of different biological, emotional, behavioral, interpersonal, and situational characteristics.

DEVELOPMENTAL COURSE

As with all disorders, trauma symptoms may present differently depending on the age of the child. Indeed, the DSM-5 contains a different set of diagnostic criteria for children six years old and younger. These criteria emphasize concrete symptoms, de-emphasize abstract ones (e.g., "a foreshortened sense of the future"), and include indirect symptom expression, such as through play. Children under age six are less likely than older individuals to experience emotional numbing and detachment in particular (Galano et al., 2014; Scheeringa et al., 2006), though these symptoms increase over time (Scheeringa et al., 2005). Like older traumatized individuals, these youth do re-experience details of the trauma, but in contrast to emotional numbing and detachment, re-experiencing decreases over time in young children (Scheeringa et al., 2005). Young traumatized children also often exhibit aggressive behavior, developmental regressions (e.g., toilet training setbacks), and separation or other anxiety (Scheeringa et al., 2001). In general, trauma symptoms seem to be harder to measure consistently and precisely in younger children, perhaps because of the variation in how they may be expressed (Contractor et al., 2013). However, a PTSD diagnosis in young children has been found to be more valid when developmentally sensitive criteria are used (De Young et al., 2011), whereas young children do not generally qualify for a diagnosis of PTSD when the traditional criteria are used, even when their symptoms are severe (Scheeringa et al., 2003). Despite diagnostic challenges, PTSD symptoms can be significant in early childhood. For example, young children with PTSD continue to have difficulties in functioning, such as problems with relationships and in school, one to two years after their diagnosis, even when they no longer meet the criteria for the disorder (Scheeringa et al., 2005).

Traditional PTSD symptoms increase with age, and school-aged children and adolescents experience many of the same trauma symptoms as adults (Brown, et al., 2014; Dogan-Ates, 2010). For example, by age seven, more traumatized children endorse avoidance/numbing symptoms than they did at younger ages, most likely due to cognitive and/or neural development in middle childhood (Scheeringa et al., 2006). Older children and adolescents also frequently report somatic symptoms (such as headaches, stomachaches, and difficulty sleeping) following a trauma

(Dogan-Ates, 2010). Trauma exposure in childhood and adolescence may result in lasting social impairments, including poor social skills and fewer romantic relationships (Bolton et al., 2004; McLean et al., 2013).

The developmental timing of exposure to a trauma influences the specific symptoms youth are likely to experience. In one study of girls, trauma exposure in childhood was more likely to result in depression, whereas exposure around the onset of puberty was more likely to lead to an anxiety disorder (Marshall, 2016). Changes in the developing brain are thought to underlie these different vulnerabilities across time. However, one meta-analysis found that age of exposure does not affect the likelihood of developing PTSD (Trickey et al., 2012). In addition, the course of children's responses to trauma varies dramatically over time. Some youth may display symptoms immediately following trauma exposure, whereas others may not experience symptoms until several months later, known as PTSD with delayed expression (American Psychiatric Association, 2013; Yule et al., 2000). For children who experience a single, discrete traumatic event, the duration of symptoms also varies significantly, with a large proportion of individuals recovering within one to two years following the trauma (Laor et al., 2001; Usami et al., 2014; Wang et al., 2013; Winje & Ulvik, 1998; Yule et al., 2000). Generally, as time elapses and a trauma is further in the past, the risk of PTSD decreases (Marshall, 2016). However, a significant minority of youth may continue to have symptoms for several years after trauma exposure, and some may even experience increasing symptom levels (Neugebauer et al., 2014; Osofsky et al., 2015; Wang et al., 2013). These wide individual differences in trajectories likely suggest that it is not merely trauma exposure but the interaction of exposure to a particular trauma with an individual's unique characteristics and circumstances that determines whether a trauma-related disorder develops.

In the trauma literature, special attention is paid to complex trauma, a multifaceted constellation of symptoms and impairment that occurs when children are exposed to multiple or chronic traumas early in life, particularly traumas that occur within relationships, such as being abused or witnessing domestic violence (Cook et al., 2003). Epidemiological research suggests that young children are particularly vulnerable to traumas involving interpersonal violence, namely maltreatment and domestic violence (Fantuzzo & Fusco, 2007; US Department of Health and Human Services, 2013). Furthermore, youth who experience one interpersonal trauma frequently experience multiple traumas, including instances in which one trauma actually leads to another (e.g., a child who is physically abused inadvertently chooses abusive dating partners as an adolescent) or different types of trauma co-occur (e.g., a youth is both emotionally abused and neglected; Grasso et al., 2013). Children who experience complex trauma have been found to have difficulties in seven domains: attachment (e.g., interpersonal boundaries, relationship formation), biology (e.g., sensorimotor problems, somatic symptoms, medical problems), emotion regulation (e.g., trouble labeling, expressing, and regulating emotions), dissociation (e.g., amnesia, dissociative experiences), behavioral control (e.g., aggression, impulsivity, substance use), cognition (e.g., problems with planning and attention, learning difficulties),

and self-concept (e.g., poorly developed sense of self, low self-esteem; Cook et al., 2005). Ongoing trauma that occurs at the hands of the very individuals (e.g., caregivers) whom children rely on to provide safety and security may be particularly disruptive to the development of a healthy sense of self, positive interactions, and appropriate behavior, as children do not have the secure relationships that allow for developmentally appropriate exploration and growth. Indeed, youth who experience complex trauma may meet the diagnostic criteria for PTSD as well as a number of other disorders, but their symptoms are more varied and severe than what is seen in individuals exposed to traumas that are not chronic or begin later in life (Cloitre et al., 2009; Cook et al., 2005; Wamser-Nanney & Vandenberg, 2013). It has been argued that this multifaceted set of difficulties that results from multiple traumas but is broader than a PTSD diagnosis should be categorized as a new diagnosis, known as developmental trauma disorder (D'Andrea et al., 2012; van der Kolk, 2005).

ASSESSMENT

Since many youth experience traumatic events, and the symptoms of PTSD can be significantly distressing and impairing, it has been recommended that all youth who present for psychiatric or psychological treatment should be screened for trauma symptoms (Cohen et al., 2010). Unfortunately, this is not necessarily common practice; it is suspected that many cases of PTSD in youth may be missed during the standard assessment that occurs in emergency rooms and inpatient units (Havens et al., 2012). Trauma symptoms screening may be appropriate in other settings as well. For example, it has been recommended that large-scale screening for PTSD be conducted in communities that have experienced a potentially traumatic event; ideally, this screening would occur one month after the trauma so as to best identify youth whose symptoms are longer lasting (Cohen et al., 2010). Youth whose screenings suggest that they have symptoms of a trauma disorder should then undergo a fuller assessment of symptom presence, severity, and effect on functioning.

Fletcher (2007) recommends beginning with a full history, including exposure to major and minor stressors, previous treatments, and any previous presenting problems. The clinician should also ask about parental exposure to trauma and family history of trauma disorders. Once it is apparent that the child has been exposed to one or more traumas, the clinician should seek to understand the details of the trauma and the child's experiences (Fletcher, 2007). Given the role of trauma type and exposure intensity in predicting the severity of symptoms, these factors must be included when assessing traumatized youth (Balaban, 2009). Aspects of the trauma that may be useful to assess include the type of event, the intensity and duration, whether the trauma was discrete or chronic, whether the event resulted in the death of a loved one (potentially leading to grief as well as trauma), and the child's actions or lack thereof during the event (and associated feelings of guilt; Nader, 2008). This information may come from youth themselves, parents, and other sources that may have covered an event, including news reports and emergency personnel. In addition, a number of standardized tools exist for assessing exposure to common stressors/traumas and their perceived impact

or significance (see Fletcher, 2007, and Nader, 2008, for overviews of these instruments).

Of course, children's responses to trauma exposure are extremely varied, and knowledge about the trauma itself is important but does not provide individualized information about symptoms. Several instruments have been designed to formally assess trauma symptoms in youth, including both structured interviews and questionnaires. For young children, the PTSD Semi-Structured Interview and Observation Record for Infants and Young Children (Scheeringa et al., 2003) is a developmentally sensitive interview designed to be used with parents of young children who have experienced a trauma. For youth ages seven and older, the Clinician-Administered PTSD Scale for DSM-5—Child/Adolescent Version (CAPS-CA-5; Pynoos et al., 2015), a modified version of the original adult instrument, is a structured interview administered to youth themselves. Questionnaires assessing PTSD symptoms in youth also exist. The UCLA PTSD Reaction Index for DSM-5 (PTSD-RI; Kaplow et al., 2020; Steinberg et al., 2013), which includes versions for younger (age six and below) and older (age seven and above) children, assesses trauma history as well as symptom severity and effect. The Trauma Symptom Checklist for Young Children (TSCYC; Briere et al., 2001) can be used to assess the symptoms of children ages three to twelve via parent report. Self-report questionnaires, including the Child PTSD Symptom Scale for DSM-5 (CPSS-5; Foa et al., 2018) and the Acute Stress Checklist for Children (ASC-Kids; Kassam-Adams, 2006), can be used with older children (generally eight years and above) and adolescents. When choosing assessment instruments, clinicians should pay attention to whether tools were developed using DSM-IV or DSM-5 diagnostic criteria and symptom presentations, especially with young children, for whom the newer criteria are notably different. It is also important to interview both children themselves and their parents about trauma symptoms, as disagreement between reporters is common (Oransky et al., 2013), and relying on the report of only one or the other may result in underdiagnosis (Levendosky et al., 2013; Scheeringa et al., 2001, 2006).

In addition, a thorough assessment should include questions about symptoms of other disorders, as a significant number of youth with a trauma disorder meet the criteria for a comorbid diagnosis (Balaban, 2009), which can both confound the diagnostic process and complicate treatment. Therefore, in order to increase the likelihood that a child's diagnosis is accurate, clinicians might consider using a semi-structured interview or questionnaire that assesses a broad range of symptoms, such as the Kiddie Schedule for Affective Disorders and Schizophrenia for School Aged Children (K-SADS-PL DSM-5; Kaufman et al., 2016) or the Child Behavior Checklist (CBCL; Achenbach, 1991a, 1991b). Given the nature of complex trauma, clinicians might consider assessing a wider variety of domains of functioning (e.g., attachment, emotion regulation) in children who have experienced traumas that occurred early in development, are chronic, and/or are interpersonal in nature (Brown et al., 2014; Cook et al., 2003). Finally, clinicians should take care to assess thoroughly enough to differentiate true ASD or PTSD from symptoms of other disorders (Cohen et al., 2010). For example, trauma symptoms such as restlessness, hyperarousal,

and agitation can be mistaken for attention-deficit/hyperactivity disorder (ADHD). Oppositionality and aggression in young traumatized children might be misdiagnosed as a disruptive behavior disorder. Especially when they are extreme, certain symptoms of PTSD can be mistaken as representing an anxiety disorder, depression, bipolar disorder, or even psychosis. Therefore, as with all disorders, assessment should be thorough and developmentally appropriate and elicit information from multiple sources about a variety of areas of development and functioning.

TREATMENT

Cognitive-behavioral therapy (CBT) has received the most empirical support as an effective treatment for PTSD in youth (Cohen et al., 2010; Leenarts et al., 2013; Morina, Koerssen, & Pollet, 2016; Silverman et al., 2008). Both trauma-focused CBT (TF-CBT), administered in individual format, and school-based group CBT have been found to be effective in reducing trauma symptoms; TF-CBT is considered a well-established treatment, and school-based CBT is categorized as probably efficacious. Several other interventions, including resilient peer treatment, child-parent psychotherapy, and eye movement desensitization and reprocessing (EMDR) have limited research support (Leenarts et al., 2013; Racco & Vis, 2015; Silverman et al., 2008). One set of practice guidelines characterizes effective treatments for childhood trauma as containing three common elements: (1) direct trauma work, (2) parent involvement, and (3) an emphasis on improving functioning or enhancing development rather than solely reducing symptoms (Cohen et al., 2010). In general, any psychological treatment is better than no treatment in reducing PTSD symptoms (Morina et al., 2016), though the effect of treatment is often smaller for younger children and clients with more severe symptomatology (Miller-Graff & Campion, 2016). Finally, psychotropic medications such as selective serotonin uptake inhibitors (SSRIs), mood stabilizers, and stimulants may be helpful additions to therapy in the case of severe or comorbid problems, but they do not appear to be an effective treatment for trauma disorders on their own (Birmaher & Sakolsky, 2013; Donnelly, 2009; Keeshin & Strawn, 2014). TF-CBT and one example of a school-based cognitive-behavioral intervention are discussed in detail below.

Trauma-focused cognitive-behavioral therapy (TF-CBT). TF-CBT (Cohen, Mannarino, & Deblinger, 2006, 2017) aims to address the myriad symptoms that youth ages three to eighteen with PTSD often experience. Traumatized youth experience symptoms in several domains, including cognitive (e.g., maladaptive thought patterns), relationship (e.g., poor social skills, difficulty trusting others), affective (e.g., extreme negative emotions and problems regulating them), family (e.g., poor family relationships or communication), behavioral (e.g., avoidance, aggression), and somatic problems (e.g., trouble sleeping, headaches or stomachaches, hyperarousal). The intervention is also appropriate for children who are experiencing childhood traumatic grief (CTG) following exposure to traumatic elements of the loss of a loved one. TF-CBT is not designed to specifically address externalizing behavior problems, as these symptoms are not considered a core feature of PTSD (Cohen et al., 2017); it is recommended that comorbid disruptive behavior problems are treated using interventions designed to address these behaviors explicitly (see chapter six).

TF-CBT includes not only traditional cognitive-behavioral elements of treatment but also elements informed by biological, psychodynamic, humanistic, and family systems theories of disorder and treatment; as different areas of functioning are assumed to influence one another, it is assumed that addressing symptoms from a variety of different angles will be most effective. There are five main goals/themes emphasized throughout TF-CBT. These goals are (1) improving stress management skills in order to alleviate trauma symptoms, (2) using exposure to decrease avoidance, (3) processing the emotional and cognitive components of the child's response to trauma, (4) improving current and future safety, and (5) including parents in treatment as much as possible. Through treatment, there is an emphasis on promoting healthy relationships, including the therapeutic alliance and relationships between the client and her family members. Supporting this goal, TF-CBT aims not only to alleviate the client's symptoms but also to help parents address their own difficulties following a child's trauma so that they may better support their child as she recovers (Cohen et al., 2017). To that end, the treatment includes both joint parent-child sessions and parallel individual sessions (meetings with children and parents separately). It is typically completed over the course of eight to twenty sessions, but more time may be necessary to cover all of the components of the intervention thoroughly and to address co-occurring problems. In addition, though the treatment is manual based, it is designed to be adaptable and flexible, such that therapists can apply the intervention components in ways that best suit the needs of unique and diverse clients.

The acronym PRACTICE is used to represent the nine components of TF-CBT (the P represents two components; Cohen et al., 2017; Kliethermes et al., 2013). The first five components are skill based, while the last four are more trauma specific. Psychoeducation, which occurs throughout treatment, is included to help families understand the nature of trauma and typical reactions to traumatic events (i.e., symptoms and functional difficulties) in order to normalize their experiences and reduce the sense of being alone. Clinicians may use handouts with facts about trauma, examples from their own clinical experience, and children's books to provide information to families. Exposure and non-avoidance are promoted even during this first stage of therapy through direct and accurate naming of children's traumatic experiences and symptoms rather than using euphemisms to discuss them. Information about TF-CBT itself, as well as concrete strategies for managing current symptoms (such as sleep problems), are also provided early in treatment. Next, Parenting skills are taught to help parents manage their own reactions to trauma and respond appropriately to their children's symptoms. This component aims to promote the use of positive parenting skills to help decrease the problematic behaviors (e.g., aggression, oppositionality) that may accompany trauma symptoms in children, bolster a healthy parent-child relationship, and minimize the negative effects of the parents' experiences of trauma (which sometimes occur vicariously through their children) on youth. Parents learn skills such

as using effective praise and behavior charts to reinforce desired behaviors and using selective attending (ignoring) and time-out to remove potential reinforcers for problem behaviors. Relaxation skills, such as deep/mindful breathing and progressive muscle relaxation, are taught to help children and parents decrease their own trauma- and anxiety-related physiological arousal. Enjoyable activities (e.g., listening to music, playing sports, drawing, praying) that can be relaxing are identified as well. Different scenarios and settings in which youth may encounter trauma reminders are discussed, and therapists work with families to identify a variety of relaxation techniques that can be used when a child begins to experience distress or other symptoms in these settings. Through this work, avoidance is addressed during this component of treatment.

During the Affective modulation component, the focus of treatment is on helping children identify and appropriately express the feelings that they may have learned to suppress following a traumatic experience. Youth are encouraged to expand their emotional vocabulary and make links between feeling words and their own physiological experiences, cognitions, and triggers. Youth learn a variety of emotion regulation techniques—such as negotiating, seeking social support, thought interruption/stopping, positive self-talk, and problem solving—through creative activities such as drawing and playing games. Once youth have gained emotion recognition and regulation skills, they work with therapists to apply them in real-life situations (e.g., recognizing their emotional reactions, recognizing when they need to be regulated, selecting an appropriate strategy, using the strategy effectively). In parallel work, the therapist works to provide parents with a supportive environment in which to express their own emotions around the trauma. Parents also learn to listen reflectively, validate their children's emotions, and praise them for expressing their feelings. The final general component focuses on the traditional CBT intervention of Cognitive coping, or techniques for managing negative emotions and behaviors through focusing on changing thought processes. Youth are first taught to identify the connections among thoughts, feelings, and behaviors. Next, they learn to identify distorted cognitions, unhelpful or inaccurate thoughts that are likely to produce negative emotions and/or maladaptive behaviors, such as black-and-white thinking, a focus on negative outcomes, and catastrophizing. Clients and therapists then work to identify alternative thoughts that are more helpful and/or accurate and to replace their distorted thoughts with these new ones in order to change their emotions and behaviors. For example, an adolescent who experienced a serious car accident may believe that any time he drives on the street where the incident occurred, he will get into another accident. This thought may lead to anxiety and avoidance of the location of the accident, which could be particularly impairing if it is a street he needs to travel on or if his avoidance expands to other locations. If the client is able to replace this distorted belief with the belief that another accident is extremely unlikely to occur, and he comes to truly believe this, he will feel calmer and be able to work his way toward driving near the site of the accident again.

In order to explore the trauma more specifically, youth create a Trauma narrative in which they write (or draw) the story of their trauma experience over the course of several sessions. As the child and therapist delve into more and more details about the traumatic event, the creation of the trauma narrative serves as a type of gradual, stepwise exposure that helps desensitize the client to reminders of the trauma and reduce resulting anxiety and avoidance. The narrative contains information about the child before the trauma occurred, the details of the trauma and how it has negatively affected the child, and the story of how the child has changed and grown in the aftermath of the trauma. For children who have experienced complex or multiple traumas, it may make more sense to frame this activity as a life narrative that covers both positive and negative events over the course of the child's lifetime. Some children may have difficulty talking about or writing many details about the trauma. For these youth, it is important to proceed slowly and may be helpful to begin by having children relay non-traumatic personal experiences. Reading developmentally appropriate books written about a trauma similar to the client's experience can also serve as a model and an encouragement. Once the narrative has been created, the client and the therapist review it and add details about thoughts and feelings in order to help identify distorted cognitions and facilitate cognitive coping, as learned earlier in therapy. The therapist should encourage the client to include any fears or mental images about future traumas that they may be experiencing as well as to include the "worst" aspects of the trauma story (worst memory or moment). Sharing this information with appropriate support from the therapist (including implementation of relaxation techniques when necessary) helps expose particularly distressing cognitive distortions and gives the child the opportunity to learn to cope adaptively with (rather than avoid) strong negative emotions.

Following the imaginal exposure that occurs through the discussion and remembrance of the trauma, In vivo exposure and desensitization is utilized to help children overcome their anxiety and avoidance of places and situations that remind them of the trauma and cause distress and impairment but are not truly threatening. (It is important to note that in vivo exposure should only be used when it does not endanger the child; for example, this would be an inappropriate intervention for a child whose fear revolves around a sexual assailant who still attends her school and is present in the situations that trigger her anxiety in avoidance. In this case, the therapist and parents should work with the school to promote the client's true safety instead.) During in vivo exposure, the child puts herself in increasingly anxiety-provoking situations related to the trauma, using her emotion regulation and cognitive coping skills to manage her reactions in each situation until she can tolerate them. Exposure desensitizes the child to the situation or stimulus that is viewed as threatening and teaches her that there is nothing to truly be afraid of or avoid. Furthermore, it allows the child to practice her skills and gain a sense of mastery, which may be especially important for youth who have lost their sense of control and competence following a trauma. Throughout the course of treatment, Conjoint child-parent sessions facilitate communication within the family as well as parental support of the child's treatment gains. During these sessions, therapists encourage children to share their trauma narratives with their parents (and facilitate supportive parental responses), teach families skills for communicating openly about topics that are difficult to discuss, and facilitate safety planning, the final treatment component. For youth who have been traumatized, Enhancing safety is an important part of preparing for the end of therapy and healthy development in the future. Parents and therapists discuss ways to create and protect safe environments for children, and youth themselves learn personal safety skills, such as awareness of danger, assertiveness, appropriate help seeking, and problem solving. For example, a child who has been maltreated might discuss with the therapist the best way to respond to a similar situation in the future, including leaving the house or telling a safe adult. In this component, children are empowered as they are taught safety skills as well as accurate vocabulary and effective communication to help them connect clearly with adults who can help promote their safety.

TF-CBT has been found to be effective for reducing PTSD symptoms as well as several other types of problems commonly experienced by traumatized youth, including depressive symptoms, behavior problems, and social difficulties; treatment gains are seen in clients ranging from preschool-aged to adolescence and are maintained at six-month and one-year follow-ups (Cohen & Mannarino, 1996; Cohen et al., 2004; Deblinger et al., 1996; Mannarino et al., 2012; Scheeringa et al., 2011; Webb et al., 2014). Examples of culturally sensitive adaptations of TF-CBT can also be found in the literature (BigFoot & Schmidt, 2012; de Arellano et al., 2012).

Cognitive Behavioral Intervention for Trauma in Schools (CBITS). Originally developed through collaboration between researchers and the Los Angeles Unified School District, the Cognitive Behavioral Intervention for Trauma in Schools (CBITS) was designed as a school-based approach for treating trauma symptoms in diverse inner-city youth (Stein et al., 2003). CBITS is a ten-session intervention that is delivered to small groups (five to eight youth) of fourth- through eighth-grade students by mental health professionals in a school setting. To reduce barriers to treatment, appropriate clients are identified via a brief screening process, and the intervention is designed to be implemented by appropriate school personnel within the confines of the regular school day (rather than after school; Kataoka et al., 2014). The intervention program also includes one to three individual sessions as well as two optional psychoeducational sessions with parents and one with teachers. The program consists of six components: (1) psychoeducation, (2) relaxation training, (3) cognitive restructuring, (4) exposure and coping skills training, (5) exposure via trauma narrative construction, and (6) social problem-solving skills training (Jaycox, 2004; Nadeem et al., 2014; Stein et al., 2003). As these components overlap significantly with those of TF-CBT, they are described in less detail below.

In the first session, before psychoeducation begins, group members are introduced to each other, group rules, and the links among thoughts, feelings, and behaviors. The subsequent nine sessions cover the six main treatment components. First, *psychoeducation* is provided about common reactions to trauma in order to normalize students' experiences and provide them with hope for recovery (i.e., other people have experienced these symptoms before and have gotten better). The group format can be helpful in this component, as clients can share their symptoms with one another if they choose, providing a more in-the-moment, peer-based normalization and comradery of experiences. Second, students are trained to use *relaxation skills* to cope with anxiety and trauma symptoms. Deep breathing, guided imagery, and progressive muscle relaxation are included. Third, therapists introduce the group to the basic tenets of *cognitive therapy*, which revolve around the idea that inaccurate and unhelpful thoughts (distorted cognitions) underlie problematic behaviors and feelings and must be changed in order to produce improvement in symptoms. Students learn strategies for identifying and challenging their distorted cognitions. A "hot seat" activity can be useful in which one child is assisted by the rest in the group to identify positive thoughts to counter cognitive distortions around a given scenario. Fourth, in vivo *exposure* is used in order to reduce the avoidance behaviors that many individuals with PTSD display and which often interfere with functioning. Students identify situations or stimuli that they have begun to avoid following trauma exposure; each student then constructs a fear hierarchy related to the situation/stimulus he has identified. Through the rest of the intervention, students and therapists plan ways for students to work through the hierarchy, being exposed to increasingly fear-provoking (but actually safe) situations while using the relaxation and cognitive restructuring skills learned earlier to manage their anxiety. As with other trauma interventions, this component must include communication and collaboration with parents and other school officials to ensure that exposure does not truly endanger the student. Fifth, students work with therapists individually and in the group setting to create a *trauma narrative* in which they talk, write, and/or draw the story of their trauma. The trauma narrative construction and telling provides opportunities for students to process the event and their reactions, to use coping skills to manage their anxiety, and to allow anxiety to diminish naturally through the process of exposure. Therapists use a "feelings thermometer" to help students identify their level of distress during these sessions and to chart anxiety reduction. Sixth, students learn *social problem-solving skills* in order to improve their ability to manage difficult situations they may encounter in the future. Connections are made with the material learned earlier in therapy about the role of cognitive distortions, which may affect students' identification and choice of the best plan of action in a social situation. Youth then work to identify possible solutions to a social situation and pick the one that is likely to produce the best outcome. Both general and trauma-related social situations are explored; an example of the latter would be if a friend told a client's peers about her traumatic experience without her permission.

CBITS has been found to be effective in reducing symptoms of PTSD and depression in traumatized youth (Jaycox et al., 2010; Kataoka et al., 2003; Stein et al., 2003). One notable finding is that the intervention may have a higher participation rate when it is delivered in the school context rather than through a community mental health center (Jaycox et al., 2010). CBITS has been success-fully implemented with youth from a variety of cultural backgrounds, with researchers and clinicians adapting specific intervention elements and examples for different cultural contexts (Goodkind et al., 2010; Morsette et al., 2009; Ngo et al., 2008)

INTEGRATIVE APPROACH TO TREATMENT

There has been a limited amount of theoretical and empirical work exploring cognitive-behavioral interventions for traumatized youth that include explicit spiritual and religious elements (e.g., Walker, Quagliana, Wilkinson, & Frederick, 2013; Walker et al., 2010; Wang et al., 2016). It is encouraging that there is recognition of the importance of addressing these elements of clients' lives, which evidence suggests may help improve both psychological symptoms and spiritual well-being (Wang et al., 2016). In this section, we will build on this work as we draw from a variety of Christian biblical and theological sources. We will discuss Christian integrative considerations for the five common components of treatments for childhood trauma, which are psychoeducation, coping skills, trauma narratives, cognitive restructuring, and future planning (Black et al., 2012).

Psychoeducation. Unfortunately, given its often challenging aftermath, trauma is not an uncommon part of the human experience. The Bible describes a wide variety of traumatic experiences, including the enslavement of the Israelites (Exodus 1); Saul's vengeful pursuit of David (1 Samuel 19–23); the destruction of Israel's holy city and the people's subsequent captivity (2 Chronicles 36); God's destruction of sinful nations and peoples, sometimes through Israel's military action (Joshua 10;

Isaiah 13); the execution of the longed-for Savior (Matthew 27); and the persecution and even murder of some of Jesus' early followers (Acts 7; 2 Corinthians 11). We also see in Scripture the responses of communities and individuals (including Jesus) to various traumas, such as sadness or sorrow (Lamentations 1:16; Mark 14:34, John 20:11-13), anger and aggression (Exodus 2:11-12), anguish and terror (Job 9:34; Isaiah 13:8; Ezekiel 7:18), physical expressions of distress (Lamentations 1:13; Luke 22:44), frightening dreams and visions (Job 7:14), groaning and crying out (Psalm 57:2; Lamentations 1:21), and even expressions of regret that one ever lived (Job 3). (Scripture also contains many examples of growth and joy despite or even because of trauma and suffering, which we will discuss in more detail later.) It has even been argued that traumatic events shaped the history of the Jewish and Christian communities out of which the Bible developed and without which the themes of suffering, community, and redemption could not have been fully illustrated (Carr, 2014). In light of these biblical portrayals of trauma and its aftermath, Scripture can be a useful tool for normalizing both the experience of trauma and the deep suffering and distress that may follow, even for God's faithful followers. Of course, the Bible is not meant to be a diagnostic instrument or a case manual, nor was it written with modern understandings of trauma in mind. Therefore, it is important not to limit the discussion of typical reactions to trauma to biblical material; rather, these examples can be a helpful complement to symptoms and illustrations that are drawn from the DSM, research, and clinical experience.

Walker and colleagues (2010) point out that it may also be important to specifically nor-malize the spiritual doubts and difficulties youth experience following a trauma. It is important for youth and families to understand that because we are holistic beings, and trauma often has a far-reaching impact on one's well-being and functioning, it can impact not only physical, emotional, cognitive, and behavioral aspects of life but also spiritual ones. Furthermore, our spiritual nature interacts with and manifests itself through these other aspects of our functioning. For example, emotional manifestations of spiritual struggles following a trauma could include feeling stagnant in one's faith, lacking a sense God's presence, feeling angry at God, or feeling emotionally numb during spiritual activities or gatherings that were previously sources of joy, such as prayer or corporate worship. Cognitively, children or parents may doubt God's goodness or power, since he did not stop the trauma from happening, or even doubt their own salvation. From a CBT perspective, these emotional and cognitive experiences impact one's behavior; traumatized clients may stop attending church, stop engaging in personal spiritual practices such as reading the Bible or praying, or act out in ways that they consider inconsistent with their values, such as drinking heavily or being aggressive toward others. Though some Christian clinicians may be hesitant to engage in a discussion of these difficulties for fear of encouraging or contributing to them, normalizing them in a caring manner and listening empathically are actually likely to have the opposite effect. Clients who are ashamed of their spiritual difficulties following a traumatic experience and do not have a source of support with whom to share them may have trouble working through their struggles, which may further contribute to their symptoms (including not only trauma symptoms but also depression and anxiety).

Coping skills. The coping skills element of trauma-focused treatments includes practical skills for managing symptoms and problems, such as relaxation training, emotion regulation work, and problem-solving skills training. From a theological perspective, working with traumatized youth to build these types of coping skills acknowledges both their full personhood and their agency, as it testifies to the importance of enabling children to effect change in themselves and their environments (agency) and their ability to learn and grow and gain skills (as full persons; Miller-McLemore, 2003). Traumatized youth may especially benefit from mastering coping skills and seeing themselves implement these skills effectively, given the loss of a sense of agency and control that has been linked to worse posttraumatic symptoms (Zhang et al., 2011). Youth who can manage formerly overwhelming emotions and work through possible solutions in types of situations in which they formerly felt helpless are likely to shift to a more internal sense of control, which can contribute to symptom reduction and improvements in overall well-being.

In addition to these general implications, there are some specific ways in which biblical and theological ideas can be used to enhance skill training for Christian youth. Walker and colleagues describe examples of such integrative practices with traumatized youth, such as having clients repeat a simple prayer ("Lord Jesus, have mercy on me") during deep breathing or progressive muscle relaxation (Walker et al., 2010; Walker, Doverspike, et al., 2013). They also suggest utilizing spiritually oriented imagery to enhance relaxation. Clients might picture God sheltering them in his sacred tent (Psalm 27:5), God's wing wrapping around them as protection (Psalm 57:1), God fighting for them while they rest (Exodus 14:14), God rejoicing over them with singing (Zephaniah 3:17), or any other images that help the client be comforted by God's care, protection, and power. Prayer and meditation on Scripture can also enhance youths' emotion regulation efforts by providing comfort, hope, and a shift in focus off themselves and their difficulties and onto God and his characteristics. In trauma treatment, strategies for regulating emotions are often closely linked to strategies for replacing distorted cognitions with accurate and helpful ones, a process that is also informed by theological and biblical ideas.

Trauma narrative creation and cognitive restructuring. Because the integrative material we will discuss here is highly relevant for both the process of cognitive restructuring and the creation of the trauma narrative (which involves some work with cognitive distortions), we have combined these important elements into one section. It is clear that God does not desire for us to live in fear or to believe lies, which is essentially what cognitive distortions are. Such distortions about one's own guilt or weakness, the unsafe nature of the world and other people, and/or hopelessness about the future may come to dominate an individual's (sometimes automatic) thoughts following a traumatic experience. Scripture is a useful tool for combating certain cognitive distortions, as it is a source of truth that can be used to address inaccurate or unhelpful thoughts (Tan, 2007). For example, an adolescent who has experienced an interpersonal trauma might experience the recurrent thought that she is permanently "damaged" and unworthy of love following her experiences. In order to combat this belief, the therapist and the client might explore Scriptures that describe God's love and our resulting worth, such as Psalm 139:13-14 ("For you created my inmost being; you knit me together in my mother's womb. I praise you because I am fearfully and wonderfully made; your works are wonderful, I know that full well"), Luke 12:6-7 ("Are not five sparrows sold for two pennies? Yet not one of them is forgotten by God. Indeed, the very hairs of your head are all numbered. Don't be afraid; you are worth more than many sparrows"), Romans 5:8 ("But God demonstrates his own love for us in this: While we were still sinners, Christ died for us"), 2 Corinthians 5:17 ("Therefore, if anyone is in Christ, the new creation has come: The old has gone, the new is here!"), and 1 John 3:1 ("See what great love the Father has lavished on us, that we should be called children of God! And that is what we are!"). These passages and many others offer truths that a client can speak to herself when she recognizes the distorted thoughts that contribute to her trauma and other symptoms.

A limited knowledge or understanding of Scripture may actually contribute to negative or unhelpful thoughts for youth who have experienced a trauma. There are many biblical passages, particularly in the Psalms, that speak about God keeping the righteous or faithful safe from harm but punishing the wicked (Psalm 4:8; Psalm 32:6-7; Psalm 37:18-20). Following the experience of an assault, abuse, or natural disaster, some youth may come to believe that God is punishing them or does not truly love them (or, alternatively, that God's Word is untrue); in other words, if something bad has happened to them, they must be among the wicked. From a theological point of view, it is important to help these youth understand such passages within a fuller understanding of both God's nature and human nature. While we know that God is faithful to his promises and that the wicked will be punished and the righteous prevail, we recognize that we may not see these outcomes in this life. Punishment, reward, and triumph can be eternal consequences. Furthermore, as believers living under the new covenant, we understand that we gain righteousness only through Christ's substitutionary atonement—Jesus' taking on our sins and imparting to us his righteousness through his death and resurrection—not through our "right" behaviors. Therefore, as Christians, we can be assured that traumatic experiences are not God's punishment for our unrighteousness but rather must be understood in light of the fallenness of a broken world, in which natural disasters occur and people sometimes use their free will to harm others. Our trust, then, is in a God who uses everything for his purposes and will ultimately enact justice and re-creation.

One spiritual purpose for trauma and suffering is our refinement and growth. Throughout Scripture, we see that the growth of our faith and character—as well as the revealing of God's power and glory—can come through suffering (Romans 5:3-5; 2 Corinthians 12:9-10; James 1:2-4; 1 Peter 1:6-7). Suffering creates a situation in which our illusions of power and control are stripped away and we recognize our need for a powerful, glorious, and wise God to work through our weakness (our human imperfection and inadequacy; see chapter two). The challenge of navigating suffering and the negative emotions that accompany it also facilitates personal growth and self-examination in a way that situations that are easy and joyful do not; we rarely learn to persevere, to focus only on what is most important in our lives, and to exhibit deep faith without trying, difficult experiences. Psychological literature recognizes the phenomenon of posttraumatic growth (PTG) as encompassing the positive changes that can also emerge following a traumatic event. Such changes can include gaining a more positive view of oneself and one's abilities, seeing new possibilities for one's life and direction, experiencing enhanced interpersonal relationships and closeness with others, and developing a stronger faith and sense of meaning (Tedeschi & Calhoun, 1995, 1996; Tedeschi et al, 2017). Even those who experience negative psychological outcomes following trauma may experience this growth. Indeed, there is a positive association between trauma symptoms and PTG, at least at lower levels of symptomatology, and the relationship between PTSD and PTG seems to be stronger in youth than in adults (Shakespeare-Finch & Lurie-Beck, 2014). For example, adolescents who reported that their core beliefs were challenged by their experiences in an earthquake had higher levels of both trauma symptoms and PTG than those whose beliefs were not affected by trauma exposure (Zhou et al., 2015).

For clients who are Christians, there are some therapeutic applications for these ideas. The idea of PTG or God's unique use of suffering to refine us can undergird the process of cognitive restructuring. For example, meditation on passages that describe the purpose or benefit of suffering may provide encour-

agement and hope that can help counter predominantly negative thoughts about oneself and the future. For example, clients and therapists might work to replace the belief that "the event happened because of the sort of person that I am" with the thought that "God is able to use the event to help me to grow to be more like him, and I can glorify him in that process." For some clients, working to reframe their trauma story as a source of not only pain and suffering but also growth and positive change may be an important process in therapy. Clients and therapists might spend time thinking about the growth that either has already occurred or might occur in the future as the result of the trauma. Therapists can encourage clients to think about the answers to questions such as, How am I a different person following the trauma? In what ways have I grown? What relationships in my life are stronger as a result of this experience? How has my faith grown through the trauma and its aftermath? How have I come to understand God and his nature better? An emphasis on growth and positive change that would not have occurred without the traumatic experience will especially help clients change the tone and hopefulness of their trauma narrative. Furthermore, the child's construction of her trauma narrative is a way to impart agency and an increased sense of power. Individuals who have experienced trauma may lack a sense of control or power in their own lives, and for children, who are inherently less powerful and more vulnerable than adults, that sense may be especially overwhelming. Helping a child write her own trauma story in her own words, and communicating that her view of her experience is important, can begin to return her sense of agency, which is both psychologically and theologically important, as we have discussed previously (chapter two, this volume; Miller-McLemore, 2003).

In addition, youth might explore the stories of people in biblical or Christian history who experienced suffering, especially through trauma, and positive changes as a result of their experiences (even as they may also have experienced significant pain and distress). This activity may be helpful both in restructuring cognitive distortions and in creating the trauma narrative. For example, Lachs (2002) suggests that the traumatic experience of nearly being sacrificed at his father's hands shaped Isaac's closeness to his mother and his introverted and self-reflective personality. Jacob's son Joseph experiences traumas at the hands of multiple people, including his own brothers, as he is thrown into a well, sold into slavery, and falsely imprisoned, yet we see how God uses Joseph's experiences for good. The book of Lamentations is an expression of lament following the destruction of Jerusalem and has been understood as a collective response to trauma (Boase, 2014). German theologian Dietrich Bonhoeffer was imprisoned in a Nazi concentration camp in 1945, where he was executed later that year (Bethge, 2000). It is hard to imagine a circumstance more full of traumatic experiences. However, during his imprisonment, Bonhoeffer wrote a poem to his mother which was later set to music for use as a hymn (Watson, 2002). His assurance of God's goodness despite his horrific circumstances is evident:

> And when this cup You give is filled
>   to brimming
> With bitter suffering, hard to understand,
> we take it thankfully and without trembling,
> out of so good and so beloved a hand. (p. 402)

Future planning. At the same that we recognize God's sovereignty, we also recognize that, in many realms of life, there are active roles that God calls us to play. For example, God alone can save (Ephesians 2:8-9), but we are clearly instructed to share the gospel with nonbelievers (Matthew 28:19-20), and God uses the church to make himself known (1 Corinthians 3:5-11). In the parable of the talents, a master praises the servants who invested the money he gave them while he was away and rebukes the one who did not (Matthew 25:14-30 NRSV). In this parable, the money (talents) is commonly understood to represent our God-given gifts, and the main message of the story is that we are responsible for actively using the abilities we are given to serve God and others (France, 1994). With regard to trauma interventions, we believe it is not only appropriate but necessary to recognize the complementary roles that God and people play in promoting our own and others' safety. As we explored earlier, God is a powerful protector, capable of rescuing us even in situations in which defeat appears inevitable (1 Samuel 17; Psalm 27:1-3). The care and presence of our sovereign Lord is an important source of comfort and assurance. At the same time, we recognize that we have a responsibility to actively promote the safety of the vulnerable, such as children, particularly those who are at heightened risk. Parents who cover electrical outlets and put up baby gates when their infants begin crawling are not dismissing or failing to trust in God's protection; rather, they are recognizing their active role as God's agents of protection over the vulnerable individuals in their care. Similarly, the safety planning and skill building that are important components of moving toward terminating trauma-focused treatment do not invalidate earlier messages about and images of God's protection but complement them. In addition, the safety planning component of treatment includes active work on the part of adults (e.g., clinician, parents, teachers or other school officials) as well as youth themselves. Some safety actions are more appropriately taken by parents or others adults in power; for example, if a child has been assaulted by a peer at school, it may be appropriate for the child's class schedule to be rearranged so that he does not come in regular contact with the assailant or even for the assailant to be removed from the school. However, there are other safety-promoting actions that can best be enacted by the youth himself. Children need to know how to communicate with adults when they have been harmed or are in danger; they also need to possess the skills to accurately assess whether a situation might be dangerous (which can be particularly challenging for traumatized individuals) and to effectively problem solve how to remove themselves from dangerous situations when possible. Theologically, we see the illustration of the complementary ideas that children are gifts to be celebrated and protected and that they are individuals with agency who play an active role in their own lives (Miller-McLemore, 2003). Recognizing both of these elements of a holistic view of youth can help us understand the importance of both taking an active role as adults and guarding the active role that is appropriate for youth to take themselves.

Finally, effective planning for the future must be based on a sense of past and present success in gaining skills and reducing symptoms. For youth, explicitly celebrating those accomplishments in the final session (as is included in CBITS, for example) will help bolster them to meet future challenges. We see the importance of joining together in community to rejoice with those who rejoice as a part of the body of Christ (Romans 12:15; 1 Corinthians 12:26-27). All clinicians should include a celebratory element during the final session, and those working with Christian families might explore with clients how they might celebrate their growth and the termination of therapy with other members of the body of Christ. Depending on whether other people know about the trauma and its aftermath as well as how comfortable the child is sharing about therapy, youth or other pastors, friends from within the church community, youth groups, Sunday school classes, and even the larger church body might join with the child in celebration and support. This expression of support not only marks past and present achievements but, hopefully, provides a source of hope and help in future times of trouble, including the return of trauma symptoms.

CASE STUDY

Pertinent history. Kate Reeder is an eleven-year-old Caucasian female in the fifth grade. Her parents sought therapy due to their concern about her apparent anxiety and frequent nightmares. They were referred by a local children's advocacy center following a founded investigation of sexual abuse by her paternal grandfather on three occasions. The children's advocacy center had gotten involved with the family, and the abuse had come to light, due to Kate's inappropriate sexual behaviors with a younger male cousin at a family gathering. Before the allegations of sexual abuse, the family was very close with their extended family. However, after discovering what had happened, family members had differing reactions to the allegations, which were causing additional stress for the family. Kate's parents' goal for therapy is for Kate to receive support and help her process the abuse she has experienced so that past experiences will not negatively impact her currently and in the future. They would also like to bring healing to their family.

At the time of the initial intake, Kate's primary diagnosis is posttraumatic stress disorder. Kate presents with difficulty sleeping, often feeling tired and having some nightmares in which she is alone in the dark with "something bad" coming to get her. She also worries that something bad might happen to her. She displays somatic complaints, including stomach pains, chest pain, and feelings of nausea. She tries not to think about her grandfather to avoid her feelings of sadness and anger, and becomes upset when thoughts about what happened "pop into her head," especially when she is at school or trying to sleep. Kate feels nervous when she visits with extended family now because she feels like she is to blame for what happened and that she is a "bad kid" for the incident with her cousin. She also has begun avoiding areas of her house and settings to which her grandfather took her, including her favorite extracurricular activity, soccer. She also does not want to attend church because her extended family attends the church and her grandfather attended special church events with them on occasion. Kate is described as "very smart" and earns good grades at school. She participates in several extracurricular activities and enjoys hanging out with friends.

Kate lives with her parents, older brother (age sixteen), and younger sister (age six). Her family is highly religiously and spiritually oriented and evangelical Protestant Christian in affiliation. They requested explicit spiritual interventions from the onset of therapy. Their family environment is characterized by a consistently high degree of love and support for one another. In particular, her parents have a warm and accepting parenting style and a strong marital relationship. They place an emphasis on kindness and display a lighthearted sense of humor. Kate's parents are highly supportive of her and the therapeutic process. They have a strong, affectionate relationship with Kate. However, they have difficulty discussing negative affect or thoughts and tend to minimize or dismiss pain in their focus on optimism and gratitude. At times her parents seem to excuse the behavior of Kate's grandfather in a desire to decrease their felt guilt and to avoid conflict.

Course of treatment. Following an intake interview with Kate's parents in which background information is gathered and therapy is explained, the therapist meets with Kate alone for an initial individual session. The purpose of therapy and how children use therapy is explained, and they read a short book about therapy. They also play a game to get to know each other and to help Kate become comfortable with the therapist. Kate is given two measures, a general measure of behavioral and emotional functioning and a specific measure of trauma symptoms, to be reviewed at the next session. Based on Kate's interest and strengths in creativity and visual learning, she and the therapist decide that art will be used throughout therapy to process her emotions, relationships, and her past experiences. They decide on a predictable structure for each session which will include talking about "highs" and "lows" of the past week, learning (psychoeducation), practice of skills, and an art activity with discussion.

In the second session, the therapist meets with Kate and her parents together to provide psychoeducation about trauma and children's typical reactions to traumatic events. The measures Kate completed are reviewed. She is demonstrating clinically significant anxiety symptoms (e.g., often worries, is easily stressed, and is nervous) and clinically significant somatization (e.g., often complains of being sick when nothing is wrong, gets sick, and complains of stomach pain). The trauma measure is used to explain Kate's specific response to her experience, including the following: feeling afraid something bad might happen; remembering things that happened that she did not like and difficulty stopping thoughts about what happened to her; intrusive, distressing memories about the events and distressing dreams; efforts to avoid distressing memories, thoughts, or feelings about the abuse, and efforts to avoid external reminders about the abuse; displaying uncharacteristic irritable behavior; distorted cognitions about the cause of the abuse that lead to self-blame and negative beliefs about herself; physiological reactions to cues regarding the abuse (e.g., her heart rate increases and she feels sick to her stomach when she walks down to their basement family room because the abuse occurred there, and when her grandfather is mentioned); feelings of detachment from others and withdrawn behavior at home; and distress about these emotional experiences and memories of the abuse that sometimes impede her ability to have fun

with her friends and pay attention in school. The therapist and the family set specific goals for therapy, which include: Kate will be able to identify her emotions and thoughts, and clearly communicate them; Kate will develop awareness of what happens in her brain and body when she is triggered; Kate will implement adaptive emotion regulation strategies and cognitive challenging; Kate will process her past history of abuse into a more comprehensive understanding of herself; Kate's parents will be able to identify and utilize parenting strategies that promote her expression and her sense of safety; and Kate will articulate her spiritual questions and utilize adaptive spiritual practices. The therapist then closes the session in prayer and asks for guidance for therapy and God's comfort.

In the next session, the therapist meets individually with Kate. She is guarded but becomes more comfortable after talking about age-appropriate topics for the first ten minutes according to the predictable structure of sessions decided on in the first individual session. Kate and the therapist read a children's book about trauma (*A Terrible Thing Happened*). Kate is uncomfortable talking about her grandfather or the abuse. Utilizing an emotions visual, the therapist helps Kate identify and express her feelings without talking explicitly about the abuse. Kate also is helped to name the trauma, and she decides she wants to call it "Evil Dark." During this session, she draws a storm cloud with herself portrayed in the middle of the cloud. The feelings she associates with the drawing are scared, alone, angry, confused, and lost. She is asked to create a second drawing representing what she wants her future to look like. She draws herself spinning in the middle of a field of flowers with arms outstretched. She links the drawing with the feelings of happy, carefree, safe, strong, and calm.

Kate and the therapist again meet for an individual session. One aim of the session is to help Kate become aware of the physical sensations in her body that are related to her emotions, and to help her find strategies to manage these feelings. Outlines of the human body are used to identify the physical experiences she has for different feelings. The therapist and Kate then engage in a breathing exercise and a relaxation exercise. She is assigned to practice these exercises at least once a day, and is provided a daily log for recording them. Another purpose of this session is to assess Kate's emotional security within her family and within her relationship with God. Kate draws herself and her parents with adjoining statements from each ("Love you," "Love you, too"). The many ways she knows her parents love her are discussed. Interestingly, she also draws a box in the picture. In discussion about the picture, she explains that Evil Dark is in the box and she and her parents are not looking at or talking about it so it will not come out of the box. Kate's drawing of God includes herself with flat affect, a figure behind her in the sky (God), a dark cloud in between herself and the God figure, and a small church with a sun and rainbow above it in the distance. Kate has difficulty explaining the picture but notes that she feels "bad" and does not know how God could still love her. A feelings chart is used to help her identify "embarrassed" and "lonely" as her bad emotions. The therapist does not want to end the session with Kate focused on her negative emotions and so asks Kate to draw one more picture— how she would have drawn God before the

Evil Dark. Kate draws herself and God in a heart under a rainbow with rain falling in the background. The therapist observes that she looks happy in the "before" picture and asks Kate to complete the following sentence, "When I think about God, I think . . ." Kate provides the following thoughts: that he comforts people, how he knows everything, that he is loving to everyone, about how God gave his only Son, he is always near, and he wants us near him and to worship him. They reflect that these concepts of God do not include judgment, anger, or punishment; rather, they represent God as a helper and caregiver. The therapist then offers the verse "And the peace of God, which transcends all understanding, will guard [your heart and your mind] in Christ Jesus" (Philippians 4:7) with a hand gesture for a heart for Kate to use to remember he offers her peace in her heart and mind.

A parenting session is held to discuss the use of positive parenting strategies to decrease Kate's withdrawn behavior at home. With Kate's permission, the therapist verbally shares Kate's concept of God. Her parents are asked to complete the same sentence prompt, and their similar views of a caring and loving God are linked to her concept of God and to their parenting style. They express gratitude for the reminder of the values that guide them. They discuss Mr. and Mrs. Reeder's observations of the strengths of their family and what they could develop to support Kate. The therapist observes that Kate has a secure relationship with them and truly feels their love for her. The use of this strong parent-child relationship to bolster her sense of self and her healthy emotional expression is discussed. They each identify a weekly time when they can spend time one-on-one with Kate doing something she enjoys with them, as well as a daily time when one of them checks in with Kate about her feelings; even if Kate does not want to share her feelings right away, it is important for her to know that her parents want to know. They acknowledge they struggle to discuss difficult emotional content and worry they minimize Kate's feelings. The therapist takes this opportunity to discuss the need to create safety for Kate to experience and express the different emotions she is experiencing. Kate's parents are guided in how to provide verbal reflection for Kate and validate her emotions when she expresses them through both nonverbal and verbal responses. They agree to focus on this in their daily interactions with Kate in order to practice these skills around positive emotions, which may feel easier.

The therapist begins the subsequent individual session with Kate with mindful breathing, a review of her practice of breathing and relaxation, and discussion of the week's "highs" and "lows" with a focus on identifying emotions and thoughts. She then is provided with psychoeducation about the relationship among thoughts, emotions, actions, the body, and the environment. They practice understanding these relationships with the use of worksheet activities and discussion of typical experiences Kate has throughout the day. Kate and the therapist examine what happens when thoughts change. Kate then is asked to share the most difficult thought she has right now, and she identifies the thought "I am bad" as one that keeps "popping up" randomly or when minor things happen (e.g., her teacher seems upset at her class for being too loud, her friend talks to another classmate instead of her at recess). The therapist gently inquires

about the foundation of this belief, and Kate quietly states, "Because of my cousin." Kate is challenged to give herself advice on how to replace or change this thought, which she has difficulty doing. The therapist reviews the characteristics of God that Kate identified in the past individual session and asks her to complete a drawing of God challenging her thought. She depicts God's face with a voice coming from heaven with the words, "I forgive you, Kate." These words are associated with Kate's feelings of relief and happiness. She notes that her body feels calm with this thought and that she would potentially be able to have more energy and interact with others differently if she holds onto the thought that she is forgiven. Because Kate has expressed the heaviness of her guilt for her own actions, they discuss the following verse as a truthful tool for combating unhelpful thoughts: "Finally, I confessed all my sins to you and stopped trying to hide my guilt. I said to myself, 'I will confess my rebellion to the LORD.' And you forgave me! All my guilt is gone" (Psalm 32:5 NLT). (Note: The New Living Translation is used for wording that is easier for Kate to understand at her age.) They then discuss forgiveness, and in this case the decision to choose self-forgiveness, as an example of a change of thought, feeling, and behavior. They take a few minutes to pray silently before ending the session with a check in about Kate's feelings and thoughts. She is asked to keep a log of her emotions and thoughts along with her practice of breathing and relaxation.

Kate and the therapist meet for another individual session. After talking about her past week, they review her log of thoughts and feelings. It is clear Kate frequently experiences feelings of anxiety (worried, scared, nervous). She is given instruction on how to do a mindful body scan throughout the day to recognize her arousal level and her need to regulate emotions through the use of coping strategies. From a list of coping strategies, Kate selects the use of seeking social support, positive self-talk, and visualization as options in addition to breathing exercises. They practice the use of visualization, and it is added to her weekly practice log. Through a drawing of self-forgiveness, the therapist checks in on Kate's thought of "I am bad" as discussed in the past session. She draws herself getting unstuck from "the muck" of self-unforgiveness. Kate is asked to draw or write the thoughts, feelings, and behaviors that are part of this "muck." Kate opens up about her interactions with extended family members since beginning therapy. She wants to be able to apologize to her parents, as well as to her cousin and his parents, so they can trust her again and so "things can go back to normal." They decide to schedule another session with Kate's parents and a family therapy session for the next week to discuss this topic.

The therapist meets next with Kate's parents. Mr. and Mrs. Reeder first review their attempts at providing reflection for Kate to increase her safety in expressing emotions, to help her better understand her emotions, and to validate these emotions. They express feeling even closer to Kate than they have in the past, and indicate she is spontaneously opening up to them about her feelings more often. Mr. and Mrs. Reeder describe their difficulty grappling with how evil has impacted their family and how Kate herself carried on the evil introduced to her toward a family member. The therapist facilitates their understanding of this symptom of trauma for a child Kate's age and explains how her reenactment of her own abuse is a mirror to what she experienced. Kate's parents express guilt for reporting the abuse, but they are able to hear and accept that if they had not reported it then they potentially would be failing to protect other children who are vulnerable. They express comfort in looking from beyond their fear of their family's animosity and the negative effects on their family to the bigger picture of calling out evil inflicted on the vulnerable. Mr. and Mrs. Reeder's confidence in their decision to address instead of hide the truth about the abuse also is rooted in a sense of justice. The therapist and Kate's parents discuss how they cannot control family members' responses. They feel they may have sacrificed their family members' sense of comfort; however, even with that outcome, they would choose again to confront evil and protect children in their family. The therapist asks Mr. and Mrs. Reeder to draw a picture for Kate expressing their forgiveness and their view that she is not bad, which they will present to her in the following family session.

The main focus of the family therapy session is to first process the difficulty of forgiving herself and to discuss her desire to make amends with her cousin. In order to facilitate emotional forgiveness, the therapist's goal is to help Kate experience the forgiveness her parents would like to offer her. The therapist provides psychoeducation about apologies —what they consist of, how they impact our well-being and others' well-being, and the possibility for interpersonal forgiveness (though that depends on the victim's response, which cannot be predicted or controlled).

Kate and her parents discuss how they could ask to meet with her cousin and his parents. To prepare for this meeting, they process how her cousin felt during and after the incident. Kate draws herself apologizing to her cousin. Her character says, "I'm sorry for what I did," and her cousin responds, "I forgive you." Kate demonstrates empathy for her cousin and what he felt but has difficulty showing the same kind of empathy for her own experience. The therapist gently provides a preview that Kate will better understand herself in the context of exploring her experiences with a trauma narrative later in the therapeutic process. To close the session, the therapist checks in on Kate's use of coping strategies identified in the last individual session (breathing, social support, positive self-talk, and visualization) and encourages Mr. and Mrs. Reeder to continue to support her use of these strategies throughout the day.

In the next individual session, Kate brings a picture she drew of her parents saying to her, "We love you no matter what." She describes a sense of "lightness" and trust that her parents still do love her and have forgiven her. Her log of emotions and thoughts is reviewed. It is clear that Kate is continuing to experience anxiety with trauma reminders. The therapist provides psychoeducation about avoidance and how it maintains anxiety. Kate is asked to list places she is avoiding, which include settings her grandfather took her to and settings in which the abuse occurred. She lists the family room in her basement, the local park and soccer field, and the river that flows through their town where her grandfather took her fishing. This avoidance is affecting her functioning as she does not utilize the family basement, she and her family used to

love walking alongside the river in the evening, she will not go to the park with her friends when they invite her, and soccer will be starting soon. Her log also indicates she becomes anxious when alone with an adult male (e.g., riding in the car with her maternal grandfather, in the kitchen with her brother). The therapist and Kate need to engage in breathing and relaxation exercises to manage her anxiety during this discussion as it is difficult for her to talk about these triggering settings. Her motivation to address this avoidance is assessed through an interview, and Kate expresses a desire to overcome her anxiety because the activities she would like to engage in are ones she used to love. The therapist presents information about engaging in brave behaviors that result in decreased anxiety responses over time with the use of visual graphs about the links between anxiety and avoiding or facing trauma-related stimuli. The therapist explains that they will take small brave steps that move Kate toward her goal of being able to feel comfortable in these settings and situations. To assist her in being brave, they meditate on a verse about God's wing wrapping around them as protection: "Have mercy on me, O God, have mercy! I look to you for protection. I will hide beneath the shadow of your wings until the danger passes by" (Psalm 57:1 NLT). Kate draws a picture of large wings shading her figure as she places one foot on the first step of a staircase.

Over the next few sessions, Kate and the therapist work with her parents to engage in exposure therapy. Kate and the therapist first set up an exposure hierarchy for the park, as Kate would like to begin the soccer season without anxiety about this setting. Kate first draws a picture of the park, and then a picture of herself at the park. Kate and the therapist discuss her emotions and thoughts while monitoring her arousal level and practicing breathing. They then engage in imaginal exposure, with Kate describing the park and herself approaching and then playing there. In a family session, Kate's parents learn about the use of exposure therapy for the settings that trigger Kate's trauma responses. The family practices using breathing and body scan during imaginal exposures in therapy. Kate and her parents are instructed to stay within the setting until her anxiety decreases. They also decide they will pray at each step and ask for God's blessing on the settings she is avoiding. Kate and her parents are then assigned "brave work" of driving past the park, sitting in the adjacent parking lot, sitting in the park, and finally playing at the park. She identifies a couple of friends with whom she feels secure and comfortable to play soccer with for the final step. A similar hierarchy is developed for the family's basement and the riverwalk. Through these exposures, Kate learns these trauma-related settings and the associated feelings and memories she experiences do not need to be avoided. Throughout the exposures, Kate is given encouragement by the therapist and her parents about how much growth has occurred in and outside of therapy. Kate draws herself with these adults verbalizing encouragement to her ("You are really brave!").

In a parenting session, Kate's parents talk about their own emotions about the trauma. They indicate difficulty talking about it for several reasons. Mr. and Mrs. Reeder feel a sense of shame that abuse occurred within their family. They also feel uncomfortable talking about it because they want to avoid questioning God's protection of their daughter. They are willing to talk about the problems associated with shame and secrecy, and consider offering themselves compassion. Through discussion, they identify they would rather have openness about the subject in order to prevent something like it from occurring again, to validate Kate's experience so she can better cope with the thoughts, feelings, and sensations she has about the trauma, and to promote Kate's self-esteem and confidence so she does not feel ashamed or damaged. They acknowledge that they have felt closer to each other and more willing to share emotions throughout the therapy process. The therapist models support and kindness to Mr. and Mrs. Reeder and encourages them to treat themselves in the same way. Just as they would not blame Kate for what happened to her, they understand that the abuse is not a reflection on them as parents or as a family. Mr. and Mrs. Reeder's feelings about God and his care of their family are explored. They identify conflicting feelings and beliefs about God's nature prior to and after the abuse. Just as Kate will be exploring the effects of the abuse, Mr. and Mrs. Reeder are encouraged to reflect on how the abuse has affected them with a focus on their relationship with God. They are also encouraged to confront God with their feelings through prayer by being honest and to speak openly with their pastor whom they trust.

The next phase of therapy involves talking about the trauma over the course of several sessions. The therapist reviews the brave steps Kate has taken and the progress she has made facing her anxiety through her exposures. The process of sharing her story and how trauma experiences have influenced her is presented.

Kate expresses a seven out of ten for anxiety when thinking about discussing her grandfather and the abuse she experienced. The therapist reflects these feelings and asks Kate to again reflect on her exposures. Kate is able to acknowledge her own strength but states that she does not know if she is strong enough for this part of therapy. The therapist discusses how God has called us to "carry one another's burdens," (Galatians 6:2) including the box that she has placed the trauma (Evil Dark) in, and thus the therapist will be supporting her throughout the process. The therapist also reviews the psychological benefits of approaching rather than avoiding the Evil Dark so it does not have power over her. The next four individual sessions with Kate focus on slowly increasing her exposure to discussion of the trauma. Kate and the therapist decide to make a book similar to the one they read at the beginning of therapy.

Kate first draws herself and the therapist carrying the box together and opening it up. She then provides a narrative of the trauma as if it was a nightmare with vague details. Before the next session, Kate's mother reads Psalm 91 with Kate, and Kate immediately finds solace in the psalm. She lets the therapist know she can face the trauma with God's protection. The therapist reads the psalm with her in therapy and asks Kate to draw a picture during the reading. Kate draws herself sheltered under wings with words that represent God's promises surrounding her body (peace, comfort, mercy, rescue, hope, protection), and snakes well below her feet. The therapist asks Kate to also think about what skills God has provided over the course of therapy that she can use during the trauma narratives. They review the use of body scan and relax-

ation while engaged in the narratives, as well as identifying unhelpful or untrue thoughts (distorted cognitions). With each subsequent session, Kate provides more details and concludes each story with God's presence being with her.

During the narratives, several themes are discussed regarding how the trauma affected Kate, how she has changed and grown after the trauma, and how she understands her relationship with others. The therapist supports Kate in examining her beliefs and expectations about how she should be reacting emotionally to the abuse, as well as typical emotional responses to such experiences. The narratives provide a chance to acknowledge and process Kate's anger at her grandfather and the fear the abuse instilled in her, which they relate to the anxiety already addressed in therapy. For example, she describes her realization that she struggles to manage emotions when in an argument and begins to hyperventilate when being disciplined. She is able to identify the thought that there is something wrong with her during these instances. Kate expresses feelings of not being in control and unsafe at times because she did not have power to stop the abuse. By identifying these feelings, she can understand her own suffering and recognize an opportunity to offer compassion to herself and allow compassion from others. Kate also grieves the losses she experienced as a result of the abuse and expresses increased acceptance of feeling sad about the abuse being part of her life story. She discloses that she often feels self-conscious, as if everyone knows and is looking at her. She describes feeling different from her friends and defective in some way. Unfortunately, during these sessions, Kate overhears peers at church gossiping about what happened to her. Kate and the therapist explore her reactions to this experience, and again focus on the love, compassion, and understanding others have shown her. By telling her story, Kate realizes she does not feel alone or to blame for the abuse, which she attributes to the support she has received from her parents and in therapy. She is thankful that she can see and accept God's view of her as valuable, loved, and beautifully and wonderfully made no matter what happens in her life.

Kate and her parents meet for a parent-child session to share some of Kate's selections from her narratives. Emphasis is placed on communication about emotions. Kate and her parents name the many ways Kate has shown growth in skills that will help her be resilient throughout her life. Kate shares with her parents some ways the abuse has affected her with which she could use their help. For example, she has stopped babysitting a neighbor without a clear reason. She realizes she is avoiding interactions with men (the father in this case). Kate and her parents engage in problem solving to identify ways to help Kate feel safe and prevent avoidance. They identify ways Kate can comfortably tell her parents if something makes her nervous or if something were to happen to her again. The spiritual growth of each of them through this process is discussed. They listen to the hymn "It Is Well with My Soul," and discuss what is means for things to be well with their souls. Mr. and Mrs. Reeder express amazement and gratitude that they can actually see good from this evil in their family. The therapist affirms their provision of consistent encouragement and affirmation over the course of Kate's treatment and their willingness to address things when

it was difficult for them to do so. They provided a safe space for Kate to ask questions, express her emotions, and rebuild her sense of safety. With Kate, they discuss her more positive view of herself and her abilities, their improved relationships and closeness, and how they are developing a stronger faith and sense of meaning. They see new possibilities for the future. Kate and her parents review ways they have supported each other and will continue to support each other, and with the therapist, decide that therapy can conclude.

For a celebration session (termination), Kate engages in an art activity to represent her process through therapy. Kate illustrates a triptych that is placed in a three-panel picture frame. Her first panel uses dark colors and depicts a girl sitting alone with her head in her hands and a box in front of her. The second panel depicts broken chains and rainbow colors entering the sides of the picture. The final panel is similar to a picture she drew earlier in therapy in which she is in a field of flowers with her arms outstretched, and her parents and the therapist are cheering in the forefront. While engaged in the art activity, they explore strategies to manage her distress and triggers in the future and create a plan for reinitiating services in the future if needed.

Additional considerations from a developmental psychopathology framework. Kate reports some triggers at school, so the therapist works with the school counselor to identify ways Kate could communicate when she feels overwhelmed or in distress. The school counselor initiates and develops a relationship with Kate in order to be a resource should she experience distress at school. It is important for Kate to feel like she has a support system in place at school that she could utilize in the event of increased difficulties in the future. The school is open to setting up a care system for her with requested breaks as needed. Kate needs these at the initiation of therapy but quickly utilizes coping strategies learned in therapy within the school setting. The therapist also helps Mr. and Mrs. Reeder discuss Kate's history with Kate's teacher with appropriate disclosure that was acceptable to them and to Kate. The best situation for children who have experienced trauma is placement within a classroom that is trauma-informed and with supportive peers. Further, training should be provided to teachers to ensure they understand the effects of trauma and how to support children's regulation. In this case, school leadership has emphasized trauma training over the last two years to ensure an informed understanding of the effects of trauma and how to develop a supportive culture for students. Thus, Kate's teacher is open to understanding triggers for Kate that lead to anxiety (e.g., high expressed emotions, disappointments by adults). Further, Kate has strong social skills and is in a classroom with close friends.

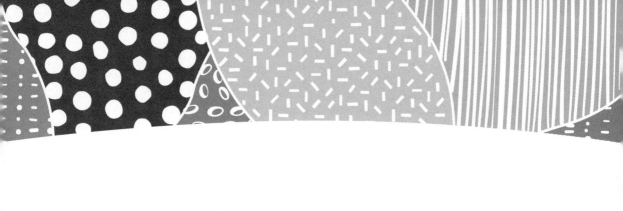

Part Three

Externalizing Disorders

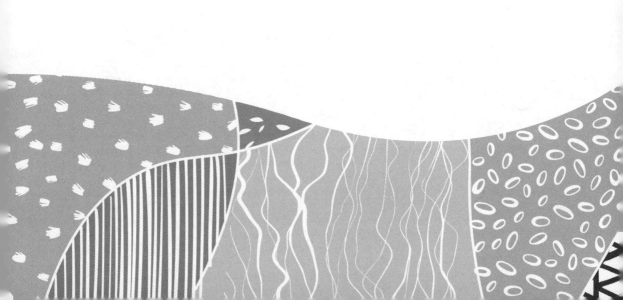

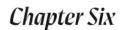

Chapter Six

Disruptive
Behavior Disorders

ISBEHAVIOR IS normative in childhood and even common in young children. However, when misbehavior is extreme in frequency or intensity, interferes with individual or family functioning, or manifests in unusual ways (e.g., cruelty to animals), it may be of clinical concern and categorized as a *disruptive behavior disorder* (DBD). DBDs are the most common reason that young children are referred for psychological services (Zisser-Nathenson et al., 2018). Two specific DBDs are recognized in DSM-5. *Oppositional defiant disorder* (ODD) is characterized by anger and irritability as well as behavior that is argumentative, defiant, and/or vindictive toward others (American Psychiatric Association, 2013). Youth must exhibit at least four of eight possible symptoms, including losing one's temper, being easily annoying, being angry and resentful, arguing with authority figures (such as parents), defying authority figures, purposefully annoying others, blaming others,

and being spiteful or vindictive. Noncompliance or defiance can include the refusal to begin or follow through with the behaviors that fulfill an adult request as well as failing to obey previously established rules, such as telling the truth or staying at the dinner table (Barkley, 2013). The symptoms of ODD are most frequently evident at home but may also occur in other settings, such as school, and must be evident not only in interactions with siblings. In addition, symptoms must occur most days (for children under age five) or at least once a week (for youth age five and older) over a period of six months, cause distress or negatively impact functioning, and be developmentally inappropriate. *Conduct disorder* (CD), generally considered the more severe of the two DBDs, involves "a repetitive and persistent pattern of behavior in which the basic rights of others or major age-appropriate societal norms or rules are violated" (American Psychiatric Association, 2013, p. 469). In order to be diagnosed with CD, youth must display at least three of fifteen possible symptoms over a twelve-month period; symptoms include bullying/intimidating others, starting physical fights, using a weapon, physical cruelty toward people, physical cruelty toward animals, robbery that involves confronting a victim, sexual assault, fire setting, destruction of others' property, breaking in (e.g., to a house or car), lying to obtain a desired item/outcome, theft, staying out past parental curfew, repeated running away from home, and frequent truancy. ODD is estimated to occur in 3.3% of youth, with CD affecting a similar percentage of the population (4%; American Psychiatric Association, 2013). Boys are more likely than girls to be diagnosed with a DBD (Maughan et al., 2004), though this gender difference may not appear until after the preschool years (Keenan & Wakschlag, 2000; Lavigne et al., 2009).

Finally, DBDs are commonly comorbid with other clinical conditions. Between one-third and one-half of children with a DBD also meet the criteria for at least one comorbid disorder (Maughan et al., 2004). ADHD is strongly associated with DBDs (Angold et al., 1999; Maughan et al., 2004), and the presence of ADHD predicts a longer duration of ODD symptoms (Biederman, Petty, et al., 2008). Parental variables, including parenting skills and parental psychopathology, significantly affect the pathway from ADHD to concurrent ODD (Goldstein, Harvey, & Friedman-Wieeneth, 2007; Harvey et al., 2011). Children with a DBD are also more likely to experience depression and anxiety (though in boys, the relationship between DBDs and anxiety appears to be accounted for by the relationship between each of these disorders and depression; Maughan et al., 2004). The links be-

tween DBDs and depression appear to be reciprocal, with DBDs increasing risk for future depression and vice versa (Blain-Arcaro & Vaillancourt, 2019).

RISK/CAUSAL FACTORS

Biological factors. Though the environmental effects on disruptive behavior appear to be stronger than the biological effects, biology does influence the development of DBDs. There are genetic underpinnings of both aggression and delinquency, with genetic factors appearing to have a stronger influence on the former (Deater-Deckard & Plomin, 1999). In addition, twin studies show that externalizing symptoms that begin in childhood are affected by genetic factors, whereas disruptive behavior that first appears in adolescence is more strongly predicted by environmental factors, as discussed later (Eley et al., 2003; Taylor et al., 2000). These findings suggest that genetic factors have a more significant effect on (1) aggressive behavior and (2) early-onset disruptive behavior than other aspects of DBDs.

Youth with DBDs show a variety of neuro-anatomical and functional differences as compared to their peers. For example, eight-year-old boys with DBDs have thinner cortices and decreased gray matter in the cingulate, prefrontal, and insular cortices, patterns thought to affect the ability to inhibit aggression and impulsive urges (Fahim et al., 2011). Adolescents with DBDs do not show normal age-related decreases in gray matter in the anterior cingulate cortex and have higher levels of connectivity between the limbic system and certain parts of the frontal lobes than nondisordered teens, suggesting that emotions may have a stronger than normal influence on decision making (Hummer et al., 2015). In addition, boys with DBDs show reduced activity in several regions of the anterior cingulate cortex (Gavita et al., 2012), a pattern that has been linked with difficulty using one's cognitive abilities to regulate emotion (Ochsner & Gross, 2005). Abnormal brain development in youth with externalizing behavior problems may occur very early in development (White et al., 2013), highlighting the complex roots of disruptive behavior.

Finally, a small body of research has examined the neuroendocrine factors that may play a role in DBDs. Hormonally, youth with DBDs show abnormalities in the activity of the hypothalamic-pituitary-adrenal (HPA) axis, including lower levels of cortisol in the morning and slower decreases throughout the day than their peers (Locke et al., 2009; Popma et al., 2007; Susman et al., 2006). Such abnormal cortisol activity may indicate a biologically based difference in how these children react and respond to stressors in their environments; for example, consequences for behavior may feel less aversive for these individuals than for youth without DBDs.

Psychological factors.

Cognitive processes. Youth with DBDs appear to process information differently than their peers during several parts of the process of encoding, interpreting, and responding to social interactions; that is, there are distinct differences in their social information processing. For example, they are more likely to inaccurately perceive others' emotional expressions as angry (Orobio de Castro et al., 2005). These children also show a hostile attribution bias, meaning that they interpret peers' ambiguous behaviors as threatening or aggressive (Crick & Dodge, 1994), which often leads to aggressive responses to others (Orobio de Castro et al., 2002). Indeed, such biases are related to aggressive behavior and violent crime commission in juvenile offenders (Dodge et al., 1990). Adolescents have been found to display similar levels of hostile attributions to those of their friends (Halligan & Philips, 2010), suggesting either a social influence on inaccurate attributions or the tendency of youth with similar attributions to associate with one another, potentially reinforcing these beliefs. In addition, the hostile attribution bias and subsequent aggressive responses may be learned from parents who model these beliefs and behaviors for their children (Healy et al., 2015; MacBrayer et al., 2003). Finally, stemming from their perceptions of others' intents as hostile, these youth view aggressive responses to social situations as beneficial, generate more potential aggressive responses, and, in turn, are more likely to respond aggressively to peers (Dodge et al., 2003; Orobio de Castro et al., 2005; Ziv, 2012). Such findings point to the importance of including cognitive interventions for aggressive children as well as their parents.

Behavioral and emotional regulation. Children with externalizing behavior problems show difficulties with self-control and self-regulation. They have difficulty regulating their behavior (e.g., delaying gratification, inhibiting emotional responses) and are more impulsive than their peers (Eisenberg et al., 2000; Lengua et al., 1998). Poor self-control during the preschool years has been found to predict aggressive behavior and even violent crime commission in adolescence (Henry et al., 1996; Robson et al., 2020). In addition, children who exhibit disruptive behavior perform poorly on executive functioning tasks, particularly those that require emotional as well as behavioral regulation (Griffith et al., 2019; Toupin et al., 2000; Woltering et al., 2016; Xu et al., 2017). In contrast, high levels of effortful control may protect at-risk youth from developing conduct problems (Morris et al., 2002; Thompson et al., 2020).

Children with DBDs also have trouble managing their emotions in appropriate or effective ways (Cole et al., 2009). Across childhood and adolescence, difficulties with emotion regulation have been linked with higher levels of externalizing symptoms such as aggression (Duncombe et al., 2013; Hall, 2014; Herts et al., 2012; Mitchison et al., 2020; Ramsden & Hubbard, 2002; Silk et al., 2003). Children who are not able to regulate their emotions well are more likely to behave in inappropriate, anger-driven, and impulsive ways. In contrast, children and adolescents who use emotion regulation strategies that are more effective at decreasing negative emotions, such as self-distraction, have lower levels of later externalizing symptoms, a link that may be mediated by peer relationships (Gilliom et al., 2002; Trentacosta & Shaw, 2009). In other words, highlighting the interactions among risk factors, youth who are able to regulate their emotions adaptively in social situations have higher quality relationships with their peers, which in turn predicts lower levels of externalizing symptoms. In addition, parenting practices such as emotion coaching that promote skillful emotion regulation in children may be protective against certain risk factors for the development of DBDs (Dunsmore et al., 2013).

Youth with externalizing symptoms display higher levels of negative emotions than their peers (Zastrow et al., 2018). Preschoolers who display disruptive behavior show more negative emotions in their interactions with their best friends than do nondisruptive children (Hughes et al., 2000). High levels of anger as well as difficulty regulating positive emotions predict externalizing behaviors in school-aged children (Rydell et al., 2003). A temperamental predisposition toward experiencing negative emotions may interfere with children's emotion regulation abilities, and poor emotion regulation may result in more negative emotions. However, it is important to note that it may not just be high levels of negative emotions that are problematic. When they were alone following a disappointment task, boys with high levels of oppositionality showed higher than normal levels of negative emotions, especially anger, whereas girls who displayed conduct problems showed lower levels of anger and sadness than their healthy peers (Cole et al., 1994). Both unusually high and unusually low levels of negative emotions may be indicative of difficulties with emotion regulation, and this finding suggests that there may be important gender differences in children with disruptive behavior problems.

Environmental factors.

Context. Low family socioeconomic status (SES) is predictive of childhood disruptive behavior problems (Boden et al., 2010; Loeber et al., 1995; Knutson et al., 2005; Mazza et al., 2017). Boys from economically disadvantaged families appear to be more likely than other children not to show the normative age-related decline in aggression from early childhood onward (Côté et al., 2006). Indeed, as many as 35% of children in low-income families may display clinical levels of conduct problems (Webster-Stratton & Hammond,

1998). Unfortunately, poorer families are less likely to show improvement with treatment and more likely to drop out (Reyno & Mc-Grath, 2006), so SES is a risk factor that must be assessed and addressed during treatment. Several potential explanations have been offered for this link between low SES and externalizing behavior problems. First, parents in low-SES families are less likely to parent sensitively and monitor their children's activities well and more likely to discipline harshly and inconsistently, perhaps because of the high level of stress they are under (Capaldi & Patterson, 1994; Knutson et al., 2005; McLoyd, 1998). Second, low SES may reflect genetic or biological risks that have either predisposed parents to living in an economically strained environment or been acquired by children who grow up in poverty, which in turn may affect parenting behaviors as well as children's well-being directly (Côté et al., 2006).

Low SES may also lead to more instability in a child's environment, which is itself a risk factor for externalizing behavior problems. Family instability (i.e., changes in parenting due to divorce, death, foster placements, etc.) and exposure to violence, including both direct abuse and exposure to domestic violence, are predictive of more severe DBD symptoms and an increased likelihood of arrest in adolescents (Boden et al., 2010; Capaldi & Patterson, 1994). Indeed, eighteen-year-olds who have been convicted of a crime are more likely than their non-offending peers to have experienced early instability in parenting and/or residence, a link that is stronger for youth who display poor self-control (Henry et al., 1996).

Finally, other youth affect children's levels of disruptive behavior. This link begins in the home; very young children who have older siblings with high levels of externalizing problems are more likely to display these behaviors themselves (Olson et al., 2020). As children age, the focus of influence moves to peers, and as early as kindergarten, children who show higher levels of conduct problems spend more time with peers who engage in disruptive behavior, which in turn predicts increases in externalizing symptoms (Snyder et al., 2005). Affiliation with deviant peers also predicts more severe conduct problems in adolescents (Boden et al., 2010). Peers appear to play an especially influential role in the development of conduct problems that begin in adolescence, as discussed later. Furthermore, peer influences do not act in isolation; for example, children who grow up in communities with a high concentration of poverty have more opportunities to associate with deviant peers, suggesting that the risk factors of low SES and negative peer influences may cluster together (Capaldi & Patterson, 1994).

Parenting. As with many other disorders, one of the most significant environmental influences on children's outcomes is parenting, which may also explain the link between other contextual risk factors, such as SES, on outcomes. Parenting variables appear to play a particularly strong role in the development of disruptive behavior. Children with DBDs are more likely than their peers to have parents who discipline inconsistently and/or harshly, display insensitivity and overly controlling behavior toward children, express negative emotions toward family members, and report higher levels of family conflict (Di Giunta et al., 2020; Duncombe et al., 2012; Healy et al., 2015; Lavigne et al., 2019; Waller et al., 2018;

Webster-Stratton & Hammond, 1998). Overall, the patterns of parenting that have been linked with externalizing behaviors in children involve inconsistent discipline (e.g., the same behaviors are not consistently punished/rewarded, parents give in to children's misbehavior, expectations and consequences change unpredictably, there is significant variation between the disciplinary responses and expectations of two caregivers in a family), irritable and explosive discipline (e.g., parents yell and hit, parent-child conflicts are long and intense, parents use more intense and frequent punitive discipline), inflexible and rigid disciple (e.g., parents use the same disciplinary strategy for all types of misbehavior, parents do not explain consequences and their causes to the child, parents don't adjust their responses based on the context or severity of the misbehavior), and low parental involvement (e.g., parents rarely engage with children, parents are unaware of children's peers and activities, parents do not provide supervision for children who are associating with negative peers; Chamberlain et al., 1997). While these parenting practices are generally understood to contribute to children's behavior problems, there is some evidence that the links are reciprocal, with interactions between children and parents becoming more negative as externalizing symptoms worsen (Liu et al., 2018; Rolon-Arroyo et al., 2018). Finally, on the extreme end of the parenting spectrum, maltreatment appears to play a causal role in increasing antisocial behavior in children and adolescents, particularly when it occurs early in development (Calhoun et al., 2019; Docherty et al., 2018; Jaffee et al., 2004).

The pattern of parent-child interaction that is generally seen in DBDs has been termed coercive family process (Patterson, 1982; Forgatch & Patterson, 2010). A coercive interaction may unfold as follows. First, the child misbehaves in some way, such as throwing a tantrum when asked to clean up her toys. The conflict between the parent and the child escalates as the parent repeats the command more loudly, the child ignores the parent and continues to tantrum, and the parent becomes more upset and forceful with the command. The interaction generally ends when one party "gives in" to the other; in this example, as in many cases of the coercive cycle, the parent may stop attempting to get the child to clean up and instead end the unpleasant interaction, likely leading the child to stop tantrumming. Through such patterns of interaction, the behavior of both the child and the parent are shaped by the principles of operant conditioning. The child's misbehavior (tantrumming) is reinforced when parental attention increases and the child ultimately gets her way (avoiding cleaning up); the parent's attempt to elicit the child's compliance is punished by the beginning/intensifying of the child's tantrum, and the parent's giving in to the child is reinforced by the end of the child's tantrum. Therefore, in a future interaction, both the parent and the child are likely to repeat their respective behavior, creating a cycle of coercion. In families seeking treatment for children's behavior problems, these conflictual cycles occur, on average, every sixteen minutes (Patterson, 1982).

A number of other parental factors, which likely affect parents' interactions with their children, predict externalizing symptoms. Children with parents who have psychological problems or abuse substances are more likely to develop conduct problems

(Baker & Kuhn, 2018; Breaux et al., 2014; Clark et al., 2004; Loeber et al., 1995). In addition, children show fewer improvements in DBD treatment when their mothers have psychological disorders, and maternal depression is a predictor of treatment dropout as well as poorer treatment outcomes (Muratori et al., 2015; Reyno & McGrath, 2006). Illustrating the transactional nature of the impact of child and parent variables on one another, there is also evidence that coercive interactions between mothers and young children increase mothers' depressive symptoms (Hails et al., 2018). Therefore, assessing and intervening in parental variables, including both parenting techniques and the factors that affect parenting styles, is an important component of treatment.

DEVELOPMENTAL COURSE

ODD is the most common disorder in early childhood (Lavigne et al., 2009), with one study of a nonclinical sample of two- to five-year-olds finding a prevalence rate of over 16%, though only half of these children displayed impairment because of their symptoms (Lavigne et al., 1996). According to the Oregon model (Forgatch & Patterson, 2010), DBDs generally begin with overt behaviors such as tantrums, hitting, and biting that are unknowingly reinforced by parents' responses to them (see full discussion of coercive family process above). Indeed, the most common symptoms of ODD in preschool-aged children are defiance, losing one's temper, arguing, and annoying others, whereas young children diagnosed with CD commonly start fights, bully others, use objects to hurt others, and lie (Keenan & Wakschlag, 2000).

Because oppositionality and noncompliance are common behaviors in early childhood, peaking during the toddler years and then declining (Côté et al., 2006; Lavigne et al., 1996), it is important to compare a child's symptoms to normative levels of these behaviors in order to understand whether they are truly elevated (American Psychiatric Association, 2013). Furthermore, reports of clinically significant behavior problems in early childhood are fairly unstable (NICHD Early Child Care Research Network, 1998), which may suggest that clinicians should be especially cautious in diagnosing children younger than three to four years of age, after which there is more diagnostic stability (Bufferd, Dougherty, Carlson, Rose, & Klein, 2012). However, the commonality of misbehavior in early childhood does not mean that problem behavior should be ignored or assumed to be transient, as externalizing symptoms at age two predict future difficulties in some children (Keenan et al., 1999), and a valid DBD diagnosis can be made using developmentally sensitive methods in preschool-aged children (Keenan & Wakschlag, 2002, 2004). Whereas some externalizing behavior is typical in young children, there are certain behaviors that are seen in preschoolers with conduct disorder but not in healthy populations, including high-intensity defiance, aggression toward people and animals, severe destruction of property, and high levels of lying and stealing (Hong et al., 2015). Accurate early identification is important because some treatment protocols are designed to be utilized in early childhood in order to address risk factors and ameliorate their effects before they become entrenched (e.g., The Incredible Years; Webster-Stratton & Reid, 2010).

Many children outgrow their externalizing behaviors as they age. Even during the preschool years, only a small portion of children who are diagnosed with a DBD will still meet criteria for the disorder two years later (Lavigne et al., 1998; Kim-Cohen et al., 2005). For others, these problem behaviors will continue or even worsen. There appear to be essentially two groups of children: those who display clinically significant levels of disruptive behavior throughout development and those whose externalizing symptoms are limited to either early childhood or adolescence. As in early childhood, disruptive behaviors become more normative in adolescence (Atherton et al., 2018; Patterson & Yoerger, 2002). However, of the adolescents who display antisocial or disruptive behavior, some of them continue to display these behaviors into adulthood (frequently leading to legal trouble), whereas others desist by the end of adolescence (Patterson & Yoerger, 2002). Youth whose disruptive behavior begins in childhood and continues through adolescence are sometimes described as having "life-course-persistent" antisocial behavior (Moffitt, 1993). The roots of this early-onset, persistent disruptive behavior likely take hold at a young age. Life-course-persistent youth frequently have neuropsychological deficits, such as problems with executive functions, low IQ, and developmental delays (Moffitt, 1990; Moffitt et al., 2001), as well as cognitive patterns characterized by impulsivity, aggression, and suspicion toward others (Moffitt et al., 1996). In addition, youth with early-onset disruptive behavior are more likely than their adolescence-limited peers to experience early family dysfunction, including ineffective parenting, family conflict, parental antisocial behavior and mental

health problems, and parental unemployment, which suggests that patterns of family interaction and instability may promote persistent disruptive behavior (Capaldi & Patterson, 1994; Patterson & Yoerger, 2002). These individuals also have more social difficulties and lower self-esteem.

A larger number of adolescents display problem behaviors beginning in adolescence and ending by early adulthood, known as "adolescence-limited delinquency" (Moffitt, 1993). For these youth, antisocial behavior is less violent and appears to emerge as a response to the immediate environment (specifically, peer demands) and end when it no longer serves a clear function (Moffitt et al., 1996). It appears that involvement with peers who are engaged in and encourage delinquent activities leads to increased antisocial behavior, a phenomenon known as "deviancy training" (Dishion et al., 1996). It is thought that associations with deviant peers play a strong role in the development of behavior problems in this group of adolescents. Indeed, youth who display problem behavior beginning in adolescence have better peer relationships than youth whose antisocial behavior begins in childhood (Patterson & Yoerger, 2002), which may suggest that they adapt their behavior to the demands of the proximal social situation. These youth are also closer with their parents (Moffitt et al., 1996) and have fewer coercive interactions with them (Patterson & Yoerger, 2002), suggesting that the lack of reinforcement for antisocial behavior in the family setting may help explain the time-limited nature of the behavior. Across both types of delinquency, DBDs in adolescence are more likely to be characterized by covert or surreptitious behaviors—

such as stealing, lying, running away, truancy, and substance use—than by overt activities such as aggression and open defiance (Forgatch & Patterson, 2010; Maughan et al., 2004).

Assessment

In addition to an evaluation of the risk or causal factors that may play a role in the development and maintenance of symptoms for a given client, the assessment of DBDs must include a focus on (1) the child's behavior and (2) the child's interactions with significant others in her life (e.g., parents, teachers, siblings, peers; McMahon & Estes, 1997). Therefore, clinicians should begin the assessment process with interviews with parents and the child to begin to understand the target problem behaviors. The clinician will also generally find it helpful to ask the child's parents and teacher (and the child herself, if she is older) to complete questionnaires that include scales assessing oppositional and aggressive behavior (see McMahon & Frick, 2005, for a list of assessment tools for DBDs). Finally, given the likelihood of coercive interactions within the family, assessment also needs to include an observation of the parent-child dyad or triad, which can take place in the office or in the family's home. During the observation, the parent and child may be instructed to engage in a variety of activities, including free play, child-directed play, parent-directed play, cooperative tasks, and compliance tasks (Schroeder & Gordon, 2002). The clinician may want to pay particular attention to certain aspects of the parent-child interaction, such as how frequently and in what manner the parent asks questions, praises the child, gives commands, and pays attention to the child's behavior. It is also valuable to note the child's response to parent-initiated activities, especially compliance tasks, and the parent's reaction to any child noncompliance.

A functional analysis of behavior is a key component of understanding how an individual child's disruptive behavior is being inadvertently created and/or maintained by interactions with adults. Clinicians often explain the nuances of these interactions as the "ABCs": antecedents (A), behaviors (B), and consequences (C; Kazdin, 2005). Antecedents are any stimuli or contexts that precede or influence behavior before it occurs, and consequences are events that follow a behavior and can reinforce (i.e., increase the likelihood it will occur again) or punish it (i.e., decrease the likelihood of recurrence). Although families are generally interested in changing the child's behaviors themselves, behavioral interventions target the antecedents and consequences of behavior because they are alterable by others and can in turn influence behavior; thus, the therapist and parents can effectively impact the child's behavior by changing the stimuli or contexts that influence, reinforce, or punish the behavior. Therefore, the events and situations that precede and follow a child's misbehavior must be thoroughly assessed. An analysis of antecedents and consequences leads to a better understanding of the function or purpose of a child's behavior (e.g., Why is the child behaving disruptively? How is he benefiting from the misbehavior?). Functional analysis of behavior can be based either on clinical observations of the family or detailed parental report of the child's behavior in other settings.

For example, consider a five-year-old child who throws a tantrum at bedtime every day. A functional analysis of behavior might reveal that most evenings she is wrestling with her siblings until 9:00 p.m., at which point her parents tell her it is time to go to bed. She ignores them until they pick her up and carry her to her room, at which point she begins to kick, scream, and cry. One or both parents spend an average of two hours in her room trying to calm her down, after which she falls asleep in their arms out of exhaustion. In this situation, antecedents to the bedtime resistance include playing actively and enjoying her time with siblings, being given no warning that bedtime is approaching, and having a late bedtime. The consequences that follow the tantrum include individual attention and physical comfort from her parents as well as falling asleep in their arms, which she may have come to depend on in order to soothe herself to sleep. This example offers a number of potential targets for intervention, in terms of both antecedents and consequences, that are likely to reduce the child's tantrums at bedtime.

It is also important to assess whether the child's problem behavior is indeed at a level that requires clinical intervention. Because all children misbehave, and oppositional behavior is common during certain developmental periods (such as early childhood and adolescence; Côté et al., 2006; Patterson & Yoerger, 2002), it is possible that parents or teachers with unrealistic expectations for children's compliance could view normative levels or types of misbehavior as problematic (McMahon & Frick, 2005). The use of questionnaires with age- and gender-normed data, as well as a thorough assessment of impairment, is helpful in distinguishing between normative and problematic levels of conduct problems. Finally, as with the assessment of

any disorder in youth, it is important to evaluate both the presence of any comorbid disorders and the specific risk factors and developmental pathways that have shaped the child's current maladaptive behavior in order to design the best possible treatment for a client (McMahon & Frick, 2005).

TREATMENT

A number of behaviorally based, family-focused treatment approaches have been found to be effective for treating youth with DBDs (Kaminski & Claussen, 2017; McCart & Sheidow, 2016). There is variance among approaches, but effective treatments for these disorders are generally highly structured and share certain components. Garland et al. (2008) outline the common elements of effective treatments for DBDs; we will describe these common elements according to their categorizations and then give examples of treatment programs that utilize them.

Before we begin to describe these treatment elements, it is important to note that there are a variety of factors that impact how effective an intervention is for a particular youth with a DBD. Such factors include aspects of the family environment and characteristics that may reduce parents' ability to engage consistently in the often-taxing components of treatment, such as changing disciplinary techniques; for example, parental unemployment, a parent's depressive symptoms, and low family income are each associated with a poorer response to treatment (Shelleby & Kolko, 2015). In addition, racial, ethnic, and/or cultural minority families may respond differently to these interventions than white families, with whom most of the treatment development and research has been conducted

(Forehand & Kotchick, 2016; McNeil et al., 2002). The behaviorally based parenting interventions most commonly used in the treatment of DBDs are inherently based on a particular set of values, assumptions, and norms for family dynamics and child socialization goals; it is possible that if these underlying ideas are inconsistent with a family's parenting-related values, including those that are culturally based, an intervention will be less acceptable or effective for a particular client. For example, Neal-Barnett and Smith (1996) argue that traditional behavioral approaches do not take into account the values of relationality, extended family and social networks, and culturally normative expressivity that are inherent in an Afrocentric view of development and behavior. A clinician who is unfamiliar with black culture, then, runs the risk of overemphasizing the centrality of the individual over the community, failing to include family members outside of the home in the assessment and intervention process, and/or misinterpreting verbal or physical expressions out of context. These mistakes can lead to a lack of trust between the clinician and the family, who may feel that their views are misunderstood or even dismissed, as well as to attempts to encourage families to implement parenting practices that may not fit well with their community's parenting practices and views of youth. Therefore, it is important for clinicians working with culturally different families to take the time to understand a particular family's unique goals for parenting and for their child's development as well as the role of each family and community member in supporting those goals.

Common treatment elements.

The parent-child relationship. Changes in discipline and parenting strategies are un-
likely to be effective without the foundation of a positive relationship between the child and the parent in which warmth, sensitivity, and care are evident (Zisser-Nathenson et al., 2018). Therefore, many DBD interventions begin with activities aimed at promoting positive parent-child interactions. One such activity involves the parent spending purposeful time each day focused on the child, known as "child-directed activity" (CDI; Zisser-Nathenson et al., 2018) or "special time" (Barkley, 2013). During this period (typically twenty minutes or so), the child leads the interaction and chooses the play activity, while the parent follows the child's lead. The parent uses skills such as praising specific child behaviors, reflecting the child's verbalizations, and narrating the child's play in order to purposefully attend to the child's behavior, reinforce positive behaviors, and spend time engaged positively with the child (Barkley, 2013; Zisser-Nathenson et al., 2018). In contrast, parents are instructed to be careful not to speak to the child in ways that may inadvertently take the lead from the child or introduce a negative tone to the interaction; specifically, parents should avoid giving commands, asking questions, or speaking critically to the child. Minor misbehavior, such as yelling, should be ignored by the parent during these interactions. Parents should end the child-led time, however, if the child engages in more major disruptive actions, such as hitting or breaking objects, and begin it again at a later time. (At this point in most treatment protocols, parents have not yet worked with the therapist on discipline techniques, which will come after positive parent-child interactions are more consistent, as described below.) Though many interventions focus on describing

special time with young children, it is also valuable to use with adolescents, with whom it may take the form of engaging in a fun activity together (e.g., playing video games, baking, going for a walk, playing basketball, going out for coffee or ice cream, going shopping) or having a conversation around a topic selected by the child during which the parent listens, supports, and expresses empathy but does not challenge or argue.

Positive reinforcement. Parents are encouraged to pay purposeful attention to children's positive behaviors (e.g., listening to the parent, sharing, playing quietly) and reinforce the behaviors they want to see continue or increase, which can also have the effect of reducing negative behaviors (Kazdin, 2005). Child-led time introduces these skills to parents, though their application is expanded to other times and types of interactions, including times when the child is playing appropriately and independently (Barkley, 2013). Desired behaviors can be positively reinforced through nontangible means, such as verbal praise or hugs, or through material rewards, such as stickers or privileges. The Parent Management Training—Oregon Model (PMT-OM), for example, teaches parents to pair social reinforcers with material rewards. Families create incentive charts (or "sticker charts") to reward children for completing routine behaviors, such as chores, and to help visually track their positive behaviors over time, which can be rewarding in itself for children. Within a token economy system, tokens (e.g., points) can be exchanged for candy or small toys; this system allows parents to reward discrete positive behaviors, such as staying beside a parent in the grocery store, with points on an immediate basis without

having to carry around rewarding items. When a child is materially rewarded as well as praised for a positive behavior, even children who do not initially respond to social reinforcers will come to desire them (Forgatch & Patterson, 2010). Reinforcement will be most effective when it is only provided when the desired behavior occurs, immediately following the behavior, after every instance of the behavior, and in a form that is truly appealing to the child (Kazdin, 2005).

Some programs (e.g., Barkley, 2013) teach parents to utilize "compliance training periods" to allow parents to practice giving effective commands and children to practice (and be reinforced for) obeying them. Compliance training periods are brief chunks of time (three to five minutes) that are implemented two to three times per day when the child is otherwise unoccupied. During this time, the parent gives the child a series of simple commands requiring minimal effort and which the child will find easy to follow. Parents might use commands such as, "Hand me the glass," and "Put the crackers on the table." Children, even defiant children, are likely to obey these simple, easy commands. Following the completion of each task, the parent should explicitly reward the child's compliance with tangible rewards (for younger children) and/or praise. The parent is "training" the child to comply with simple tasks in order to increase the likelihood of compliance with more complex or difficult tasks at other times.

Zisser-Nathenson and colleagues (2018) outline several guidelines for giving effective commands. First, commands should be clear and direct, communicating that the child is being given an instruction and not a choice (e.g., "Put the toy on the table" rather than "Can you put the toy on the table?"). Second, commands should be specific so that the child knows exactly what is expected (e.g., "Sit down in your chair" rather than "Be careful"). Third, commands should be phrased positively, so that the child is clearly being instructed on what they should do (e.g., "Keep your hands in your lap" rather than "Don't touch your sister"). Fourth, commands should be given one at a time so that the child does not forget what she is supposed to do (e.g., "Brush your teeth" rather than "Brush your teeth, put on your pajamas, and pick out a book"). Fifth, commands need to be age appropriate (e.g., "Put the apple in this bowl" rather than "Put the produce in the right drawer in the refrigerator" to a young child). Sixth, parents should not explain the rationale for the command immediately after it is given (such as when the child asks "Why?" before complying). Otherwise, children may use explanation seeking to avoid obeying a command, and an explanation given at this time is not likely to be heard. Rather, the reason for a command can be explained either before it is given (e.g., "Someone could trip and fall on the blocks. Please put them in the blue basket") or after it is obeyed (e.g., "Thank you for putting your plate in the sink. It is helpful to Daddy to not have to carry everything by himself"). Finally, parents should use a polite and respectful tone when they give commands, which helps the child learn that calm statements (not just angry-sounding ones) need to be obeyed and models appropriate interactions with others for them.

Many interventions (e.g., Webster-Stratton & Reid, 2010) emphasize the importance of improving the parent-child relationship and increasing parenting skills during positive interactions as the initial focus of treatment. Misbehavior can be significantly reduced through the use of child-directed time, reinforcement, and effective commands. Parents and children generally also enjoy the time spent working on these skills, as they engender a positive relationship and a sense of warmth, care, and success within the family. Once these parenting skills have been mastered, significant misbehavior may still remain, at which point the focus of treatment shifts to developing effective disciplinary techniques.

Limit setting and punishment. In addition to reinforcing positive behavior with the goal of decreasing negative behavior, disruptive actions generally need to be directly addressed in treatment. The first step in implementing effective disciplinary techniques involves setting clear limits and communicating these clearly to the child. Rules and expectations should be made explicit and communicated in a developmentally appropriate manner; some families may choose to display a written version of rules targeting misbehavior in a common area of the home. For example, families or parents might create rules such as, "You must obey the first time Daddy or Mommy asks you to do something," "Keep both feet on the floor when you're sitting at the table," or "You must get Mom or Dad's permission before you leave the house." In addition to making rules and expectations explicit, the consequences for breaking rules need to be determined and communicated clearly to the child before the infraction occurs. Consequences will vary depending on the rule (and, therefore, the severity of breaking it) and perhaps even be different for each child (depending on age), but children should be aware of and able to identify the consequences for misbehaviors that are being targeted by parents. Before entering a situation in which misbehavior has occurred in the past, the parent can remind the child about the rules and consequences and ask the child to repeat them back to assess understanding (e.g., "We are going to story time at the library now. If you scream or yell while we are there, we will come home. What happens if you scream while we are at story time?"). As parents must be prepared to follow through with the consequences that are explained to children, families should think these through ahead of time to make sure they are feasible and agreeable to the parent; otherwise, consequences may become empty threats and have no impact on or even worsen a child's behavior. (One classic example of a consequence that is rarely followed through with is when a parent yells to children arguing in the car on a family road trip, "If you don't stop fighting, I'll turn this car around!")

Some misbehavior is minor, without direct disobedience or the potential to harm people or objects and done mainly for attention. For example, some parents report that their children play quietly until they are on an important phone call, at which point the child begins to make a lot of noise or approach them with requests. At the dinner table, a child might start flipping his peas onto the table with his fork when his parents are both talking to his sister and not attending to him. Such behaviors are best addressed by ignoring (i.e., not reinforcing) them, which serves in operant conditioning terms to extinguish them (Kazdin, 2005). If the main purpose of the minor misbehavior is truly parental attention, then consistent ignoring will remove

the reinforcement, and the child will eventually stop the behavior. It is important to note, however, that it may require some trial and error in order to determine the purpose of the child's behavior and, therefore, the most effective response (ignoring, punishing, reinforcing an alternative behavior, etc.).

When a child disobeys a clear command or misbehaves in other significant ways, punishment is used to decrease the likelihood that the behavior will occur again in the future. One form of punishment that is commonly taught in the treatment of DBDs is time-out, which is sometimes known as "time-out from reinforcement" (e.g., Kazdin, 2005). A child who does not comply with a parental command is given a warning (e.g., "If you don't put the blocks away, you will get a time-out."), followed by a brief (e.g., five-second) waiting period by the parent. If the child still does not obey the command, a time-out is initiated, and the child is told why he is receiving a time-out in a simple statement (e.g., "You are going to time-out because you did not put the blocks away like I asked"; Zisser-Nathenson et al., 2018). The time-out should take place in a designated spot that is separate from the main area of family activity but still within view of the parent (e.g., on the bottom step of a staircase, in a chair in the corner) and not in a place where inadvertent reinforcement is occurring. For example, time-out should not take place on the couch in front of the television that others are watching or in a child's room where she can play. Parents should ignore misbehavior that occurs during a time-out. Different interventions teach different methods for determining the appropriate length of a time-out, but they are consistent in establishing that the parent should be in control of communicating when the time-out ends (rather than saying, "You can get up when you are ready to obey"; Zisser-Nathenson et al., 2018). Time-out might last for a certain amount of time, such as three minutes plus five seconds of quiet (Zisser-Nathenson et al., 2018) or one minute for each year of the child's age plus thirty seconds of quiet (Barkley, 2013). During the time-out, no one should engage with the child verbally or physically, as these activities can serve to reinforce the misbehavior with one-on-one attention. Once the predetermined time is over, the child should be told that time-out can end if he is ready to obey the original command. If the child responds that he is not ready to obey, then the time-out begins again. If the child complies with the original command, the parent should factually acknowledge the obedience but not be overly reinforcing. The parent may then give another simple command, which the child is likely to obey, after which she may more enthusiastically praise the child for the compliance. This distinction in parental response occurs so as not to be overly reinforcing of a behavior that is part of the time-out sequence (Zisser-Nathenson et al., 2018). If the child leaves the time-out chair or spot repeatedly, the parent may send her to a time-out room (Zisser-Nathenson et al., 2018) or her bedroom, provided all toys and games have been removed from the latter (Barkley, 2013), until the time-out conditions (elapsed time, quiet, and compliance) have been met. Parents who prefer not to utilize a time-out room can use other forms of punishment for leaving the time-out chair.

The removal of privileges is another form of discipline that can be useful. A child who misbehaves might have his cellphone, video-game use, or outdoor play time taken away for a short time (fifteen to thirty minutes) following the disobedience (Forgatch & Patterson, 2010). Kazdin (2005) notes, however, that parents and clinicians should be mindful of the long-term negative effect of punishing through the removal of activities that promote healthy development, such as playing outside or spending time with friends. Finally, punishments such as fines or extra chores can be imposed on youth, especially as a consequence for covert or serious misbehavior. When possible, therapists and parents should select natural or logical consequences for a child's misbehavior. For example, a child who becomes angry and throws a toy against the wall, breaking the toy, no longer has a whole or working toy. The parents should not fix or replace the toy, as having a broken toy is a naturally occurring consequence for throwing it. An adolescent who lies to her parents about where she was on Saturday night must be accompanied by her parents whenever she leaves the house the following weekend, which is a logical consequence for untrustworthy behavior. Natural and logical consequences help children better understand the impact of disruptive or destructive behavior and develop more adaptive behaviors in the long term.

It is important to note that punishment can have a number of negative side effects on children, including distress, aggressive responses, and the modeling of punishing behavior. In addition, it often feels unpleasant for parents to administer, though some parents of children with DBDs will come to therapy using harsh and ineffective methods of punishment out of desperation to change their child's behavior. For these reasons, a focus on discipline is necessary in therapy, and clinicians might aim to help parents utilize punishment only in situations in which the child's behavior is dangerous and needs to be stopped immediately, the positive alternative behavior cannot readily be reinforced, and in which it is viewed as a temporary measure to decrease negative behavior while reinforcement is being used to increase desired behaviors (Kazdin, 2005). In addition, clinicians should work with parents on how to administer punishment without yelling or arguing with the child, which often delay the implementation of consequences and make the disciplinary interaction more unpleasant than necessary for parents and youth. Finally, though the discussion and implementation of disciplinary techniques may be a significant focus during certain phases of treatment, and punishment may need to be used frequently when it is first introduced, parents should be made aware of the importance of using punishment sparingly in the long run so as to minimize the potential for negative effects on the child and the parent-child relationship.

Problem-solving skills. Children with DBDs often display distortions in the way they view situations and other people, such as the hostile attribution bias (Crick & Dodge, 1994), which lead to aggressive and hostile behaviors. Therefore, teaching children how to select more appropriate responses to social situations can help reduce problem behavior. Problem-solving skills training has several core steps that are taught to children in sequence (Kazdin, 2010). First, children are taught to identify a problem situation that requires a response or solution. Second, children are taught to generate possible solutions and,

third, how to evaluate potential consequences of each solution. Fourth, children are taught that they need to choose and carry out the solution that appears to be best based on possible consequences. Fifth, children learn to evaluate how well the response actually worked and to go back to the selection of a different response from step two if necessary. Creative applications of these skills can include role-playing with the therapist or parents, practicing these skills in vivo in a group therapy setting, videotaping problem-solving vignettes, or creating cartoons or comic books that illustrate successful problem solving (e.g., Lochman et al., 2010).

For example, a ten-year-old client might be exhibiting aggressive behavior toward his classmates on the playground. In exploring his thoughts and behaviors, the clinician learns that he perceives his classmates to be excluding him from their basketball games at recess. When he comes out onto the playground and sees a basketball game in progress, he becomes angry and tries to take the ball away from the child who is holding it, resulting in a negative reaction from his peers and the consequence of spending recess inside with the teacher. During the course of problem-solving skills training, the client learns to put into words that the problem is that he would like to play basketball on the playground, but the game has always already started by the time he walks outside. The clinician helps him identify the solution he usually implements (grabbing the ball) as well as the consequences that occur (being excluded, spending recess inside). The child and the clinician then brainstorm other possible solutions (asking the other children if he can join the game, asking an adult on the playground to ask the other children to include him, starting another game on the other basketball court, finding another fun activity) as well as their potential consequences. With the clinician's guidance, the child decides to try to start another game of basketball on his next day of school, as this does not necessitate confronting his peers and will not result in negative consequences from adults. However, when he comes in to therapy the next week, the child tells the clinician that he discovered that his class only has one basketball, so he was unable to use the solution they selected. The client and the therapist then go back to the list of possible solutions and consequences, add new ones if desired (such as using a soccer ball instead of a basketball), and select a solution for the child to implement the next time the situation arises.

Emotion understanding. Accurately interpreting the physical and cognitive signs associated with different emotions, as well as understanding the effects of emotions on behavior, are skills with which youth with DBDs may struggle (Kimonis et al., 2014). Therefore, before emotions such as anger can be effectively managed, therapists may need to work with children on emotional understanding. One approach that focuses on coping with anger teaches children to view the physiological signs of anger as the body's "early warning system" about the need to be aware of and cognitively manage one's behavior in the face of emotion (Larson & Lochman, 2011). Therapists working with children around emotion understanding should focus on one emotion at a time, and though children with DBDs may have trouble understanding a variety of emotions, anger will almost always be a target of intervention.

Emotion understanding sessions generally aim to help youth define the emotion, recognize their own bodily signs of the emotion, recognize expressions of the emotion in others, and explore their thought patterns when they experience the emotion. In addition, it is important to help children understand what situations, particularly social situations, evoke various emotions for them. Discussion, videos, photos, and role-playing are useful tools for helping children explore these different aspects of emotional experience and expression. Older children and adolescents can be encouraged to keep a journal of their emotion experiences, documenting the triggering event, the location, the emotion and its intensity, their behavioral response, and an evaluation of how well the situation was handled (Larson & Lochman, 2011). As emotion understanding work progresses, helpful and unhelpful self-talk during emotional experiences can also be a useful component of a feelings journal.

Anger regulation. Children with DBDs, particularly those who are aggressive, often struggle to manage their anger itself as well as their behavior when they are angry (Lochman et al., 1997). Therefore, while parents play a role in shaping behavior, an important component of treatment involves helping youth themselves learn to regulate their anger in ways that promote positive behavior. Once children learn to better understand the physiological signs of anger and their own anger triggers, as discussed earlier, they can also begin to understand the cognitive processes that often accompany anger. It has been suggested that aggressive children encode details of interactions with others differently than their nonaggressive peers, such that they pay attention to fewer overall cues and are more likely to remember aspects of the interaction that might signal hostility (Lochman et al., 1999). Furthermore, these children are more likely to interpret others' ambiguous behavior as hostile (Crick & Dodge, 1994). Therefore, these cognitive distortions must be addressed in order to help aggressive children regulate their anger and respond more appropriately in social situations.

One method for reducing misinterpretations of others' intentions is to improve children's perspective-taking skills. In one group therapy approach (Larson & Lochman, 2011; Lochman et al., 1999, 2010), children are asked to interpret ambiguous interactions between characters in a picture. The children then role-play the ambiguous scenarios and share their perspectives on the situation from the point of view of the different characters. Each "character" is asked to share what he noticed about the situation, what he was thinking about, what he was feeling, and how he thought others might be thinking and feeling. The therapist leads a discussion of the differences between individuals' responses in order to help clients understand that people have different views of the same situation and that it is difficult to know what other people are thinking.

Children may be taught other anger management techniques as well. Puppets can be used to model self-talk, in which children coach themselves verbally (often internally) to respond to anger-evoking stimuli in a more adaptive manner. For example, a child who is being teased might say to himself, "I'm starting to get mad, and I want to be careful not to get too angry and lose my temper. I think I'll ask them to stop and see if that works" (Larson & Lochman, 2011, p. 99).

Children can also be taught to distract themselves from the anger-provoking situation by shifting their visual or cognitive focus elsewhere. Finally, diaphragmatic breathing, in which a child takes slow, deep breaths, can serve as both a distraction and a tool to reduce the physiological signs of anger, decreasing the intensity of the child's anger so that she can respond to the situation more appropriately. If therapy is done in a group setting, children may even practice their anger management skills in vivo while they are being taunted by other members of the group (Lochman et al., 1999).

Preparation for setbacks and relapse prevention. Each session should begin with a review of the previous session's content as well as the child's progress during the time between sessions in order to reinforce the implementation of skills learned in therapy and address problems and frustrations as they arise rather than at the end of the treatment program. In addition, it is important to explain to parents that disruptive behavior will generally increase when disciplinary methods such as time-outs are initially implemented. As described by the coercive family process theory (Patterson, 1982), children with DBDs have learned over the course of hundreds of interactions with their parents that they can "get their own way" if they persist in their misbehavior. Therefore, children will often escalate their misbehavior when discipline is introduced, as this behavior has been reinforced in the past. In conditioning terms, this is known as an "extinction burst" and is actually a sign that the change in discipline is beginning to work (Kazdin, 2005). For this reason, it is very important for the parents to understand that "things may get worse before they get better," to be consistent in their implementation of time-out and other disciplinary techniques, and to follow through with all treatment components until the goal (e.g., child compliance) is accomplished; otherwise, parents risk actually increasing problem behavior by intermittently reinforcing it and teaching children that disruptive behavior is an effective method of achieving their goals.

Barkley (2013) recommends providing parents with specific steps for addressing new or reoccurring problem behaviors. Parents are encouraged to keep a written record of the misbehavior, including the circumstances around it, in order to assess why it is occurring and how it might best be addressed. Parents should then review the skills they have learned—including nurturing the parent-child relationship though "special time," giving effective commands, rewarding positive behaviors consistently, and using time-outs and other punishments immediately and effectively—and assess whether they need to improve the implementation of any of these skills. Finally, parents are instructed to set up and explain to the child the plan for addressing the problem behavior, continuing to keep a written record of the child's behavior and how it is addressed, and to follow up with the therapist if additional support is desired or improvement does not occur. Therapists may prepare parents for this process by introducing hypothetical scenarios toward the end of the intervention and providing support while the parents assess the situation and make a plan to address the potential problem behavior. Clinicians may also want to schedule a booster session with parents about one month after the final treatment session in order to assess the family's progress and address any new questions or problems before they become more significant (Barkley, 2013).

In summary, the common components of effective treatments for DBDs include parent-focused components aimed at improving the parent-child relationship, the use of positive reinforcement, effective limit setting and punishment, and relapse prevention, as well as youth-focused elements that address problem-solving skills, emotion understanding, and anger regulation. It is important to note that while these treatments are often manualized and the skills they teach standardized, care must be taken to tailor the intervention to the needs and problems of an individual client and his family. For this reason, there is flexibility within each treatment component as well as a number of specific treatment approaches that have been developed to include these common core elements as well as other unique components. A number of specific behavioral interventions that have been found to be effective for treating DBDs are summarized below, and clinicians may select different treatment protocols for different clients depending on age, developmental level, family strengths and challenges, and the main risk or causal factors that have been identified in the assessment process.

Specific treatment approaches.

Defiant Children. Barkley's (2013) treatment program focuses on changing the coercive interactions that have developed between oppositional children (ages two to twelve) and their parents. After a thorough assessment—including evaluation of development, symptoms, impairment, and family risk factors—parents are taught the basic principles of operant conditioning and the impact of risk factors on parent and child behavior. Parents then learn techniques to increase their positive interactions with their children and reward desired behavior, such as "special time," the use of praise, giving effective commands, and using token reward systems. Once parents have mastered these skills, they work with the therapist to implement effective and consistent punishments for misbehavior, including time-outs and token system "fines." The Defiant Children approach also includes a component in which parents work with the therapist to develop a plan to specifically prevent and address misbehavior in public places. The Barkley program has been found to effectively treat oppositional behavior in children with DBDs as well as those with ADHD (Curtis, 2010; Danforth et al., 2006).

The Incredible Years. The Incredible Years program (Webster-Stratton & Reid, 2010) uses a multifaceted approach that includes parent, child, and teacher components to address the many risk factors that lead to the development of conduct problems. The Incredible Years program utilizes interactive video instruction in which positive skills are explained and modeled for clients, who engage with the video material with a therapist. The parent component of the program teaches the parenting skills typically covered in DBD interventions; however, it also includes material to assist parents with other personal skills (e.g., positive-self talk, anger regulation, communication skills, problem-solving strategies, giving and receiving social support) in order to decrease barriers to effective parenting. In addition, an optional, adjunct component of parent training focuses on school-related variables and interactions, such as promoting children's academic self-confidence, facilitating reading and language skills in early childhood, supporting homework completion, setting academic goals and motivating children, communicating with teachers, and helping teachers implement interventions for problem behavior at school. Another unique aspect to the Incredible Years parenting component is its division into a focus on four separate age ranges: infancy (zero to one years), toddlerhood (one to three years), preschool years (three to six years), and school age (six to thirteen years). Tailoring the program to the child's age allows for age-appropriate vignettes and applications as well as instruction about normal child development and individual variation.

Due to the frequency of behavior problems that affect learning and classroom engagement in these children (Webster-Stratton & Reid, 2010), the Incredible Years program also includes a teacher training component. The teacher intervention is administered in a group format and includes instruction and skill building in areas such as classroom management strategies, strengthening positive relationships with students, promoting students' social and emotion regulation skills, clear communication between teachers and parents, and sensitivity to individual student differences. Finally, the child training component of treatment is designed to parallel the parent component and address areas of difficulty that often accompany (exacerbating and/or being caused by) behavior problems. Targets of the child training include social skills, conflict management, self-control, emotion awareness and regulation, perspective taking, self-esteem, and school readiness and academic skills. Interactive videos show vignettes of children interacting with adults and peers, which are supplemented by the use of life-sized puppets to model appropriate behaviors and thoughts for children. Child clients discuss the scenarios and select and role-play appropriate responses and behaviors, which are reinforced through creative activities (e.g., games) as well as homework. The Incredible Years program has significant research support and indicates that all of the treatment components (parent, teacher, and child) play a role in promoting improvement (e.g., Beauchaine et al., 2005; Webster-Stratton, 1994; Webster-Stratton et al., 2004).

Parent-Child Interaction Therapy (PCIT). PCIT is based on the theory and research linking authoritative parenting, high in both warmth and firmness, with positive outcomes in children (Baumrind, 1966; Steinberg & Silk, 2002). PCIT is administered in two phases. In the first phase, the emphasis is on child-directed interaction (CDI), in which the child leads the play and the parent positively attends to, praises, and verbally reflects on the child's behavior. The second phase focuses on parent-directed interaction (PDI), which entails the parent directing and/or correcting the child's behavior when necessary (Zisser-Nathenson et al., 2018). At the beginning of each treatment phase, the therapist teaches the phase's skills to the parent through verbal instruction and modeling. The bulk of each phase consists of coaching sessions, beginning with a five-minute observation of the parent-child interaction that guides the target of the remainder of each session. Following the brief observation, the parent spends the session playing with the child while the therapist coaches the parent on the use of CDI or PDI skills, giving praise for skill use as well as suggestions for changes in the moment. Ideally,

the therapist is coaching the parent while watching through a one-way mirror in an adjacent room, with the parent listening through a "bug-in-the-ear," but it can also be done with the therapist in the same room as the parent and child. After the coaching portion of the session, the therapist and the parent review the observations from the beginning of the session. PCIT emphasizes the use of weekly rating scales and charts to monitor progress. A number of studies have found PCIT to have both short- and long-term effects on parenting skills and children's behavior (Boggs et al., 2004; Eyberg et al., 2001; Schuhmann et al., 1998).

Parent Management Training—Oregon Model (PMT-OM). The focus of PMT-OM is the promotion of five "positive parenting practices" that break the coercive cycle typically seen in these families rather than directly changing parental discipline strategies within conflictual interactions. It is assumed that parents who are knowledgeable and practiced at the use of positive methods of parenting will shift toward such techniques and away from a reliance on coercive strategies. Parents are taught *skill encouragement*, in which they utilize techniques such as scaffolding and reinforcement to increase children's desired behaviors. Parents also learn how to *set limits*, establishing rules prohibiting negative behaviors and appropriate consequences when rules are broken. The importance of *monitoring* and supervising children's behavior, in and outside of the home, is discussed. Families are taught the steps of *problem solving* in order to help them plan effectively and manage challenges to their plans. Finally, parents learn how to display affection and interest toward their children, the skill of *positive involvement.* PMT-OM has been found to be effective in a wide variety of formats and settings (see Forgatch & Patterson, 2010, for a review).

Problem-solving skills training (PSST). PSST was developed as a child-focused treatment approach in response to concerns about the prognosis of youth whose parents could or would not participate in treatment (Kazdin, 2018). The main purpose of PSST is to address the cognitive processes that often distort aggressive and defiant children's views of social situations and other people and, therefore, lead to maladaptive responses. The first stage of treatment focuses on teaching youth the steps of effective problem solving, particularly in interpersonal scenarios. Games and role-playing are introduced as methods of practicing solving problems and evaluating their solutions. In later sessions, children and therapists concentrate on the application of these skills in the child's real-life interactions with parents, siblings, teachers, and peers. Tokens that can be redeemed for small prizes are awarded to the child for prosocial applications of the problem-solving steps (and, less often, taken away for negative behavior). When possible, PSST is often administered in combination with parent-focused approaches, such as PMT-OM. PSST has been found to positively impact child, parent, and family functioning (see Kazdin, 2018, for a review of studies).

Multisystemic therapy (MST). MST was developed as a family-based treatment for adolescents whose disruptive behavior was severe enough to lead to juvenile justice system involvement (Henggeler & Schaeffer, 2017; Henggeler et al., 2009; Henggeler et al., 2002). This intervention is designed to address the

risk factors associated with delinquent behavior, including individual youth characteristics, family dynamics, peer relationships, academic problems, and neighborhood characteristics, as well as the interactions between elements of the environment (e.g., adolescents and parents, family and school). The emphasis is on the role of parents or caregivers in facilitating change in these areas based on their work with the clinician. MST consists of multiple contacts each week between the treatment team and various systems and individuals (e.g., youth and family, school, justice system) over the course of three to five months, totaling sixty hours or more of therapeutic contact between the clinician and the family. Clinicians are also available around the clock to respond quickly to crises as they arise. The treatment emphasizes nine main principles: (1) understanding how the adolescent's disruptive behavior "fits" within the environmental context; (2) identifying and building on family strengths; (3) increasing responsible behavior by family members, even in the context of difficulties and challenges; (4) selecting interventions that are present-focused, action-oriented, and clearly defined; (5) targeting the sequences of interactions (e.g., coercive family processes, interactions with delinquent peers) that maintain antisocial behavior; (6) applying interventions in a developmentally appropriate manner; (7) encouraging continuous effort on the part of all individuals to implement changes on a daily basis; (8) evaluating progress continuously using objective measures; and (9) empowering family members to generalize skills and treatment gains to other current and future problems. Intensive training for clinicians, organizational-level support, and regular quality assurance assessments to ensure that clinicians maintain fidelity to the main principles of the treatment are also emphasized. MST has been found to decrease adolescents' antisocial behavior, improve family functioning, decrease the likelihood that youth will be removed from their homes, and reduce recidivism, especially when clinicians adhere very closely to all elements of the treatment (Borduin et al., 1995; Curtis et al., 2004; Smith-Boydston et al., 2014; Vidal et al., 2017). Youth treated with MST are also less likely to be involved with the criminal justice system well into adulthood (Sawyer & Borduin, 2011; Wagner et al., 2014).

INTEGRATIVE APPROACH TO TREATMENT

The parent-child relationship and positive reinforcement. Children are gifts and blessings to their parents (Genesis 15:4-5; Psalm 127:3-5), and the relationship between parents and children is to be highly valued. Parents also have an important role in caring for and loving their children. Parents are instructed not to "exasperate" or "embitter" their children (Ephesians 6:4; Colossians 3:21) at the same time that children are expected to obey and honor their parents (Exodus 20:12; Ephesians 6:1), highlighting the intended reciprocal nature of the parent-child relationship. In DBDs, we see coercive family process as reciprocal interactions that have gone awry, leading to maladaptive responses on the part of both the child and the parent and disrupting the positive tone that a healthy relationship is designed to have. Therefore, the centrality of correcting these interactions in interventions for DBDs emphasizes the importance of a warm and positive parent-child relationship for sub-

sequent changes to parenting techniques as well as children's well-being.

As fellow members together in the body of Christ, our relationships with our children, as with everyone, should be characterized by love, empathy, kindness, patience, and forgiveness (Mark 12:31; 1 Corinthians 13:4-7; Hebrews 13:3; James 1:19-20). Indeed, the parent-child relationship is a commonly used analogy for the relationship between God and his people, and one aspect of that relationship involves love, care, and mercy (e.g., Psalm 103:13). Theologian David Jensen (2005) discusses Horace Bushnell's (1908) emphasis on the relational aspect of human nature as it applies specifically to children: "True human being is being-with, and this is especially apparent in the relation between parent and child" (p. 55). In addition, parental care involves instruction in right living, including seeking wisdom and knowing God's commands (e.g., Genesis 18:19; Deuteronomy 4:9; 6:6-9; Proverbs 2). Children who do not feel loved and cared about by their parents are unlikely to be receptive to their instruction. This pattern is the reason that DBD treatments generally begin with interventions that aim to promote positive interactions between parents and children. Christian parents should see the promotion of the parent-child relationship as especially important, given the biblical and theological understandings of children as gifts as well as the importance of parental influence in the development of wisdom. The central role of wisdom in right living is a pervasive theme throughout Proverbs, which portrays it as a necessary foundation for right decisions, relationships, speech, and behaviors, as well as general well-being. For youth with DBDs, the wisdom that parents provide (sometimes with the support of clinicians) might play an especially important role in their common areas of difficulties and deficits, such as countering information-processing biases and promoting accurate views of other people, supporting problem-solving skills and decision making that is acceptable to others, avoiding negative consequences, obeying authority figures, and managing strong emotions.

One method for fostering a positive parent-child relationship is play. Some theologians have talked about the spiritual implications of children's play as an act that celebrates and displays the God-given freedom that adults often neglect in the face of responsibilities and busyness (Bushnell, 1908; Jensen, 2005). Play and the exercise of imagination therein allow us to envision possibilities outside of our current reality, including the restoration of previously broken relationships, the perfection of heaven, and the new order that will come with Christ's second coming. For example, childlike imagination has no trouble visualizing a world in which predators and their prey lie peacefully together (Isaiah 11:6) and people transform their weapons into life-giving farming tools (Isaiah 2:4). Furthermore, playing with children exposes us to their imaginative worlds and can connect us to these theological truths in addition to nurturing our relationships with them. "One does not play with children to avoid responsibilities for them, but to be opened anew to children and even guided by them" (Jensen, 2005, p. 57). In families in which time for purposeful, positive parent-child interactions has been neglected, as is often the case when children's disruptive behavior dominates family interactions, designed "special time" can be

relationally and spiritually beneficial for both the child and the parent. In addition, taking the humble stance of desiring to learn from a child's play and imagination may help transform a parent's view of a child from mainly "the problem" to a source of joy and a gift to the family.

Limit setting and punishment. Another important component of the healthy relationship between parent and child involves guidance and discipline. Proverbs, in its focus on promoting the development of wisdom and right living, is rife with references to the importance of discipline in shaping children as they grow (e.g., Proverbs 5:22-23; 13:24; 19:18; 22:15; 29:17). Indeed, God is portrayed throughout Scripture as a Father who disciplines his children. God's discipline does not come out of anger or as revenge; rather, it is out of love and with the purpose of shaping his children's character and behavior so that they might repent and be sanctified, and those who experience God's discipline should see it as a blessing and a reflection of his love, even though it may not feel positive in the moment (Job 5:17; Proverbs 3:11-12; Hebrews 12:7-11; Revelation 3:19). Such truths are important reminders to parents who may feel exhausted by their children's misbehavior and be discouraged from months or even years of attempts at discipline that have been or appeared to be ineffective. These parents may have stopped disciplining their children or resorted to harsh and authoritarian methods, which are often seen in parents of children with DBDs. Reminding such parents of the importance of—as well as techniques for—disciplining out of love and care rather than anger can be helpful. On the other hand, some parents are hesitant to discipline their children for fear of causing them distress or pain. Often these parents have a hard time seeing the long-term benefits of discipline in the shaping of the children's behavior and character. They may also have difficulty recognizing the role that learning to obey one's parents at a young age has in preparing children to obey other authority figures, including the Lord. (The child who grows up in a household in which their misbehavior has no negative consequences is not likely to view obedience to God's commands, or the instructions of teachers or bosses, as important.) Indeed, the words *discipline* and *disciple* share the same linguistic root meaning, "to learn" (Gillogly, 1981); shaping our children into disciples of the Lord (in addition to healthy, productive members of society) involves discipline. When appropriate, clinicians might encourage parents by helping them remember the true purpose and importance of disciplining their children by looking at the Scriptures on discipline and its role.

From a Christian perspective, it is important to note the concerns that some writers have raised about the possibility that the very behaviorally focused interventions commonly used in the treatment of DBDs will only change children's outward actions and not their inward attitudes and orientations, sometimes dismissing behavioral interventions completely for this reason (e.g., Tripp, 1995). Has the child who has come to obey his parents and treat others appropriately because his defiance and aggression have been disciplined effectively also come to respect his parents and feel empathy and kindness toward his peers? These concerns are valid, as researchers have not generally been concerned with the internal effects on children. However,

given that the research on behavioral interventions is clear that they are effective in changing behavior as well as children's emotional and cognitive functioning, a more balanced view is appropriate. Scripture is clear that God knows us deeply and cares not only about our behavior but also about the state of our hearts and our attitudes and motivations (e.g., 1 Samuel 16:7; Psalm 139:1-4; Proverbs 16:2; Matthew 23:25-28). Therefore, Christian parents and clinicians may want to be careful to include discussions with children about the reasons for obedience and positive behaviors toward others as well as honest questions about what children are feeling and thinking during acts of positive and negative behavior, which reflects a view of the child as her own person with valid thoughts and feelings. Families might set aside time together to explore the Scriptures about interactions between parents and children as well as how God desires for us to treat others, with parents modeling an examination of their own hearts and behaviors, repentance for wrong acts and attitudes, and efforts to change their own hearts and behaviors with God's help and leading. These interactions should not occur during or immediately following children's misbehavior, when both children and parents may be highly emotional and unlikely to be able to respond thoughtfully, but might occur at a set family devotional time during the day or week. When appropriate and helpful, parents can then refer more briefly to the Scriptures they have studied with their children when they are processing disruptive behavior and its consequences in the moment.

Problem-solving skills. Good problem-solving skills are an important component of navigating social and other situations in a manner that promotes one's own well-being, the well-being of others, and the maintenance of relationships. Significant attention is devoted throughout Scripture to living in ways that honor God and others, with some instructions for specific situations given, such as in the Ten Commandments (Exodus 20:1-17) and the Sermon on the Mount (Matthew 5–7). In other cases, we are provided with commands and guidance that are more general (e.g., non-situation-specific), such as, "For if you live according to the flesh, you will die; but if by the Spirit you put to death the misdeeds of the body, you will live" (Romans 8:13) and "Be alert and of sober mind" (1 Peter 5:8). What does it mean to live according to the Spirit or to be of sober mind? As we seek to obey instructions such as these in a given situation, we use biblical and theological understandings in combination with our reasoning or problem-solving abilities to assess how to think or behave in an optimal way. As youth have cognitive abilities that are not yet fully developed, and youth with DBDs often further have social information-processing deficits, supporting the development of good problem-solving skills promotes their ability to live in a way that follows Scripture and honors God. For Christian youth, the problem-solving process can be explicitly linked to biblical principles. For example, consider a child being excluded by her peers in the school cafeteria (not an unlikely scenario for aggressive youth who may be rejected by peers). When she walks into the cafeteria and is told by a group of classmates that she cannot sit with them, she must decide what to do. Once the problem (exclusion) has been identified (step one), the therapist would work with the child to identify possible solu-

tions (step two) and evaluate their potential consequences (step three). They might brainstorm solutions such as the client yelling and throwing her food at the peers who excluded her, sitting by herself in the cafeteria, eating with her teacher in the classroom, or finding another student who is sitting alone. While all but the first option are acceptable solutions that are unlikely to have significant negative disciplinary consequences, the therapist might encourage the child to take the perspective of each of the other individuals in the situation, helping her to empathize with the other student who is sitting alone (especially since she has had the same experience) and recognize the opportunity to care for someone else who may be sad or hurting. If the child selects and tries this option (steps four and five), she and the therapist can discuss how this experience went from the child's point of view as well as how it may have honored God, perhaps even bringing in the idea that God can use our negative feelings and experiences for good purposes and outcomes (e.g., Romans 8:28).

Furthermore, working with youth with DBDs to improve their problem-solving skills recognizes their agency in their own lives, particularly in the course of an intervention that is largely focused on changing parental behavior. Given their common information-processing and skill deficits, these children may perceive themselves as having no control over their environments and how authority figures respond to them, especially if they have parents who are inconsistent, rigid, and/or harsh in their interactions with them. Therefore, presenting and practicing the steps of effectively solving a problem with these youth can give them a sense of agency and control over their environments as well as improve their self-esteem and self-efficacy as they brainstorm and implement solutions that result in positive outcomes to situations that have previously ended poorly for them. As these youth (as well as the adults in their lives) increasingly recognize their own agency, they may also better come to understand the potential impact of their actions on others and others' responses to them and be empowered to make choices that promote well-being for themselves, their peers, and their family members.

Emotion understanding and anger regulation. As a part of our human nature, God has given us the capacity to experience a wide range of emotions. However, within the church, certain emotions are often viewed as desirable and good (e.g., happiness, joy), whereas others are seen as bad and to be avoided by believers (e.g., anger, fear, sadness). A more nuanced (and biblically faithful) view of emotions embraces the idea that it is not the presence or absence of an emotion but the thoughts it reflects as well as its management that determine whether an emotional experience is desirable or undesirable for Christians (Hall, 2014). Helping children understand their emotions—including both physiological signals and causal thoughts and events—is the first step in helping them to lead an emotional life that honors God. If we cannot reflect thoughtfully and accurately on our emotions, we will not be able to know whether our anger or joy is the type that God desires or discourages. Therefore, as we take a Christian approach to working with children with externalizing behavior problems, who often have trouble with emotion understanding and regulation, we might link our discussions of feelings and their causes to a biblical picture of emotion and how we know

whether it honors God. Children with DBDs struggle especially with anger and its management, and given their symptoms, it is likely that their anger is unrighteous and harmful toward others rather than glorifying to the Lord; though both situations involve a perceived wrong, an adolescent's righteous anger at social injustice in his city is clearly different from a young child's anger and aggression toward a peer who has taken her toy. Therefore, from a biblical perspective, our work with these children will most likely aim to decrease their anger by helping them more accurately perceive social situations and regulate their emotional responses in appropriate and adaptive ways. However, God-given passion can be viewed as a gift; therefore, rather than aiming merely to dampen these youths' emotional responses, as they grow and mature, we might help them reorient their anger and passion toward causes that grieve the heart of God. For example, parents might teach the child who is quick to anger and motivated to action by her anger about the history of racial discrimination in the United States and help her use her emotions to work, pray, and advocate for change.

Preparation for setbacks and relapse prevention. If we recognize the full humanity of children, we acknowledge not only their worth and value but also their sinfulness (Miller-McLemore, 2003). While many parents of children with DBDs will have no trouble accepting this truth at the point when they seek treatment, it can be an important reminder throughout the course of treatment, as improvement is not a steady, flawless path. Just as adults do, children will experience setbacks, and misbehavior may persist or reappear, especially when children experience illness, stressors, environmental changes, and adaptation to new stages of development. It is important for parents to understand that setbacks are normal and do not indicate that treatment has failed.

In addition, just as our children are sinful, so are we as their parents, guides, and caregivers. Even the most devoted, careful parents will not execute the strategies for managing their children's misbehavior perfectly in every instance (whether the child has a DBD or not). Parents should be reminded of this truth that is inherent in their flawed, human nature. There will be times when they clearly sin against their children, disciplining out of anger rather than sensitive concern and exasperating rather than encouraging their children. There will also be instances when parents' best efforts to discipline their children fall short, not because of specific individual sins but because of our imperfect nature. God always disciplines his children wisely and perfectly; human parents do not. Caregivers need to return to this truth in order to (1) repent and ask forgiveness of God and their children when necessary, when they have failed to truly love their children through their words and actions, and (2) forgive themselves and be able to accept grace and mercy, whether their failures have been clearly sinful or not. When parents are able to examine their actions and admit to wrongdoing or mistakes (to others as well as themselves), they will be able to learn from past failures and focus fully on parenting in the present. When parents either deny their errors or ruminate on them excessively, their ability to care well for their children will be impeded, and children's misbehavior is likely to increase.

In order to prevent significant relapse, we must view ourselves and our children as imperfect, sinful people, who have been forgiven by a merciful God who is continually working for our sanctification (e.g., Philippians 1:6). Indeed, the way in which we view children affects our interactions with them and their responses to us. Smith Slep & O'Leary (1998) found that parents who view their children's misbehavior as voluntary and purposeful are angrier and discipline more harshly, which in turn increases children's negative emotions. Helping parents understand the individual risk factors and processes that have shaped their children's present behavior and functioning, from a developmental psychopathology framework, may allow parents to locate the cause of misbehavior as external rather than internal to their children (even while recognizing that their fully human children are affected by the sin nature). Such a view does not condone children's misbehavior but gives parents a framework for conceptualizing it more complexly and accurately, setting them up to be able to address the factors that have promoted and maintained problem behaviors and develop effective, sensitive methods for disciplining as well as nurturing their children.

CASE STUDY

Pertinent history. Eric Crag is a four-year, six-month-old Caucasian male whose mother, Winona Shell, requested a diagnostic evaluation due to concerns about his behavior at home toward his siblings and caregivers. Ms. Shell's major concerns for Eric include an increase in aggressive behavior toward his siblings, such as hitting, throwing objects, and spitting at them. She says he deliberately annoys his brothers and is vengeful toward them. Ms. Shell is also concerned that Eric is unable to control his anger, often becoming upset when he does not get his way and having temper tantrums about once per day. His tantrums typically entail screaming, crying, throwing himself on the floor, throwing items near him, and kicking or hitting anyone near him. In the past year, Eric has broken two windows in the family's home during more severe tantrums. The onset of these behaviors was at three years of age. Ms. Shell says she sometimes holds Eric and talks quietly to him when he loses his temper; he cries in her arms until he eventually falls asleep. Ms. Shell also says she sometimes spanks Eric on his rear end when he loses his temper. She notes she uses an open hand and does not leave a mark. At other times, Ms. Shell uses time-out and loss of toys as disciplinary strategies but reports that "nothing works."

Ms. Shell feels ineffective in disciplining Eric to calm him and notes he frequently argues with her about his punishments. He also frequently defies his mother and his grandparents when asked to do something and has difficulty following family rules even with repeated threats of punishment. Ms. Shell notes Eric's tantrums often occur soon after he awakens in the morning. Eric and his brothers share bunk beds in their one-bedroom apartment. Ms. Shell reports that Eric usually goes to bed at 9:00 p.m. but has difficulty falling asleep and frequently climbs into bed with her on the futon mattress in the family room. He awakens at 6:00 or 7:00 a.m. and takes a nap for about two hours in the afternoon. He sometimes has difficulty falling asleep for his nap, which he takes with his mother on the living room couch in front of the television.

Eric lives with his mother, his brother Marc (age seven), and his half-brother Bryant (age nine). Eric's father was not involved in Eric's life until he was six months old due to relational conflict between his parents, at which point they reconciled and Eric's father moved into the family home. When Eric was two years old, his father passed away from a heart attack following a prolonged illness. Ms. Shell works part-time hours at a retail store with variable shifts. Eric is frequently watched by a neighbor or his maternal grandparents when his mother works. She says Eric separates easily from her when she leaves for work, though he sometimes becomes agitated when she has worked long hours for two or more days in a row. Ms. Shell says Eric seems jealous of the attention she gives to his brothers. She finds it difficult to provide individual attention to all of her children, though Eric receives most of her attention because of his behavior problems. Ms. Shell describes her relationship with her son as "good," although she often feels frustrated with Eric because of his challenging behaviors. Eric's grandparents reportedly allow Eric to "do what he wants" so that he does not have outbursts at their house; however, they frequently express their frustration with Ms. Shell's parenting and her lack of control over his behavior.

Ms. Shell's responses on a parenting measure indicate she feels she is able to provide comfort during times that Eric is distressed. However, she reports challenges in determining what Eric needs or what mood he is in, making it difficult for her to respond appropriately. In addition, Ms. Shell also reports experiencing distress about controlling and understanding Eric's behaviors. She notes that they argue often, and she has difficulty communicating with him. Eric and his mother have regularly attended a large church for about two years. Eric reportedly enjoys the children's worship services, though he sometimes refuses to participate in activities. Ms. Shell notes her desire to be more involved at church and states that she has turned down other families' requests to get together with them because she was worried Eric might misbehave.

Eric is not currently enrolled in daycare or preschool, though Ms. Shell is hoping to have him attend preschool the following year. Ms. Shell reports that Eric mostly plays with his brother Marc and does not have any same-age peers with whom he regularly spends time. She notes he generally plays well with other children at neighborhood parks and is not aggressive toward them. Eric meets criteria for oppositional defiant disorder, mild severity.

Course of treatment.

Sessions 1-3: Setting the stage, behavior monitoring, and positive attending. The clinician first meets with Ms. Shell to set up expectations of therapy and review what has brought them to this point. Ms. Shell feels at her "wit's end" and is skeptical of treatment and its effectiveness; however, she feels she has nowhere else to turn. Her parents blame her for not disciplining Eric enough, and friends have provided her with a popular Christian parenting book that argues against psychology and behavioral principles, which Ms. Shell did not find useful. The clinician first focuses on psychoeducation regarding Eric's defiance and tantrums as well as the benefits of changing the environment to improve his behaviors. The clinician visually depicts the interactions that might contribute to Eric's misbehavior with an explanation of antecedents and consequences. Though the

focus is on understanding how Eric's behavior is influenced by the environment and how his behavior affects her parenting decisions, emphasis is also placed on Eric and Ms. Shell's thoughts and feelings during these interactions. Ms. Shell feels more comfortable knowing the behavioral principals will be presented along with explanations to help Eric know what is expected and why (i.e., to target internal character); thus, they also discuss how she can approach "[training] up [Eric] in the way he should go [so that] when he is old he will not depart from it" (Proverbs 22:6 ESV). A major aspect of this calling for Ms. Shell is helping Eric become a strong, kind man, but she becomes overwhelmed by fear about his future, given his present behaviors, and by the daily tasks of training, discipline, supporting his development, and modeling good behavior as required by this verse. The therapist suggests that this complex job of parenting may feel less overwhelming with a focus on one day at a time and with encouragement and problem solving (rather than the criticism she experiences from her family). They mutually decide to work on parent training with some joint parent-child sessions and individual therapy with Eric. Ms. Shell also completes a Home Situations Questionnaire (Barkley, 2013) to assess the family's home environment.

In the second session, the clinician observes Eric and his mother playing. The clinician begins to discuss how to attend to Eric's desired behavior and strengthen the positive aspects of their relationship through play. To give credence to this foundation for the parent training, the clinician presents the idea that the parent-child relationship mimics God's relationship with us, and they discuss how God *delights* in us (e.g., Proverbs 8; Zephaniah 3:17) and how this delight is mutual. This idea is appealing to Ms. Shell, as she links it to her own experience of God's love that encourages her to follow his commands. The clinician then joins in the play to model different ways to attend to Eric's play (reflection; narration; copying his play; labeled praise; and expressing enjoyment while refraining from leading the play, asking questions, or giving commands). At this point, Ms. Shell is instructed to keep the interaction brief and to ignore misbehavior. Ms. Shell is provided with a weekly tracker of "special time" as well as a behavior log to monitor the most severe problematic behaviors she would like to target, which generally occur at transition times (mealtimes, getting dressed, when asked to leave his play to do something, at bedtime). She identifies the time immediately following dinner as a reasonable time for "special time."

In the third session, the clinician reviews the problematic behaviors identified in the behavior log with Ms. Shell. She is most concerned about Eric's daily aggression toward his brothers and his daily tantrums when he does not get what he wants. Together, they identify specific positive behaviors to replace these disruptive behaviors (e.g., using gentle hands, using words instead of hands, labeling his feelings, talking to mom instead of tantrumming). The clinician discusses the importance of attending to these positive behaviors with labeled praise whenever Eric shows them, both in special time together and throughout the day. Ms. Shell is surprised but interested in the idea that it is "godly" to delight in children, to provide praise, and to acknowledge their specific assets in order to

"build [them] up according to their needs"; further, she is open to considering that children's behavior is generally good and that we want to "catch them being good" in order to build up these characteristics and behaviors. Special time is reportedly going well, as both Eric and Ms. Shell enjoy the play time, which Ms. Shell was able to include during five out of seven days. She also reports that her interactions with Eric throughout the day have felt more positive.

Sessions 4-6: Focus on emotion regulation skills and behavior modification. In session four, the clinician meets with Eric to play catch, and after enjoying the activity together, she substitutes a feelings ball to help Eric identify different feelings and the situations in which he experiences them. Anger appears to be a particularly difficult emotion for Eric to discuss. Therefore, the clinician has Eric complete a drawing worksheet about what anger feels like in his body (like a hurricane—fast and strong and like he doesn't know what will be destroyed). His mother joins the session, and they read a children's book about anger (*1-2-3 A Calmer Me*; Patterson & Miles, 2015) together and talk about how family members show anger as well as ways to manage anger. The practices of breathing, listening to each other, and identifying what family members are feeling with a feelings chart are discussed as ways to be slow to anger or at least handle the anger well when they experience it (James 1:19-20). The session ends with a ten-minute play time with feedback provided to Ms. Shell about following Eric's lead and attending to positive behavior.

In the fifth session, treatment progress is reviewed. The behavior log shows that Eric is throwing slightly fewer tantrums (five instead of seven days a week) but showing no decrease in aggression. The clinician works with Ms. Shell and Eric to identify five basic family rules and create visuals for these rules that would be placed around the house. They then develop a behavior system to motivate Eric and reinforce desired behavior. Because it is not tasks but specific behaviors Ms. Shell would like Eric to display, a point system is put in place. Eric will be provided with a small candy to put into a jar every time Ms. Shell observes a gentle reaction to his brothers, his use of words instead of aggression, labeling his feelings and using calming strategies, and acceptance of his mother's decisions instead of tantrumming. Ms. Shell also develops a point system with Eric's brothers for specific behaviors she wants to see increase (e.g., helping around the house, doing homework when asked). Further, she and Eric identify goals for Ms. Shell herself, such as using a calm voice and counting to ten instead of yelling. To promote his sense of agency, Eric is involved in identifying rewards, which include picking the dessert at dinner, going to his favorite park, and reading extra books at bedtime.

The clinician meets with Eric individually for the first twenty minutes of session six. Eric spontaneously reports that he was "really bad" and felt sad because he threw a toy at his brother which made a cut on his brother's forehead. He states his mother became upset with him and "hit my head with my toy." There were reportedly no bruises or marks on his head and none are seen by the clinician. Eric further reports that he was hit with a belt on his leg "last week" and that both he and his brothers have been hit with a belt when they are in trouble. Eric describes feeling scared during these incidents. The clinician deter-

mines that she is mandated to report these incidents to child protective services (CPS).

The clinician then meets with Ms. Shell individually for the remainder of the session. She provides praise and encouragement to Ms. Shell with regard to her effort and consistency in therapy. They discuss current dynamics in the home and Eric's report. Ms. Shell reports feeling stressed and alone because of conflicts with her extended family around Eric's behavior. She describes losing her temper and hitting Eric during the most recent incident and using a belt to spank her children on their rear ends in the past when they have gotten in trouble. She describes feeling out of control when she resorts to this discipline and ashamed about not knowing what else to do. Ms. Shell has been told that corporal punishment is the best way to disciple her children and send them the message of what is right and wrong behavior in God's eyes, and her parents modeled this method of discipline when she was a child. The clinician and Ms. Shell discuss the negative impact that spanking and anger have on her family, given their particular characteristics and referring back to the coercive cycle discussed in the first session. They discuss the importance of clear rules and consistent discipline and how genuine discipline occurs in a context of love (Proverbs 3:11-12; 13:24; Hebrews 12:4-11). Eric's fear and sadness may hinder their relationship and the development of positive behavior and strong character that Ms. Shell desires for Eric, whereas tenderness combined with discipline can help him link consequences with his behavior. Further, Ms. Shell's desire to disciple her children is supported with an emphasis on helping her identify what she wants them to learn from her discipline about themselves, relationships, and loving behavior. She is open and receptive to this discussion. The clinician also discusses her mandated reporter status with Ms. Shell and the necessity of a report to CPS, and they make the phone call together.

At the end of the session, Eric rejoins them to ensure him he is not in trouble and for the clinician to explain to him that someone will be coming to talk to him and his mother within the next twenty-four hours. Ms. Shell explains how adults sometimes make mistakes and lose their tempers; she apologizes to Eric, and the session ends with five minutes of play, with praise provided by the clinician for Ms. Shell's positive attending skills.

Sessions 7-11: Problem-solving and specific parenting skills. In the seventh session, the clinician meets with Ms. Shell individually to process the CPS investigation. Eric's mother reports having a relatively positive experience with the case worker who conducted the investigation. Ms. Shell explains that since the investigation, she has had a new "outlook" on her parenting. She realizes that her ongoing grief, life stress, and minimal social support have been negatively impacting her parenting. Ms. Shell reports that Eric's aggression and tantrums have decreased (three tantrums per week), and she is more optimistic about his ability to start preschool the following year. Ms. Shell discusses her family's disbelief about the effectiveness of her parenting and their comments that Eric is "just like his father" and needs to be disciplined; she has received the message that his will must be broken and that being tender with him will make him weak. The clinician explores Ms. Shell's feelings about these messages and her perceived incompetence.

The clinician then helps Ms. Shell identify characteristics consistent with her faith that she wants to have as a mother (e.g., patience, slowness to anger, understanding, forgiveness, joy in her children) and that also relate to the characteristics she'd like to develop in Eric. Emphasis is placed on the parenting strategies she is comfortable with and which fit her valued characteristics. She reflects on how these strategies are different from the parenting she had as a child and what her parents and others tell her she should be doing with Eric. The clinician relates her desired characteristics with the progress she has made so far in therapy and to different parenting strategies she can learn to use more (to be further discussed in the next session). Finally, Ms. Shell reports that she has enrolled Eric in a karate class in order to give him an outlet for his energy and to help him to learn self-regulation and control. He seemed to enjoy the first class.

In session eight, the clinician meets with Ms. Shell to discuss two specific parenting skills: giving effective commands and the use of natural/logical consequences and time-out. The clinician provides handouts about these skills and facilitates discussion about Ms. Shell's skepticism that they would work. These strategies are linked to her values and vision for her parenting and her relationships with her children. They discuss her children's free will and their need to learn from their choices and the world around them as balanced with Ms. Shell's opportunity to respectfully and effectively speak into their development with her values and priorities through how and what she chooses to discipline. Obedience is one characteristic of following the instructions of the Lord, and Ms. Shell hopes her children will grow in generosity, responsibility, and respect for themselves and others, among many other areas. Ms. Shell and the clinician role-play many different scenarios in which she can implement these parenting skills and practice how to respond to Eric's probable responses.

In the ninth session, Ms. Shell and the clinician engage in problem solving around the ways in which Ms. Shell has found it difficult to implement the behavior plan consistently. She identifies two additional problematic behaviors she wants to target and updates the behavior system accordingly. Ms. Shell also discusses her ongoing sadness and lack of social support. The clinician helps her identify a friend from church with a child the same age as Eric whom she can call for support and company, and Ms. Shell plans to invite this family over for lunch the upcoming Saturday.

The tenth session focuses on updating the behavior plan with Ms. Shell, who continues to share her underlying fear of what the future holds for Eric. Both the clinician and Ms. Shell have individually been focused on the same Bible verses over the last couple weeks: "The steadfast love of the LORD never ceases; his mercies never come to an end; they are new every morning; great is your faithfulness" (Lamentations 3:22-23 ESV). To Ms. Shell, these verses speak to the continual grace God offers despite our failures; God is steadfast in his provision to her and to Eric in his future, and she wants to meet him every morning with that knowledge. She found greater freedom in remembering that her son is God's and that she can accept him and help him grow but does not need to be fearful of failure.

In session eleven, Ms. Shell notes Eric and the family are doing much better. She wants

to enroll Eric and his brothers in more extracurricular activities (including karate classes) and to develop her own social support network. She expresses more confidence in her own parenting skills and her ability to observe her children's behavior, develop and implement a behavior plan, and make changes accordingly. Ms. Shell and the clinician plan a termination session to discuss what she and Eric have learned as well as the option of having "booster sessions" at a later time.

Additional considerations from a developmental psychopathology framework. While they are not the main focus of treatment for Eric's DBD, a variety of other risk factors and co-occurring difficulties are explored throughout treatment. Ms. Shell reports a normal pregnancy and uncomplicated delivery. She denies any substance use during her pregnancy but reports experiencing a stressful pregnancy due to relational conflict with Eric's father. This difficulty in their relationship coupled with his sudden death led to complicated grief for Ms. Shell, with weeklong periods over the last two years of crying, hopelessness, and low motivation to get out of bed. The clinician mentions the possibility of Ms. Shell seeking individual therapy, but she is resistant at first. The clinician watches for opportunities to provide positive feedback to Ms. Shell about her gains in therapy as well as opportunities to link her personal struggles with effects on her parenting and the suggestion of individual therapy. Ms. Shell speaks with her physician and is prescribed antidepressant medication. She is still considering the feasibility of individual therapy for herself at the end of treatment.

Two years prior to beginning therapy, Eric was found to have high blood lead levels, for which he received medical treatment. Though Eric's lead levels have normalized, his pediatrician continues to monitor them. While Eric was receiving medical treatment, a health department inspection of the family's apartment found that the window frames contained lead. However, the building management had not replaced the windows. During therapy, Ms. Shell and the clinician discuss her desire to advocate more for her family by getting the windows in their apartment fixed. They explore ways Ms. Shell might organize the other apartment tenants to petition the landlord. They then link this proactive step toward caring for her family's health and asserting herself with her sense of efficacy as a single mother. By the fourth session, Ms. Shell has taken Eric to his physician, who recommends a sleep hygiene plan and possible sleep study should his sleep continue to be poor. Eric also starts treatment for constipation. After these steps Eric seems less irritable at home.

Finally, in order to develop Eric's prosocial behavior, it is also recommended Eric begin to participate in group settings (e.g., preschool, Sunday school, library programs, extracurricular activities) that would provide supervised social interactions with same-age peers as well as physical activity. As noted, he joins karate classes, and his mother also initiates social interactions with other families.

Conclusion

DBDs are characterized by defiant, oppositional, aggressive, and rule-breaking behavior, and are common reasons that youth present in therapy. There are a variety of risk factors that interact to produce a DBD, with research emphasizing the role of environmental and family variables, particularly coercive family process. Therefore, effective interventions have focused on behavioral methods for reducing children's misbehavior, including promoting a positive parent-child relationship, effective parental use of reinforcement and punishment, and emotion regulation and problem-solving skill building work with youth themselves. There are a number of manualized treatment protocols that utilize these elements, which can be informed by an integrative perspective on children and families.

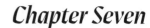

Chapter Seven

Attention-Deficit/
Hyperactivity Disorder

THE DIAGNOSIS OF attention-deficit/ hyperactivity disorder (ADHD) in children and adolescents has risen dramatically around the world in recent years, leading to questions about the cause of this apparent increase (Boyle et al., 2011; Conrad & Bergey, 2014). Some professionals assert that increases in diagnosis are due to more youth being accurately diagnosed; others raise concerns about overdiagnosis and the pathologizing of poor attention and high activity levels that are actually within the normal range. Though it is difficult to tease apart the various factors that contribute to the rising rate of diagnosis, it is clear that clinically significant inattention and hyperactivity affect some youth and interfere with their ability to learn, relate to others, and function well in daily life. In order to be diagnosed with ADHD, an individual must display a variety of symptoms of persistent inattention and/or hyperactivity (American Psychiatric Association, 2013). There are two categories of symptoms within ADHD. Symptoms of inattention include not paying close attention or making careless mistakes at schoolwork or other work, having trouble paying attention for long periods of time, appearing not to hear when spoken to, failing to complete tasks, having poor organizational skills, avoiding or disliking tasks that require a lot of focus and effort, losing items, becoming distracted easily, and being forgetful during everyday activities. Symptoms of hyperactivity and impulsivity include fidgeting or squirming in one's seat, getting up when one is expected to stay in one's seat, running or climbing when not appropriate (which may manifest as a sense of restlessness in adolescents or adults), being noisy while playing or engaging in other quiet activities, acting as if "driven by a motor" or having trouble being still for very long, talking excessively, blurting out answers when inappropriate, having difficulty waiting one's turn, and interrupting or intruding on other people and their activities or belongings.

Youth who display at least six symptoms in each category are diagnosed with the combined presentation of ADHD. Youth who display at least six symptoms of inattention but not hyperactivity/impulsivity have a predominantly inattentive presentation; youth who display six or more symptoms of hyperactivity/impulsivity but not inattention are diagnosed with the predominantly hyperactive/impulsive presentation of the disorder. For all individuals, symptoms must begin before the age of twelve, be present in at least two different settings (such as home and school), and interfere with functioning or development.

Estimates of the prevalence of ADHD in US youth vary widely, ranging from as low as 5% to as high as over 15% (Oehrlein et al., 2016; Merikangas et al., 2010; Rowland et al., 2015; Wolraich et al., 2014). Boys are diagnosed with the disorder around three times as often as girls (Willcutt, 2012). Youth with ADHD frequently also meet the criteria for other disorders. The most commonly comorbid disorders are conduct disorder (CD) and oppositional defiant disorder (ODD), which co-occur in half or more of youth with ADHD and affect boys at a higher rate (Angold et al., 1999; Gaub & Carlson, 1997). Internalizing problems such as depression and anxiety may also co-occur with childhood ADHD, especially in girls (Angold et al., 1999; Chronis-Tuscano et al., 2010; Levy et al., 2005). Comorbid internalizing disorders do not generally persist into adolescence (Bagwell et al., 2006), but childhood ADHD does appear to raise the risk for substance use disorders in adolescence, especially among youth with comorbid conduct problems (Wilens et al., 2011). Finally, autism spectrum disorders and traits may co-occur with ADHD (Ronald et al.,

2014, 2008), and youth with both ADHD and ASD traits have more severe symptoms (Cooper et al., 2014). Youth with ADHD are at heightened risk for a variety of other associated problems, including poor school performance (Martin, 2014; Zendarski et al., 2017), language impairments (Korrel et al., 2017), emotional dysregulation (Graziano & Garcia, 2016; Morris et al., 2020), poor relationships with peers (Hoza, 2007; Stenseng et al., 2016), health problems (Jameson et al., 2016; Kutuk et al., 2018; Sciberras et al., 2016), sleep difficulties (Becker et al., 2019; Cortese et al., 2009), and accidents resulting in injury or death (Bonander et al., 2016; Dalsgaard et al., 2015).

RISK/CAUSAL FACTORS
Biological factors.

Genetics. Familial studies of ADHD suggest that genetic factors play a strong role in risk for ADHD, with high heritability estimates (70-80%; Chang et al., 2013; Chen, Brikell, et al., 2017; Faraone et al., 2005). The presence of a number of specific genetic markers, mostly on genes related to the regulation of serotonin or dopamine, have been linked with increased ADHD risk (Gizer et al., 2008; Mohamed et al., 2017; Shang et al., 2018; Williams at al., 2012). Genetic risk appears to be transmitted through effects on brain structure and function (Albrecht et al., 2014; Bralten et al., 2013; Franke et al., 2009; Nymberg et al., 2013). However, genetic factors account for only a very small amount of variation in the occurrence of ADHD, so while they may be useful in identifying some youth who are at heightened risk, they are far from explanatory. One reason genetic markers may explain limited variance in the disorder is that they interact with environmental factors to predict risk for ADHD (discussed below).

Neurological factors. Youth with ADHD evidence both structural and functional brain abnormalities. Beginning in early childhood, individuals with ADHD have lower brain volume overall as well as in some specific brain regions, including parts of the corpus callosum, cerebellum, parietal lobe, caudate nucleus, and right prefrontal cortex (Castellanos et al., 2002; Giedd et al., 2001; Jacobson et al., 2018; Kumar et al., 2017; Seidman et al., 2005; Vetter et al., 2020; Wyciszkiewicz et al., 2017). Among other functions, these structures play a role in planning, impulse control, goal-directed action, motor control, and integration of information (Nigg, 2017). Functional imaging studies reveal certain patterns as well. Youth with ADHD have reduced brain activity in multiple areas of the prefrontal cortex (PFC) and in the pathways connecting the PFC to the basal ganglia and the parietal lobes (Dickstein et al., 2006; Janssen et al., 2015). This neural circuitry has been implicated in the regulation of attention, behavior, and emotion, areas in which youth with ADHD often display deficits.

Psychological factors. Executive functions (EF) are complex mental tasks that involve the regulation and control of attention and action (Barkley, 1997; Nigg, 2017). They rely on an individual's ability to harness the functions of a variety of brain regions in the service of performing challenging tasks of self-control that help them achieve future goals. EFs include tasks such as planning, time management, organization, emotion regulation, and self-monitoring. Research suggests that youth with ADHD struggle with two particular executive functions, response inhibition and working memory, beginning as early as age three (Skogan et al., 2014, 2015), though significant heterogeneity exists in the EF abilities of individuals diagnosed with ADHD (Roberts et al., 2017). Response inhibition, also known as inhibitory control, is the ability to suppress a prepotent or automatic behavioral response in order to behave appropriately and meet social or other goals. Youth with ADHD perform more poorly than their peers on measures of response inhibition (Alderson et al., 2007; Amorim & Marques, 2018; Atherton et al., 2019; Dimoska et al., 2003; Sartory et al., 2002; Willcutt et al., 2005). With regard to symptoms, difficulties with response inhibition may underlie both impulsivity and inattention/distractibility (Nigg, 2017).

Working memory involves remembering information while manipulating it or performing another task (Nigg, 2017). Difficulties with both verbal and nonverbal (visuospatial) working memory are common in individuals with ADHD (Cockcroft, 2011; Martinussen et al., 2005; Willcutt et al., 2005). Furthermore, among youth with ADHD, those with working memory deficits display poorer academic performance (Fried et al., 2016), whereas those with better working memory have lower symptom levels (van Lieshout et al., 2017). Working memory deficits are theorized to underlie the symptoms of ADHD by interfering with an individual's ability to focus on information at hand and resist attending to distractions, which may account (in part) for associated inattention and academic difficulties (Barkley, 1997). Interestingly, demands on working memory have also been theorized to impact behavior, as youth with ADHD who are faced with overly challenging (and perhaps frustrating) working memory tasks may either display disorganized behavior or redirect their behavior toward other sources of environmental stimulation (Rapport et al., 2001). Indeed, boys show higher levels of activity during and after tasks that place a high demand on their working memory, a pattern that is amplified in youth with ADHD (Hudec et al., 2015; Patros et al., 2017).

Environmental factors.

Prenatal and birth factors. Brain development begins in utero, and prenatal variables and perinatal experiences can affect the developing brain and predispose an individual to later disorder. In the case of ADHD, certain prenatal patterns have been linked with children's symptomatology through their effect on brain development and neuropsychological functioning (Hatch et al., 2014; Morgan et al., 2018; Wiggs et al., 2016). For one, being born early and/or small interrupts normal brain development and raises a child's risk for ADHD. Babies born preterm (before thirty-seven weeks) are more likely to develop symptoms of ADHD, and the earlier in gestation a child is born, the higher the risk for the disorder (Galéra et al., 2011; Johnson et al., 2016; Sucksdorff et al., 2015). Furthermore, preterm birth is often associated with low birth weight (less than 5.5 pounds), which is itself linked with heightened risk for ADHD (Galéra et al., 2011; Hatch et al., 2014; Mick et al., 2002). Even in twin pairs in which one twin is smaller than the other at birth, there is a negative correlation between birth weight and ADHD symptoms, suggesting that birth weight itself plays a unique causal role that cannot be explained by other factors (Lim et al., 2018; Pettersson et al., 2015).

Prenatal exposure to certain teratogens may also play a causal role in ADHD. Prenatal nicotine exposure, via maternal smoking, appears to raise the risk for ADHD two- to fourfold (Galéra et al., 2011; Linnet et al., 2003; Zhu et al., 2014). Two main explanations for this link have been suggested. First, prenatal nicotine exposure may affect the developing brain, specifically the dopaminergic system, leading to structural and/or functional changes that affect behavior (Ernst et al., 2001; Pagani, 2014). Second, maternal prenatal smoking is linked with certain environmental and family factors which may also increase the child's risk for ADHD, suggesting that though smoking does have a unique effect on children's outcomes, confounding factors may account for a large proportion of the variance (Brion et al., 2010; Knopik et al., 2016; Skoglund et al., 2014). The impact of prenatal alcohol exposure on later ADHD symptoms is less clear, with some studies finding drinking during pregnancy raises ADHD risk and others finding no association (Galéra et al., 2011; Linnet et al., 2003). However, prenatal alcohol exposure has been consistently linked with poorer executive functioning in children (Kodituwakku et al., 2001; Rasmussen & Bisanz, 2009).

Parental psychopathology and family dynamics. The aggregation of ADHD within families is due to both genetic factors and shared environmental factors, suggesting that family experiences may play a role in risk for ADHD (Chen, Brikell, et al., 2017; Peng et al., 2016). The literature links two main family-level variables, parental psychopathology and family dynamics, with ADHD in youth. First, there is a consistent association between parental psychopathology, including depression, bipolar disorder, anxiety, antisocial behavior, and substance-related disorders, and higher rates of ADHD in children (Cheung & Theule, 2016; Galéra et al., 2011; Park et al., 2014). Additionally, in youth with ADHD, parental psychological disorder is associated with the persistence of ADHD symptoms as well as worsening conduct problems over time (Agha et al., 2017; Chronis et al., 2007; Law et al., 2014). Parental psychopathology is generally understood to affect children's outcomes through its impact on parenting behavior, adversely affecting factors such as warmth, sensitivity, communication, and effective discipline (Berg-Nielsen et al., 2002; Tung et al., 2015; Vera et al., 2012; Wymbs et al., 2015). For example, when a parent has ADHD, families report higher levels of conflict and lower levels of cohesion (Biederman et al., 2002a).

Even in the absence of parental pathology, certain patterns of dynamics emerge in families with a child with ADHD. Families of youth with ADHD display higher levels of conflict and lower levels of cohesion (Biederman et al., 2002b; Counts et al., 2005; Elmore et al., 2016; Pheula et al., 2011). These families also tend to have poorer communication and display less affection, and parents provide less consistent discipline, display more coercive parenting behaviors, and are more overprotective of youth (Galéra et al., 2011). Other child-level variables may affect this relationship; for example, depression and conduct problems in youth with ADHD are linked with poorer family functioning (Garcia et al., 2019; Sollie, Mørch, & Larsson, 2016).

It is likely that the causality between children's ADHD and dysfunctional family dynamics are bidirectional or reciprocal (Breaux & Harvey, 2019; Cheung & Theule, 2016; Deault, 2010). On the one hand, family variables may increase the risk for ADHD and

associated problems by disrupting the system of support for the development of self-regulation that exists within healthy family interactions across development (Carlson et al., 1995; Johnston & Mash, 2001). Longitudinal studies that assess early environmental risk as predictive of later ADHD support this theory (e.g., Carlson et al., 1995; Østergaard et al., 2016). Similarly (though conceptualized differently), for youth at risk for ADHD, being raised in highly sensitive, communicative, and cohesive family environments may actually attenuate predispositions toward the disorder as children learn to adaptively self-regulate their impulsivity, hyperactivity, and inattention (Crea et al., 2013; Johnston & Mash, 2001). Alternatively, the effects of the child's symptoms may drive family dysfunction. The impulsivity, high levels of activity, distractibility, and frequently comorbid conduct problems associated with ADHD can be disruptive to healthy family functioning and lead to negative emotions and responses from other family members as they interact with the child and one another (Johnston & Mash, 2001). Indeed, parents of youth with ADHD report higher levels of parenting-related stress than parents of children without the disorder (Hutchison et al., 2016; Leitch et al., 2019; Theule et al., 2013), and interviews with parents and children reveal that interactions around homework and managing children's ADHD-related misbehavior are experienced as stressful for families (Wong & Goh, 2014). Such findings support the idea that there may be child-to-parent effects in the relation between ADHD and family dynamics. Indeed, one study of reciprocal interactions between parenting and children's behavior found worsening conduct problems in youth with ADHD to predict decreases in positive parenting over time, rather than changes in parenting causing children's behavior to worsen (Burke et al., 2008).

In contrast, in youth with ADHD, positive parenting has been linked to better social and behavioral outcomes. When parents have higher levels of warmth and lower levels of anger, youth display more prosocial behavior and have fewer problems with peers (Bhide et al., 2017). In addition, positive parent-child interactions (characterized by parental praise and expression of positive emotions) appear to be protective against the later development of conduct problems in youth with ADHD (Chronis et al., 2007). Positive, prosocial parent-child interactions may model appropriate behavior and social interactions for these youth, help avoid situations that elicit escalating conflict with parents and others, and help families to be more open to working together to ameliorate the symptoms of ADHD on children's functioning.

Other environmental influences. It is important to consider a wide variety of environmental influences on ADHD, as the more environmental adversity that is present, the greater the child's risk of developing the disorder and associated problems (Biederman et al., 1995; Pheula et al., 2011; Østergaard et al., 2016). We will briefly review two additional environmental factors associated with heightened ADHD risk in youth. First, exposure to certain toxins has been linked with ADHD (Banerjee, Middleton, & Faraone, 2007). For example, lead, a heavy metal, is a neurotoxin which can affect children's brain development and functioning even at very low levels (World Health Organization, 1995). Children with higher blood lead levels, a mea-

surement of lead exposure, have higher levels of ADHD symptoms (Chiodo et al., 2004; Nigg, Nikolas, Knottnerus, et al., 2010).

Second, socioeconomic status (SES) appears to affect risk for ADHD. Children born into low-SES families (identified by low levels of parental educational, occupational status, and/or income) have rates of ADHD that are more than double their higher SES counterparts (Østergaard et al., 2016; Russell et al., 2016). Furthermore, for youth with ADHD, living in low-SES families may affect the course and severity of the disorder. For example, low-SES youth with ADHD have more persistent symptoms, display poorer overall functioning, are more likely to have problems at school, and are diagnosed with comorbid learning disabilities at higher rates than their more financially well-off peers (Biederman et al., 2002b; Law et al., 2014). Various mechanisms may explain the link between SES and ADHD. One possibility is that other factors that heighten a child's risk for ADHD (e.g., genetic disposition, prenatal smoke exposure, parental psychopathology) disproportionately affect low-SES families and children; thus, the link between SES and ADHD is actually accounted for by these associated variables (Russell et al., 2014, 2016). The home learning environment may also help explain the association between SES and ADHD symptoms (Schmiedeler et al., 2014). Children whose parents promote a learning environment at home—through activities such as reading and playing interactive games—and who have access to educational resources such as newspapers and libraries have better outcomes, such as better self-regulation, stronger social skills, and lower levels of hyperactivity (Sylva et al., 2007, 2008). Youth with ADHD may particularly benefit from a family environment that promotes self-regulatory skills (Johnston & Mash, 2001), and those raised in lower SES families may be less likely to experience such learning-rich environments. Therefore, interventions aimed at ameliorating the effects of low SES on ADHD in youth might be most effective when they examine and target a variety of associated causal factors.

Interactive risk factors. While it is clear that ADHD is somewhat heritable, there has been limited success in identifying specific genetic markers of risk, perhaps because genetic risk generally only leads to ADHD when environmental risk is also present. Indeed, in youth with markers of genetic risk, psychosocial risk factors are more strongly linked to ADHD symptoms than in controls (Elmore et al., 2016; Nigg, Nikolas, & Burt, 2010; van der Meer et al., 2014, 2016). For instance, youth with one genetic risk marker (a particular genotype of the dopamine D4 receptor gene) are only at heightened risk for ADHD when they experience inconsistent parenting (Martel et al., 2011). The field of epigenetics, which explores the interaction between genetic and environmental factors in directing outcomes, may hold the key to understanding and predicting which youth are likely to develop ADHD (Nigg, 2017). This field suggests that exposure to certain environmental variables may trigger the expression of underlying vulnerability via mechanisms such as gene expression or direct physiological or neurological changes. For example, stress exposure is more strongly predictive of decreases in gray matter in certain areas of the brain for individuals at genetic risk for ADHD (via a particular serotonin transporter genotype) than controls (van der Meer et al., 2015).

Therefore, a child with genetic risk for ADHD may have certain vulnerabilities related to serotonin and/or dopamine transport. That child may also have a genetically based pattern of brain abnormalities, including in the prefrontal cortex, that make it more difficult for him to exhibit self-control and perform other executive functions well. If the child's parents are economically disadvantaged, he may also be more likely to be exposed to nicotine prenatally and/or lead as a young child. If the genetic risk passed to the child via his parents is expressed as ADHD or other psychopathology within his mother or father, a family environment characterized by low cohesion and high conflict may interact with genetic vulnerability to lead to ADHD symptoms, which might otherwise be attenuated within a family context that promotes self-regulation. When the child presents for assessment and treatment of ADHD, his symptoms have developed through the complex interaction of genetic and environmental factors, a pathway which is important to consider in the intervention process.

DEVELOPMENTAL COURSE

Although ADHD cannot be reliably diagnosed in very young children, some early patterns may indicate risk for later symptoms. High levels of negative emotional expression in infancy, including prolonged crying and expressions of anger when restrained, are associated with risk for later ADHD (Sullivan et al., 2015; Wolke et al., 2002); in addition, six-month-olds who display higher activity levels than their peers are more likely to display symptoms of ADHD later in childhood (Meeuwsen et al., 2019). As infants and young toddlers (seven to twenty-five months), boys with high levels of familial risk for ADHD have higher levels of activity and anger and poorer attention-shifting abilities and inhibitory control, characterized more globally as difficult temperament (Auerbach et al., 2008). Other cognitive and behavioral characteristics—such as motor delays, language impairment, cognitive abilities, sleep problems, and internalizing and externalizing symptoms—measured during the first two years of life predict ADHD symptom severity in elementary school (Arnett et al., 2013; Gurevitz et al., 2014). Though they may not be reliable enough for diagnosis, these patterns may help families and clinicians identify youth at heightened risk for hyperactivity and attention problems.

By age three to four, ADHD symptoms in their traditional form become more apparent and can be reliably diagnosed. Most preschool-aged children with ADHD display significant symptoms of both inattention and hyperactivity/impulsivity, though they are more likely to meet the criteria of the combined or predominantly hyperactive/impulsive subtype than the predominantly inattentive subtype of the disorder (Egger, Kondo, & Angold, 2006; Lahey et al., 2004, 2005). There is a high level of diagnostic continuity during this period of development, particularly for children with higher levels of symptoms and more functional impairment (Bunte et al., 2014). These symptoms differ from the developmentally normative limited attention span and high activity level of children at this age, as they are not a sign of development immaturity but truly heightened levels of problematic behavior (Biederman et al., 2014). However, accurate diagnosis at this age may still be challenging, as symptom presentation may change over time, and the diagnosis or ADHD subtype that best characterizes a given youth often changes across the preschool years (Biederman et al., 2014; Lahey et al., 2004). Further, symptoms of other disorders that are still developing (e.g., the inattention of an anxious child, the poor regulation of a traumatized child) may present as ADHD symptoms, leading to misdiagnosis. By the preschool years, ADHD is already associated with a variety of areas of impairment, including lower levels of independence, poor motor and communication skills, academic problems and preschool expulsion, and social difficulties with peers and parents (Egger, Kondo, & Angold, 2006; García, Grau, & Garcés, 2015).

Most young children (75-80%) with a diagnosis of ADHD will still meet the criteria for the disorder in elementary school (Lahey et al., 2004, 2005). As children age, symptoms of hyperactivity and impulsivity decrease, whereas inattention increases (Curchack-Lichtin et al., 2014; Galéra et al., 2011; Narad et al., 2015). The latter pattern may be observed because of a true increase in inattention or because attention is difficult to measure accurately in young children. Children are most likely to receive their first ADHD diagnosis during the elementary school years, when their symptoms often interfere with classroom and/or academic functioning as they struggle to complete assignments, plan ahead, organize their work well, meet deadlines, and interact in prosocial ways with friends (Cherkasova et al., 2013; Nigg & Barkley, 2014). Although ADHD is associated with academic and social difficulties in school-aged children, there is significant heterogeneity, with children's impairment in these areas ranging from low to high (DuPaul et al., 2016).

Many youth who experience ADHD as children will continue to meet the criteria for the disorder into adolescence and beyond, though continuity estimates from childhood to adolescence vary from 30% to 90% (Anixt et al., 2016 Molina et al., 2009). Not surprisingly, given earlier patterns, adolescent ADHD is more likely to be characterized by symptoms of inattention than hyperactivity or impulsivity (Biederman et al., 2000; Molina et al., 2009). ADHD is more likely to persist into adolescence for children with more severe symptoms (Anixt et al., 2016) as well as those with more widespread psychosocial problems, such as social communication problems, poor language skills, and conduct problems (Riglin et al., 2016). Youth with ADHD are also at risk for academic, occupational, relational, and legal problems as they become adolescents and young adults, including poor social skills, difficulties with time management and planning, high school dropout, antisocial behavior, arrest, and unemployment (Behnken et al., 2014; Cadman et al., 2016; Hechtman et al., 2016; Kofler et al., 2015; Sasser et al., 2016; Sibley et al., 2014). Estimates of the prevalence of ADHD in adults vary, suggesting that anywhere from half to two-thirds or more of youth with the disorder will still experience at least some symptoms in adulthood (Cherkasova et al., 2013; Cheung et al., 2015; Kessler et al., 2006; Merikangas et al., 2010). In other words, most youth do not outgrow their symptoms as they age. Instead, they may manifest in problems in multiple arenas of life. This pattern highlights the importance of early and effective intervention for improving both current and future functioning.

ASSESSMENT

Assessment for ADHD must be multimodal and include elements such as interviews with parents, symptom rating scales completed by parents and teachers, and observations of the child and family (Pelham, Fabiano, & Massetti, 2005; Schroeder & Gordon, 2002; Smith, Barkley, & Shapiro, 2007; Sowerby & Tripp, 2009). Interviews with parents should include questions about symptom occurrence, impairment, developmental history, medical history, parent-child interactions, and family dynamics and characteristics. It is important to note that even individuals with ADHD can display sustained attention in certain situations, particularly those that are highly engaging or rewarding (American Psychiatric Association, 2013). We have encountered numerous parents who report that their children have significant inattention and hyperactivity but can sit and play video games for hours on end. Therefore, clinicians must elicit information about children's behavior around a wide variety of stimuli. Clinicians can choose to administer unstructured interviews or to utilize structured or semi-structured interviews that systematically elicit symptom information. Structured interviews for children generally focus on a wide range of symptoms and disorders, which can be useful for screening for comorbid problems. Examples of structured interviews that assess ADHD and other symptoms include the Kiddie Schedule for Affective Disorders and Schizophrenia (K-SADS; Kaufman et al., 1997) and the Diagnostic Interview Schedule for Children (DISC-IV; Shaffer et al., 2000). For younger children, the Preschool Age Psychiatric Assessment (PAPA; Egger, Erkanli, et al., 2006), a parent interview designed to assess symptoms in youth two to five years old, may be a useful tool.

In addition to conducting parent interviews, clinicians should solicit information from multiple informers across multiple settings, which is most easily done via the use of questionnaires or rating scales. Because the diagnostic criteria specify that symptoms must be present in at least two settings, information about children's behavior must be provided by individuals who have seen them in a variety of settings (American Academy of Pediatrics, 2011; American Psychiatric Association, 2013). In most cases, different individuals can provide the best reports of a client's behavior in different settings, such as parents at home, teachers at school, child care providers at daycare, and Sunday school teachers or youth leaders at church. The youth himself may be able to report about his own behavior in these settings as well. Symptom presence and severity is likely to vary depending on the reporting source. For example, adolescents' and young adults' self-report of ADHD symptoms is much lower than parent-reported symptoms (Barkley et al., 2002; Du Rietz et al., 2016). In addition, teacher ratings may be especially important in capturing symptom severity and impairment in functioning (Efron et al., 2016). Rating scales are either narrowband, assessing information about a specific category of symptoms, or broadband, including questions on a variety of types of problems. Clinicians may choose to focus on ADHD symptoms through the use of rating scales such as the ADHD Rating Scale-IV Preschool Version (for children ages three to five; McGoey et al., 2007) or the ADHD Rating Scale-5 (for youth ages five to seventeen; DuPaul et al., 2016). Alternatively, broadband

measures provide information about ADHD symptoms as well as other possible comorbid conditions in order to rule out comorbid diagnoses or determine whether apparent ADHD symptoms are better accounted for by another disorder. Examples of broadband measures include the Conners, Third Edition (Conners 3; Conners, 2008) and the Behavior Assessment System for Children, Third Edition (BASC-3; Reynolds & Kamphaus, 2015).

For externalizing symptoms such as those that characterize ADHD, clinician observations are often a useful tool. During the assessment phase (as well as throughout treatment), clinicians may want to observe children's activity level, impulsiveness, level of self-control, distractibility, focus, and sustained attention. Such observations can be made informally during child and family sessions or via the use of standardized observational measures such as the Disruptive Behavior Diagnostic Observation Schedule (DB-DOS), which has been found to be a reliable and valid tool for assessing symptoms of inattention, hyperactivity, and impulsivity (Bunte et al., 2013).

Once the appropriate assessment tools have been selected, a few additional cautions and recommendations are in order. As in the assessment of any childhood disorder, symptoms must be assessed in a developmentally sensitive manner. For example, gathering information about the dynamics of symptoms (e.g., frequency, intensity, and duration) rather than merely their presence or absence will help clinicians distinguish true problem behavior from developmentally normative patterns (Sowerby & Tripp, 2009). Furthermore, since hyperactivity decreases and inattention increases as youth with ADHD age, different symptoms may be more central to accurate diagnosis during different developmental periods. For example, for younger children, symptoms of hyperactivity are most helpful in diagnosing ADHD, but by ages five to six, clinicians are likely to find reports of inattention to be more central to diagnosis (Curchack-Lichtin et al., 2014; Harvey et al., 2015). Accordingly, assessment should be developmentally sensitive, with attention paid not only to symptoms levels relative to other children but to which symptoms are likely to best distinguish ADHD from other diagnoses (or normal development). Finally, given the high rates of comorbidity, assessment of any childhood disorder must include screening for co-occurring conditions (AAP, 2011). Children with symptoms of ADHD should be assessed for symptoms of depression, anxiety, and conduct disorders; assessments of adolescents should include questions about substance use. Thorough assessment and treatment planning should also include questions about associated problems, given the association between ADHD and heightened rates of physical, social, and academic problems (Pelham, Fabriano, & Massetti, 2005). Clinicians should assess medical history, sleep problems, academic performance, language abilities, emotion regulation skills, and social skills and peer relationships in order to acquire a fuller picture of the child's functioning than may be apparent from symptom measures alone.

TREATMENT

Both medications and psychosocial treatments have been found to be effective in the treatment of ADHD in youth. Psychostimulant medications are generally considered the first-line treatment for ADHD in youth over age six (AAP, 2011; Southammakosane & Schmitz, 2015). These medications are understood to reduce ADHD symptoms through their effect on prefrontal cortex functioning via dopaminergic and noradrenergic pathways (Arnsten & Pliszka, 2011; Spencer et al., 2015). Around 75% of youth who are prescribed a stimulant for ADHD experience a reduction in symptoms (Barbaresi et al., 2006). Stimulant medication also reduces aggression, oppositionality, conduct problems, and sleep disturbances in youth with ADHD (Pringsheim et al., 2015; Solleveld et al., 2020). Stimulants are less effective in reducing ADHD symptoms in youth with comorbid internalizing problems than their peers (MTA Cooperative Group, 1999b; Say et al., 2015). Studies suggest that 25-50% of youth taking stimulants for ADHD experience significant side effects, including poor appetite, weight loss, trouble sleeping, emotional lability, and irritability (Barbaresi et al., 2006; Storebø et al., 2016; Wigal et al., 2006). More serious side effects, such as high blood pressure or heart problems, are reported in a small number of youth taking stimulants for ADHD (Dalsgaard et al., 2014). Findings have been mixed as to whether long-term stimulant use in youth leads to reductions in growth across development (Harstad et al., 2014; Hinshaw & Arnold, 2015; Powell et al., 2015).

Stimulants reduce ADHD symptoms in preschoolers, but their effectiveness appears to be more limited than in older children (Greenhill et al., 2006). Long-term follow-up studies suggest that treatment gains resulting from stimulant use in preschool do not persist and that most children continue to experience significant symptoms several years later

(Riddle et al., 2013). In addition, little research has examined the effects of taking stimulants, which are generally prescribed for only a few months, over a long period of development, which may be especially likely to occur when medication use begins in early childhood (Storebø et al., 2016). Furthermore, though they are often prescribed "off label," most stimulants are not approved by the FDA for use in children younger than six (Southammakosane & Schmitz, 2015). For these reasons, it is often recommended that clinicians implement psychosocial treatments first for young children and add medication only if therapy alone is insufficient (AAP, 2011; Tandon & Pergjika, 2017).

Though stimulants are the most commonly prescribed medications for ADHD, others may also be effective. Some clinical trials have found that guanfacine, an alpha 2 adrenergic agonist that affects dopamine and noradrenaline, is also effective in reducing ADHD symptoms, producing improvement in 50-75% of youth (Biederman et al., 2008; McCracken et al., 2016; Sallee et al., 2009; Wilens et al., 2015). Like with stimulants, some youth taking guanfacine experience side effects; the most common complaints are sleepiness, headaches, fatigue, and stomachaches (Biederman et al., 2008; Sallee et al., 2009; Wilens et al., 2015). Guanfacine is commonly prescribed to young children with ADHD, but its effects in that population are not well researched (Black et al., 2016). The combination of guanfacine and a stimulant produces larger improvements than either medication alone, perhaps due to the greater effects resulting from two medications that target dopamine and noradrenaline (McCracken et al., 2016). Finally, atomoxetine has also been found to be effective in reducing symptoms of ADHD in youth, though as with other medications, a significant minority of patients experience side effects and/or continuing symptoms (Schwartz & Correll, 2014).

The most effective psychosocial treatments for ADHD tend to be behavioral in nature. Specifically, parent training, classroom management, peer interventions, and combinations of these approaches are behaviorally based interventions that are considered well established in the research on ADHD treatments; organizational training is also well established as an intervention (Evans et al., 2018). After a discussion of the research comparing the effectiveness of medication and psychosocial interventions, we will describe each of these well-established psychosocial treatments and also present a multimodal treatment program for ADHD in children and adolescents that combines elements of multiple approaches to intervention.

The question about which treatment is the most effective is more complex, as the research comparing different types of treatments (medication, psychosocial interventions, and combined treatments that include both medication and psychosocial treatment elements) on ADHD have produced mixed results. Smith, Barkley, and Shapiro (2006) propose that ADHD should be understood as a chronic condition, with multiple treatment elements necessary to address both the ongoing underlying (neuropsychological) dysfunctions and the resulting impairments in social, academic, and other realms of functioning. Therefore, they predict that treatments that combine biological and psychosocial elements are most likely to be successful. Treatment studies produce less clear results, however.

In general, medication and combined treatments both produce bigger effects on symptoms than psychosocial treatments alone (Chan et al., 2016; MTA Cooperative Group, 2004b; Van der Oord et al., 2008). Some research has found that combination treatments are as effective in reducing ADHD symptoms as medication alone; in other words, adding psychosocial intervention components creates no benefit above and beyond the effects of medication (Abikoff et al., 2004a, 2004b; Duric et al., 2017; Ercan et al., 2012; MTA Cooperative Group, 2004a; Van der Oord et al., 2008). In other studies, combination treatments have been found to lead to greater symptom reductions than medication alone (Amado et al., 2016; Milea & Cozman, 2012; Pelham et al., 2005). One possible reason for this difference in findings is described and analyzed by Conners and colleagues (2001), who reassessed the results of the Multimodal Treatment Study of Children with ADHD (MTA) that originally suggested that combination treatment was no more effective than medication. These authors note when examined separately, many outcomes (e.g., hyperactivity, impulsivity, inattention, global functioning, social skills, parent-child interactions) showed statistically nonsignificant trends toward combination therapies producing greater change. When these separate variables are combined into a single treatment outcome, analyses show combination treatment to be more effective than medication alone in promoting symptom reduction and improvement in functioning in youth with ADHD.

Psychosocial interventions and combined treatments are more effective than medication alone in improving other aspects of func-tioning beyond merely symptom levels, such as academic and organizational skills, social skills, and family dynamics (Chan et al., 2016; Hinshaw & Arnold, 2015; MTA Cooperative Group, 1999a). In addition, when outcomes are assessed among clinic-referred youth (as compared to those recruited for treatment research), many youth who take stimulant medications continue to have ADHD symptoms and resulting impairment (Sollie & Larsson, 2016). Furthermore, treatment gains resulting from medication use generally decrease over time (MTA Cooperative Group, 2004b). Taken together, these findings indicate that medication, psychosocial, and combination treatments may have different impacts on youth with ADHD, and the choice of which type of intervention to pursue for a particular client depends on targeted outcomes, youth age, accessibility of various treatment options, and family and youth preferences.

Behavioral parent training. Parent training interventions teach parents to use behavioral principles, focusing on the antecedents and consequences of behaviors, to modify children's behavioral symptoms (Fabiano et al., 2009). They are generally effective in reducing externalizing symptoms in youth, including symptoms of ADHD (Evans et al., 2018; Fabiano et al., 2009; Mulqueen et al., 2015), though some research has not found these interventions to result in widespread or lasting changes in symptoms (Abikoff et al., 2015; Chacko et al., 2009). The parent training programs that are used in the treatment of ADHD are the same programs that are effective for treating disruptive behavior disorders (e.g., Barkley, 2013; Kazdin, 2005; Zisser & Eyeberg, 2010). Because we have previously reviewed these programs in detail (see chapter six), we will briefly summarize their content here and refer readers to the chapter on treating disruptive behavior disorders for more detail.

Behavioral parent training programs generally have three common treatment elements that focus on enhancing parents' skills to manage children's behavioral symptoms (Garland et al., 2008). First, clinicians begin with tasks aimed at improving the quality of the *parent-child relationship* through the institution of "child-directed activity" or "special time." Second, parents are taught to *reinforce desired behaviors* using attention, praise, and tangible rewards; some interventions also aim to help parents give commands more effectively. Third, clinicians and families develop a plan to implement effective *limit setting and punishment*, including making expectations and consequences clear, ignoring minor misbehavior, and using time-out and the removal of privileges as consequences for problem behaviors. Together, these elements contribute to an environment in which appropriate limits and feedback help support a child with ADHD to behave in more appropriate ways.

Behavioral classroom management. Some interventions focus on the management of children's behavior in the classroom. A parallel to parent training, classroom management interventions focus on helping teachers utilize behavioral principles to promote positive behaviors and reduce negative behaviors in the classroom setting. These interventions are also designed to facilitate communication between teachers and parents and the implementation of appropriate consequences at home for behaviors that occur at school. Some approaches also involve a paraprofessional aide who works directly with the

child (Arnold et al., 1997). It is important to note that behavioral classroom interventions are more effective with the assurance of certain practices (DuPaul & Stoner, 2014). For instance, parental participation is important, as is clear communication between parents and teachers. In addition, if they are old enough, students should participate in identifying acceptable intervention strategies, goals, and consequences, and teachers should provide clear, consistent feedback to students about their performance. Finally, daily and weekly goals should address both behavioral and academic issues, and only a few goals should be targeted at a given time.

Behavioral classroom management interventions have several main components, many of which parallel the components of behavioral parent training (DuPaul & Kern, 2011; DuPaul & Stoner, 2014; Fabiano et al., 2010; Pelham, Massetti, et al., 2005). First, *school-wide rules and expectations* are developed and communicated to teachers and students. Ideally, rules should be developmentally appropriate and phrased positively (e.g., "Keep your hands to yourself" rather than "Don't touch other people"). Second, *behavioral reinforcers* for desired behaviors should be identified and implemented. Social reinforcers such as praise are commonly used. In addition, for children over the age of five, a token economy can be established, in which youth receive either a physical item (e.g., a poker chip) or a sticker or mark on a chart for each previously identified positive behavior. Tasks may be given different token values based on different levels of difficulty or completion time, and complex behaviors can be broken down into smaller parts, with the completion of each part leading to the rewarding of a token. Once a child has earned multiple tokens, she can redeem them for rewards whose "costs" have been previously established and communicated, such as toys or privileges. Some programs encourage parents to allow children to redeem tokens earned at school for rewards at home, enhancing the link between the settings. Teachers may also record children's achievement of specific behavioral goals on a "daily report card" that is then sent home to parents. Third, teachers and staff identify and consistently implement *consequences* for behavior that breaks the rules established earlier. These consequences should be age appropriate, instructive, flow naturally or logically from the misbehavior when possible, and be clearly communicated to students. For significant misbehavior, more impactful consequences may be necessary to identify in a student support plan. Finally, some children may require *individually tailored behavioral plans*. For these youth, school staff (often in collaboration with parents) will identify a child's problem behaviors in addition to discerning the function served by the behaviors or the environmental contingencies (antecedents and consequences) maintaining the behavior. Next, rewards and consequences that are likely to be effective for an individual student can be established, communicated, and implemented. These youth may also benefit from more frequent verbal feedback about their behavior as well as skill-building instruction that teaches them alternative, appropriate behaviors. Behavioral school interventions are generally viewed positively by teachers and parents and are effective in reducing ADHD symptoms and disruptive behavior, increasing on-task behavior, reducing disciplinary referrals and suspensions, and increasing homework completion (DuPaul & Weyandt, 2006; Fabiano et al., 2009; Pelham, Massetti, et al., 2005; Langberg et al., 2010).

Behavioral peer interventions. As youth with ADHD often struggle to form peer relationships and interact appropriately with others, and general behavioral treatment programs do not typically produce improvement in these areas, some interventions focus specifically on social skills training (SST) for youth with ADHD (Frankel et al., 1997; Hinshaw, 2005; Mikami, 2015; Mikami, Lerner, et al., 2010). These interventions are typically administered in a group format in which youth meet weekly for sixty to ninety minutes; each session includes instruction from a clinician about specific social skills as well as the opportunity to practice these skills with the other youth in the group. The socials skills taught to youth may include how to have a conversation (speaking at an appropriate volume, smiling, and respecting others' personal space), how to enter a group (observing the group, engaging verbally with the group, deciding when to attempt to enter the group, and responding appropriately to rejection), how to interact with peers during one-on-one time (praising the other person, avoiding criticism, staying engaged with the other person during the entire play time, following the rules of games, taking turns), and how to respond to teasing by peers (reacting neutrally or with humor) and handle confrontations with adults (be respectful, avoid arguing). Some SST programs also include an element focused on emotions, including managing a child's own emotions appropriately during interactions with peers and reading others' emotions accurately.

Some interventions include or are even centered on parent-led coaching of the child's social behaviors and interactions. The Parental Friendship Coaching intervention (Mikami, 2015; Mikami, Lerner, et al., 2010) teaches parents to facilitate positive peer interactions for their youth with ADHD. Over the course of group and individual sessions, parents learn to build up the positive parent-child relationship, use behavioral principles to shape children's social behavior, and teach youth how to play appropriately with peers. Parents are also instructed on how to set up playdates for their children that are likely to be successful, including choosing peers with whom the child is likely to interact appropriately (e.g., peers who seem to like the child, who have similar interests, and who seem to be tolerant of the child's symptoms), selecting a playdate setting/activities that will promote prosocial behavior and avoid boredom, and monitoring their children during the playdate and redirecting their behavior when necessary.

Finally, one novel approach involves training youth to be socially inclusive of peers with ADHD in the classroom through teachers' modeling and reinforcement of inclusive behavior (Mikami et al., 2013). In this intervention, teachers purposefully develop positive relationships with children with ADHD to model that they are worthy of social attention, use clear classroom rules and a token system to reward socially inclusive behavior and punish ostracism of peers, and highlight the strengths of children with ADHD by acknowledging them with daily classroom awards. Each of these types of SST has limited but promising support as effective

ways to improve the peer relationships and social skills of youth with ADHD (Frankel et al., 1997; Mikami, Lerner, et al., 2010; Mikami et al., 2013).

Organizational skills training. The main goal of organizational skills training (OST) is to improve the difficulties youth with ADHD often have with organization, time management, and planning (OTMP) skills, which represent deficits in their executive functions and interfere with their functioning at home and school (Gallagher et al., 2014). OST directly targets these areas of difficulty using behavioral principles to provide youth with the knowledge and skills that underlie successful performance in these areas. It is recommended that before beginning this treatment, children diagnosed with ADHD should be screened for difficulties with OTMP skills, since not all children with ADHD exhibit the deficits addressed by this intervention. OST was designed for use with children in late elementary school (grades three to five) and is administered as twenty twice-weekly, hourlong, after-school sessions. The intervention consists of four skill modules sandwiched between an introduction and a program summary. Parents meet with the therapist at the beginning and end of each child-focused session in order to review progress, discuss the skills the child is learning, and plan ways for the parent to encourage and reinforce the child's skills implementation at home using both social (e.g., praise) and tangible (e.g., objects and privileges) rewards. Teachers are also asked to participate by monitoring and praising the child's use of OTMP skills at school.

In the first module, children learn how to *track assignments* using a daily assignment record and a test calendar to record in detail each day's homework and materials needed to complete it as well as keeping track more broadly of all assignments and exams over the course of a several-week period. Children are taught about the importance of these tracking tools for defeating the "glitches" in our minds that interfere with our ability to remember important information (the "Go-Ahead-Forget-It Glitch"), distract us from keeping track of items (the "Go-Ahead-Lose-It Glitch"), make us lose track of time and due dates (the "Time Bandit"), and interfere with our ability to think ahead (the "Go-Ahead-Don't-Plan Glitch"). The second module focuses on *materials management*, which includes organizing school papers, books, a backpack, and the child's work areas. Children learn to use a binder with labeled tabs and a file box to organize school papers, assignment trackers, and therapy handouts. They also create and learn to use a checklist to make sure they have everything in their backpacks (or other bags, such as gym bags) they need to take from school to home and vice versa. In addition, therapists teach children how to organize their work spaces at home and school so that they contain all the necessary materials, do not contain unnecessary or distracting items, and have clear space to work. The third module teaches skills designed to improve *time management*. Therapists work with children to help them use calendars and clocks to keep track of time, estimate the amount of time needed for a given task, track the time they spend doing homework, create a daily homework schedule in which they plan to devote the right amount of time to homework completion each day, and address issues that may interfere with good time management (e.g., distractions,

tiredness). Finally, module four focuses on *task planning*. Children learn to identify the goal of a specific task or situation; to prepare to work on a task or goal by breaking it down into smaller steps and gathering necessary materials; to manage their time by planning the order in which they will complete the steps identified earlier, estimate the amount of time needed for each step, and identifying specifically when they will complete each step; and to assess their performance. The task planning module incorporates and builds on the skills learned in previous modules as children apply these steps to both short- and long-term goals and projects.

OST has been found to be effective in improving organization skills, academic performance, homework completion, and even family dynamics in children with ADHD (Abikoff et al., 2013). The intervention has been adapted for use with young adolescents (grades five to eight) and been found to improve organizational skills, homework skills, planning, and academic achievement in this age group (Langberg et al., 2008, 2012).

Multimodal treatment (MTA). The most comprehensive multimodal treatment study is the NIMH Collaborative Multisite Multimodal Treatment Study of Children with Attention-Deficit/Hyperactivity Disorder. In this study, almost six hundred children with the combined presentation of ADHD were randomized into one of four groups (MTA Cooperative Group, 1999a, 1999b). The control group received treatment as usual, the medication management group received only a psychostimulant, the behavior therapy group received a variety of behavioral interventions (listed below), and the combination group received both medication and the behavioral interventions. The behavioral interventions provided to two of the groups consisted of twenty-seven group parent training sessions, eight individual parent training sessions, eight weeks of intensive summer treatment, twelve weeks of classroom behavioral intervention, and ten teacher consultation sessions. The summer treatment program (STP) component of the intervention consisted of six to nine weeks of all-day programming, which youth attend in groups (Fabiano et al., 2014; Pelham et al., 2017). Throughout STP classroom sessions and recreational activities, youth received instruction, feedback, and behavioral management, with counselors implementing reinforcements for positive behaviors, time-out and other consequences for problematic behaviors, social skills and problem-solving training, and communication with parents via daily report cards. As reported earlier, the medication management and combination intervention groups experienced the greatest symptom reductions by the end of the treatment period (MTA Cooperative Group, 1999a). Two years later, the youth taking medication had fewer symptoms than those in the other treatment groups (Abikoff et al., 2004b; MTA Cooperative Group, 2004a). Unfortunately, a long-term follow-up indicated that treatment gains had essentially disappeared for all the treatment groups by six to eight years later (Molina et al, 2009). These findings suggest that, particularly without continued treatment, youth with ADHD may continue to experience symptoms and resulting impairment. More long-term intervention research is needed in order to understand how to best treat ADHD over the course of development.

INTEGRATIVE APPROACH TO TREATMENT

As is true for all youth with psychological disorders, we have both a professional and a biblical responsibility to provide youth with ADHD the best possible care. As Christian clinicians, we strive to integrate our applications of effective treatments with biblical and theological principles. There are many ways in which Christian thought informs our application of behavioral principles of intervention, which we discuss in detail in chapter six and encourage readers to review because of the relevance in the treatment of ADHD. Because we have already discussed integrative considerations for each of the elements of behavioral treatment of externalizing problems, we focus in this section on ways that biblical and theological ideas might inform our conceptualizations of the symptoms of ADHD, their effects on youth, and the importance of treatment.

Self-control is clearly portrayed in Scripture as a positive personal characteristic and even a fruit of the Spirit (Proverbs 25:28; Galatians 5:22-23; 2 Peter 1:5-8). How, then, do we understand youth who display a lack of self-control, such as those with ADHD? Is impulsivity a sign of moral failure? Most clinicians who work with youth with ADHD would be quick to observe that these children's behavior is not voluntary or the result of a failure to apply skills that they have; rather, these youth have underlying problems with sustaining attention, impulse control, and hyperactivity that may make it impossible, particularly without intervention, for them to behave in a societally acceptable manner. Recall our earlier general discussion in chapter two about the idea of weakness or individual predisposition toward certain difficulties or problems (Johnson, 1987). This concept is particularly relevant here, as the research we have reviewed clearly points to a number of genetic, neuroanatomical, and neuropsychological underpinnings of the behavioral difficulties displayed by youth with ADHD. We must recognize that while self-control is a valued characteristic, we cannot hold these youth to the same expectations as those without a predisposition toward distractibility, inattention, impulsivity, and hyperactivity. Their susceptibility to difficulties in these areas should be seen as a weakness or vulnerability but not an expression of sin as we might interpret poor self-control in an individual who is fully capable of controlling his impulses.

Indeed, it may even be helpful to think about behavior of youth with ADHD in the same way we would think about the behavior of a younger child. We do not expect very young children to display self-control; we fully expect them to fail to have the impulse control and planning abilities necessary to keep themselves safe, which is why we install baby gates and furniture anchors, hold their hands tightly in parking lots, and supervise them closely in the bathtub. At the same time, we recognize self-control as an important virtue and work to support and encourage it in ways that are developmentally appropriate as children grow. A toddler might be allowed to choose how much of each food on her plate she wants to eat but not to determine what is served; a preschooler who is not tired during nap time is given the freedom to play quietly in his room but not to roam around the house. In addition, we set limits and provide consequences that create expectations for right behaviors and correct wrong behaviors, and we provide the support to develop skills that will

make these desired behaviors attainable; in implementing these structures, we provide the framework in which a child learns self-control. The child who raises his arm to throw a toy, is warned by an adult of the consequence if he does so, and lowers his arm without releasing the toy has just displayed self-control supported by parental limit setting. By the time they reach mid to late childhood, we expect children to have developed improved self-control skills such that they can regulate their own behavior with less adult intervention. However, youth with ADHD still need extra support and structure. Thus, it may be helpful to think about these youth as akin to being in an earlier developmental period when it comes to the ability to control their impulses and focus for longer periods of time. When we approach them with the understanding that these abilities have not yet developed, we are more likely to be able to be empathic and to view their lack of self-control as not a moral failure but a developmental task yet to be accomplished.

Theologian Catherine Stonehouse (1998) writes about ministry to children in light of their developmental abilities and stages. In describing typically developing toddlers, she notes, "In this stormy period of life, children must be protected from themselves by firm outer limits. . . . Young children need limits that provide a sense of security and guidance. But those limits must give enough space for free and healthy expressions of autonomy" (p. 54). Based on Erikson's (1985) psychosocial theory, Stonehouse explains that optimal development in early childhood is promoted by the balance of limit setting and appropriate freedom that allows children to learn self-control as well as a sense of control and effectiveness in their own lives. Viewing youth with ADHD as being at an earlier stage of development with regard to their self-control and related abilities, while still validating the many age-appropriate strengths that they possess in other areas, may help us provide them with the most sensitive and helpful structure. We are more likely to be able to empathize with their difficulties, rather than blaming them, and to see the importance of supporting their development. Of course, youth with ADHD are not just "behind" developmentally; though their impulsivity and attentional abilities may be more similar to those of younger children, they will not naturally "catch up" over time. These youth need additional, individualized assistance to address their symptoms, which may come in the form of medication that enhances focus and self-control at a neurobiological level as well as behavioral interventions that provide the environmental structure that facilitates the development of positive behaviors and skills. Treatment outcome research suggests that this structure and support may need to be intensive and long-term, as the symptoms of ADHD are likely to return without continuous treatment (particularly in cases for which medication is an important component of treatment). From a theological perspective, we might consider this a specific application of our call to care for the weak and vulnerable among us (James 1:27), as the deficits displayed by these youth put them at heightened risk for a variety of negative health, safety, and psychological outcomes.

In addition, the symptoms of ADHD have the potential to interfere with spiritual development and well-being. Youth who struggle to sustain attention may find it difficult to listen well to a sermon, read lengthy passages of Scripture, or quiet their minds of distractions in order to listen for God in prayer. High levels of impulsivity may interfere with the ability to form close relationships with other believers or engage in spiritual disciplines. Furthermore, when youth "fail" at their attempts to engage in these spiritually significant activities, they may feel discouraged by the frustration of adults around them as well as implicit messages that are sometimes promoted in churches that their difficulties are due to personal shortcomings and that they just need to "try harder." Particularly when youth lack relationships with mature believers, these messages and the resulting discouragement may lead youth with ADHD to stop trying to implement spiritual practices into their daily lives and even eventually to give up on their faith altogether. Therefore, youth with ADHD can benefit from support from sensitive adults who work with them to develop ways to engage in faith practices that come more easily to them. For example, parents might engage with their children throughout a church service to ensure their understanding and attention and to assist in their self-monitoring, ideally with support and understanding from the broader church community about the communication that might occur between parent and child during otherwise quiet moments. Sunday school teachers or youth group leaders could provide youth with hands-on activities during lessons, allow them to move around or draw what they are being taught in order to facilitate focus and minimize distractibility, or pair them with a peer who can assist them in maintaining attention. At home, parents might help youth brainstorm more physically active ways to connect with God and grow their faith, such as praying while walking or running outside. As Christian clinicians, we may also find it useful to engage in explicit conversations with adolescent clients of faith about their experiences of their symptoms within the context of their spiritual lives. In what ways have their symptoms affected their spiritual growth and shaped the ways that they find it easy or difficult to worship, read the Bible, pray, and pursue fellowship with other believers? How might they use their perceptions of their own strengths and challenges to set them up for success in their spiritual endeavors? Through this conversation, we might also help youth explore their beliefs and feelings about the impact of their symptoms on their own spiritual practices and to dispel any inaccurate self-blame or discouragement.

However, even as we understand that youth with ADHD have predispositions toward difficulties with attention and self-control, we recognize that these youth have the capacity to behave in ways that do or do not exercise the self-control they do possess. A child with ADHD may be able to sustain attention during a boring (but brief) experience, to refrain from hitting his sister when he is angry with her, or to complete and turn in a homework assignment. Of course, the abilities of different children to behave appropriately or complete tasks will vary depending on individual symptomatology, the specific situation, and the children's circumstances at the time of the task (e.g., whether he is tired, hungry, or already being asked to exercise self-control in other areas). For several reasons, though, we do youth with ADHD a disservice when we assume that they are not capable of completing any tasks that require self-control, restraint, or focus. First, recog-

nizing youths' ability to display these characteristics acknowledges their agency. If children and adolescents with ADHD are presumed to be unable to ever restrain their behaviors or impulses, we essentially reduce their functioning to being a result of their disorder. In contrast, when we encourage these youth to manage challenging situations and behaviors in ways that are sensitive to their individual abilities and difficulties and then rejoice with them in their successes, we build up their own sense of agency and ability. This encouragement may be especially important for youth with ADHD who have spent years struggling with or failing at the tasks put before them by parents, teachers, and peers. Second, and relatedly, it is crucial to be aware of youths' abilities and give them opportunities to succeed at tasks that require self-control and/or focus in order to observe and encourage treatment gains. Youth are likely to encounter these tasks in their daily lives, as they are asked to sit still in class, complete chores before playing at home, and act in ways that benefit their friends in peer interactions. However, for some children with ADHD, parents and teachers may have adjusted their expectations over time such that they assume these youth will fail at these types of tasks and, as a result, do not present them with opportunities to display the skills and characteristics with which they may struggle. These adults need to adjust their expectations so that youth are given developmentally appropriate tasks in which they can apply the skills learned in behavioral interventions and/ or have the opportunity to display improved attention and self-control supported by medication-based improvements in functioning. Third, if we truly view youth with ADHD as fully human, we recognize that there may be ways in which their conscious choice to not employ the self-control of which they are capable can and should be understood as sin. We need to help these youth understand how and when their choices reflect not a lack of ability but poor (even sinful) decisions and actions. This recommendation comes with a caution about the importance of discernment about whether an individual child's behavior in a specific situation is best understood as reflecting weakness or sin. If we assume that a behavior that a child cannot control is sin, we risk adding inappropriately to a sense of guilt and taking away from the child's developing sense of agency. Indeed, it has been suggested that one of the mechanisms linking early ADHD to the development of conduct problems is the harsh assertion of parental authority, leading to conflict and oppositionality (Beauchaine et al., 2010) that may be an expression of a child's sense of frustration and powerlessness. However, on the contrary, if we fail to accurately identify behaviors that result from sinful choices, we run the risk of enabling youth to view their behavior as out of their control and fail to help them understand their ability to make godly choices, even within the context of their symptoms and predispositions, and the important role of our actions within the Christian life (cf. James 2).

Finally, as we consider how we might best help youth with ADHD, we refer back to the links between ADHD and family dysfunction that suggest that the presence of this disorder is particularly stressful for families. It often interferes with family cohesiveness and parental sensitivity and is likely to increase (perhaps already existing) parental stress and family conflict. Therefore, as we seek to best care for our clients, it may be especially important in the case of youth with ADHD to address the impact of the disorder on parents and siblings. How are a child's symptoms negatively impacting other family members? How might we best support parents and siblings and help them manage their stress well? What interventions are necessary for promoting godly interactions and dynamics within families? How, in turn, might enhancing family functioning positively affect the child's ADHD symptoms? We encourage clinicians to think in a dynamic and multifaceted way about what research-based care for youth as well as their families looks like in the presence of ADHD.

Case Study

Pertinent history. Dylan Wright is a twelve-year-old boy in the sixth grade who lives primarily with his mother, Cassandra Logan. He was referred for a psychosocial evaluation due to concerns regarding his inattention and behavioral struggles at school and his poor grades. His mother reports a chronic history of these school difficulties, including immature behaviors (e.g., blurting out answers, disruptive behavior in class). He needs frequent reminders to stay on task, especially in the morning when getting ready for school and when they are in a "time crunch." He also has difficulty following directions because he misses steps. Dylan avoids tasks that require effort, such as homework, chores, and helping his parents with tasks when they ask him. He makes careless mistakes "all the time," and has difficulty completing tasks he starts. He loses items and is disorganized, with his bookbag and bedroom described as "danger zones." Dylan is often overly active and has trouble sitting still, though he can sit still quietly when he is reading. At school, he tends to be off-task and disruptive, including having difficulty staying seated and joking around with his classmates when he finishes his work quickly. He fidgets and plays with material at his desk. Dylan talks constantly and has had to move desks frequently because of his talkativeness. He often interrupts others and at times he has difficulty waiting his turn. At school and home, Dylan frequently and abruptly changes moods when he does not get his way and has difficulty managing his anger at times. This past year, he started to refuse to follow adults' requests and became disrespectful to teachers, more frequently arguing with them.

Despite starting middle school off strong (i.e., "great grades"), his grades worsened as the school year progressed due to frequently not completing his homework or failing to turn it in. He does well on tests; however, he is described as a "very smart boy who is down on himself and his abilities." Ms. Logan notes Dylan "knows he's the kid who gets in trouble." Dylan's self-report indicates a negative view of himself. He wants to do better in school and argue less with adults, but he is often disappointed by his grades and behavior and feels like things are getting worse for him. No other symptoms of depression or anxiety are reported. Dylan describes school as boring and explains that his mind wanders so he sometimes misses material. His teachers confirm these reports of his grades and his behavior in school. Dylan is receptive to positive feedback from adults at school and the use of incentives.

Dylan's mother describes him as "friendly, inventive, energetic, sociable, and loving"; his strengths are his academic capabilities, his in-

tuition, his creativity, and his friendships. Dylan frequently spends time with his friends at their homes or his. Typical discipline for Dylan's behavior includes verbal reprimands, time-outs, removal of privileges (usually loss of electronics), or yelling at him. Ms. Logan notes she "gets on Dylan" about things and will "lose her cool" after a while. Dylan's parents are divorced; Ms. Logan has full parental rights. Dylan lives with his father, Jeff Wright, every Wednesday and every other weekend; Mr. Wright is remarried with two children (ages four and six). Ms. Logan describes a good co-parenting relationship with Dylan's biological father, though she is often the one making decisions and "trying to get his father onboard." They try to get along and not bicker in front of Dylan. According to both Dylan and his mother, they are struggling with defining their parent-child relationship and coping with changes in this relationship over time as Dylan approaches adolescence. Dylan sometimes does not feel understood and struggles with accepting rules, and thus quickly becomes frustrated and angry when limits are placed on him or when he feels that his perspective is not taken into account. He becomes upset when he gets in trouble and sometimes lies to get out of trouble.

Dylan is diagnosed with attention-deficit/hyperactivity disorder (ADHD) with a combined presentation of symptoms of inattention and hyperactivity/impulsivity. It is recommended that Dylan's mother consult with his physician or a psychiatrist to evaluate whether psychotropic medication would be beneficial in reducing his ADHD symptoms. Individual therapy for Dylan is also recommended to help him gain insight into his emotions and impulsive behavioral reactions. Additionally, therapy can help

Dylan understand the diagnosis of ADHD and his current executive functions, and help him develop skills for the future. The therapeutic setting will also provide him with a comfortable, secure outlet in which he could discuss any troubling issues (e.g., conflict with family members, adolescent transitions). It is also recommended that Dylan and Ms. Logan participate in family therapy to improve their relationship. Sessions should help them better understand each other's perspectives, learn more effective communication, and identify rules and expectations. A collaborative approach and inductive parenting may be the most beneficial. Inductive parenting involves relationship enhancement by providing clear limits, rules, and expectations alongside open communication, understanding, and negotiation; it values a child's perspective while also communicating the effects of a child's behavior and reasoning with the child to promote logic and social competence. Dylan's father should also be involved in Dylan's treatment to ensure consistency across caregiving settings and to strengthen the co-parenting relationship.

Course of treatment.

Individual and parent-child sessions. The first session is used to build rapport and provide psychoeducation about ADHD. Because he enjoys reading, a few books regarding ADHD are presented to Dylan, and he chooses one to read at home. The therapist presents and implements a clear structure for each session to encourage Dylan's active participation in therapy, understanding of therapy goals and material, and self-monitoring of attention and behavioral inhibition during the session. In the second session, Dylan discusses the book's presentation of ADHD as a "special brain." The therapist reflects his apparent intrigue about this definition of ADHD but also his skepticism. Dylan describes his frustration with himself and asks why God made him the way he did. Dylan and the therapist work through what he likes and dislikes about himself. Dylan identifies the valuable aspects of characteristics with which God made him; for example, he recognizes his energy, athleticism, spontaneity, wit, and ability to hyperfocus on things he is passionate about. Through the therapist's supportive questioning, Dylan discusses what he perceives his parents want for him, and identifies what he wants for himself in terms of behavior, treatment of others (mainly adults), and growth (self-control, achievement of goals) in a way that does not make him feel he is flawed. The therapist leads a reflection on 2 Corinthians 12:9, and Dylan finds solace in the idea that God's grace is sufficient for him in a way that does not feel shaming of his weaknesses but rather views it as an opportunity to rely on God, as he uses this opportunity God has given him to work directly on his skill development in areas of weakness.

Dylan and the therapist talk about difficulty sustaining attention, and the therapist helps Dylan describe what feeling distracted is like. He is introduced to self-monitoring strategies (e.g., setting an alarm on his phone to beep every five minutes to remind him to ask himself, "Am I paying attention?") as ways to bring his attention back to the task at hand. The clinician works with Dylan to help him accept that his mind will wander but there are things he can do to keep his mind engaged; for example, he often daydreams at church but could bring a notepad to take notes or doodle on during the sermon to remain engaged, or he could choose to read the Bible or song lyrics during repetitive routine parts of the church service. Subsequent therapy sessions will provide a time for Dylan to practice recognizing when his attention wanders and how to bring attention back to the present moment, with decreased support from the therapist over the course of therapy.

During the second session, the therapist also sought to understand Dylan's specific executive function strengths and weaknesses in order to identify skills Dylan would like to work on during therapy. Deficits in Dylan's application of executive function skills within the home and school settings were reported by Dylan, his mother, and his teachers. Specifically, concerns regarding his inhibition of impulses, his self-monitoring of behavior, his initiation and completion of tasks, his ability to manage task demands and his everyday environment, and his capacity to hold information in mind in order to complete tasks were reported. These difficulties, particularly with cognitive regulation, are likely to be exacerbated within the academic setting, and when his mood is negative.

The clinician uses a semi-structured interview to better assess Dylan's executive functions and the impact of his ADHD symptoms on his everyday functioning. He denies any difficulty with task initiation. He reports difficulty remembering his assignments, and notes he does not write them down or remember them by the time he gets home. He also forgets to turn in his homework. Dylan explains that whether he is able to work on homework long enough to get it done depends on the subject. He also becomes distracted by other things he would rather be doing and by his siblings when he does his

homework at his father's house. Regarding long-term projects, Dylan reports difficulty choosing a topic, developing a timeline, breaking the assignment into smaller parts, and sticking with a timeline. He typically finishes the project by the deadline. However, he often forgets to review the rubric and thus loses points for not completing parts of the project unless his teachers allow him to correct his mistakes. This causes him stress because he has a book report due every two months. He does not review his work to proofread or catch mistakes but believes he is able to edit his own work if he tries. Dylan says he generally does not study for tests but knows what to study and how to study. Dylan describes a range of daily chores he is responsible for; however, he sometimes does not do them when he is supposed to, and his parents "bother [him] until it's done." He is able to complete his chores once he starts and do them thoroughly. Finally, Dylan describes his difficulties with organization, leaving his belongings (e.g., coat, backpack, binder) all over the house and other places and not keeping them tidy. Based on this interview, it is decided that Dylan and the therapist will target his organization and work completion, as these difficulties cause the most distress for Dylan due to the impact on his academic functioning. During the second half of the session, Dylan's mother joins him and the therapist for the discussion of which executive function skills he would like to target.

In the third session, the therapist and Dylan identify a tracking system that Dylan is motivated to use. His class schedule, his typical homework assignments, the ways teachers notify him of homework, and the materials he needs to complete the homework are discussed. After reviewing several options and reasons he does not think he would be able to utilize these systems, Dylan elects the use of a homework app on his phone. The therapist and Dylan set up the app to reflect his schedule. Dylan's mother joins them at the end of the session so Dylan can describe to her how he will keep track of his assignments. They identify how she will support him in this goal: prompting him prior to school to remember to use the system, monitoring his use by checking the app after school each day, and rewarding him for its completion (e.g., watching a television show together from a series they enjoy).

In session four, the therapist and Dylan first engage in problem solving regarding tracking assignments. He reports feeling a sense of pride and relief the first time he had turned in his homework in every class. These positive feelings helped him to be more engaged during the class period as well. He missed writing down a couple of assignments and identifies talking to friends rather than listening to the teacher as the reason. Dylan and the therapist role-play how long it takes to note the assignment (less than twenty seconds, which surprises Dylan!) and how to prioritize this behavior over socializing. Dylan brought his backpack and binder to the session as planned. He has been shoving his papers into his binder without using individual folders for classes, and has not cleared out his backpack during the current school year. The therapist and Dylan spend time organizing his papers, clearing out old papers, identifying specific folders for each class, and identifying additional materials he needs to carry (e.g., calculator, pencils, pens, highlighters, colored pencils). Dylan has fun by

giving classes different colored folders to represent what he likes or dislikes about each class. Dylan believes he can implement this organization system effectively, in addition to tracking his homework assignments.

His mother again joins the session and is encouraged to check his backpack twice during the week (a timeline Dylan identifies as acceptable) to ensure that the organization system is maintained during the first few weeks of its implementation. They discuss the difficulty of setting priorities and maintaining them with discipline but also the benefits associated with self-control (e.g., less anxiety, positive feedback, reward of good grades). In the context of developing skills, self-control is identified as a virtue that can be practiced and strengthened.

Following arguments between Dylan and his parents over the past week, the therapist and Dylan decide to work on routines for specific adaptive skills at home in session five, as this causes the most conflict with his mother and father. Dylan and his mother are given guidelines for the session to ensure their respectful, collaborative communication about this problem. Value is placed on Dylan's perspective and his role as an agent of change in his own life. Basic expectations are identified with Dylan's mother, including a daily shower, picking up dirty clothes and wet towels off his floor, helping at dinner in some manner, and brushing his teeth twice a day. The therapist facilitates collaborative problem solving between Dylan and his mother. Dylan agrees these are reasonable daily requirements but communicates a desire to shower in the morning instead of the evening as his mother prefers, and to set the table instead of clearing dirty dishes. He also expresses that he can respond calmly to his mother with one reminder as long as there is no follow-up "nagging." Dylan and his mother make a visual for what is required in setting the table. Ms. Logan agrees to provide one reminder without frustration, and Dylan agrees to respond to the reminder or receive a consequence. Ms. Logan is reminded to notice his compliance with these expectations and provide frequent praise to Dylan.

In the next session, the therapist first checks in with Dylan about his thoughts regarding his symptoms of ADHD, as they have been meeting for almost two months now. He shares that he had heard in church "God does not make mistakes," which he keeps thinking about. He tries to remember this when he forgets something or when someone calls him out on a mistake. He expresses that he does not think his parents understand that God loves and works through imperfect people, which the therapist explores with him. He is able to identify ways his mother and father show their love but focuses mostly on their frustration with him. They decide to talk about his feelings at the next parent-child session, and the therapist invites both of his parents to the session. This sixth session then focuses on helping Dylan plan and complete academic tasks. Because he has a book report due in a week, the therapist and Dylan go over the rubric. Dylan is instructed on how to use a highlighter to read through the instructions and pick out important aspects of the instructions. He then is supported in using a time sheet and a calendar to estimate the amount of time each task should take and to set deadlines for himself for each task. Ms. Logan joins the session to review these timelines and to identify how she can help him review his completed project to ensure each part of the rubric is addressed.

Dylan and both his parents attend the seventh session together. The therapist first checks in with Dylan and his mother about completion of daily expectations at her house, and the prompting and monitoring of his tracking of assignments and organization. This conversation also provides an opportunity to review these skills and systems with Dylan's father. Dylan and Ms. Logan report his increased consistent use of the assignment tracker, work completion, and organization. They also report less conflict at home, though Ms. Logan needs a reminder to focus on the identified daily requirements and not additional behaviors that have been bothering her. Dylan is helped in expressing his feeling that he fails a lot in his parents' eyes and that he is misunderstood.

The therapist keeps in mind during this discussion the goal of helping the family move their interactions from conflict and low levels of communication toward greater cohesion and communication. The family is first helped to identify the ways they express love and warmth between Dylan and both his mother and father. Their engagement in activities together over the last several weeks provides a helpful basis for this discussion and illustrates their motivation to engage each other respectfully. Dylan's parents reflect on skills they needed to learn when they were Dylan's age and how they have grown since then. They talk about the dialectic of how to accept mistakes while also seeking to change and develop skills. Dylan and his parents agree to work together to identify clear rules and expectations across home settings to address high conflict communication. They identify ways they can show each other they are listening, how to disagree respectfully, and how to share emotions verbally instead of reactively. Dylan and his parents also reflect on how instructions are given to him for chores that are asked outside of the daily expectations. Dylan acknowledges he either does not fully attend to or "blows off" most of their requests. He identifies that it would be helpful to have the requests written down with a reminder to look at the note. His parents are willing to write things down for him, provide one reminder without frustration, and limit the number of requests to a reasonable amount. They are encouraged to apply this collaborative problem-solving approach to other problems that arise in their relationships in the future.

In session eight, Dylan reports continued application of skills addressed in therapy with resultant strong grades at the end of the quarter. He and his parents still have some arguments but they feel more comfortable in working out disagreements without intense anger. Dylan's hopes and dreams for the future are discussed. He wants to be able to do well in high school in order to go to college. The therapist encourages him to view these three years of middle school as learning opportunities for self-understanding, development of executive function skills, and identification of strategies that will help him succeed. He and his mother are referred to several resources through the CHADD website (chadd.org) for strategies to manage ADHD symptoms. Monthly booster sessions are planned to check in with Dylan about his application of skills and his relationships with his parents.

Parenting sessions. In the first session, Ms. Logan is provided with information about ADHD and space to ask questions. She ex-

presses many misconceptions about ADHD and what it will mean for Dylan's future. She is helped to identify Dylan's strengths and to interpret his symptoms in a new light—not as behavior problems under his control but as opportunities to develop skills he is lacking. For example, Ms. Logan can see Dylan's forgetfulness as being present in the moment to what is around him, his loss of items as not being beholden to material things, and his hyperactivity as boundless energy and creativity that can be channeled in beautiful ways. She is also introduced to the idea that she and Dylan's father can take the role of coaches to develop the skills that are difficult for him in preparation for addressing specific executive functions over the course of therapy and beyond. Aspects of this coaching are presented, including setting goals collaboratively with Dylan and targeting only one or two skills at a time, developing compensatory strategies for specific executive function difficulties, providing environmental supports while he develops the skills, praising efforts and small improvements in behavior or gains in skills (i.e., reinforced practice and shaping) to keep Dylan motivated to work together with his parents, providing multiple opportunities to correctly execute desired behaviors, and decreasing or removing supports once Dylan demonstrates attainment of targeted skills.

In the second parenting session, Ms. Logan describes "constant conflict" with Dylan; she cries when discussing her desire to enjoy being with him again and her frustration with his behavior and her "constant nagging" due to his lack of following through with instruction. She worries about his future and wonders when he "is going to get it." She is receptive to discussing how she feels most connected to Dylan (e.g., cuddling on the coach while watching television, playing games, laughing and joking, working together on a project). As a first line of intervention, times that work in their family schedule for them to have positive interactions are identified. The therapist also provides psychoeducation about mindful parenting, to have a clear, calm mind focused on the present moment in a nonjudgmental manner. Ms. Logan reports feeling comfort that she can acknowledge both his strengths and his need for improvement without taking his behavior personally (a dialectical perspective).

The therapist also helps her apply these approaches to herself, to be attentive to her own emotions and thoughts in interactions with Dylan, and to accept she is doing the best she can yet also wants to grow in her parenting skills just as her son is doing the best he can but has skills he needs to learn still. The therapist facilitates her reflection on the characteristics of God that speak to her heart the most. Ms. Logan identifies patience, being slow to anger, and grace as characteristics she would like to embody and recognizes her high emotional arousal in parenting. Ms. Logan is given homework assignments to practice mindfulness and to engage in breathing before responding. The therapist also calls Dylan's father to offer a session in which to provide psychoeducation about ADHD. His father chooses to ask questions about ADHD over the phone. He is also encouraged to identify positive interactions he can implement during Dylan's time with him. Dylan's parents choose not to put him on medication without first trying behavioral interventions.

In the third and fourth parenting sessions, the therapist and Ms. Logan review Dylan's functioning and her coaching of Dylan in the specific targeted executive function skills. They discuss foundational behavior management strategies to help develop Dylan's skills. For example, she learns how to reinforce desired behaviors using attention, praise, and a tangible reward system for target behaviors. She also learns how to effectively give commands and instructions after she has ensured Dylan's attention to her. The therapist also provides information about limit setting and discipline, including making expectations and consequences clear, ignoring minor misbehavior, and using time-out and the removal of privileges as consequences for disrespect and not doing what he is asked.

Ms. Logan shares she has been praying for the words to speak with Dylan to connect with him and to help him when he is upset. She expresses that she is hard on herself when she gets frustrated with him. She wants to focus more on the use of attention, praise, and rewards to counter the negative cycle that has developed between them. Through discussion, Ms. Logan recognizes the frustration stems in large part from worry about his future and a desire for him to be successful. Ms. Logan and the therapist discuss how trust in God for Dylan's future would impact her parenting in the present. Ms. Logan explores what it means to her to trust in God to work through what is happening in Dylan's life and to trust in God's plan for Dylan. She realizes her frustration feels less necessary when she takes a proactive parenting approach and recognizes that whatever Dylan's trials, God is able to work through them.

Additional considerations from a developmental psychopathology framework. Dylan's parents are against putting Dylan on medication at the beginning of therapy. However, Ms. Logan identifies her fears about medication and reads information provided to her. She also speaks with a good friend at her church who takes medication for ADHD and explains the benefits, which helps Ms. Logan begin to view medication not as something against God's plan but as a possible tool to help Dylan reach his potential. The therapist facilitates a phone conference with Dylan's parents to help them come to a joint decision about whether to seek medication management. About halfway through therapy, Dylan is prescribed Vyvance by his pediatrician. His symptoms are monitored through administration of measures to two of his teachers at two time points during therapy. Their reports indicate a decrease in inattention problems and impulsivity. Specifically, his teachers and his mother report he seems to be listening better to directions, taking more time and care in the completion of work, and noticeably off-task less often, even at baseball practice after school.

Given Dylan's symptoms of ADHD and specific executive function weaknesses, and their impact on his functioning at home and at school, it is suggested he be provided with environmental supports at school until he has developed skills in the areas of concern. He has responded well to supports in the past and in the current academic year, and has difficulty achieving to the level he should without these supports. The therapist, Ms. Logan, and Dylan meet with his team of teachers and discuss skills Dylan is focusing on to improve his functioning in the school setting. The therapist emphasizes the need to encourage Dylan as he begins to practice these skills at school. As Dylan is provided with direct instruction and support of these skills, Dylan

will also need to learn to advocate for himself, particularly when he enters high school and in more difficult courses. Thus, his teachers are encouraged to work collaboratively with him, and Dylan is encouraged to approach teachers and ask for support or accommodations as needed.

Dylan and his teachers select specific supports from the following list of recommendations reviewed together that are feasible and fit with this school setting: establish appropriate times and places for Dylan to move around (e.g., walking to back of classroom, standing to stretch) through scheduled breaks in the school day, and alternative seating (e.g., a standing desk) to accommodate for his need to move; provide alternative, nondistracting sources of activity to help keep Dylan active but attentive (e.g., a fidget, doodling); implementation of a system in which homework assignments can be accessed at home to assist Dylan in work completion; increase in academic rigor to challenge Dylan; a system for checking work (e.g., teachers identify peer "monitors" whom Dylan can check in with to ensure that all assignments are noted in the software program chosen to manage his assignments); allow him to carry his backpack during school to assist with organization; provide him with immediate feedback regarding his accuracy and work completion; allow him to correct his mistakes; teach note-taking strategies to increase his attention during academic instruction; provide him with rubrics and go over the rubric with him to help him break it down, particularly with more complex or lengthy assignments or material; break longer assignments into smaller parts so Dylan can see an end to the work, and provide established deadlines for each short task; when possible, his parents or teachers should go over the plan he develops for work completion to help him make changes when needed; permit Dylan to engage in self-talk while completing assignments at a level appropriate to the setting (e.g., whispering) or allow him to complete work in a separate location; and testing in a separate location upon Dylan's request when he is particularly distracted.

It is also recommended that Dylan's mother consistently remain in close communication with his team of teachers throughout the school year in order to help the teachers understand Dylan's specific skill deficits and identify and ensure effective strategies are utilized across home and school settings. After individual sessions with Dylan that targeted specific skills pertinent to his academic functioning, the therapist provides information to his team of teachers about the skill Dylan was targeting. The therapist also emphasizes the effectiveness of positive feedback and a personal relationship with Dylan on his behavior. The teachers occasionally ask questions about the skills or engage in problem solving with the therapist over the course of therapy.

Finally, the therapist provides consultation twice to Dylan and Ms. Logan's church ministry at the request of Ms. Logan, who perceive adults working with Dylan as struggling to understand his behavior. The therapist begins the consultation by presenting ADHD as a brain-based disorder and not a spiritual problem. The consultations are interactive with common misconceptions about ADHD presented first to facilitate questions about the disorder. In coordination with the youth pastor (with whom the therapist had talked on the phone prior to the first consultation), a

discussion is facilitated regarding what acceptance and encouragement of Dylan and other children with ADHD symptoms could look like, as members of the body are called to do. In discussion about the gifts these children bring to the church, just as every other child does, staff reflect on Dylan's enthusiasm and creativity during engaging tasks. His contributions to creative ideas for outreach events for the youth group, for which he seems to have a particular passion, are also recognized as is his willingness to communicate his thoughts during group discussion and take on certain roles (e.g., reading in church, introducing the youth group to others).

The group then reviews the structure of youth group and engages in problem solving about ways the church could better serve and support youth with ADHD. The children's ministry identifies the need to have a clear, consistent structure to each meeting with activities that last no more than ten minutes each before a movement break of some kind. During youth group in particular, structure and guidelines for discussions are developed to encourage listening to each other and to prevent any one child from taking over the discussion. Adults working with children with behavior problems also decide to address concerns and provide feedback to children in private rather than in front of the group. It is decided that children will be permitted to engage in activities during "talk times" without worry that it prevents their engagement (e.g., doodling on provided paper, holding a fidget). In general, it is emphasized that children want to be in the setting but may be restless. Children also will be allowed to move around or stand at their seat or on the rug during "talk times" (e.g., when reading a

Bible story, during discussions). Leaders' questions and difficulties regarding implementation of these decisions and additional concerns they identify are discussed in the second consultation. At the end of treatment, Dylan's mother reports he loves going to youth group. Dylan's reflection indicates he feels he belongs and is accepted at church. He reports higher self-esteem and happiness.

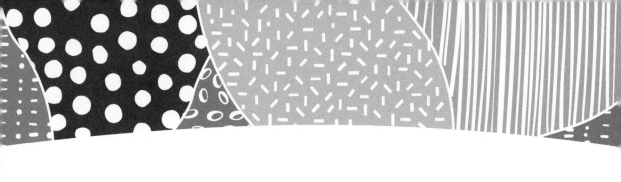

Part Four

Other Disorders in Childhood and Adolescence

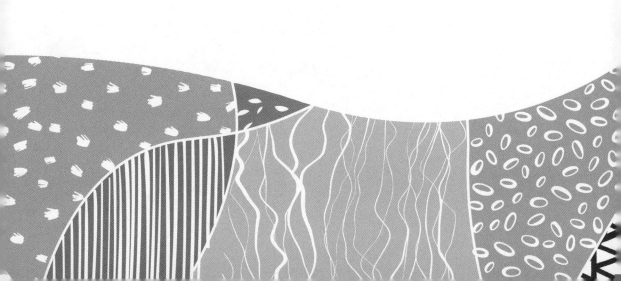

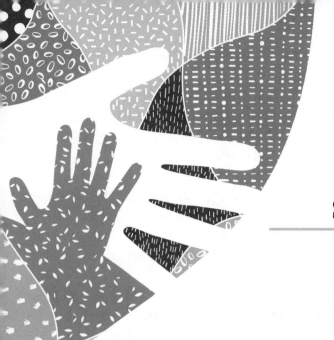

Chapter Eight

Autism Spectrum Disorder

THE TERM "AUTISTIC" (from the Greek *autos*, or self) was first used in 1911 to describe the withdrawing into oneself sometimes seen in schizophrenia (Moskowitz & Heim, 2011). Since its initial inclusion in the DSM-III as its own diagnosis (American Psychiatric Association, 1980), autism spectrum disorder (ASD), or autism, has become both better understood and more frequently diagnosed. In the most recent edition of the diagnostic manual, DSM-5 (American Psychiatric Association, 2013), several previously separate diagnoses (autistic disorder, Asperger's disorder, childhood disintegrative disorder, and pervasive developmental disorder not otherwise specified) have been subsumed under the broader category of ASD based on research that failed to find consistent differences among these subtypes (Gibbs et al., 2012). The number of youth diagnosed with ASD has increased dramatically over time from one in 3,000 in the late 1980s to one in 150 in 2000; the most recent data

indicate that approximately one in every 54 youth in the United States has been diagnosed with the disorder (Maenner et al., 2020). This change in the rate of diagnosis is thought to be due mainly to a combination of improved detection of symptoms, improved public and professional awareness, successful practices and policies for early identification of developmental disabilities, and broadening of diagnostic criteria, though these factors do not fully explain it, and the remaining causes are unclear (Faja & Dawson, 2017; Maenner et al., 2020).

ASD is characterized by two main areas of deficits (American Psychiatric Association, 2013). First, individuals with ASD have difficulty with social interaction and communication. These deficits may manifest themselves in the areas of social-emotional reciprocity (e.g., difficulties with social interaction, shared affect, or conversational participation), nonverbal communication (e.g., lack of eye contact, difficulties using or interpreting body language or gestures, or lack of facial expressiveness), and relationships (e.g., difficulties making or keeping friends, lack of shared play, difficulty behaving appropriately in different social contexts, or lack of interest in peers). Second, ASD is characterized by patterns of stereotyped or restricted behaviors or interests, such as repetitive motor movements (e.g., hand flapping), repetitive speech (e.g., echolalia), rigidity in routines and rituals (e.g., insistence on eating the same foods every day), abnormally intense preoccupation with specific topics or objects, and sensory abnormalities (e.g., hypersensitivity to certain aspects of clothing, hyposensitivity to pain or temperature, or excessive touching/smelling of objects). In order to be diagnosed with ASD, symptoms must interfere with functioning and have been present early in development even if they are not fully apparent until youth are older.

It is important to note that ASD is exhibited along a spectrum, with youth ranging from very high to very low functioning, and it is important for clinicians to identify the particular areas of strength as well as impairment for each client. To help communicate variations in functioning and impairment, several diagnostic specifiers exist, including two that allow clinicians to formally express whether individuals have accompanying intellectual and/or language impairment. In addition, youth with ASD may display a variety of commonly co-occurring signs and difficulties that are not considered a formal part of the diagnosis, including motor abnormalities, clumsiness, self-injury, and aggression (American Psychiatric Association, 2013). Boys are diagnosed with ASD four times as frequently as girls (Maenner et al., 2020; Shaw et al., 2020). Studies of families with genetic risk for ASD show that siblings of youth with autism are more likely to develop ASD if they are female, suggesting this gender difference may be due to differences in vulnerability to genetic risk (Ozonoff et al., 2011; Werling & Geschwind, 2015). However, girls with ASD tend to have higher levels of behavioral and social problems and lower intellectual abilities (Dworzynski et al., 2012; Maenner et al., 2020).

Seventy percent of youth with ASD meet the criteria for a comorbid disorder, and many youth have multiple disorders that co-occur with autism symptoms (Kerns et al., 2015; Simonoff et al., 2008; van Steensel et al., 2011). Many youth with ASD (42-44%) also meet the criteria for an anxiety disorder, such as specific phobia, social anxiety disorder, or obsessive-compulsive disorder. Other common comorbidities include attention-deficit/hyperactivity disorder (28-31%) and disruptive behaviors disorders (30%). The associations between ASD and other disorders do not appear to be due to common causal or risk factors, and though the explanations for comorbidity are unclear, they may have to do with how the symptoms of ASD predispose youth to difficulties in other areas of functioning. For example, a child with ASD who is easily overwhelmed by sensory stimuli and has difficulty communicating his needs and his distress may act out aggressively; an adolescent who feels socially isolated and lonely may develop an anxiety disorder. In addition, about one-third of youth with ASD also have an intellectual disability, generally defined as an IQ at or below 70 (Christensen et al., 2016; Maenner et al., 2020), with this co-occurrence higher among girls than boys. Youth with ASD have higher rates of physical or medical problems as well, including sleep disturbances, gastrointestinal problems, and epilepsy (Ballaban-Gil & Techman, 2000; Buie et al., 2010; Doshi-Velez et al., 2014; Herrmann, 2016; Richdale & Schreck, 2009). It is important to note that there are likely complex links among the various difficulties youth with ASD experience; for example, there is evidence that sensory sensitivity may contribute to sleep problems, which may in turn increase externalizing behavior problems (Mazurek et al., 2019).

RISK/CAUSAL FACTORS
Biological factors.
Genetics. Heritability estimates for autism spectrum disorder range from 38% to 90% (Bai et al., 2019; Bailey et al., 1995; Caglayan, 2010; Hallmayer et al., 2011; Tick et al., 2015). Youth with an older sibling with ASD are thirty times more likely to be diagnosed with the disorder than youth without an affected sibling (Miller et al., 2018). While the specific relative genetic and environmental contributions are still unclear, it is apparent that genetic factors significantly influence the development of ASD. The frequent co-occurrence of ASD with a variety of chromosomal abnormalities, such as Fragile X syndrome and Down syndrome, is considered further evidence of the role of genetic factors in its etiology (Caglayan, 2010; Gillberg & Billstedt, 2000). Variations in over twenty-two chromosomal regions have been linked with heightened risk for ASD (Xu et al., 2004). Specific genes implicated in ASD risk include genes involved in GABA reception, oxytocin reception, serotonin transport, growth factors, gastrointestinal functioning, and language (An et al., 2018; Yoo, 2015). In addition, individuals with ASD are more likely to have

certain types of copy number variations (CNV) that reflect unusual genetic deletions or repetitions (Girirajan et al., 2013; Marshall et al., 2008). These variations generally occur de novo within an individual's genome, resulting from mutation within a sperm or egg cell that was not present within the parent's other cells, though a very small number appear to be inherited (Levy et al., 2011). Sex differences in CNV have been offered as an explanation for the higher rate of ASD in males (Pinto et al., 2014). It is important to note that while genetic vulnerability has a clear influence on ASD risk, there is significant variability among genetic risk factors even between members of the same family with ASD, indicating that it is a genetically heterogeneous disorder (Yuen et al., 2015).

Brain development. Genetic predispositions may translate into neuroanatomical differences between individuals with and without ASD. ASD is sometimes associated with macrocephaly, abnormally large head circumference caused by rapid brain growth in early development (Sacco et al., 2015). Research suggests that abnormalities in various neurotrophic factors, such as brain-derived growth factor (BDNF), lead to atypical connections among neurons and/or neuronal pruning (Nickl-Jockschat & Michel, 2011). Indeed, youth with ASD are more likely than healthy controls to have certain neuroanatomical abnormalities, including increased gray matter in regions of the parietal, temporal, and occipital lobes and decreased gray matter in the cerebellum, patterns which have been linked with social cognitive deficits (Liu et al., 2017; Rojas et al., 2006). In childhood, ASD is associated with an enlarged amygdala, but this difference disappears by adolescence, suggesting that the amygdalae of youth with ASD grow more rapidly than normal in childhood but then fail to grow as expected into adolescence (Schumann et al., 2004; Sparks et al., 2002). Larger amygdalar volume is associated with higher levels of internalizing symptoms and lower levels of social and communication skills in youth with ASD (Juranek et al., 2006; Munson et al., 2006). Functional magnetic resonance imaging (fMRI) studies suggest that individuals with ASD also process information differently than their typically developing peers. For example, they display slower reaction times and decreased activation in certain parts of the brain during face processing tasks, abnormalities which may contribute to the social deficits in ASD (Dawson et al., 2005; Stigler et al., 2011). Other research suggests that dysfunction within the mirror neuron system, which supports our understanding and imitation of others' actions (Rizzolatti & Craighero, 2004), may underlie theory of mind deficits (difficulties inferring others' mental states) that frequently occur in this population (Chien et al., 2015; Dapretto et al., 2006).

Environmental factors.

Toxin and medication exposure. Because genetic risk does not always translate into disorder, ASD is generally understood to result from the complex interaction of environmental and genetic factors, with environmental experiences influencing the expression of genetically based risk (Mandy & Lai, 2016). Exposure to a number of xenobiotic factors, chemicals and toxins that originate outside the body, are thought to increase a child's risk for developing ASD. ASD has been associated with higher levels of exposure to air pollutants (especially in the third trimester of pregnancy and the first year of life), certain types of volatile organic compounds (VOCs) released by paints and cleaning solutions, metals (e.g., mercury, chromium, and nickel), and pesticides (especially in the first trimester of pregnancy; Kalkbrenner et al., 2014). The specific manner in which exposure to these toxins may raise the risk for ASD is yet unknown but is proposed to affect the development of the immune or endocrine systems, alter processes involved with genetic expression, change the microbiome (i.e., gut bacteria), and/or affect the functioning of mitochondria.

Maternal medication use during pregnancy may also raise the child's risk for ASD. In utero exposure to certain anticonvulsant medications, used to treat epilepsy as well as bipolar disorder, has been linked to heightened risk for ASD (Christensen et al., 2013; Wood et al., 2015). Findings on the link between the use of selective serotonin reuptake inhibitors (SSRIs) in pregnancy and the development of ASD in the child are mixed; some studies point to a higher incidence of ASD in children whose mothers took SSRIs while they were pregnant (Croen et al., 2011; Gidaya et al., 2014), while others find no effects of SSRIs on ASD risk (Malm et al., 2016; Viktorin et al., 2017). It has been suggested that these inconsistent findings may be due to the risk for ASD being raised by maternal psychopathology (and its associated genetic and other contextual risk factors) rather than medication use itself.

Other prenatal and birth factors. In addition to prenatal toxin exposure, other prenatal and perinatal variables are thought to contribute to the development of ASD. Research has consistently linked increased parental age of both mothers and fathers with a child's heightened risk for ASD (Hultman et al., 2011; Kolevzon, Gross, & Reichenberg, 2007; Merikangas et al., 2017; Sandin et al., 2016). The most commonly proposed explanation for this finding is that the sperm and eggs of older parents are more prone to spontaneous genetic alterations, such as CNV, that may underlie the disorder (Hultman et al., 2011; Umbarger, 2017). In addition, a number of maternal and infant characteristics that are associated with suboptimal fetal growth or nutrient deficiency have also been linked to ASD risk; these factors include being born small for gestational age (SGA) and the presence of maternal metabolic conditions such as obesity, high blood pressure, and diabetes during pregnancy (Hultman et al., 2002; Krakowiak et al., 2012). Finally, birth complications, including breech position, Rh incompatibility, respiratory distress, oxygen deprivation (in males), and jaundice (in females) have been linked to heightened risk for ASD, likely via their effects on brain development and functioning (Froehlich-Santino et al., 2014; Gardener et al., 2011).

Developmental Course

ASD is generally conceptualized as a set of developmental delays, with symptoms representing abilities and functioning that are delayed compared to peers without the disorder. However, manifestations are heterogeneous, and ASD is considered a "spectrum" because there is a wide range of severity levels and symptom manifestations depending on a child's age and developmental stage (American Psychiatric Association, 2013). Researchers conceptualize ASD as having two main patterns of onset: early onset and regressive onset (Goin-Kochel et al., 2015). Most children display early-onset ASD, with symptoms appearing within the first year of life. Since ASD is not diagnosed in infancy, long-term prospective studies of very young children have been used to link early signs with later ASD. Motor delays are apparent as early as six months of age (Flanagan et al., 2012; Nickel et al., 2013), and social deficits can begin to occur even earlier. At two months of age, infants who will later be diagnosed with ASD are indistinguishable from their peers in the amount of time they spend looking at other people's eyes (a socially adaptive and normative behavior), but this behavior declines drastically by the time they are six months old (Jones & Klin, 2013). Observations of eleven- to twelve-month-old infants show that they are less socially engaged with their parents during play, look at other people as well as objects held by others less frequently, are less responsive to their own names, and display more repetitive movements than typically developing babies (Campbell et al., 2015; Osterling et al., 2002). Delays in both receptive and expressive language are also observable by one year (Zwaigenbaum et al., 2005). Other children display a regressive onset, developing typically for a period of time and then showing a loss of previously established skills and functioning. This regression occurs most frequently around the middle of the second year of life and involves a loss of language, social, and/or adaptive skills (Barger et al., 2013; Goldberg et al., 2003). Despite the concept of two separate patterns of onset, the lines between them often blur. For example, even for children who display the early-onset pattern, social and behavioral symptoms generally worsen during the second year of life, as children with ASD become increasingly different from typically developing peers (Estes, Zwaigenbaum, et al., 2015; Landa & Garrett-Mayer, 2006). In addition, some studies suggest that regression is actually quite common in ASD (Thurm et al., 2014), and some youth display a "delays-plus-regression" pattern of onset in which symptoms are apparent from early development but regression also occurs (Ozonoff et al., 2005). By three years of age, type of onset does not affect symptom presence or severity (Werner et al., 2005).

Regardless of early versus regressive onset, ASD symptoms are observable within the first two years of life. These symptoms include deficits in verbal communication, use of gestures, social orientation to others, and typical play with objects (see Jones et al., 2014, for a review). As early as twelve months of age, children who will later be diagnosed with ASD show deficits in joint attention (Osterling et al., 2002). Joint attention is two people's shared focus on the same object or situation (Bakeman & Adamson, 1984). Evidence of joint attention can be seen visually (e.g., directing another's attention to an object by looking at it), verbally (e.g., discussion of an object), or through gestures (e.g., pointing at an object). A child can either respond to an adult's bid for joint attention or initiate one herself (Yoder & McDuffie, 2006); in both cases, the function of joint attention is shared communication about the object or situation on which both individuals are focused. Young children with ASD are less likely to look where an adult is looking or pointing and trying to direct the child's attention and less likely to point at desired or interesting objects, indicating deficits in both responding to and initiating joint attention (Stone et al., 1997; Sullivan et al., 2007). Difficulties with joint at-

tention have been linked with language deficits in children with ASD (Shumway & Wetherby, 2009; Toth et al., 2006). Although it is clear that targeted intervention can improve joint attention in children with ASD (Yoder & McDuffie, 2006), the evidence is mixed as to whether these deficits resolve naturally by age four (Dawson et al., 2004; Naber et al., 2008).

Though symptoms are frequently apparent within the first two years of life, many youth are not diagnosed until after their fourth birthday (Christensen et al., 2016; Shaw et al., 2020). This delay may be due to parents' failure to recognize and report early signs of ASD, lack of recommended early screening by care providers, and systemic variables such as low socioeconomic status, which can interfere with access to evaluation and intervention services (Daniels, Halladay, et al., 2014; Daniels & Mandell, 2014). Further, although there are no differences in the early identification of autism among white and black young children, which suggests that gaps across racial groups have decreased over time, the overall prevalence for Hispanic children is lower, which may represent continued disparities in early identification (Shaw et al., 2020). Early identification is important for children to receive necessary services as soon as possible; thus, early developmental monitoring and screening is recommended for all children (Johnson & Myers, 2007). Without intensive early intervention, there is a high level of continuity in ASD diagnoses across childhood, with symptoms persisting as youth age (Lord et al., 2006; Woolfenden et al., 2012). However, significant individual variability exists (Ben-Sasson & Gill, 2014), and some youth who display early potential signs of ASD may not meet the diagnostic criteria as they age (Spikol et al., 2019). In addition, different types of symptoms show different developmental patterns. Verbal communication and repetitive behaviors and mannerisms appear to be stable across childhood; social interaction and nonverbal communication increase, as does insistence on sameness (Moss et al., 2008; Richler et al., 2010; Thurm et al., 2007). Mothers report that youths' overall ASD symptom severity increases across childhood and into adolescence (McStay et al., 2014).

Although the majority of children diagnosed with ASD continue to meet criteria into adolescence, parents report improvements in adaptive behavior, social skills, repetitive behaviors, and empathy, particularly in youth without a comorbid intellectual disability (McGovern & Sigman, 2005; Seltzer et al., 2004). However, symptoms plateau after these youth leave high school; this halt in progress is thought to be due to the ending of support and services offered through the school system as well as a decrease in overall stimulation (Taylor & Seltzer, 2010). Very few of these young adults are employed in a traditional, "competitive" position; some work in low-skilled, supported positions, and many attend sheltered workshops or day activity centers (Taylor & Seltzer, 2011). Young adults without intellectual disabilities are more likely to be competitively employed or continuing their education. Overall, outcomes in adulthood vary, but longitudinal studies begun before intensive early intervention was common find continuing symptoms and impairment, particularly in social and sensory realms, for most adults diagnosed with ASD in childhood (Billstedt et al., 2007; Howlin et al., 2004). Consistent with other research, better early communication abilities (specifically, the presence of speech before age five) and the absence of cognitive impairment predict better adult outcomes (Billstedt et al., 2007; Howlin et al., 2004).

ASSESSMENT

Given the importance of early intervention, early screening for ASD is critical. The American Academy of Pediatrics recommends that all children be screened for ASD symptoms at eighteen- to twenty-four-month primary care visits (Zwaigenbaum et al., 2015). If concern about ASD exists following routine screening, children should be referred to a specialist for further assessment. Several tools for assessing ASD have been developed and include questionnaires, interviews, and observational measures. Briefer questionnaires that can be used as screening tools include the Modified Checklist for Autism in Toddlers (M-CHAT; Robins et al., 2001), designed to be completed by parents of sixteen- to thirty-month-olds, and the Social Communication Questionnaire (SCQ; Rutter et al., 2008), for use with individuals ages four and older. The Gilliam Autism Rating Scale, Third Edition (GARS-3; Gilliam, 2014) is a 56-item questionnaire that can be completed by parents, teachers, or other caregivers of three- to twenty-two-year-olds. Gaining information about symptoms and functioning from parent interviews is also an important component of the assessment process. The Autism Diagnostic Interview—Revised (ADI-R; Lord et al., 1994) is a semi-structured interview for parents of children forty-two months and older who display symptoms of ASD. Questionnaires are selected based on the child's verbal ability and assess social communication, restricted interests, and repetitive behaviors. The ADI-R is long (ninety minutes or more) but has good specificity and sensitivity (Lord et al., 1997).

Clinician observation is also an important component of assessment and diagnosis, and a number of structured observational measures of ASD exist. The Autism Diagnostic Observation Schedule, Second Edition (ADOS-2; Lord, Rutter, et al., 2012) is often seen as the "gold standard" in ASD assessment; clinicians choose one of five developmentally based modules to administer to a client depending on his age and language ability. The clinician then interacts with and observes the client during a series of structured and unstructured activities (e.g., free play, pretend play, and discussion of hypothetical social situations), coding a wide variety of behaviors related to the main categories of ASD symptoms (e.g., social engagement, joint attention, emotional reciprocity, and engagement with objects). The ADOS-2 can be used with nonverbal to verbally fluent individuals and includes a Toddler Module designed specifically for children twelve to thirty months old (Lord, Luyster, et al., 2012). The instrument has very good diagnostic sensitivity and specificity (Lord et al., 2000; Luyster et al., 2009). The Childhood Autism Rating Scale, Second Edition, (CARS2; Schopler et al., 2010) provides a rating system for clinicians to use during unstructured observations of youth. Clinicians observe clients in the setting and activities of their choice, take detailed notes, and rate clients' behavior in fifteen areas of functioning, such as verbal communication, emotional expression/responses, and adaptation to change. CARS2

contains two versions of rating scales for use with younger/lower functioning and verbally fluent/higher functioning individuals, both of which have good reliability.

In addition to assessing the presence of ASD symptoms for diagnostic purposes, it is often useful to include tools that evaluate children's adaptive skills in various domains and contexts. For young children up to forty-two months old, the adaptive behavior subtest of the Bayley Scales of Infant and Toddler Development, Third Edition (Bayley-III; Bayley, 2006) may be useful; for individuals of any age, well-established tools include the Adaptive Behavior Assessment System, Third Edition (ABAS-3; Harrison & Oakland, 2015) and the Vineland Adaptive Behavior Scales, Second Edition (VABS-II; Sparrow et al., 2005). The VABS-II is an interview- and questionnaire-based caregiver report measure of five domains of adaptive behavior: communication abilities, daily living skills, social interactions, motor skills, and maladaptive behavior. The Verbal Behavior Milestones and Placement Plan (VB-MAPP; Sundberg, 2008) is a task-based protocol designed to assess the developmental milestones and skills of language-delayed children ages zero to four. The clinician uses caregiver questions and tasks given to the child to assess the child's milestone acquisition (e.g., language, listening, motor, social, academic abilities), barriers to learning language and other skills (e.g., poor listening, lack of responsiveness to operant conditioning, poor eye contact, self-stimulating behavior), and progress toward attendance in a regular school setting as well as supports needed in school (e.g., IEP planning). Both adaptive behavior and developmental milestone assessments are useful for gaining more detailed and specific information about a child's abilities in different realms as well as assessing areas of strength and weakness. Using adaptive behavior assessment tools in combination with other measures of ASD symptoms improves diagnostic accuracy above the evaluation of symptoms alone (Tomanik et al., 2007). Given the common occurrence of intellectual disability in ASD, clinicians may find it helpful to administer a cognitive ability test to assess cognitive functioning and degree of impairment. The Stanford-Binet Intelligence Scales, Fifth Edition (SB-5; Roid, 2003) can be used with individuals ages two and up. The Wechsler family of intelligence tests assess cognitive functioning using tools designed for particular development periods; specifically, the Wechsler Preschool and Primary Scale of Intelligence, Fourth Edition (WPPSI-IV; Wechsler, 2012) can be used with children from two years, six months to seven years, seven months; the Wechsler Intelligence Scale for Children, Fifth Edition (WISC-V; Wechsler, 2014) is normed for children age six through sixteen years, eleven months; and the Wechsler Adult Intelligence Scale, Fourth Edition (WAIS-IV; Wechsler, 2008) was developed for use with adolescents and adults age sixteen and older. Finally, a comprehensive assessment of ASD should include the evaluation of developmental milestones, medical history, attention impairment, executive functioning, academic abilities, comorbid conditions such as anxiety disorders, the child's functioning in school, and the family and community context (McCrimmon et al., 2016; Ozonoff et al., 2005; Tarbox et al., 2016). Additional assessment of relevant functioning by a speech pathologist and an occupational therapist are ideal

(Campbell, Ruble, & Hammond, 2014; Johnson & Myers, 2007). Exploration of each of these variables allows for a better understanding of the child's functioning and impairment, other comorbid diagnoses that may need to be addressed, and how he can best be supported in various contexts.

TREATMENT

There is one very clear consensus from the research on treating autism spectrum disorders: early intervention is critical (Fettig & Fleury, 2017; National Research Council, 2001). The American Academy of Pediatrics (Zwaigenbaum, 2015) recommends that primary care providers screen all children for "red flags," or early signs, of ASD between eighteen and twenty-four months. Treatment should begin as soon as these early signs are apparent but ideally no later than twenty-four months. Specific effective psychosocial treatments for ASD fall into two categories (Smith & Iadarola, 2015). Applied behavior analysis (ABA) uses the principles of operant conditioning to shape children's behavior based on the view that these youth need specialized, targeted interactions in order to learn effectively from their environments. Developmental social-pragmatic (DSP) interventions aim to improve the impaired joining and social interactions of youth with ASD by targeting caregivers' sensitivity and responsiveness to their children, which in turn improves children's social skill and engagement. Comprehensive treatment models (CTM) combine elements of both ABA and DSP programs. Finally, some youth with ASD also benefit from supplemental speech and language, occupational, and/or physical therapy that helps them build skills and overcome deficits in communication and physical functioning (Fettig & Fleury, 2017). In the next section, we will describe ABA and DSP interventions in detail and discuss an example of a program that combines them.

Applied behavior analysis (ABA). ABA was originally developed as a treatment for ASD in the 1960s by Ivar Lovaas, a behaviorist at UCLA (Leaf & McEachin, 2016). Lovaas applied the operant conditioning principles of reinforcement and punishment to shape the behaviors of young children with ASD, with the goals of decreasing problematic behaviors and increasing desired behaviors. Early research on ABA produced stunning long-term results, with almost 50% of the treatment group scoring average or above average on an IQ test and being placed in a regular education classroom (compared to 2% of the control group; Lovaas, 1987). Based on the high level of effectiveness of this approach, early and intensive behavioral interventions (EIBI) have been developed and manualized and continue to produce significant improvement in the symptoms and functioning of youth with ASD. EIBI differs from the original applications of ABA with youth with ASD by (1) beginning the intervention when children are very young, (2) implementing the intervention in naturalistic settings, such as the child's home and school, and (3) focusing on the use of reinforcement and extinction rather than punishment (Leaf & McEachin, 2016; Smith, 2010). EIBI is a long-term treatment in which children receive twenty to forty hours per week of ABA instruction over the course of two or more years (Eikeseth, 2011; Green, Brennan, & Fein, 2002; Smith, 2010). EIBI is by necessity intensive, as youth with ASD do not learn adaptive be-

haviors from their environments like their typically developing peers, who are being constantly "trained" by their surroundings. Furthermore, EIBI is most effective when it begins in early childhood, when maladaptive behaviors have not existed for a lengthy period of time and the developmental gaps between youth with ASD and their peers are smaller. In EIBI, ABA-trained professionals work one-on-one with youth to shape their behavior and also train parents to serve as cotherapists who continue to reinforce desired behaviors outside of therapeutic sessions.

Several principles of operant conditioning are central to the methods of ABA/EIBI (Eikeseth, 2011; Kearney, 2008; Smith, 2001). Consequences are events that occur immediately after a behavior and make it more or less likely to occur again in the future. There are three main types of consequences. First, *punishments* are aversive consequences that decrease recurrence of the behavior; because they are controversial and less effective than the other types of consequences for changing behavior, they are no longer commonly used in ABA. Second, *reinforcements* are events that follow a behavior and make it more likely to reoccur; these are one of the main tools of ABA therapists. For example, an infant's use of the sign language for "more" is reinforced when his mother refills his bowl with the desired food; an adolescent's friendly text message to a new classmate is reinforced when the classmate responds in kind. Reinforcers can be primary, reinforcing in and of themselves because of innate drives (e.g., good-tasting food); secondary, rewarding because of their association with primary reinforcers (e.g., verbal praise that is initially offered alongside food); social, involving positive attention or praise from others; automatic, occurring without intervention from others (e.g., the enjoyable self-stimulation created by hand flapping); generalized, rewarding because they are linked with many other reinforcers (e.g., money or tokens); or backup, able to be "bought" with the use of generalized reinforcers (e.g., toys, games, privileges). In ABA with young children, commonly used reinforcers include food, physical touch (e.g., hugs, playful tickling), praise, and small tokens (e.g., stickers). These are all examples of positive reinforcement, in which a behavior is encouraged by the presentation or addition of a desired reward. Negative reinforcement can also be used in ABA. In the process of negative reinforcement, an aversive stimulus or situation is removed as a consequence of the behavior, thereby rewarding the behavior and increasing the likelihood it will be repeated. Negative reinforcement can change behavior via escape, in which an individual performs a behavior in order to end the aversive stimulus (e.g., a child who screams until his parents turn off the music he dislikes), or avoidance, when an individual behaves in a particular way in order to avoid an undesired outcome before it starts (e.g., a child who learns to use the toilet because she does not like the feeling of wearing a dirty diaper). The third type of consequence is no response from the environment, which leads to the *extinction* or elimination of a behavior over time. In the context of ABA, extinction is usually facilitated by ignoring problematic behaviors, such as when a child throws a tantrum.

Another important operant conditioning principle involves antecedents, events or circumstances that precede a behavior and affect the likelihood of its occurrence. There are multiple types of antecedents. *Stimulus control* or *discriminative stimuli* refer to signals in the environment that trigger or suggest a particular behavior. ABA therapists use stimulus control or antecedents to elicit certain behaviors only under certain conditions. For example, observing a peer raise his hand and say, "High five!" is the stimulus which indicates that one should hit his hand with yours; when this stimulus is absent, hitting is not a desired behavior. Therapists frequently use *cues* or *mands* (a common ABA term short for command), verbal requests for a particular behavior, as discriminative stimuli designed to elicit that behavior. This is essentially the same technique that parents and teachers use for all children when they want them to follow an instruction (e.g., "Put the napkins on the dinner table," or "Get out a pencil"). For youth with ASD, these mands are not enough to elicit a behavior themselves, at least at the beginning of treatment; reinforcement of the desired behavior is what truly shapes it, but the mand makes the desired behavior clear to the child. A cue is often accompanied by a *prompt*, in which the therapist supports the child in responding to the cue, such as by modeling the behavior or physically guiding the child. Another type of antecedent is an *establishing operation* (EO) or *motivating operation* (MO), a situation that makes a reinforcer more or less rewarding. Hunger would be an example of an EO that makes a cookie a more effective reinforcer; not having played with her favorite toy all day could be an EO that makes the desired toy a particularly effective reward for a child. Antecedents are often combined with consequences, such that a behavior is cued beforehand by an antecedent and rewarded afterwards by a reinforcer.

ABA therapists use antecedents and consequences to change the behaviors of an individual with ASD so that they behave in more appropriate and positive ways and perform fewer maladaptive behaviors. Some additional behavioral training concepts explain how more complex behaviors are taught. *Shaping* is used to train an individual to perform a more complex behavior or series of behaviors. In shaping, successive approximations of a particular behavior are reinforced, while other behaviors are ignored, so that the individual's behavior becomes closer and closer to what she is being trained to do. For example, if you are training a child to clean up toys, you might first reward her for touching the toy she is supposed to clean up. You would then reward her for picking up a toy off the floor, then for taking one step toward the toy box, then for moving even closer to the toy box with the toy in hand, then for touching the toy box, and finally for putting the toy in the toy box or even in a specific spot in the toy box (while ignoring off-task or undesired behaviors throughout the processes). *Chaining* involves teaching a child a step-by-step behavior by rewarding the child for the performance of each step. Chaining can start with either the first or the final step in the process (the latter is known as reverse or backwards chaining). For example, chaining could be used to teach a child how to wash her hands by rewarding her for performing each of the steps of the process (e.g., turn on water, wet hands, squirt soap on hands, rub hands together, rinse hands, turn water off, dry hands), teaching her a new step once she is consistently displaying the one previously taught. Once a behavior has been learned, a therapist can use *response differentiation* to shape that

behavior further. In this process, only the performance of the behaviors in a particular desired manner is reinforced, while others are extinguished. To build on our previous example, once a child has been trained to follow the steps in washing her hands, a therapist might teach the child to wash her hands in a manner that is effective for killing germs. To do this, he might only reinforce the child's behavior when it meets certain criteria (e.g., she makes the water hot but not too hot, uses the right amount of soap, scrubs her hands for twenty seconds, and dries her hands thoroughly). Finally, once a behavior has been trained to the desired standard, *fading* can be used to slowly eliminate the use of artificial prompts and reinforcers which will not be present in real-world settings. If fading is successful, the child will continue to perform the behaviors she has been taught based on natural cues or commands (e.g., washing her hands when they are dirty or an adult tells her, "It's time to wash your hands") even when she is not directly imitating the therapist or being reinforced as she was during therapy.

In addition to symptom assessment that directs diagnosis, some approaches (e.g., applied behavior analysis) emphasize the importance of beginning treatment with a *functional analysis of behavior* or *functional behavioral assessment* (FBA; Cautela & Kearney, 1986; Kearney, 2008). The purpose of an FBA is to assess why a child is performing a certain behavior; in other words, what function or purpose does the behavior serve for this child? The answers to these questions revolve around understanding the context or features of the environment in which the behavior occurs. To conduct an FBA, clinicians begin by identifying the specific and detailed target (problematic) behavior and keeping track of how often it occurs. Then, they identify the antecedents of the behavior, the situations or events that most frequently immediately precede it, as well as the place and time when the behavior occurs. Next, the consequences of the behavior are identified; what happens immediately following a child's behavior that may be rewarding it, often inadvertently? Finally, the clinician and parents work to identify the rewards and punishments that are likely to be effective for a particular child. Performing an FBA at the beginning of treatment might help parents and clinicians understand, for example, why a child with ASD hits his head on the wall repeatedly. They might discover that this behavior usually happens toward the end of the school day after the child has been asked by his teacher to perform challenging academic tasks and generally results in the child being removed from the classroom and talking to an adult one-on-one. This pattern could suggest that the behavior occurs when the child is tired and stressed and serves the purpose of reducing his stress by avoiding the requirement to complete the difficult schoolwork. Effectively addressing the behavior in treatment, then, involves considering the role of these antecedents and consequences in addition to helping the child develop a more adaptive way of getting his needs met (e.g., managing stress and/or communicating his feelings). Below, we describe one example of an ABA intervention.

The UCLA Young Autism Project (YAP), which grew directly out of Lovaas's early work, is one example of an intervention for youth with ASD that systematically applies these behavior change principles (Cohen, Amerine-Dickens, & Smith, 2006; Smith, 2010). As with other ABA interventions, it is considered ideal for children to begin this intervention at age three or younger, though it has also been implemented with four- and five-year-olds. Treatment begins with thirty-five to forty hours per week of one-on-one intervention (twenty to thirty hours for children younger than three) and is designed to last for roughly three years. During the first year of treatment, intervention takes place mainly in the child's home; as treatment progresses, training is expanded to school and peer settings. In addition to the clinician's direct contact with the child, regular team meetings include therapists, parents, and higher-level supervisors and project managers who work collaboratively to assess the child's development and progress and to tailor the intervention accordingly. Parents are also trained in the principles and techniques of ABA so that they may serve as co-therapists for their children, participating in therapy sessions as well as working with children to help generalize skills to other areas of functioning.

Following a one- to two-hour intake interview, the UCLA YAP model divides treatment into five stages. Stage one focuses on *establishing a teaching relationship* over the course of two to four weeks. During this stage, professional team members and parents begin the process of discrete trial training (DTT), a significant component of training throughout the intervention. In DTT, the principles of operant conditioning discussed earlier are applied through one-on-one interaction between the child and an adult in an environment that is free from distractions. Individual instructional interactions in DTT are referred to as trials. Each trial has five parts: (1) a cue (the child is given clear and simple instructions about a desired behavior), (2) a prompt (the therapist models the behavior or guides the child in performing it), (3) a response (the child responds to the cue, correctly or incorrectly), (4) consequences (if the response is correct, the behavior is immediately reinforced; if not, the therapist says "no" or looks away and does not reward the behavior), (5) intertrial interval (one- to five-second pause between the consequence and the next cue; Smith, 2001). The aim of DTT in the first stage of the intervention is to train the child to perform simple behaviors at the request of parents and clinicians, who give clear instructions and reinforce the desired behavior. Negative behaviors such as crying and hitting, which young children with ASD may display in order to avoid performing requested tasks, are ignored in order to extinguish them. During early DTT, the child is asked to perform behaviors that are likely to be easy for her (e.g., putting a block in a container), as the main goal is not to teach the child new behaviors but to train the child to respond appropriately to the therapist's commands and requests. In essence, the child is being trained to learn. Though this training is generally very effective, even over the course of the initial session, it is often challenging at first. Because these children have often learned previously that they can escape an undesired situation by misbehaving, when their misbehavior is not initially reinforced in DTT, it will generally escalate. Behaviorists refer to this common pattern as an extinction burst. However, if the behavior is consistently not rewarded (i.e., the command is repeated to the child until it is followed, despite the child's attempts to avoid complying), it will stop occurring and will be replaced by the behavior that is reinforced.

In the second stage of the UCLA YAP model, *teaching foundational skills*, the focus on the intervention shifts to teaching adaptive behaviors that form the basis for life skills. Over the course of one to four months, therapists work intensively with children, administering three to eight trials at time, with sets of trials separated by brief (one- to two-minute) breaks, for fifty minutes per hour. After fifty minutes of DTT, ten minutes is spent in structured play or other less formal activities designed to help generalize the skills children have learned. Some of the types of skills that are taught during this phase include receptive language (i.e., following commands), imitating actions, matching and sorting (which can support language development), self-care skills (e.g., getting dressed), and play skills. Parents and therapists use positive reinforcement, extinction, mands, establishing operations, shaping, chaining, response differentiation, and fading to shape children's behavior. Once a child has mastered a behavior in DTT, they are instructed by different adults in different settings to perform it in order to further facilitate generalization.

During *beginning communication*, the third stage of the UCLA YAP intervention, DTT continues as children learn additional skills in the areas previously taught, and a focus on expressive language skills begins. Modeling is central to the teaching of expressive language, as therapists teach children to imitate speech sounds, words, and strings of words through DTT. Therapists help children learn the meanings of words by labeling objects and events and then prompting children to do the same. Children who struggle to speak may be taught to use visual communication systems (e.g., holding up a picture of an apple rather than saying the word "apple"). Because this stage of the intervention is more challenging, it can last for six months or longer. Once children have mastered simple words and phrases, stage four, *expanding communication and beginning peer interaction*, can begin. In this stage, children learn more advanced concepts, such as color, shape, and size. They also learn to connect words with emotional expressions and to speak in full, grammatically correct sentences. In addition, children work on new developmental skills, including pretend play, social skills, and toilet training. During this stage of treatment, children begin to go to preschool, ideally attending a regular education program accompanied by an aide who provides continuity in training across settings. The child's time in the classroom may be brief at first (five to ten minutes) and gradually lengthened as the child adjusts to and succeeds in the preschool setting. Once children have mastered certain social skills (e.g., responding to questions, taking turns), parents may set up playdates with peers from school during which a therapist facilitates activities and prompts the child to use skills appropriately. By one year into the intervention, children average twenty-six to thirty-one hours of individual in-home intervention, six to nine hours of preschool, and three to five hours of peer play per week.

In stage five, *advanced communication and adjusting to school*, the time spent in one-on-one intervention decreases as participation in treatment groups increases. In both settings, children are learning more advanced language skills (e.g., prepositions, pronouns, past tense), conversation skills, perspective taking, reading nonverbal cues (e.g., body language, facial expressions), social problem solving,

appropriate help seeking, school rules, and independent self-care. As children are spending more time in group settings, they are encouraged to learn from their peers and teachers, so that the role of the aide decreases over time. This stage generally continues until children enter elementary school, at which point the intervention ends. This typically happens at age five, though some children will benefit from repeating preschool and continuing to work on communication, social, and school-readiness skills in familiar group and one-on-one settings. Children who still are not successful in a regular education classroom at this point are likely to need additional ongoing support, including continued one-on-one DTT (McEachin et al., 1993). Educational support for these children can range from placement in a regular education setting with collaborative teachers and peers to placement in a behavioral or special education classroom.

The UCLA YAP intervention decreases ASD symptoms in young children with ASD, including producing improvements in receptive and expressive language, intelligence, adaptive functioning, and social skills (Cohen, Amerine-Dickens, & Smith, 2006; Eikeseth et al., 2002, 2007, 2012; Hayward et al., 2009). Analyses of ABA interventions more broadly find that they positively impact IQ, social functioning, daily living skills, and expressive and receptive language, with the greatest improvements occurring in communication skills (Virués-Ortega, 2010). However, significant individual variation in treatment response exists, with some children ("rapid learners") showing significant intellectual, language, and academic gains, whereas others ("moderate learners") continue to show a great deal of impairment (Lovaas, 1987; Sallows & Graupner, 2005). Some studies have found a high percentage of youth treated with ABA to be "indistinguishable" from their typically developing peers posttreatment (McEachin et al., 1993), whereas others have found significant delays in communication and IQ to remain even among youth who improve with treatment (Smith et al., 1997). Two main patterns may help explain these variations. First, treatment that is more intensive (i.e., longer in duration and/or for more hours/week) produces larger effects on children's functioning, particularly in the areas of language and adaptive functioning (Virués-Ortega, 2010). Second, variation in responses to intensive treatment may be explained by individual differences. For example, youth with higher levels of pretreatment skills, including imitation and language, are more likely to have better treatment outcomes than their peers (Sallows & Graupner, 2005; Smith et al., 2010). Additional research is needed to best understand for whom and under what conditions ABA produces the best results for youth with ASD.

Developmental social-pragmatic interventions (DSP). DSP interventions, which are somewhat newer than ABA interventions, focus on promoting healthy interactions between youth with ASD and their caregivers. Developmental interventions assume that children learn social communication skills through their reciprocal relationships with sensitive, responsive adults rather than through discrete operant conditioning trials (Ingersoll et al., 2005; Prizant et al., 2000; Sandbank et al., 2020). DSP interventions, therefore, aim to help parents respond to children's social behaviors and communication attempts in an encouraging, responsive

manner in a naturalistic environment. Such interventions focus less on eliciting very specific, adult-directed behaviors or communication attempts (e.g., particular phases or signs), as ABA interventions do, but rather create an environment designed to elicit communication from the child but then follow the child's lead in initiating interaction. The child is viewed as motivated and capable of connecting and communicating with caregivers when provided with the right structure and opportunities. Emotional expressiveness and reciprocity are also emphasized in DSP interventions. There is a growing body of evidence that indicates DSP interventions are effective in the development of social communication skills, improvements in the synchrony of parent-child interactions, and thus long-term developmental outcomes (Sandbank et al., 2020). Below, we describe a specific example of a DSP intervention.

The Focused Playtime Intervention (FPI; Siller et al., 2013) is a DSP protocol designed to teach responsive parental communication to families of youth ages six and younger with ASD. The twelve-week, in-home intervention comprises weekly ninety-minute sessions in which the therapist and parents spend the first thirty to sixty minutes applying the topic of the session while the therapist both demonstrates the interaction strategies and coaches the parent in her interactions with the child; the remainder of each session is spent without the child present, as the therapist and parent further discuss the topic, go through a parent workbook, review videotape of the parent-child interaction from earlier in the session, and discuss homework for the following week. Sessions target eight topics, phrased in the form of questions parents might ask; three coaching sessions and a wrap-up session are also included in the intervention.

Topic one focuses on the question, *When and how does my child communicate?* After introductions, the parent is then asked to spend ten minutes playing with the child (using toys provided by the clinician if the child is interested) while the interaction is videotaped. The parent-child interaction is videotaped in every session in FPI; most interactions will be reviewed and discussed by the parent and clinician together, but this initial videotape is created mainly as a baseline. The parent and clinician then spend the rest of the session discussing (1) the nature of the intervention and (2) the child's strengths and difficulties in communication (e.g., in the areas of verbal language, social interactions, making needs known, and joint attention). During topic two, *What do I hope to accomplish during play?* the therapist aims to get a sense of the parent's goals for the child during play time and to connect these goals to the goals of FPI. To begin the session, both parent-child and therapist-child interactions are videotaped and discussed. Play times involving the therapist and the child serve several purposes, including helping the therapist understand the child better, allowing the therapist to test the effectiveness of different strategies with the child, and modeling strategies for the parent. (All remaining sessions begin with videotaped interactions between the child and each adult that are then reviewed as a way of discussing the session topic.) Subsequent discussion focuses on the parent's goals for the child during play, including prompting communication, decreasing problematic behavior, connecting emotionally with the child, allowing the child

to enjoy himself, and teaching the child to play correctly with toys; the therapist and parent then review the videotape from earlier in the session in order to connect these goals with the parent's strategies in interacting with the child. Topic three addresses the question, *How do I develop a special play time routine?* The videotapes of the child's interactions with the parent and therapist are used to discuss the importance of elements of a routine in play. Parents are taught how to structure a consistent, predictable play time that promotes positive behavior and growth in the child by establishing a routine (e.g., starting and ending with consistent cues, such as getting toys out and putting them away), choosing a setting and toys that support the child's focused attention and build desired skills (e.g., a ball to promote social interaction, a book to promote language development), and ending the play time on a positive note. Parents are encouraged to keep a journal of their reflections on each day's play time in order to hone their routine over time. Establishing this special play time routine prepares the dyad for the skill-building activities and interactions that will take place during play over the course of the intervention.

The goal of topic four, *How to tackle play one step at a time?* is to help the parent promote joint or shared attention due to its role in social and language development. Videotape review focuses on identifying moments when the parent and child are focused on the same object, and parents are encouraged to add observations about shared focus to their play time journals. Topic five, *Who gets to pick the toys?* continues the work focused on promoting joint attention. Through discussion and videotape review, the therapist teaches the parent how to (1) follow the child's lead by paying attention to his gaze and interest, (2) effectively direct the child's attention to a particular toy or activity, and (3) change her strategy when the child is not responding to it. The idea of flexibility is emphasized; parents must be sensitive to a child's needs and discern whether to lead or follow and how to best promote shared attention (e.g., joining in the child's play when it is constructive; introducing a new toy in a way that encourages the child to engage with the parent, such as stacking a few but not all blocks; removing distracting toys that promote solitary, repetitive play; beginning with a game focused on social interaction and gradually introducing a toy into it). Topic six, *Who decides the "correct" way of using the toys?* addresses the issue of how the parent and child should play together once shared focus on a particular toy has been established. In order to help the child learn that interacting with others can be fun and to establish a tone that facilitates teaching, parents learn to play with a toy at (1) the same level of complexity as the child and (2) the same pace as the child (before moving on to a new activity). These skills require the parent to pay close attention to the child's behavior and to respond sensitively and flexibly based on the child's signals. The therapist might encourage the parent to practice imitating the child's play for a short period of time in order to better understand the child's approach to the toy and pace of play. In discussing this topic, therapists might also remind parents that children sometimes play with toys in unconventional ways and that they may play repetitively with a toy for a long time as they are figuring out how it works and what they like about it; parents, then,

should be patient and flexible and follow the child's lead in play.

Topic seven asks, *How do I speak to my child during play?* Once shared attention has become a part of dyadic play, the focus of the intervention shifts to verbal interactions. Parents are encouraged to use descriptive language during play interactions. This technique accomplishes several goals, including connecting emotionally with the child, joining unobtrusively in the child's play, attributing positive intent to the child's behavior, and seeking to understand the child's point of view. In order to facilitate connection and understanding, parents are encouraged to use language that is warm and exciting, give the child time to respond, use short sentences, and highlight important words. Topic eight, the final subject in the intervention, addresses the question, *How do I make play more balanced between me and my child?* The aim of this intervention element is to help encourage the child to become more responsive to the parent, who has been focused on responding to the child throughout the intervention. Videotape review focuses on two patterns. First, parents are encouraged to pay attention to ways that the child actively attempts to engage the adult in his play, including watching the parent play, joining the parent in her play, becoming interested in a toy the parent has introduced, trying to imitate the parent, making eye contact during play, or pointing to/ showing the parent something he likes. Second, parents learn strategies to encourage these behaviors, such as showing the child simple new ways to play with a toy, making a big deal out of unexpected experiences with toys, imitating the child's actions in order to get his attention, creating opportunities for the child to join in an activity or game, creating games that involve pointing at objects the child is already looking at, and offering only the child's favorite toys at first. Finally, three coaching sessions are used to elaborate on topics five, six, and eight; they typically occur following the sessions on each of these topics but can be moved around in the schedule. Each coaching session begins with a videotaped parent-child interaction, which is then reviewed in order to target specific parental behaviors identified ahead of time by the therapist, who uses two techniques to teach the parent. First, the therapist models both effective and ineffective techniques in interactions with the child. Second, the therapist coaches the parent during her interactions with the child, providing praise to reinforce specific effective behaviors, gentle correction to discourage counterproductive strategies, and specific direction to prompt the use of particular behaviors.

FPI has been found to improve parent-child interactions, including maternal synchronization (i.e., sensitive reciprocity to children's behavior), children's emotional and social reciprocity, and secure attachment (Siller et al., 2013, 2014). Expressive language skills also improved for children with poorer pretreatment communication abilities. It is suggested, therefore, that FPI may be particularly useful for young children with significant communication and social impairments, though the long-term effects of the intervention (beyond twelve months) are not known.

Comprehensive interventions.

The Early Start Denver Model (ESDM; Rogers & Dawson, 2010) is a comprehensive intervention for children with ASD between twelve and sixty months. It is a younger adaption of the Denver Model, which originated as a preschool-based program for two- to five-year-olds, and is based on an understanding of ASD as based in a lack of responsiveness to social rewards. Therefore, the ESDM is designed to increase these children's social motivation in order to provide a forum for the teaching of social, emotional, and communication skills. The intensive, two-year intervention is delivered in the child's home or school by a trained therapist for fifteen to twenty hours per week. The ESDM curriculum combines principles and strategies from ABA, DSP, and pivotal response training. The ESDM draws from ABA in the use of functional analyses of behavior, antecedents, consequences, prompting, fading, shaping, and chaining. Pivotal response training (PRT; Koegel et al., 1999) is based on ABA principles but offers a more interactive alternative to discrete trial training that emphasizes the role of motivation in children's ability to learn. The ESDM incorporates PRT principles such as reinforcing effort and not just success, alternating easy and difficult skills, using natural or logical reinforcers, providing opportunities for the child to lead as well as follow, giving children choices when possible, and reinforcing spontaneous or child-initiated behaviors. Finally, the ESDM includes elements of DSP interventions as well, such as using positive affect and tone, responding sensitively to the child's emotions and expressions, using play as a teaching context, and offering the child a variety of opportunities for communication.

Teaching occurs during play-based interactions that are initiated by the child. The therapist follows the child's lead, matching her tone and speed. The child and the therapist take turns and develop the play activity together; the therapist then directs the play and interaction in a way that facilitates progress toward desired skills. The ESDM targets ten domains of functioning: receptive communication, expressive communication, joint attention, imitation, social skills, play skills, cognitive skills, fine motor skills, gross motor skills, and self-care skills. Every twelve weeks, the therapist selects two to three goals within each domain to inform treatment; as the twelve-week period progresses, adjustments to the targets of the intervention are made based on the child's progress. Each goal that is selected is broken down into a series of concrete "learning steps" that shape progress toward the overall goal. In each session, then, the therapist uses ABA, PRT, and DSP principles to help the child practice each most recently mastered step and learn the next one. The child's level of mastery of each step is recorded every fifteen minutes on detailed coding sheets in order to track progress over time.

For example, one goal for a young child with ASD might be to increase his expressions of shared affect (one application of joint attention). The overall goal could be for the child to indicate his desire to share positive affect with an adult at least three times in ten minutes during play with a toy. The learning steps toward this goal might be: (1) occasional eye contact, (2) consistent eye contact, (3) occasional eye contact with smiling, (4) consistent eye contact with smiling, and (5) alternating smiling at adult and looking at toy (Rogers & Dawson, 2010). The therapist would follow the child's lead in selecting a toy to play with together and work to build shared enjoyment of the toy and the play by

introducing activities with it that the child enjoys. The therapist would both model smiling and looking at the toy for the child and reinforce his eye contact and smiling by continuing to play with the object in the way the child desires. As the child took initiative to play with the toy in a different manner, the therapist would imitate the child and continue to reinforce the child's bids for attention and shared affect.

The ESDM has been found to improve symptoms, IQ, language abilities, adaptive skills, and social behavior in young children with ASD (Dawson et al., 2010, 2012). Furthermore, a two-year follow-up found that these gains persist even after the intervention has ended (Estes, Munson, et al., 2015). School-based group interventions as well as parent-delivered interventions based on the ESDM also show promise for improving ASD symptoms (Eapen et al., 2013; Rogers et al., 2014; Vivanti et al., 2014).

Integrative Approach to Treatment

Conceptualizing ASD and interaction with individuals with the disorder are challenging tasks that raise many questions for Christian scholars, clinicians, and parents. The nature of the disorder itself is likely to challenge us to examine our assumptions about humans and about God. Therefore, before we talk about an integrative approach to treatment, we must address some of the implications of a Christian perspective of the disorder itself. We frame this discussion around Miller-McLemore's (2003) themes of children as (1) gifts, (2) full persons, and (3) agents, including within each theme some reflection on the implications of the theme for ABA and DSP interventions.

Valuing children as gifts. In scriptural and theological conceptualizations of children as gifts (see chapter two, this volume; Flanagan & Hall, 2014), this gift nature is not based on whether a particular child has certain positive characteristics or is experienced as a gift in others' subjective, affective evaluations of them. Rather, children are gifts because God has chosen to make them a blessing, a sign and fulfillment of his promises to his people. It is particularly important to keep these truths in mind when we consider children and adolescents whose gift nature can sometimes be overshadowed by their personal characteristics and difficulties. As we have discussed, youth with ASD can face challenges in nearly every arena of their lives and functioning: physical, emotional, social, communication, and academic. Unfortunately, this myriad of difficulties and challenges, particularly for youth with severe symptoms and low levels of functioning, runs the risk of masking the truth that they are gifts from the Lord. Explicit and implicit feedback and exclusion of youth with ASD from full community participation can also be discouraging to families who sense that their children are seen as "less than" typically developing youth. In the midst of the challenges of caring for these youth, we need to remain steeped in Scripture, prayer, and truth-seeking Christian community that reminds us daily of who God is and who he has created us (and our children) to be. God knitted the child with ASD together in her mother's womb; he knows her deeply, including her strengths and limitations; he loves her and calls her; and he desires her praise and worship (Psalm 139; 150; Romans 8:39). These reminders are an encouragement that our work with youth

with ASD is important and valuable; they are gifts who deserve our attention, care, and love, by which the Giver of the gift is honored. The time and monetary investment in early and intensive intervention, which may involve over six thousand therapeutic hours for a single young child with ASD, is a reflection of the view of these youth as gifts whose development is worth a great deal of attention and resources.

Another manifestation of our view of these youths as gifts is professional and community support for their direct, day-to-day caregivers (e.g., parents). Research suggests that parents of youth with ASD find parenting more stressful and experience higher levels of overall psychological distress than parents of typically developing youth (Baker-Ericzén et al., 2005; Davis & Carter, 2008; Estes et al., 2009). Therefore, if we truly understand children to be gifts from the Lord, we will seek to be a part of the wider community who cares for them and seeks to help them thrive (Miller-McLemore, 2003). For youth with ASD, this care likely entails supporting and caring for their families, especially their parents. Therapists might take special care to ask parents how they are doing and to offer parents opportunities to talk about their experiences of parenting and the associated stressors; family, friends, and the church community might offer emotional support as well as practical help to these parents, such as providing meals and creating opportunities for couples to spend time alone. These supportive efforts do not eliminate the difficulty of caring for youth with ASD, of course, but they can provide temporary respite and communicate a recognition of the burden that these parents frequently feel alone in carrying. The psychological literature recognizes the importance of caring for parents of youth with ASD; how much greater should the support of the church be, given God's special concern for the suffering and our responsibility to care for one another as brothers and sisters in Christ (Job 36:15; Galatians 6:2; 1 Peter 3:8)?

Finally, youth with ASD are a gift in the way they teach us about ourselves and about human nature. In his memoir about raising a son with ASD, Michael Blastland (2006) comments on his fascination with his son's nature and what it reveals about humanity. He notes that his son's limitations contribute to his own amazement at the ability of typically developing individuals to understand and navigate the complexities of social interactions. "He makes much that we take for granted appear suddenly luminous, and we see equally starkly where we would be without it" (p. 5). The social, communication, and functional skills with which many individuals with ASD struggle remind us not to take for granted the myriad abilities on which most of us depend every day. Individuals with ASD may also possess abilities and perspectives that their unique characteristics facilitate. For example, artist Jeremy Sicile-Kira, who has ASD and synesthesia and is nonverbal, credits his ability to perceive stimuli such as faces and emotions as colors as integral to the creation of his unique paintings (Sicile-Kira, 2017). Satoshi Tajiri's desire to share his childhood love of collecting insects with others led to the creation of the wildly popular video game Pokémon (Tobin, 2004). Animal scientist Temple Grandin has used her unique perception of the world to design humane livestock containment systems that provide calming pressure and to write insightfully

about the implicit norms and rules that govern human social interactions (Grandin, 2006; Grandin & Barron, 2017). (We do want to be careful to guard against the temptation to see individuals with ASD merely through the lens of what they can contribute to us and, therefore, reduce their gift nature to its impact on the recipients of the gift. The other two theological themes we will discuss, children as fully human and as agents, can help us maintain an appropriately complex view of youth with ASD.)

In addition, caring for youth with ASD can help us better understand truly sacrificial love. Many parents would agree that raising children is one of the most challenging tasks they have faced, but for most parents, it is also one of the most rewarding. The infant who wakes up in the middle of the night smiles at the mother who feeds her; the toddler who has often struggled to share offers his last piece of candy to his younger sibling; the adolescent initiates a heartfelt discussion with her parents about how she navigated a difficult situation with peers. Events such as these occur frequently for families with typically developing youth and often reinforce and encourage parents in their efforts to persevere in the challenging task of raising children. Parents of youth with ASD, however, particularly when the child's symptoms and impairment are severe, may not experience these same rewarding moments and interactions. The child with ASD may rarely respond socially or emotionally to their parents. Blastland (2006) describes his son Joe's inability to understand the world from his perspective, which means that Joe sees and interacts with other people solely on the basis of what they can do for him. "I'll . . . resign myself to the notion that I am more machine-like to Joe than human; . . . when he wants something from me, I must support that I am nature's universal vending machine" (p. 100). For many parents of youth with ASD, the love they experience and enact for their children is highly sacrificial, as the task before them is more challenging and less rewarding than for many parents of typically developing youth. As Christians, then, caring for youth with ASD may give us a unique glance into the sacrificial love of God for his people, which is not based on and does not depend on our nature or response but rather flows out of God's character (Romans 9:16-18; Titus 3:4-5).

ABA interventions. One of the implications of viewing youth with ASD as gifts is that we take seriously the responsibility to support their development and promote their thriving. The relatively long history of research into ABA and its effectiveness in improving the functioning of youth with ASD in a wide variety of areas makes it an extremely useful means toward these ends. ABA has the potential to enable youth with ASD to gain language, cognitive, and social skills. Furthermore, it can improve their adaptive functioning skills such that they are much more likely to be able to care for themselves and live independently, be able to learn in regular education settings as youth, and seek postgraduate education and hold traditional independent jobs as adults. Before Lovaas's foundational work applying ABA to the treatment of ASD, it would have been unimaginable for many youth with more severe symptoms of ASD to lead what is often considered a "normal" life, thriving socially and cognitively; pervasive developmental delays such as ASD were seen as lifelong conditions

that significantly impeded development and functioning for nearly every diagnosed individual (American Psychiatric Association, 1994). Recognizing the gift nature of these youth should lead us to a willingness to commit our time, resources, and attention to the interventions that promote their thriving, of which research suggests ABA is at the forefront.

DSP interventions. Like ABA, intensive DSP interventions involve a significant investment in a child. One of the emphases of DSP interventions such as the Focused Playtime Intervention (FPI) is the exploration of the child's characteristics, strengths, and weaknesses via the review of videotaped interactions between the child and the parent and therapist. Each weekly session involves this videotape review, which then informs the direction of the rest of that session's work. This focused evaluation of the naturalistic interactions between the child and each adult facilitates deeper understanding of who the child is, what abilities he possesses, how he best connects with other people and the environment, and the ways in which he is trying to communicate. Seeking to understand—and base treatment on—the child's natural abilities and difficulties recognizes that he is a gift, purposefully created with value and strengths and deserving of investment and attention. Other specific aspects of FPI embrace the view of children with ASD as gifts. First, flexibility by the parent and clinician as they respond to the child is emphasized; sensitivity to the child's needs and leadings enables us to meet them at the developmental stage and emotional state that they are currently in. We do not expect them to meet the requirements we set for them; we respond to them sensitively and lovingly as we express our care for them. Second, the special play time routine that is developed early in treatment and utilized throughout the intervention communicates to the child that he is valued by and important to his parent. This play time is structured to be enjoyable to the child in addition to being a forum for the development of communication and social skills, and for a dyad in which interactions may have previously been experienced as stressful and conflictual (with one-on-one play time even being completely absent for some families), there is great value for both the parent and the child in regular, positive interactions that build up their relationship.

Respecting children as persons. Children, including those with ASD, are fully human. But what does it mean to be human? We have noted that as Christians, a central feature of our consideration of the humanity of children is their possession of the *imago Dei*. The most important aspect of our nature is that we are created in the image of God, which imbues us with immeasurable worth. However, it is also commonly understood to reflect certain aspects of the nature of God, including creativity, emotionality, the capacity for moral and rational thought, and relationality (see chapter two). How, then, do we conceptualize the humanity of a child who does not appear to have the capacity for abstract thought or deep connection with other people? Blastland (2006) notes that if we rely on traditional philosophical and scientific definitions of the characteristics that distinguish humanity— such as sophisticated self-awareness, complex language use, and the ability to reason abstractly—he faces the "chilling verdict" that his son is not considered human (p. 7). Macaskill (2017) addresses these questions by

emphasizing the central role of Christ as the utmost human manifestation of the image of God (Colossians 1:15). Jesus, in his perfect oneness with the Father, possesses the "strongest" image of God in human form; in contrast, all other humans represent "weaker" imaging of our Creator (Tanner, 2010). The image of God in each of us is lesser than that of Christ, but we are no less human; our human reflection of God's nature is imperfect and incomplete, just as Christ's is full and perfect. Therefore, distortions in characteristics that we consider to reflect the image of God in people, such as a lack of relationality or reduced reasoning abilities, are just some of the wide variety of ways in which we depart from being flawless manifestations of the *imago Dei*. In this perspective, youth with ASD are no less human—and no less in possession of the image of God—than any other created person. There is, in fact, a growing movement among individuals diagnosed with ASD who find a powerful identity in their diagnosis and view ASD as a form of neurodiversity among many human differences (den Houting, 2019).

However we understand the implications for understanding ASD and the *imago Dei* in light of one another, we recognize that youth with ASD are fully human beings. As such, they have unique and valid views and experiences of the world. Furthermore, we must seek to understand each individual's unique perspective in order to have a better sense of who they are and how they experience the world around them. This is especially important for youth with ASD, who may interact with and see other people and their environments in ways that are dramatically different from typically developing individuals. For example, a young child with ASD might draw a high level of pleasure from an activity (stacking and unstacking blocks) which would not appeal to most other youth, whereas an activity that is traditionally thought of as "fun" for many children (pretending to cook a meal with a peer in a play kitchen) might be frustrating and hard to understand. Standing in line at the grocery store, an activity that might be experienced as mundane by a typically developing adolescent, might be overwhelming to one with ASD (due to the bright lights, variety of smells, and anxiety associated with interacting with the checkout person). Seeking to understand the unique perspectives of youth with ASD both validates their experiences (which, in turn, validates their humanity) and helps us empathize with their feelings and reactions in various situations; furthermore, it helps build a foundation of the knowledge and understanding that is crucial for supporting these youth and helping them manage their emotions and behaviors adaptively. Even some secular sources speak to these truths. The Center for Autism and Related Disorders (CARD), which has developed a comprehensive intervention, outlines several core assumptions about ASD and treatment (Granpeesheh & Tarbox, 2014). These include the belief that all human beings, including those with ASD, have the ability to learn; that the dignity of individuals with ASD must be respected by integrating opportunities for independence, self-expression, and self-determination into treatment; that youth with ASD are unique, whole people, for whom treatment must be individualized; and that these youth have the right to receive effective treatment.

Respecting the humanity of youth with ASD involves the willingness to explore the dialectic and tension of opposing ideas. For example, to what degree do we consider a child's behavior intentional versus the uncontrollable result of autism? Do we judge the behavior of the youth with ASD by the same moral standards of other youth? For example, how do we respond to the youth with ASD who is so happy to be at church that he knocks over an older woman as he runs into the building (Walsh, 2016)? Should he be scolded, forgiven, charged with assault, or dismissed as incapable of changing his behavior (or some, all, or none of these)? Another set of ideas that we must hold in tension are the desire to treat/eliminate the symptoms of ASD and the importance of accepting and supporting youth as they are, especially in the church. We can validate both of these ideas as true. On the one hand, we recognize the full humanity of these youth by promoting their well-being and the achievement of the full potential. On the other hand, we acknowledge that being truly human involves being limited, whether we are limited by mental illness, developmental disability, or other personal characteristics and experiences. Therefore, we must seek to care for our image-bearing youth with ASD even as we seek to promote change and improvement.

Unfortunately, youth with ASD are much less likely than either typically developing youth or those with chronic physical health problems to attend religious services, which may result from a variety of organizational and congregational barriers that make it difficult for these youth to participate fully in religious communities (Whitehead, 2018). This finding suggests that churches may need to make a special effort to include these children and their families in the life of the body of Christ. In a wonderful resource for churches on how to be truly welcoming and inclusive of individuals with ASD, Newman (2011) gives specific suggestions for soliciting information about individuals' characteristics and needs, and setting up the church environment in a way that supports the growth and participation of youth and adults with ASD. She offers ideas such as supporting differences in sensory sensitivity (e.g., providing a way for individuals to take a break from bothersome light or sound), using mentors to pay attention to and advocate for individuals' needs in the moment, providing visual representations of lessons and routines, and supporting a wide variety of communication abilities (e.g., explaining figures of speech, using sign language or communication devices when helpful). Other writings on how to better facilitate inclusion for youth with ASD in religious communities and activities emphasize the role of flexibility (McGee, 2010), experiential learning (Swanson, 2010), and continual evaluation of whether programming and accommodations are meeting the spiritual and practical needs of youth and families (Goldstein & Ault, 2015).

ABA interventions. Despite their clear effectiveness in reducing symptoms and improving functioning, concerns have sometimes been raised about some of the underlying assumptions of ABA. Behavioral interventions are sometimes criticized as being reductionistic, focusing on the many small behaviors and environmental interactions that contribute to human functioning to the point that a larger sense of complex personhood is lost (Jones et al., 2011). To what degree does ABA train a child to behave in certain ways merely because they have been reinforced to do so, creating a sort of robotic operational response (Devita-Raeburn, 2016)? Furthermore, is the focus on reinforcing only desired behaviors and extinguishing undesired ones in intensive trials inhumane? Crying and other escape behaviors are generally ignored during ABA in order to extinguish them in favor of a desirable response to a prompt, a task which can feel difficult or even cruel to some therapists and parents. Is this type of seemingly insensitive response to young children dehumanizing, denying them the dignity they deserve as people? Responses to such criticisms argue that the clear effectiveness of ABA therapy for improving the well-being of many youth with ASD far outweighs these time-limited and theoretical downsides, but the concerns remain valid for some critics.

Weighing the drastic nature of intensive behavioral therapy with the outcomes it can produce presents us with another question: What does it mean to be a healthy, productive person? What is central to "the good life" that we desire for our children? Like much of society, the goals of ABA are based on a certain understanding of how we want people to live and behave: socially interested and skilled, able to communicate effectively, free of unusual behaviors, thriving in educational and occupational settings, and able to live independently and take care of themselves. Though few people would argue that these are negative outcomes, more might wonder whether they are the only outcomes that can be considered positive and of value. Is being "normal" inherent to healthy functioning or to the way that God desires us to live? Phrased differently, do the symptoms of ASD interfere with the fulfillment of one's full human potential? Does the ABA approach, which emphasizes changing behaviors so that youth are more typical in their functioning and behavior, inherently demonize anything that is unusual or different from the norm (Parker, 2015)? Or, is there diversity in the form of a healthy, productive life that can encompass both traditional presentations of success and well-being and the life of an individual with ASD? Theologically speaking, how do we distinguish between who God made us to be and how sin has distorted that creation? These are difficult questions, with many individuals praising ABA for the positive change it has enabled in their lives or their children's development, and a small but vocal minority raising concerns that intensive therapies aim to change the very nature of who children are in a way that denies them dignity and respect (Parker, 2015).

DSP interventions. In many ways, DSP approaches are built on assumptions that contrast with the foundation of ABA that there is one prescribed way to train children to be successful people who conform to a certain desired outcome. Rather, DSP interventions aim to build on the naturally occurring interactions between parent and child in the development of adaptive, social, and communication skills. This emphasis is consistent with the common Christian emphasis on the centrality of our relational nature to our personhood and, thus, validates the fully human nature of youth with ASD. The DSP approach also aims to build on the child's existing skills rather than assuming that many of their maladaptive tendencies need to be extinguished before progress can be made (as ABA often begins), again validating the idea that these youth have foundational characteristics and

abilities by virtue of their human nature, on which treatment can build. Furthermore, DSP interventions are more consistent with certain views of ASD that are becoming more commonly expressed and celebrated, that the behaviors and characteristics of individuals with ASD represent variations within the full range of human functioning that should not inherently be considered disordered or problematic (Prizant, 2016; Silberman, 2016).

Viewing children as agents. We sometimes run the risk of considering youth with conditions that significantly impair their functioning, such as ASD, primarily according to what they are incapable of—speaking, making eye contact, reciprocating socially, using toys in traditional ways, or functioning well in a regular education classroom or competitive job. However, the theological concept of agency reminds us that all youth, including those with ASD, have the capacity to effect change and to express their desires and needs. In order to fully recognize their agency, we may need to adjust our assumptions about the ways in which agency is expressed. For example, Walsh (2016) notes that it is a "moral imperative to listen to the voiceless," including individuals with ASD who do not communicate verbally but rather through their behavior (p. 345). Their "voices" are often more difficult for us to hear and interpret, but they are as important and valid as those of the most eloquent speakers. For very young children and/or low-functioning individuals, we may need to play close attention to what they are communicating through their behavior and other nonverbal signs. When a child with ASD throws a tantrum or becomes extremely upset, what is he communicating? What emotions is he feeling, how might those emotions be affected by his environment as well as his interpretation of his experiences, and how can we support and care for him in light of those understandings? When a child is exhibiting repetitive (e.g., hand flapping) or even self-injurious (e.g., head banging) behaviors, what might she be experiencing or trying to communicate? What do those behaviors tell us about the child's experiences and needs? Is the child overstimulated, bored, or frustrated? Seeking to pay close attention to the circumstances under which a child exhibits particular behaviors will help us better understand their purpose and respond to them appropriately, which is perhaps the most important way that we can respect the child's agency.

Youth with ASD have spiritual agency too. A diagnosis of even severe ASD does not eliminate the potential for these youth to thrive spiritually. In fact, some writers have noted that ASD may enhance some individuals' spirituality. It has been suggested that the heightened sensitivity to stimuli sometimes associated with ASD could also heighten these individuals' perception of spiritual realities (Stillman, 2006). In addition, youth with ASD may find unique ways to understand and connect with God when they are supported and viewed as capable of such growth. For example, we may limit God if we view prayer as performable only by individuals who are verbal (Dearey, 2009); rather, our creation in the image of God, whose Son is the living Word (Genesis 1:27; John 1:1), and the intercession of the Holy Spirit (Romans 8:26-27) suggest that prayer is more complex than merely people speaking words out loud to God. Finally, we must recognize that God is Lord over all of our abilities and inabilities and can use anyone he wants for any of his

purposes. Moses, who was an integral instrument in God's fulfillment of his promise to make Israel into a great nation with a land of their own, was "slow of speech and tongue" (Exodus 4:10). Yet, God chose to use him in a powerful leadership role, perhaps using Moses' limitations to further showcase his own power and glory: "The LORD said to him, 'Who gave human beings their mouths? Who makes them deaf or mute? Who gives them sight or makes them blind? Is it not I, the LORD? Now go; I will help you speak and will teach you what to say'" (Exodus 4:11-12). God can use youth with ASD to achieve his purposes as well, of course, and encouragement of their agency entails communicating this truth to them and expecting God to work in and through them rather than being surprised when this occurs.

In assessment and treatment for ASD, then, recognizing children's agency means providing opportunities for their (literal or figurative) voices to be heard and to allow for self-direction. For the very young or nonverbal child, a thorough analysis of the function of their behavior (e.g., what need is it communicating?) is important. As children age and grow in their communicative abilities, we want to be careful to validate their emerging attempts at language, not just in a perfunctory or shallow manner but in a way that truly recognizes what they are saying and seeks to respond in sensitive ways. Into later childhood and adolescence, especially for higher functioning youth, we may involve them in more of the treatment planning. What areas of their own functioning do they see as weaknesses which they would like to improve? What do they like and appreciate about their own strengths and unique characteristics, and how might they use these qualities to succeed in self-care, relationships, and school? Throughout development, we can also make space in the treatment context for youth to take initiative; this might occur in choosing where to direct their attention for young children, in creating games and activities for older children, and for selecting conversation topics for adolescents.

ABA interventions. Similar to points we discussed in relation to the personhood of children, ABA has been criticized for not respecting children's natural tendencies and bents but rather aiming to aggressively shape them into who adults want them to be. If we regard children's nonverbal behaviors (e.g., crying, self-stimulating) as expressions of their needs and feelings, then what do we make of ABA therapy that ignores these "undesired" behaviors so that they are extinguished in favor of behaviors that are more desired by parents and therapists? Furthermore, who decides which behaviors are "best" for the child? Do ABA interventions that prescribe a particular set of abilities and behaviors as desirable mean that we are really only validating the agency of those who decide which behaviors are desirable (the creators of the intervention as well as the parents and clinicians who set goals for individual youth)? Do we see these means and goals of ABA as completely dismissive of the child's agency?

On the other hand, does ABA, which can dramatically improve a child's functional adaptive and communication skills, actually respect the child's agency by facilitating its long-term growth? Longitudinal research suggests that the child with severe ASD who does not receive early intervention may never learn to speak normally, have reciprocal social relationships, or live independently. It is likely that this individual will have few opportunities to express his agency in his own life, which will instead be more heavily directed by parents and other caregivers. In contrast, if the same child receives intensive ABA intervention beginning by the age of twenty-four months, he has a much higher chance of developing complex speech, better cognitive abilities, positive social skills, and the ability to live and work independently. In this second scenario, this youth is likely to have a greater sense of his own agency and to interact with an environment that respects his agency and self-determination, as he may be better able to express his thoughts and desires and to have the social and functional tools to seek the fulfillment of his needs. Therefore, even if ABA is seen as dismissive of the child's agency during the intervention itself, is the child's long-term development and improved agentic ability more important?

DSP interventions. Although the improved outcomes of youth treated with DSP interventions are not quite as dramatic, the assumptions and techniques of these approaches are generally more validating of a child's agency and self-direction. DSP interventions often explicitly assume that children with ASD are capable of communication and social relationships, motivated to interact with others, and deserving of opportunities for independence and self-determination. Furthermore, they view all communication attempts as purposeful, even for youth who are nonverbal and/or severely impaired by their symptoms. Such assumptions highlight the child's agency and emphasize the importance of respecting it in the therapeutic context. The techniques of DSP interventions are faithful to such assumptions, creating opportunities for the young child with ASD to express her agency. For example, in the FPI, there are a number of therapeutic principles that respect the child's signals, such as encouraging the parent to match the child's pace and level of complexity in play, recognize and validate the child's efforts to communicate or engage the parents in play, and attend to the child's signals about whether she is ready to respond to a parent-led change in the manner of play. In addition, many intervention elements involve creating opportunities for the parent and the child to take turns. The child is given opportunities to both follow and lead the parent in choosing games and activities as well as initiating joint attention. This turn-taking emphasis provides opportunities for the parent to teach and lead the child, which is crucial for change to occur, balanced with opportunities for the child to enact her agency and gain confidence in her growing abilities, which are in turn reinforced and built on by a sensitive parental response.

CONCLUSIONS

A truly deep commitment to view youth with ASD as gifts, full persons, and agents can radically change our understanding of them and their symptoms as well as our approach to treatment. Both ABA and DSP interventions have areas of strength with regard to each of these theological commitments. Perhaps, then, comprehensive interventions may represent the best way to effectively address ASD symptoms in a way that honors children and helps us better know the God who made them. No matter which approach is used, it seems clear that we need humility as we listen to those who may disagree with us as to how to best understand youth with ASD and promote their well-being and sense of being valued.

CASE STUDY

Pertinent history. Hayden Schoff is a six-year, seven-month-old Caucasian male in the first grade who displays deficits in social-emotional reciprocity (e.g., difficulty engaging in back-and-forth conversation, reduced sharing of others' interests and emotions, failure to readily respond to social interactions), poor understanding of social rules and relationships (e.g., difficulty approaching peers, "just wanting to play his way" with peers), and deficits in age-appropriate peer relationships (e.g., lack of age-appropriate play with peers, difficulty adjusting his behavior to social contexts, disinterest in peers). He also displays insistence on specific routines with distress at small changes (e.g., crying, rocking, asking questions over and over), and difficulty with transitions; for example, Hayden becomes upset when the class routine changes or when he has a substitute. He also perseverates on changes in the family's schedule or routines (e.g., driving routes, disruption in caretaking due to father's absence on a work trip). Hayden displays stereotyped use of objects and speech (e.g., lining up objects, repetition of movie phrases out of context, scripting), restricted and fixated interests (e.g., towns' mottos, Thomas the Train), and repetitive behaviors (e.g., rocking, arm flapping). These symptoms have been present throughout his development and impair his social and behavioral functioning at home and school. Hayden underwent a comprehensive multidisciplinary evaluation conducted by a clinical psychologist, speech/language pathologist, occupational therapist, and developmental pediatrician. Hayden was diagnosed with autism spectrum disorder (ASD) without accompanying intellectual impairment requiring substantial support, generalized anxiety disorder, language disorder, and developmental coordination disorder.

Though he is described as a polite child who wants to please his teachers, Hayden frequently becomes upset in the regular education classroom and hides under his desk or in the boys' bathroom. Mr. and Mrs. Schoff describe Hayden as intelligent, concrete, loving, affectionate, and visually skilled. He is the only child to parents who have been married for ten years. His mother has an associate's degree and works part-time as a paraprofessional in the local school district, and his father has a high school degree and works full-time in construction. They have extended family who live nearby and frequently watch Hayden when his parents are at work.

The multidisciplinary team recommended that Hayden's parents seek family therapy for guidance on how to better understand his current level of functioning, and how they could help him develop skills for his future through effective parenting strategies to address symptoms of ASD, language delays, and anxiety. It was also recommended that Hayden participate in therapy to develop his social communication skills and address his anxiety. Hayden's mother expresses her specific concern regarding his anxiety, which he experiences in response to changes in routine and transitions and which presents as aggressive behaviors, as this symptom has the most negative impact on his daily functioning. Given Hayden's strengths (intelligence, verbal skills, ability to learn from the environment, relationship with parents, desire to please adults) and his older age, a specific program is not utilized; rather, treatment incorporates behavioral principles from empirically supported treatments to address Hayden's communication skills, social skills, and regulation skills through naturalistic play and parent-child interactions.

Course of treatment.

Sessions 1-6. The first few sessions focus on building rapport with Hayden and his parents. The first and fourth sessions are held with Hayden's parents alone. The therapist also seeks to set up collateral contacts with the team of service providers working with Hayden in the school setting.

The therapist sets up a visual schedule for therapy sessions and introduces it to Hayden. Hayden responds positively to his mother using a visual clock with a timer to transition from the waiting room to the therapy office and to indicate the end of the session. During these initial sessions, the therapist first gets to know Hayden's preferred interests and utilizes these to build rapport and introduce therapy content. That is, the therapist seeks to understand what Hayden draws pleasure from. For example, playing with train tracks and Thomas the Train characters can be used as an incentive at the end of each session over the course of therapy.

During play, the therapist reflects Hayden's play to promote social communication and emotion awareness; for example, the therapist provides a running narrative of his play and labeling of his emotions and how he shows them nonverbally. Instruction and positive feedback is provided to Hayden's mother during her play with Hayden. The therapist models and reinforces responding flexibly to Hayden's distress during the session. Hayden's mother and the therapist use distraction and redirection (e.g., drawing emojis on the whiteboard, playing with the Lego table, telling knock-knock jokes) when he becomes distressed to help him engage in preferred activities. During the third session, Hayden is also taught that he can say "No, thank you" to an activity (rather than screaming or hiding behind the couch) and choose from two other activities presented as alternative options. This more adaptive manner of letting the therapist and his mother know his preferences verbally rather than through maladaptive behavior is first role-modeled for him, and then acted out by him prior to the time he may want to use it.

Parent consultation sessions first help Mr. and Mrs. Schoff understand the ASD diagnosis and identify next steps in helping Hayden's development. The therapist utilizes the 100 Day Toolkit for School Age Children from the Autism Speaks organization website that was developed to help families of newly diagnosed children. Mr. and Mrs. Schoff discuss their grief and fears about the future; for example, they report their worry about Hayden's behaviors and whether he can learn requisite skills to cope with his environment. They also express their worry about whether he will be happy if he struggles with social relationships. Their feelings and experiences are reflected and validated. Mr. and Mrs. Schoff want to discuss God's sovereignty in their lives and their son's life. They express their faith in God's ability and desire to comfort them but their inability to experience God's shelter right now. Writings by other parents of children with autism that explained their process following diagnosis are introduced. Through open-ended questioning, they are encouraged to recognize the gift of their son. The therapist helps them explore their belief in whether God is present in and works

through Hayden as through all children. For example, they are able to identify that Hayden brings out the best in those around him, and that he is affectionate and loves when others show interest in him and his specific interests, which in turn brings joy to others.

Mr. and Mrs. Schoff then want to discuss how to help close family and friends understand Hayden's strengths and deficits. For example, they experience embarrassment and a strong desire to explain his behaviors to others when Hayden throws a tantrum during family gatherings or in public. However, they do not know how they can explain it to people who know very little about autism or have misconceptions about autism. Mr. and Mrs. Schoff are provided with information about helping close family and friends understand Hayden and his behaviors.

Mr. and Mrs. Schoff also discuss the unhelpful though well-intentioned things close friends and family as well as acquaintances have said to them over the last month, as well as the demeaning things others say (e.g., a school staff member who does not believe in his capability). They feel that others express pity for them and Hayden rather than viewing his life as a blessing. Following the diagnosis, they had been reflecting together on Psalm 139:13-14. They express frustration that their friends' children could have these verses applied to them, but it seems to them that they are not permitted to also have their child seen as "fearfully and wonderfully made." The clinician problem solves with Hayden's parents how to best respond to others' pitying or hurtful comments while expressing their love for Hayden and his strengths.

Sessions 7-12. Two of these six sessions are held with Hayden's parents alone. First, the therapist normalizes the stress they feel as they work to obtain Hayden the services and environment he needs and to manage his maladaptive behavior, which continue to include at least three to five extended tantrums per day. Parenting is extremely challenging for them every day, and they often feel overwhelmed by everything they need to do to provide Hayden support and instruction. Through structured problem solving, the clinician normalizes Mr. and Mrs. Schoff's feelings and helps them identify two problem behaviors to target (fighting to get out of bed in the morning, aggression toward them when things do not go as he wants) and two skill areas to focus on (emotion regulation, acceptance of changes).

The therapist teaches Mr. and Mrs. Schoff how to track aggressive behavior and analyze these data in one parent session. They then engage in analysis of these behaviors in the subsequent parent session to identify the antecedents and consequences for these behaviors. After tracking the behavior, a plan is developed to provide preemptive praise to Hayden for accepting the "no" they are about to give him with a reminder of the appropriate response they would like from him to convey his frustration ("You've been working hard to stay calm when you don't get your way. Remember to use your words"; "Good job accepting our 'no' even though you are angry"). They also are directed to refrain from giving Hayden attention for aggression but rather to respond calmly and direct him to a more appropriate behavior. A social story is used in session to teach emotion regulation and acceptance of "no" to Hayden. Finally, because Hayden is getting to bed too late after watching streamed video games, the bedtime routine is

changed to permit Hayden time to settle down at night to fall asleep. A visual for the morning routine is also developed with reinforcements (rewards) built into the schedule (e.g., time to eat a favorite cereal while watching a television show).

The therapist and Mr. and Mrs. Schoff also reflect on the use of play and naturalistic situations in which they can focus on the two skill areas (emotion regulation and acceptance of change) to reinforce Hayden's skills and desired responses. The couple also identifies their specific family values and their hopes for Hayden's development. The importance of maintaining focus on what is important to them and having faith in their child's potential is reinforced. Mr. and Mrs. Schoff are receptive to considering the bidirectional, dynamic interactions between themselves and Hayden. They identify the ways Hayden shapes their behavior, and are encouraged by thinking about the many ways throughout the day that they provide particular experiences for Hayden that affect his development. Discussing and identifying the many chances they have to respond flexibly to Hayden's behaviors (the many "touch points") while also developing his skills helps his parents feel less overwhelmed by the challenges of caring for Hayden. Mr. and Mrs. Schoff join an autism support group which is farther away than they would like, but they feel the benefits outweighed the cost. They hope to start a local group themselves once they understand how a group functions.

During joint parent-child sessions, a visual schedule continues to be used to help Hayden understand the structure of the appointment. Hayden refers to this schedule throughout the session, and responds positively to the use of a clock to engage in an activity and then transition from one to the next. The therapist presents interactive toys (people and cars) to engage Hayden and provide opportunities for appropriate social communication and behavior and emotion awareness. The therapist and Hayden's mother reflect his play in order to promote these skills, including sharing toys, verbally interacting, responding to joint attention, and identifying emotions. Session content also focuses on emotions and regulation strategies. Education about emotions is provided by utilizing Hayden's preferred interests. For example, Lego emoji faces help with the identification of emotions in actual photographs of people. The therapist also uses "emotion stations" to explore emotions (e.g., visually depicted train tracks for each emotion with "stations" being the physical aspects of the emotion, thoughts, and situations that cause the emotion, and ways to cope with it).

Further, the therapist reviews information provided by Hayden's school regarding the Zones of Regulation (Kuypers, 2011), which provides a framework to help Hayden become more aware of his emotions by identifying his level of arousal, how his behavior affects others, and things he can do to regulate his arousal. This system is discussed broadly and with regard to specific situations in which Hayden becomes upset (e.g., when told "no," when something in his routine changes) in order to reinforce the regulation system being used within the school setting. The therapist works with Hayden's mother to identify ways she can implement this system at home to facilitate consistency across settings in support of Hayden's identification and regulation of emotions. Visuals and prompting from this system are also used with Hayden during therapy sessions.

Finally, the therapist and Mrs. Schoff read a social story with Hayden about changes in routine, the emotions experienced when changes occur, and strategies to manage changes in a flexible manner. The social story is sent home with Hayden's mother for review and reinforcement of regulation strategies at home. At each parent-child session this story is reviewed. Hayden is able to tell the therapist the most pertinent parts of the social story and apply it to situations that occurred throughout the week. He places pictures from the story in order and identifies three steps that help him show flexibility. Hayden's mother reports reading the story daily with Hayden and helping him generalize the positive strategies to situations in which he is upset about changes (e.g., use of "train" language, such as a stop sign and crossing signal, to remind Hayden to stop and consider his choices). Hayden's mother also implements the visuals for being flexible when routines change in his daily life to remind Hayden of strategies to use.

Sessions 13-18. Again, two parenting sessions are held with Mr. and Mrs. Schoff. The therapist helps them engage in problem solving regarding their attempts to reinforce Hayden's emotion regulation and non-aggressive response when upset. Mr. Schoff discloses his difficulty responding with ignoring to undesired behaviors and refraining from "giving in" when Hayden is upset. When his feelings during these interactions with Hayden are explored, Mr. Schoff identifies his discomfort with seeing Hayden upset and his belief that Hayden's life is already hard enough without having his parents responding to him in ways that do not make him happy. It is clear that Mrs. Schoff is frustrated and places blame on Mr. Schoff and that Mr. Schoff feels both defensive and confused. They are encouraged to reflect on their different personalities that lead to different parenting approaches, and identify how they could complement each other while still seeking to provide consistency to Hayden. They recall the different spiritual attributes they each bring to their parenting, such as the love and discipline Mrs. Schoff shows in her parenting and the forgiveness and adaptability that Mr. Schoff provides to Hayden. They identify ways they could give each other grace and support each other in parenting, including Mrs. Schoff stepping into situations in which Mr. Schoff feels overwhelmed without resentment. Mr. Schoff identifies some activities he could do with Hayden on a regular basis to promote their positive engagement (e.g., coloring, building Legos, swinging in the backyard, walks in neighboring park) to help him feel more comfortable with the times he does not give in to Hayden. By focusing on their long-term goals for Hayden, they are able to look past Hayden's immediate emotions to the positive impact on his development over time.

Mrs. Schoff requests recommendations regarding a comprehensive approach to treat Hayden's anxiety, which had increased over the past few weeks. Mr. and Mrs. Schoff discuss Hayden's recent increased anxiety due to a change in the family's schedule with Mrs. Schoff working evenings. The therapist provides support for the stress and guilt Mrs. Schoff experiences and the helplessness Mr. Schoff feels. The therapist also normalizes Hayden's responses to these changes, including acting out and reassurance seeking, which are behavioral manifestations of his anxiety. The therapist again helps Mr. and

Mrs. Schoff work together to support each other to create and implement systems that would help Hayden cope with his mother's absence (e.g., a calendar with visuals for "Mom work nights," a goodnight phone call with his mother, bedtime routine with his father). The therapist consults with Hayden's physician about the use of medication to treat Hayden's anxiety symptoms. Finally, in these parenting sessions the therapist reviews the use of the first social story with Mr. and Mrs. Schoff, and they are encouraged to write social stories and use visuals at home to help develop Hayden's skills in other situations (e.g., starting something new at school, going to school without meltdowns, managing anxiety).

In parent-child sessions, the therapist continues to implement a visual schedule for the structure of the appointment with use of "first-then" prompts and a clock for transitions. Also, the therapist begins using a behavior chart to provide reinforcement for Hayden to "say yes to no" in session with multiple opportunities built into the session in which he is told "no." The therapist models and reinforces his use of calming techniques (e.g., breathing, sensory activities, yoga movements) when he is distressed by being told "no." The therapist and Mrs. Schoff help Hayden communicate about his current anxiety regarding changes in his routine (e.g., his mother working late shifts and not being home for bedtime). Through structured support, the therapist seeks to understand his unique perspective and how he experiences the world. Hayden cannot easily verbally express his past behaviors or the difficult situations he encounters at school, at home, and in the community. Thus, the use of drawings helps him explain his perspective and under- stand situations in which he becomes upset. In this instance, Hayden draws what he feels about his evening routine without his mother home. He identifies the thoughts and feelings of the child in his drawings, which reveal his fear that his father would not remember some things his mother does at night (e.g., sitting down for the twenty-minute reading as- signment, picking out the correct toothpaste, making a dinner he likes, selecting his pa- jamas) and his dislike of how his father ruffles his hair when putting him to bed. Hayden is helped to identify the new routine he would like with his father, and a visual is created of this routine.

During these sessions, Hayden sometimes actively participates, but at other times, he avoids therapeutic tasks. With support and flexibility from the therapist and his mother, Hayden is able to engage in therapeutic ac- tivities. Hayden displays increased prosocial behaviors during play, as evidenced by using social scripts the therapist provided; for ex- ample, when he cannot manipulate a toy in the way he wants, Hayden uses the script "I need help . . ."; when a character wants some- thing from another character, he uses the script, "I really like that. Can we take turns?"; or when one character hurts another, the characters use a script such as "Ouch. That hurts. I don't like it when you . . ." Hayden is appropriately engaged while reviewing the "say yes to no" star chart, while reading a new social story about him saying yes to no, and while reviewing the story about his flexibility in the midst of changes. Hayden is able to retell the social script for saying yes to no and being flexible with visual cues. Throughout these sessions, the therapist reflects Hayden's

play and promotes emotional awareness and prosocial behaviors by commenting on the play and the emotions and actions of ev- eryone in the room.

Sessions 19-24. During parent sessions, the therapist and Mr. and Mrs. Schoff focus on Hayden's social skills development. They re- spond well to discussion of parenting as "shepherding" Hayden through multiple areas, as many of the parents in their church com- munity discuss regarding their children's spiritual development. They feel encouraged to not only think of guiding Hayden spiri- tually but also to address many areas of his development explicitly. That is, they identify their desire to guide and encourage Hayden's understanding of others and how to be in re- lationship as well as his basic life skills and communication skills. The therapist works with Mr. and Mrs. Schoff to think through the demands of social interactions in order to set stepwise goals for Hayden. Although Mr. and Mrs. Schoff ultimately want Hayden to be ca- pable of intimate relationships and to navigate his social world, they realize his skill devel- opment needs to begin at a more foundational level, especially at six years of age! For ex- ample, a typically developing six-year-old is beginning to develop empathy, or an under- standing of others' feelings, and how to be kind and collaborate in friendships. Upon reviewing Hayden's current social skills, the specific skills of sharing and taking turns are identified. These can then be built on for the development of more complex age-associated social skills. It is discussed that just as the rules of games are easy to learn and adhere to for Hayden, his learning of social skills will also be "black and white." His parents first see this as a negative to overcome, as it causes

Hayden to seem "rigid"; however, it also allows him to learn and apply the skills he has learned. The family is shown additional resources for social skill development. In addition to social stories, the potential of using video modeling is presented. Mr. and Mrs. Schoff are excited to show Hayden videos of social interactions they find on websites that target specific social behaviors as models of these skills. They also begin to videotape Hayden successfully completing the social skill with their prompting. They then show him the video of him performing the behavior with their prompting edited out.

In the subsequent parent session, Mr. and Mrs. Schoff report that Hayden loved watching the few videos they made over and over. Finally, Mr. and Mrs. Schoff are encouraged to facilitate his interests that help him to connect with other children (e.g., building with Legos at the library and asking peers to join him, playing Lego video games on structured playdates, and using Lego sets to help him branch out to different topics of interest). Hayden is not yet ready to join an extracurricular activity, and thus other options are discussed, including engagement in activities at the local library and weekly supervised playdates. The therapist and Mr. and Mrs. Schoff also discuss options for reinforcing Hayden's social skills with same-age peers during and after social interactions.

The parent-child sessions continue to utilize the same structure and visuals with a focus on continued development of Hayden's emotion regulation and social skills. When Hayden struggles to engage in activities during the session, he is prompted to monitor his arousal level and body sensations and state his needs. Hayden engages in gross motor and sensory activities during the session (e.g., bouncing on couch, requesting the therapist put him upside down, doing somersaults, doing handstands with his feet on the office door), which help him reengage in therapeutic activities. Overall, Hayden is observed to be more willing to engage in social stories and session activities with little defiance or distress. Hayden enjoys drawing and practicing yoga poses to help him calm and regulate his body. The ability to be flexible continues to be presented to Hayden through drawing, movement activities and social stories. Mrs. Schoff reports Hayden is doing better accepting when changes occur in his day or routine.

Additionally, the therapist and Mrs. Schoff seek to help Hayden understand cause and effect and perspective taking in social situations by going through comic strips with him. The therapist prepares these comic strips prior to the therapy sessions, utilizing his interests in creating the comic strips (e.g., the characters were Thomas the Train characters, or characters from Lego movies). For example, a comic strip is developed to help Hayden understand how others may feel and what they might think (with thought bubbles) when he says he does not like their shirt (because of a nonpreferred color). During these sessions, Mrs. Schoff also reports Hayden was very anxious about attending a classmate's birthday party. A comic strip featuring birthday parties helps him understand how to interact with the classmate and the routines typically involved in birthday parties (e.g., greeting the classmate and other friends, gift opening, cake and birthday song), with the feelings, thoughts, and statements of the characters identified.

Termination. As is typical in child therapy, the therapist and Hayden's parents discuss whether booster sessions are needed. It is decided that booster sessions would be disruptive to Hayden as therapy would not be a regular enough part of his routine. However, the probability that therapy would need to be reinitiated is presented. Worsening of behavioral symptoms, stagnation in progress, or adjustment to normal developmental transitions are identified as times when therapy would be beneficial in the future. The many skills that Hayden and his parents have learned over the course of therapy and how to apply them to new situations are reviewed. Hayden's parents' efficacy is also reinforced, and the therapist helps them identify their growth in knowledge and confidence with a focus on the specific coaching skills they learned to help Hayden's development.

Additional considerations from a developmental psychopathology framework. To address Hayden's receptive and expressive skills, he receives speech/language services at school. His parents also sought private speech therapy biweekly. The therapist contacts the speech pathologist to better understand what she is working on with Hayden in order to build on it and implement the communication strategies in session (e.g., visuals, scripts). Hayden also receives occupational therapy services at school (twenty minutes per week as well as consultation to Hayden's teacher). After reviewing these services, sensory activities are built into individual sessions to help Hayden better maintain regulation. The therapist also presents to Hayden's school class about ASD and sensory differences with an age-appropriate book to promote peer understanding. This intervention is well received by his class;

Mrs. Schoff reports more initiation of interactions by Hayden's classmates, and greater support from his classmates.

During the course of therapy, Mr. and Mrs. Schoff stop attending the church they had been attending for the past twelve years. Despite the assurance that their family would be supported by the community, they were not permitted to leave Hayden in Sunday school unless one of them stayed with him, and church staff were unwilling to receive training on how to meet Hayden's needs and help him in his social interactions. During parent sessions, Mr. and Mrs. Schoff discuss their sense of loss regarding their church family and address their disillusionment regarding their perceptions of the church's hypocrisy. It is also difficult for them to understand why Sunday school leaders are provided training on how to support children with diabetes, epilepsy, and asthma, but not children with developmental disabilities or mental health problems. They express their weariness and sadness about having to advocate for Hayden at church after having advocated throughout the week in so many ways. These feelings are reflected and normalized, but through the conversation it is clear they desire and need to continue to seek out a support system and focus on their spiritual life. They are unwilling to begin visiting new places of worship as they do not feel they have the time or energy to do so, and they do not want to experience the rejection they anticipated from fellow Christians. Mr. and Mrs. Schoff are encouraged to talk with other parents in an autism support group they began attending during the course of therapy to see if there are local churches who are supportive of children with disabilities. Mr. and Mrs. Schoff find a church within thirty minutes of their home that is small but open to meeting with them and Hayden to better understand the family's experience and how they might support them. During the course of therapy, the therapist provides two consultations to the church on psychoeducation about ASD and the development of strategies to be used in Sunday school with Hayden (e.g., a clear schedule, visuals of routines, information about sensory differences and regulation strategies, naturalistic reinforcement of social communication and behavior). Church members and children's ministry staff ask questions about how to understand Hayden's behaviors, and how they could flexibly respond to his behaviors and needs. Again, a toolkit from the Autism Speaks organization is used to provide information to church members. The therapist also provides education to peers in the children's programming with the use of a book about having a friend with autism. From this training church leadership engages in an evaluation of children's ministry to identify the needs of children, the strategies currently used in children's ministry, and those that leaders want to learn.

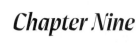

Chapter Nine

Eating Disorders

"NOTHING TASTES AS good as skinny feels." "Hungry to bed, hungry to rise, makes a girl a smaller size." Social media users promote phrases such as these using the hashtag #thinspo (short for a portmanteau of "thin" and "inspiration"), an indication of the prevalence of online messages that promote behaviors and attitudes holding weight loss in high regard. The first study of pro-anorexia, or "pro-ana," websites was published in 2006 and found that the content of these sites ranged from motivational quotes to messages about control and perfectionism to encouragement to "make a pact with Ana and sign it in blood" (Norris et al., 2006, p. 445). Not surprisingly, websites and videos such as these have been found to promote eating disordered behavior and attitudes, and they are more frequently viewed and more highly rated by users than their healthier counterparts that provide objective information about the disorders and their treatment (Rodgers et al., 2016; Syed-

Abdul et al., 2013). Concern has also been raised about the blurred lines between these pro-ana ideas and more mainstream web content (Cobb, 2017).

In this chapter, we will focus on three eating disorders (EDs): anorexia nervosa, bulimia nervosa, and binge eating disorder. We also describe the symptoms of a fourth ED that may better capture the symptoms of younger individuals but which has not yet been well studied. Anorexia has three main symptoms (American Psychiatric Association, 2013). First, individuals restrict their calorie intake to the point that their weight is significantly below normal. Low weight can be the result of weight loss or, especially for youth, the failure to gain weight appropriately as development progresses. Second, individuals display an extreme fear of gaining weight or becoming fat. This fear is irrational in that it does not improve with weight loss and may even grow as individuals lose weight. Third, distortions in one's view of weight or body shape are present; these can include an inaccurate view of one's body, a view of oneself that is overly influenced by body weight or shape, or a failure to recognize low weight as problematic. Some individuals are dissatisfied with their bodies as a whole, while others may focus on particular body parts that are disliked or problematic. Individuals with anorexia can be categorized as having either the binge eating/purging type of the disorder (if they have engaged in recurrent binge eating or purging) or the restricting type of the disorder. Disorder severity is determined by body mass index (BMI), a weight-to-height ratio; individuals with extremely severe anorexia may drop below a BMI of 15.

The first criteria for bulimia is the presence of recurrent episodes of binge eating, characterized by the consumption of unusually large amounts of food during discrete periods of time and a lack of control over one's eating behavior. An individual who purposefully and planfully eats an extreme amount of food, such as an Olympic athlete who is in training, would not meet the criteria for a binge. Individuals frequently binge eat food that they avoid under other circumstances, such as food that is high calorie or otherwise viewed as unhealthy. Individuals with bulimia report that binges are most likely to be triggered by negative emotions (especially related to food or one's body), interpersonal stressors, extreme hunger following fasting, and boredom. Second, recurrent episodes of behavior meant to compensate for increased food intake during binges are also displayed. These can include self-induced vomiting, use of laxatives or diuretics, fasting, or excessive exercise. The most common compensatory behavior is vomiting, which serves to relieve both the un-

comfortable fullness and the fear of weight gain that frequently follow a binge. Third, both types of episodes (binge eating and compensatory behavior) must occur at least once a week over the course of three months. Fourth, body shape and weight exert a problematic amount of influence on one's self-evaluation. Finally, these symptoms cannot occur within the context of anorexia; in other words, a diagnosis of anorexia takes precedence over a diagnosis of bulimia. However, as individuals with bulimia frequently restrict their calorie intake between binges, differential diagnosis can be challenging. The key difference between the two disorders is whether an individual's body weight is significantly low (anorexia) or normal to overweight (bulimia).

Individuals with binge eating disorder (BED) display recurrent episodes of binge eating, defined in the same manner as in bulimia (i.e., very large amount of food consumed, sense of lack of control). In addition, binges must be associated with at least three of the following: eating rapidly, feeling uncomfortably full, eating a lot when one is not hungry, eating alone due to embarrassment, or feelings of disgust/depression/guilt following a binge. Binge eating episodes are accompanied by distress and must occur at least once a week for three months. Finally, BED is only diagnosed when the individual does not also meet the criteria for anorexia or bulimia. Unlike in bulimia, individuals with BED do not exhibit compensatory behavior such as vomiting.

The newest edition of the DSM introduced avoidant/restrictive food intake disorder, which includes behavioral manifestations of disordered eating behavior but does not include cognitive symptoms (e.g., distorted view of body or food, undue influence of body evaluation on self-esteem); therefore, this diagnosis may capture problematic eating behavior in children who do not yet have the cognitive sophistication to describe these thought patterns. The main criteria for avoidant/restrictive food intake disorder is the restriction of food intake that results in significant weight loss (or failure to gain weight appropriately with age), nutritional deficiencies, dependence on artificial feeding (e.g., feeding tube) or oral supplements, and/or functional difficulties. An individual is only diagnosed with avoidant/restrictive food intake disorder when the above criteria are met and (1) the behavior is not due to an insufficient availability of food and (2) they do not meet the criteria for anorexia or bulimia.

Among adolescents, estimates of the lifetime prevalence of anorexia range from 0.3-1.7%, and bulimia is estimated to affect around 1% of individuals (Hoek & van Hoeken, 2013; Smink et al., 2014; Swanson et al., 2011). Binge eating disorder is more common, occurring in 1.6-7% of adolescents. Studies of community samples suggest that up to 36% of youth exhibit problem eating-related beliefs and behaviors (Jones et al., 2001; Schuck et al., 2018). The prevalence of EDs in preadolescent children has not been well studied but appears to be less common than in older youth (Nicholls et al., 2011; Pinhas, Morris, Crosby, & Katzman, 2011); children are more likely to meet the criteria for avoidant/restrictive food intake disorder than for other EDs (Kurz et al., 2015). Eating disorders, especially anorexia and bulimia, affect females much more frequently than males (American Psychiatric Association, 2013; Smink et al., 2014). This gender difference is understood to be the result of a stronger cultural emphasis on thinness as the ideal for the female body, which in turns leads to higher levels of body dissatisfaction in girls and women (Ferreiro, Seoane, & Senra, 2014; Grabe et al., 2008).

The majority of youth with an ED also meet the criteria for another psychological disorder; some research has found comorbidity rates as high as nearly 90% (Lewinsohn et al., 2000; Swanson et al., 2011). Depression, anxiety disorders, and oppositional defiant disorder commonly co-occur in youth with EDs; adolescents with bulimia or binge eating disorder are also at heightened risk for substance abuse and conduct disorder (Salbach-Andrae et al., 2008; Swanson et al., 2011). Attention-deficit/hyperactivity disorder (ADHD) is not uncommon among adolescents with EDs (Rojo-Moreno et al., 2015); however, this pattern may not reflect true comorbidity, as increases in hyperactivity have also been linked to extreme calorie restriction (Müller et al., 2009). EDs are also associated with a variety of physical problems and complications (see Müller et al., 2009, for a review). Individuals with anorexia frequently have lower bone density than their peers, which can persist and raise the risk for later osteoporosis. Other common medical correlates of anorexia include hypothermia, dehydration and constipation, hair loss, slow heartbeat, swelling, anemia, and a variety of nutritional deficiencies. Individuals with bulimia are at risk for nutritional deficiencies as well as dehydration, dental enamel erosion, esophageal and pancreatic inflammation, and electrocardiogram abnormalities. In addition, the semi-starvation that occurs within anorexia (and sometimes bulimia) can result in abnormalities in endocrine functioning, including amenorrhea and changes in hypo-thalamic-pituitary-adrenal (HPA) axis functioning, such as high levels of cortisol (Müller et al., 2009). The mortality rate for anorexia in adolescents is around 2% (Steinhausen, 2002). In long-term studies of adults with anorexia, the mortality rate rises to around 10% (Keel et al., 2003; Steinhausen, 2002). Causes of death among individuals with anorexia vary but are most commonly due to suicide or medical complications (Button et al., 2010; Keel et al., 2003).

RISK/CAUSAL FACTORS
Biological factors.
Genetic factors. The influence of genetic factors on EDs varies by gender and across development. For females, the heritability rate of disordered eating is essentially zero in childhood but rises to around 50% after puberty (Culbert et al., 2009; Klump et al., 2003, 2007, 2012, 2017). In adult females, disorder-specific heritability estimates range from 22-76% for anorexia (Bulik et al., 2006; Klump et al., 2001; Mazzeo et al., 2009; Wade et al., 2000), from 55-83% for bulimia (Bulik et al., 1998; Kendler et al., 1991; Trace et al., 2013), and from 41-57% for binge eating disorder (Javaras et al., 2008; Mitchell et al., 2010; Reichborn-Kjennerud et al., 2004). The more limited research conducted with males suggests that though the heritability rate for EDs in males is similar to or slightly lower than the rate in females, it is more stable across development, with genetic factors affecting EDs in prepubertal boys as well as adolescents and adults (Baker et al., 2009; Klump et al., 2012). Explanations for sex differences in the heritability of EDs before puberty focus on the factors that may trigger genetic risk differentially in girls

versus boys, such as exposure to high levels of ovarian hormones as well as psychosocial risk factors (Klump et al., 2010, 2012;). Studies of specific genetic factors linked to risk for EDs generally implicate genes and regions of genes involved in a wide variety of processes, including the production and transport of serotonin, encoding taste receptors, and the regulation of weight and blood glucose (Lee & Lin, 2010; Slof-Op 't Landt et al., 2011; Wade et al., 2013; Plana et al., 2019).

Neurochemical and neuroanatomical factors. Several patterns of biological functioning are thought to underlie EDs. Anatomical and functional differences between the brains of individuals with and without EDs can be conceptualized as reflecting dysregulated self-control, inhibition, and responsivity to reward (Berner & Kaye, 2017; Berner & Marsh, 2014; Friederick et al., 2013). First, adolescents and adults with bulimia display both structural and functional abnormalities within the frontostriatal circuits of the brain, which connect the prefrontal cortex (involved in executive functioning) and the striatum (involved in voluntary action). Frontostriatal circuits are understood to play a role in inhibitory control, the ability to stop oneself from performing a behavior; the binge eating and performance of compensatory behaviors central to bulimia can be conceptualized as examples of poor inhibition. Indeed, individuals with bulimia display lower levels of inhibitory control than their nondisordered peers, especially when presented with stimuli related to food or body shape (Wu et al., 2013). Interestingly, this pattern is not seen in individuals with binge eating disorder. In contrast, during cognitively challenging tasks, individuals with anorexia display higher levels of neural activity in brain regions associated with inhibitory control (Wierenga, Bischoff-Grethe, Melrose, et al., 2014; Zastrow et al., 2009).

Second, variations are seen in the anatomical and neurochemical patterns associated with responses to rewards in the environment (Berner & Marsh, 2014; Wierenga, Ely, et al., 2014). Specifically, decreases in brain volume and activity in regions associated with reward sensitivity, such as the ventral striatum and the insula, are found in individuals with anorexia. In addition, anorexia is associated with a variety of abnormalities in dopamine, a neurotransmitter associated with the experience of stimuli as rewarding (O'Hara et al., 2015). When behaviors are repeatedly associated with an environmental reinforcer, dopaminergic pathways are activated; therefore, certain behaviors may become more strongly associated with dopamine activation than others due to environmental and individual-level (e.g., cognitive) reinforcement. For example, an adolescent who experiences the rapid weight loss and sense of self-control that follow extreme calorie restriction as highly rewarding may become sensitized on a neurochemical level to the "positive" effects of these behaviors, as her dopaminergic pathways are increasingly activated by her disordered eating behavior and less sensitive to other environmental rewards. In contrast, increased activity seen in these areas in individuals with bulimia suggest a heightened sensitivity to reward (Berner & Marsh, 2014; Wierenga, Ely, et al., 2014).

Furthermore, serotonergic abnormalities in individuals with bulimia are thought to contribute to the intense negative moods that often trigger binges and compensatory behavior (Hildebrandt et al., 2010); the combi-nation of abnormalities in both serotonin transmission and reward sensitivity may lead to behavioral cycles that are very difficult to break, as symptoms are reinforced by their effectiveness in producing a sense of relief and/or reward. In addition, aberrations in the neurologically based experience of various positive (e.g., good-tasting food) and maladaptive (e.g., purging) stimuli as rewarding may be worsened by engagement in disordered eating behaviors and beliefs (O'Hara et al., 2015). It has been proposed that EDs may result from the interaction between abnormalities in reward sensitivity and problems with inhibitory control rather than the independent effects of either pattern (Wierenga, Ely, et al., 2014). For example, heightened inhibitory control combined with reduced sensitivity to rewards may lead to anorexia, whereas impairments in inhibition coupled with heightened reward sensitivity may result in bulimia.

Psychological factors.

Personality. High levels of perfectionism have been consistently linked to heightened risk for eating disorders, especially anorexia (Bastiani et al., 1995; Fairburn et al., 1999; Sutandar-Pinnock et al., 2003). Different types of perfectionism have been identified (Hewitt & Flett, 1991), and certain aspects of perfectionism are more strongly linked with EDs. Specifically, individuals with anorexia and bulimia report higher levels of self-oriented perfectionism (i.e., unrealistic self-evaluation and standards for one's own behavior and performance that originate within an individual) but not socially prescribed perfectionism (i.e., the perception that others have unrealistically high standards for one's behavior and performance) than healthy controls (Castro et al., 2004; Castro-Fornieles et al., 2007). ED risk is highest when youth display perfectionism consisting of both high standards and negative self-evaluation when those standards are not met or might not be met (Boone et al., 2010). Perfectionism in childhood that raises the risk for later EDs may be evident in a variety of domains, including schoolwork, need for order, and overall rigidity (Halmi et al., 2012). An individual's level of perfectionism may also predict response to treatment, with adult ED patients with lower levels of perfectionism having better short- and long-term outcomes following inpatient treatment (Sutandar-Pinnock et al., 2003). Perfectionism appears to impact ED risk via depression; high levels of perfectionism can lead to depression, which in turn may lead to the development of disordered eating (Drieberg et al., 2019). In addition, high levels of negative emotionality/neuroticism (Brookings & Wilson, 1994; Cervera et al., 2003; Keel et al., 1998; Lee-Winn et al., 2016) and impulsivity (Lee-Winn et al., 2016; Maganto et al., 2016; Mikami, Hinshaw, et al., 2010) have been linked with higher levels of ED symptoms in adolescents. Youth who are temperamentally prone to experiencing more frequent or intense negative emotions may be more likely to manage those overwhelming feelings maladaptively, such as through disordered eating (e.g., restricting, binge eating, purging); youth who are high on both neuroticism and impulsivity may be particularly prone to managing strong emotions in ways that can be self-damaging, such as binge eating.

View of self. Youth who view themselves more negatively are at higher risk for developing disordered eating. This negative view of self can take different forms. First, youth and young adults who have lower overall self-esteem are more likely than their peers to display restrictive eating behaviors (such as fasting or skipping meals) or binge eating and to be diagnosed with an ED (Cervera et al., 2003; Haynos et al., 2016; Sehm & Warschburger, 2018). Youth with low self-esteem may engage in disordered eating as a way to manage negative emotions or an effort to create change in their lives that they view as positive. Furthermore, the relation between EDs and self-esteem may be reciprocal, with low self-esteem contributing to the development of an ED, and engagement in disordered eating actually worsening self-esteem for some youth (Cervera et al., 2003; Wichstrøm & van Soest, 2016). In contrast, high self-esteem is linked with lower rates of EDs (Nicholls et al., 2016; Nicholls & Viner, 2009), even among youth who are at heightened risk for these disorders due to the presence of other characteristics, such as high perfectionism (Westerberg-Jacobson et al., 2010b).

A negative view of one's body, shape, and/or weight specifically has also been found to increase risk for EDs. Throughout childhood, as early as age five, youth who are more dissatisfied with their bodies display higher levels of eating disorder symptoms (Krahnstoever Davison et al., 2003; Parkinson et al., 2012). This link exists in adolescents as well, with body dissatisfaction or the desire to be thinner predicting both concurrent and future ED symptoms (Evans et al., 2017; Ferreiro et al., 2012; Keel et al., 1998 Westerberg-Jacobson et al., 2010a, 2010b). Interestingly, research examining the relationship between actual weight or BMI to eating disorder symptoms has been inconsistent, with some studies finding youth with higher BMIs to be at higher risk for EDs and others finding no link (Gardner et al., 2000; Evans et al., 2017; Lowe et al., 2019). It may be youths' *perceptions* of themselves as overweight (accurate or inaccurate), combined with dissatisfaction with how they judge themselves relative to a desired standard, that raise the risk for disordered eating (Buckingham-Howes et al., 2018). There are gender differences in the manifestations of body dissatisfaction, with adolescent boys being more likely than girls to report muscle dissatisfaction and adolescent girls being more likely than boys to be dissatisfied either with their height or with their bodies overall (Baker et al., 2019).

Body dissatisfaction interacts with other variables in the prediction of EDs. Body dissatisfaction appears to develop as youth internalize the body-related views of others around them (Keery et al., 2004). Sources of these views include the media as well as parental and peer views that provide messages about the ideal body shape/weight, a preoccupation with weight/dieting, and criticism or teasing about the youth's weight or body. Finally, youth who report higher levels of worry about gaining weight are more likely to diet, and dieting contributes to later worrying about weight gain, suggesting that when youth engage in behaviors meant to decrease negative feelings about the body, these behaviors may actually increase a negative self-view and lead to more maladaptive behaviors, creating a vicious cycle (Zarychta et al., 2017).

Environmental factors.

Family dynamics. Many aspects of family dynamics, including variables related to weight and eating as well as broader aspects of family functioning, have been linked with a higher risk for EDs in youth. First, parental views of food and the body are associated with children's ED symptoms. Maternal eating disorder symptoms and early dieting are linked with adolescent girls' ED symptoms (Pike & Rodin, 1991; Ziobrowski et al., 2019). Disordered eating behaviors, such as fasting and binge eating, are correlated between adolescents and adults living in the same household (Ferreira et al., 2013; Snoek et al., 2009). Mothers who express dissatisfaction with their own bodies have young daughters who express the same feelings about their bodies (Perez et al., 2018). Both maternal and paternal body dissatisfaction and drive for thinness (preoccupation with weight and dieting as well as fear of gaining weight) are also linked with ED risk in childhood and adolescence (Agras et al., 2007; Canals et al., 2009). Parental attitudes and behaviors related to food and weight may impact children in a number of ways, including both through pressure parents put on youth about their own weight or shape and through modeling of unhealthy attitudes and behaviors (Yamazaki & Omori, 2016). For example, mothers who are preoccupied with their own weight and dieting are more likely to restrict their daughters' dietary intake and encourage their daughters to lose weight (Francis & Birch, 2005). An experimental study designed to examine the effects of modeling measured preadolescent girls' attitudes and behavior before and after viewing advertisements promoting thinness with their mothers. Compared to a control group, daughters displayed lower levels of body satisfaction, more disordered eating attitudes, and higher levels of dietary restriction after mothers made self-critical comments about their bodies and diets while viewing the ads (Handford et al., 2018).

Interactions between parents and children that focus on attitudes and behaviors related to children's weight and eating have also been linked with ED risk. When parents perceive children or adolescents to be overweight, youth are more likely to be dissatisfied with their own weight or eating behavior, which in turns predicts higher levels of ED symptoms (Allen et al., 2009, 2015). Similarly, compared to their healthy peers, adolescent girls with EDs have mothers who believe that their daughters should lose more weight (Pike & Rodin, 1991). The degree to which mother-daughter dyads engage in "fat talk" (discussions about body dissatisfaction and negative affect) is linked to disordered eating in both mothers and adolescents (Chow & Tan, 2018). Further, mothers' dissatisfaction with their young adult daughters' body weight and shape predicts daughters' body dissatisfaction and ED symptoms (Cooley et al., 2008). In addition, parental behaviors meant to encourage weight loss in their children, such as restriction of their food intake, are linked with a heightened risk for the later development of EDs (Agras et al., 2007; Allen et al., 2009). Parental restriction or overcontrol of children's early eating behaviors likely leads to higher levels of self-restriction as youth age, with the potential for this behavior to develop into a full-blown ED (Edmunds & Hill, 1999). Finally, parental criticism of or teasing about children's weight increases body dissatisfaction, preoccupation with thinness, and risk for EDs throughout childhood, adolescence, and early adulthood (Agras et al., 2007; Cooley et al., 2008; Fairburn et al., 1998, 1999; Schwartz, Phares, et al., 1999).

Other aspects of family interactions have been found to predict disordered eating across development. In middle childhood, youth report more emotional eating when parents minimize children's negative emotions, are less emotionally expressive, and display lower levels of warmth and support (Topham et al., 2011). In adolescent girls, a higher sense of alienation from their mothers is linked with higher levels of ED symptoms (Pelletier Brochu et al., 2018). Compared to their healthy peers, women with EDs report that their parents were less affectionate, more rejecting/uncaring, more overprotective, more demanding, and generally either underinvolved or overinvolved (Fairburn et al., 1998, 1999; Pike et al., 2008). In contrast, adolescents with healthier family functioning (e.g., better communication, higher levels of affection and responsiveness), higher levels of warmth, and more parental monitoring of children's whereabouts are at lower risk for EDs (Berge et al., 2014). Higher levels of family stress and conflict throughout childhood are also linked to heightened risk for EDs in youth (Allen et al., 2009; Striegel-Moore et al., 2005). One mechanism by which these dynamics may affect youth is emotional insecurity. When marital conflict is high, young children display more emotional reactivity and behavioral dysregulation, which in turn predict higher levels of ED symptoms in adolescence (George et al., 2014). Youth who experience overwhelming amounts of family-related stress may use food and eating behavior to either express or regulate emotions in a way that serves an immediate adaptive function (e.g., feeling less sad, gaining a sense of control) but is maladaptive for long-term development. Finally, women with EDs are more likely than their peers to report having experienced sexual or physical abuse in childhood (Fairburn, 1998).

Media exposure. Exposure to unrealistic portrayals of body and appearance standards, such as thinness for females and muscularity for males, have long been understood to raise an individual's risk for developing an ED. This exposure may occur when adolescents watch television, read magazines, or view social media sites, particularly media originating in cultures in which low body weight is viewed as desirable or beautiful (Makino et al., 2004). When Western media was introduced in the Nadroga province of Fiji in 1995, rates of disordered eating behaviors and attitudes among ethnic Fijian adolescent girls jumped dramatically, and interviews with these youth directly linked television exposure to these changes (Becker et al., 2002). The link between media exposure and eating disorder symptoms has been demonstrated in an extensive body of research. A meta-analysis of seventy-seven studies revealed a consistent link between exposure to thin-ideal media and lower levels of body satisfaction as well as disordered eating behavior and attitudes in women (Grabe, Ward, & Hyde, 2008). Higher levels of media exposure also predict more internalization of the thin-body ideal, which may be the mechanism by which media exposure impacts other variables; indeed, the degree to which youth internalize societal standards of beauty, such as those presented in the media, predict body dissatisfaction and disordered eating attitudes (Francisco et al., 2015; Jones, Vigfusdottir, & Lee, 2004; Rodgers et al., 2020). In addition, youth with eating disorders may visit pro-ana and pro-mia websites that promote disordered eating behavior. Users of these sites often report that they provide help and support, though there is significant concern about the ways in which they provide misin-

formation and actually reinforce ED symptoms (Bert et al., 2016; Borzekowski et al., 2010; Gale et al., 2016). Experimental studies with non-eating disordered populations have linked viewing pro-ana content with an increase in negative affect, a decrease in self-esteem, an increased tendency to view oneself as overweight, and a large reduction in calorie consumption during the following weeks (Bardone-Cone & Cass, 2007; Jett et al., 2010).

DEVELOPMENTAL COURSE

Eating disorders are very rare in youth under the age of twelve (Lewinsohn et al., 2000). The most common age of onset for EDs is late adolescence to early adulthood, with mixed research on whether anorexia or bulimia is likely to begin earlier in development (Herpertz-Dahlmann, 2008; Stice et al., 2013). However, for a small group of youth, symptoms develop in childhood, and for individuals who do not display full-blown EDs until later in development, early signs and risk factors may be present. For example, body dissatisfaction as early as age five predicts disordered eating behaviors and attitudes in later childhood (Krahnstoever Davison et al., 2003), and children with lower levels of self-esteem at age ten are at higher risk for a variety of types of EDs by adulthood (Nicholls et al., 2009; Nicholls & Viner, 2016). Unusual early eating habits can also signal risk. Feeding problems in infancy and overeating as well as dietary restriction in middle childhood have been linked to higher rates of eating disorders later in development (Evans et al., 2017; Munkholm et al., 2016; Nicholls & Viner, 2016). These factors may represent problematic thoughts and behaviors that have become part of a child's repertoire (e.g., body dissatisfaction, restricted eating) and may develop into an ED. Alternatively, they may be an early manifestation or result of environmental risk factors that raise the likelihood of a later eating disorder, such as in cases in which infant feeding problems reflect abnormal family dynamics and pressures around eating.

Risk for the onset of eating disorders is enhanced at the onset of puberty, particularly for girls (Klump, 2013). Several explanations for this developmental pattern have been proposed. One set of theories focuses on biological factors. For example, as we have discussed previously, genetic factors appear to influence the occurrence of EDs only after puberty in girls (Culbert et al., 2009; Klump et al., 2003, 2007). This developmental change may be due to pubertal increases in ovarian hormones such as estradiol, which is associated with disordered eating (Klump et al., 2014). Indeed, the heritability of EDs is higher in pubertal twin females with higher levels of estradiol (Klump et al., 2010). Estradiol plays a role in regulating gene transcription (Östlund et al., 2003); therefore, genetically influenced differences in risk for EDs may not become apparent until increased estradiol levels during puberty affect the expression of genetic risk. Other theories emphasize the social and environmental factors that accompany puberty. For example, especially for girls, the physical changes that occur during puberty (e.g., increase in body fat percentage) may lead to heightened levels of body dissatisfaction, which some girls manage through unhealthy dieting and other maladaptive eating behaviors (Bulik, 2002).

There is a fairly high level of continuity in disordered eating across development. ED symptoms in late childhood predict symptoms in early adolescence for both boys and girls, and symptoms throughout adolescence predict EDs in adulthood (Evans et al., 2017; Ferreiro, Wichstrøm, et al., 2014; Kotler et al., 2001). Furthermore, the continuity of symptoms increases with age; symptom levels are more stable in late adolescence than earlier in development (Ferreiro, Wichstrøm, et al., 2014). However, individual variability also exists. Whereas some youth have ongoing ED symptoms, others experience worsening or improving symptoms across development. Adolescents who report drug use, higher levels of depressive symptoms, body dissatisfaction, having mothers or peers who are dieting, or being teased about their weight are more likely to move from lower to higher levels of ED symptoms; in contrast, higher self-esteem and positive family interactions are predictors of symptom improvement (Pearson et al., 2017). The specific manifestations of disordered eating may change over time as well. For some individuals with anorexia, the hunger resulting from extreme restriction may lead to bingeing; indeed, about one-quarter of individuals with bulimia have met the criteria for anorexia (Herpertz-Dahlmann, 2008). The most common changes in manifestations of symptoms within an individual is between bulimia and binge eating disorder; individuals with binge eating disorder may come to meet the criteria for bulimia if they develop a pattern of compensatory behaviors, and vice versa (Stice et al., 2013). It is uncommon for bulimia or binge eating disorder to morph into anorexia.

Finally, the course of eating disorder symptoms across development varies by gender. At age nine, boys have more symptoms than girls (Parkinson et al., 2012). However, in early adolescence, boys' average symptoms decrease, whereas girls' symptoms increase (Evans et al., 2017; Ferreiro, Wichstrøm, et al., 2014; Pearson et al., 2017). Higher rates of eating disorders in females are then seen throughout adolescence and adulthood (Neumark-Sztainer et al., 2011). Adolescents with EDs are at heightened risk for a variety of problems in early adulthood, including depression, self-harm, anxiety disorders, drug and alcohol use, and weight problems (Micali et al., 2015). Therefore, accurate assessment and effective treatment are crucial components of supporting the long-term recovery and well-being of these youth.

ASSESSMENT

Assessing (and treating) eating disorders can present unique challenges (Stice & Peterson, 2007). Caregivers are often more likely than youth themselves to characterize symptoms as problematic, and youth may not recognize the physical harm that can result from their behaviors. In addition, individuals with EDs may go to great lengths to hide their behaviors or symptoms (e.g., weight loss) from others, which can make early identification and treatment more difficult. Finally, the ego-syntonic nature (consistent with one's sense of self) of anorexia in particular may lead to resistance to assessment and treatment. Therefore, a strong working alliance with both the client and her parents is foundational for effective information gathering. Clinicians should also work to create conditions under which the client is most likely to be cooperative and honest in the process of assessment, such as during sessions in which parents are not present. The use of multiple informants is

also important, as there may be significant discrepancies between parent and youth reports, which is thought to have multiple causes; as noted above, parents may not always be aware of eating disorder symptoms (such as binge eating), but some youth (especially those with anorexia) may underreport symptoms (Couturier et al., 2007; Johnson et al., 1999; Tanofsky-Kraff et al., 2005). Ideally, the assessment of EDs should be conducted by a multidisciplinary team who is equipped to evaluate cognitive and behavioral symptoms, interpersonal functioning and context, and medical and nutritional concerns.

BMI measurements calculated during routine physicals can serve as a screener for anorexia; if youth exhibit extreme weight loss or failure to gain weight as expected, physicians should follow up with parents and youth to identify potentially problematic eating-related behaviors and attitudes (Golden & Ornstein, 2016). Once the need for further assessment has been established, clinicians will typically proceed with unstructured interviews with parents and youth (Stice & Peterson, 2007). Clinicians should ask questions designed to assess eating disorder symptoms as well as risk and maintaining factors, detailed information about core symptoms (e.g., what does the youth eat in a typical day? What is consumed during a binge? What compensatory behaviors are occurring?), the impact of symptoms on functioning, developmental history, family history and dynamics, and other environmental influences on the client's functioning. Interviews are understood to be a critical component of the assessment process, as they allow for follow-up and exploratory questions in a way that self-report surveys often do not (Fairburn & Beglin, 1994;

Stice & Peterson, 2007). One of the most commonly used semi-structured interviews for ED symptoms is the Eating Disorder Examination (EDE; Fairburn & Cooper, 1993), which was designed for use with adults but can also be used to assess disordered eating attitudes and behaviors in adolescents ages fourteen and older. The Child Version of the EDE (ChEDE; Bryant-Waugh et al., 1996) incorporates several adaptations that make it more suitable for children as young as seven, including changes in language, more concrete assessment of certain symptoms, and the assessment of intention as well as behavior (to include problematic behaviors that would be performed if the child had more control over her environment).

Once interview-based data have been collected, questionnaires can be useful for gathering information about a variety of symptoms from multiple sources that can then be compared to normative data. Several questionnaire measures of ED symptoms have been developed for use with youth, including both self-report and parent-report instruments. The Youth Eating Disorder Examination Questionnaire (YEDE-Q; Goldschmidt et al., 2007) is a 39-item self-report questionnaire for youth ages twelve to seventeen assessing restraint, eating concern, weight concern, and shape concern over the previous four weeks. The Eating Disorder Inventory, Third Edition (EDI-3; Garner, 2004) is a 91-item questionnaire for thirteen- to fifty-three-year-olds measuring attitudes and behaviors along twelve subscales. Some measures have been adapted or developed for use with younger clients, such as the Children's Eating Attitudes Test (ChEAT; Maloney et al., 1988), which is reliable with children eight to thirteen years

of age; the Kids' Eating Disorders Survey (KEDS; Childress et al., 1993), which assesses symptoms in nine- to sixteen-year-olds; and the Questionnaire for Eating and Weight Patterns—Adolescent Version (QEWP-A; Johnson et al., 1999), developed for youth ages 10-18. Questionnaires completed by caregivers include the Anorectic Behavior Observation Scale (ABOS; Vandereycken & Meerman, 1984), which assesses eating disorder symptoms with good sensitivity and specificity in youth ages 12 and up as reported by significant others, and the Questionnaire for Eating and Weight Patterns—Parent Version (QEWP-P; Johnson et al., 1999), a twelve-item questionnaire for use with children and adolescents ten to eighteen years old, which parallels the QEWP-A.

Finally, youth suspected of having an eating disorder should be assessed for comorbid presenting problems such as depression and anxiety as well as medical complications. Broadband measures completed by youth and their parents, as presented in other chapters, can be administered to assess comorbid symptoms. To ensure the treatment of any medical complications, psychosocial clinicians should refer these youth to medical professionals for a thorough assessment of physical symptoms, including cardiovascular, gastrointestinal, and endocrine problems (Campbell & Peebles, 2014). A physical examination provides information about physiological symptoms that are dangerous and need to be addressed immediately in settings ranging from outpatient to inpatient.

TREATMENT

Research generally points to family therapy as the most effective psychosocial intervention for eating disorders; however, the level of effectiveness depends on the specific disorder as well as the age of the client (Gorrell & Le Grange, 2019; Lock, 2015, 2019). Specifically, behavioral family therapy is considered a well-established treatment for adolescents with anorexia and possibly efficacious for adolescents with bulimia. Systemic family therapy and insight-oriented individual therapy are considered probably efficacious treatments for anorexia in adolescents. Unfortunately, there are no well-supported treatments for any eating disorders in children or for bulimia, binge eating disorder, or avoidant restrictive food intake disorder in adolescents. Below, we will describe both family and individual therapies for adolescents with anorexia.

Family therapy. There is significant overlap between behavioral family systems therapy (BFST) and systemic family therapy (often referred to as family-based treatment, or FBT), and despite their names, both approaches include elements of systemic and behavioral interventions. This overlap includes six elements of effective family therapy for eating disorders which appear in both approaches: (1) not placing blame for symptoms on family members (including the client), (2) emphasizing the parents' role in helping adolescents regain weight, (3) holding joint parent-child sessions, (4) directly addressing weight gain and food intake rather than taking a covert approach, (5) shifting control of eating from the parents to the adolescent as therapy progresses successfully, and (6) targeting necessary weight gain before addressing other potential therapeutic goals, such as cognitive patterns and family dynamics (Le Grange & Robin, 2017). Therefore, in order to avoid significant redundancy, we will only review FBT,

which is the more frequently researched, documented, and utilized approach. Some differences between the two approaches are discussed at the end of this section.

FBT (Doyle & Le Grange, 2015; Lock & Le Grange, 2013) originated at the Maudsley Hospital in London; therefore, it is sometimes referred to as the Maudsley approach or the Maudsley method. This family-based treatment for adolescents with anorexia combines elements of a variety of family therapy approaches, including systemic family therapy, which conceptualizes a family as a system and understands symptoms as the result of interactions among members of that system, and behavioral family therapy, which focuses on the ways in which maladaptive behaviors have been learned from the environment (mainly the family). The length of FBT varies depending on the complexity of the case and the speed of progress in therapy, but it generally involves ten to twenty sessions over the course of six to twelve months. In all cases, FBT is divided into three distinct phases.

In *Phase I,* the clinician and the family focus on directly addressing the client's symptoms, mainly low weight, during weekly sessions. The main goal over the course of this phase is to change the client's eating habits, via parent-directed intervention, so that she is gaining one to two pounds per week. Session one focuses mainly on establishing the therapeutic alliance and gathering information about symptom history as well as family functioning and dynamics. In this session, the clinician's tasks include beginning to establish a relationship with each family member, weighing the client (and establishing the first data point on a weight chart that will be used throughout treatment), and assessing family and symptom history by involving all family members. The clinician will also set the stage for the intervention by de-emphasizing blame, helping the family externalize (i.e., separate) the illness from the client, explaining the seriousness of anorexia, and emphasizing the parents' central role in weight restoration. The main focus of session two is a family meal. The family is asked to bring in a meal that they believe will be nutritionally beneficial to the client (i.e., help her gain weight). During the session, the family lays out and eats the meal while the therapist observes the family dynamics around food and eating and coaches the parents as they encourage their daughter to eat more. The clinician aims to build on the skills and knowledge that parents already possess in order to help them better understand the client's nutritional needs (e.g., what foods will contribute to weight gain) as well as to be persistently unified in their efforts to encourage eating. Both the clinician and the parents should be supportive and noncritical during this task, even as they challenge the client to increase consumption beyond her comfort level. The remaining five to ten sessions of this phase are less specifically structured and ordered; the three goals of these sessions are helping the family remain explicitly focused on symptom reduction, helping the parents continue to gain control of the client's eating behavior, and enhancing the support of other family members, such as siblings. Each Phase I session begins with the weighing of the client and the tracking of weight gain over treatment. Work during the rest of each session can include discussion of how parents can continue to promote the client's weight gain at home, how siblings can be comforting and supportive, how to reduce

family members' criticism of the client, and how to continue to separate the disorder from who the client is.

Once the client is near a normal weight and family dynamics have begun to change (e.g., the client willingly follows parental direction regarding food, parents have a subjective sense of success and empowerment), *Phase II* begins. The goal of this phase, which generally consists of two to six sessions scheduled every two to three weeks, is to transition control over eating-related behavior back to the adolescent. Parents continue to direct the client's eating until it is clear that she can manage her eating behavior in a healthy, nondisordered manner. At this point, the clinician supports the parents as they choose the specific strategies that will work best in their family for returning control of eating to their daughter; these strategies might include allowing the client to participate in grocery shopping, serve herself at meals with supervision, select or prepare her own foods, or even eat unsupervised for one to two meals per day. In addition, now that low weight has improved significantly, the therapeutic focus begins to include developmental issues in adolescence (e.g., desire for independence, importance of peer and dating relationships) and how these areas may have contributed to the development of the disorder and/or been negatively affected by it. Several of the same interventions and principles are emphasized in Phase II as in Phase I, including weekly weight tracking, improving sibling support, reducing family criticism, and externalizing the disorder. When the client reaches a healthy weight, is no longer engaging in disordered eating behavior (e.g., extreme restriction, excessive exercise), and has successfully taken back control of her eating behavior from her parents, therapy moves into *Phase III*, during which the family and clinician aim to develop healthy, developmentally appropriate dynamics and interactions between the client and her parents. This relatively brief phase generally consists of one to four sessions occurring every four to six weeks. The goals at this point in treatment include continuing to help the family communicate and navigate normal issues of adolescent development in healthy ways (so that eating disorder symptoms do not serve a purpose in the family system). Weight tracking does not take place during Phase III. Discussion of adaptive problem solving around developmental issues, planning for future difficulties, and healthy termination also occur.

Research as early as 1987, when the first randomized clinical trial was conducted at the Maudsley Hospital, shows FBT to be effective in reducing ED symptoms (Russell et al., 1987). Since then, several studies have found that FBT is more effective than individual therapy for treating both anorexia and bulimia (Le Grange et al., 2007; Le Grange, Accurso, et al., 2014; Lock et al., 2010; Schmidt et al., 2007). Differences in long-term outcomes are unclear, with some studies finding FBT to produce greater gains at follow-up and others finding no difference by treatment type (Couturier et al., 2013; Le Grange, Lock, et al., 2014). Differences in treatment response exist based on a number of client variables, with younger age, shorter disorder duration, restricting-type anorexia (compared to binge eating/purging type), and more weight gain early in treatment being associated with a better prognosis (Le Grange, Accurso, et al., 2014; Le

Grange et al., 2012). BFST has also been found to effectively reduce symptoms in adolescents with anorexia (Robin et al., 1994, 1995, 1999).

As mentioned earlier, it should be noted that some differences do exist between BFST and FBT, as the former emphasizes behavioral principles more heavily, whereas the latter focuses more on the dynamics within the family system that are not limited to behavioral principles. Specifically, five main differences exist between the two approaches (Le Grange & Robin, 2017). In BFST, a dietitian plays a central role in meal planning and documentation, whereas FBT utilizes a dietitian as a consultant rather than a part of the treatment team. In BFST, a specific behaviorally based plan for eating and weight gain is developed and followed, whereas FBT does not include a detailed, structured approach to changing eating habits and intake. BFST includes the restructuring of problem cognitions around food and the body; FBT does not directly address cognitive distortions. In BFST, only the adolescent and the parent attend sessions, whereas FBT includes all family members living in the household in sessions. Finally, during BFST, all meals take place at home, with discussion about meals occurring during sessions; FBT incorporates an in-session family meal. In addition, BFST tends to be a longer intervention than FBT.

Individual therapy. Adolescent-focused therapy (AFT) is a treatment for EDs that primarily involves work with the adolescent (Fitzpatrick et al., 2010, 2015). (In earlier research, this intervention was called ego-oriented individual therapy, or EOIT; Robin et al., 1994). AFT has its theoretical roots in psychodynamic, self-psychology approaches which understand EDs as resulting from problems with the development of the self (ego) and the inappropriate use of food-related behaviors to manage distressing developmental issues. Therefore, self-exploration, improving the strength of the ego/sense of self, and the development of healthy coping strategies are considered central components of treatment. In order to be good candidates for AFT, adolescents must be medically stable (i.e., not in need of intensive treatment) and capable of abstract thought and self-reflection. The intervention takes place over the course of twelve months; adolescents initially meet with clinicians on a weekly basis, but the frequency of sessions is often tapered closer to the end of treatment.

The relationship between the adolescent and the clinician is understood to be central to the treatment process in AFT. The therapist typically takes a "nurturant-authoritative" stance, in which the therapist is both a supportive and empathic figure and a strong leader who can motivate change for an adolescent experiencing a dangerous disorder. The role of the clinician is sometimes conceptualized as "re-parenting," not necessarily because previous parenting has been poor but because the clinician's ability to challenge and support change in the client is based on the same sense of care and support present in a healthy family. The therapist plays a parenting-type role in helping the adolescent develop the skills and autonomy necessary to function in a developmentally appropriate and healthy manner without relying on the ED. In addition to the primary therapist, the treatment team usually involves a physician and a dietitian to monitor physical health, weight gain, and nutritional planning and education. Though AFT is an individually fo-

cused intervention, it does not ignore the role of the family. Parents and other significant others participate in collateral sessions throughout treatment in order to facilitate assessment, psychoeducation, and parents' support of adolescents' healthy development and a positive home environment.

AFT is delivered over three phases. The main goals of *Phase I* are the establishment of the therapeutic alliance and case formulation. During the initial sessions of this phase, the clinician gathers historical and current information about symptoms, functioning, family and peer relationships, important life events, and methods of self-expression (e.g., art, music) from the client. Based on the information gathered, the clinician develops a case formulation centered on the client's main challenges and how anorexia serves to help the client respond to those challenges. Clinicians are encouraged to think about the ways in which clients may be experiencing regressive/independence needs (i.e., fears about becoming more independent or adultlike, which anorexia may help adolescents avoid), anger/control issues (i.e., refusing to eat as a way to express anger at or control over family members), depressive symptoms (i.e., symptoms may help combat feelings of helplessness and vulnerability by giving the adolescent a sense of control or represent a way of punishing oneself), and/or low self-esteem (i.e., anorexia may represent an attempt to gain a sense of identity, purpose, or self-worth). The formulation of a particular client's case then guides treatment planning, suggesting targets for intervention that can help eliminate the function of the symptoms. During the initial phase, the clinician also aims to educate the client about the disorder and the goals and structure of therapy as well as to help the client begin to separate herself from the disorder. Collateral sessions with parents involve gathering information, providing psychoeducation, and coaching parents in increasing the client's food intake and weight gain.

In *Phase II*, the clinician begins to help the client understand the function of her symptoms and her pattern of responses to stressors, including emotion regulation and coping skills. Treatment then focuses on helping the client develop new, adaptive, effective ways of managing negative thoughts, strong emotions, and developmental challenges (e.g., drive for individuation from family, desire for romantic relationships). Specifically, clinicians may help clients learn to identify emotions, learn to tolerate distress, find effective means of self-expression, identify techniques for coping with stressors or negative emotions, respond adaptively to challenging situations that arise in the adolescent's life, and develop a more robust sense of self not centered on the disorder. Clinicians provide support, direction, and structure, but the ultimate goal is to increase the client's self-awareness and insight, skill set, and sense of self-efficacy. Parent sessions during this phase may include discussion of how the family responds to stressors or developmental challenges, psychoeducation about adolescent development as well as recovery from anorexia, identification of sources of support within and outside the family, and ways to reinforce the skills the client is learning in session. *Phase III* involves continued work with adolescents and parents to identify and respond to developmental challenges; it also adds a focus on problem solving, relapse prevention, and

movement toward healthy termination. Research has found AFT to be an effective treatment for anorexia, producing improvements in eating behavior and attitudes, weight gain, interoceptive (body) awareness, internalizing symptoms, and family conflict (Lock et al., 2010; Robin et al., 1994, 1995, 1999).

Integrative Approach to Treatment

Valuing children as gifts. Truly viewing youth as gifts means taking very seriously the responsibility of caring well for youth with EDs, especially given the wide-reaching negative effects of the disorder on well-being and development. As we mentioned earlier, caring for these youth can be quite challenging for a number of reasons (Kaplan & Garfinkel, 1999). Comorbid disorders are often present, and treatment may need to be intensive, especially when it begins (e.g., inpatient hospitalization, intensive outpatient work). Clients may also have difficulty forming a trusting relationship with a clinician, particularly when family relationships are unhealthy, and they may even be explicitly resistant to treatment. One common pattern in individuals with EDs that makes treatment challenging is that clients may not recognize the severity of their symptoms or even that they have a disorder, they may have become very skilled at hiding their disordered eating behavior, and they may resist treatment because their symptoms are experienced (at least in part) as beneficial.

Throughout Scripture, we see children portrayed as gifts given to families (e.g., Psalm 127) and parents as having a serious responsibility to care well for these gifts (e.g., Deuteronomy 6:6-9; Proverbs 22:6). It is not only the clinician, then, whose view of youth as gifts is important in treating EDs; family members' views of and interactions with youth are also extremely influential. As we have discussed, youth are at heightened risk for ED symptoms when other people, particularly parents, are insensitive, rejecting, and critical, particularly of their body or weight. Such parenting patterns reflect difficulty truly valuing youth as gifts, as their criticism of body shape or weight in particular communicates to youth that they must change in order to be lovable, valuable, or attractive. In turn, youth develop dissatisfaction with their own bodies and their broader selves and may take drastic measures to change their bodies in order to be accepted (by themselves or by others), resulting in an ED. Therefore, valuing children as true gifts from God—valuable because they are created in his image and gifted by him—may actually serve as a protective factor against the development of disordered eating. For youth who have already developed significant symptoms, then, the central role of the family in effective treatment suggests that a change in parental attitudes and actions toward the client is an essential element of recovery.

How, then, do clinicians help family members to view youth with EDs as gifts within the context of treatment? FBT's process of externalizing the disorder is an important initial step. As they come to understand the disorder as separate from who the client truly is, family members may be able to shift negative thoughts and feelings away from the client and more toward the disorder itself (e.g., "I am angry at anorexia for interfering with my child's ability to be healthy and feel good about herself"). The more experiential components of FBT, such as the family meal, provide an opportunity for parents to learn how to enact appropriate authority in changing an adolescent's behavior without being critical or derogatory. When parents feel more empowered as progress occurs with their support, another goal of FBT, their stress levels are likely to decrease, which in turn removes another barrier to positive interactions with youth. Family therapists may also work to help parents and siblings identify positive characteristics they value in the client as well as specific ways in which they can support and care for their child and brother or sister. Clinicians working with Christian families might engage in explicit discussions of the child as a gift from God, who is valuable and worthy and who was placed by the Lord in their family to be cared for wisely and supportively. It is helpful to be careful to frame this discussion as a source of encouragement rather than a source of challenge or guilt. Finally, given the link between parents' body dissatisfaction and disordered eating behavior and EDs in youth, clinicians may also find it important to explore the severity of parents' own issues in order to determine whether they might benefit from their own treatment. Parents who view their own bodies negatively and have an unhealthy attitude toward food may have trouble disentangling their own view and experiences from their interactions with their youth with an ED. Addressing these issues in their own individual therapy, then, may be extremely important for helping them come to see their children as gifts, worthy in their own right rather than only under certain conditions (e.g., once they lose weight, if others view them as attractive).

Respecting children as persons. As we have discussed, youth, as full persons, are created in God's image and affected by sin. It is clear that God's design and desire for youth is not to starve to death or to gorge oneself and then induce vomiting or to live in a state of self-hatred. The negative effects of EDs on psychological and physical well-being, including their contribution to mortality rates, are evidence that these symptoms are not consistent with God's perfect design of our bodies as his temples (1 Corinthians 6:19-20). Therefore, we understand EDs, like all psychological disorders, to result from the impact of sin on creation and human functioning. When we think about the relation between EDs and sin, it can be tempting for some to approach this topic simplistically, reducing symptoms to the result of specific individual actions (i.e., viewing binge eating and purging as sinful behaviors because they do not "honor God with your body"). However, we remember that sin affects well-being in multiple ways, including individuals' specific sins as well as others' specific sins and the sinful state of humanity broadly. God is not honored by self-starvation or excessive exercise, but we must be careful to not reduce ED symptoms to an issue of individual sin that merely needs to be stopped by the individual, which places blame on the individual and/or the family and is antithetical to effective therapy that helps a client externalize the disordered symptoms. We have explored the wide variety of factors that contribute to the development of an ED, and it is clear that these influences come from many different sources, and as such, the role sin plays in EDs is complex. Individual sins such as sexual abuse or inappropriate parental criticism frequently play a role in the development of an ED. The sinful nature affects the genetic and hormonal factors that predispose some individuals to physical or psychological

problems, such as EDs. The role of institutional or corporate sin is also apparent when we examine the role of messages about beauty, thinness, and worth that are communicated through magazines, television, and social media. Therefore, though we recognize that sin affects EDs, we have to be cautious about drawing conclusions about the specific role of sin (including individual sin) in the life and functioning of individual clients. This caution pertains especially to the potential conclusion that ED symptoms are voluntary behaviors in which an individual can and should stop engaging when confronted. If recovery from an ED were that simple, no specialized treatment would be necessary; however, the extensive treatment literature is evidence that severe ED symptoms are not easily discontinued by clients on their own.

Rather, ED symptoms develop from the complex, dynamic interaction of a variety of factors that affect a given youth. Youths are embedded in a variety of contexts—family, neighborhood, peer group, school, church, and culture. Like adults, they are shaped by and respond to these contexts, and children and adolescents are generally understood to be especially susceptible to the influences of their environments as they develop. Furthermore, they do not come to these contexts as blank states but rather as persons with complex biological constitutions that affect how they interact with and are impacted by their environments and experiences. Indeed, in order to best understand an individual ED case, a close examination of the interaction between a youth and her contexts is important. Earlier, we discussed some of the purposes that an ED may serve for a youth, including having a sense of control, managing negative emotions, and feeling attractive. These are appropriate and common desires among youth (as well as adults) that are being met in a manner that is maladaptive. Therefore, recognizing that as full persons youth have needs and desires, an important component of therapy involves understanding how these needs and desires are being met by ED symptoms, which in turn can guide treatment. In other words, what function are the symptoms serving for the youth as she adapts to her particular contexts, and how might that need be met more adaptively? For one youth, severe dietary restriction may be a way to express control within a family who is overly involved in other areas of her life; treatment for this youth might include work with parents to reduce their involvement to developmentally appropriate levels and allow their daughter more adaptive avenues for choice and direction in her life. Another adolescent may have developed a pattern of binge eating and purging that occurs mainly when she feels overwhelmingly anxious about peer relationships and reduces her anxiety; in this case, the clinician needs to help the client identify ways to manage anxiety that are also effective but are less detrimental to her health and well-being.

For some youth, ED symptoms may be at least partially an expression or reflection of a spiritual need. Some writers have described EDs as a reflection of hunger or longing for spiritual meaning, purpose, identity, or perfection, which individuals seek to fulfill through excessive eating, dietary restriction, or other symptoms that reflect deeply powerful desires and needs (e.g., Bullitt-Jonas, 1999; Hardman et al., 2003; Lelwica, 1999). Though it can be challenging to identify and disentangle the various driving forces behind disordered eating symptoms, it may be useful for families and clinicians to explore an adolescent's spiritual well-being, including her subjective experiences of God, her spiritual practices, and her sense of meaning and fulfillment. Indeed, young college students who are wrestling with existential and faith-related issues report more disordered eating behaviors and attitudes (Boyatzis & McConnell, 2006). For youth with EDs who are grappling with these big questions and issues, treatment needs to take spiritual development and well-being into account. Once spiritual concerns have been identified, clinicians and families can work with youth to identify the ways in which symptoms may be an expression of these needs and desires as well as resources and sources of support for healthy exploration of questions of meaning and purpose. Writing about her own struggle with and recovery from binge eating, Margaret Bullitt-Jonas (1999) reflects, "It was only when I stopped attaching all my desire to food that a larger, deeper desire could flow freely through me. It was a desire for something infinite, . . . a Someone I wanted fiercely to know" (p. 249). At the same time, it is important not to overspiritualize a client's symptoms. For some youth, spiritual issues may be central to the disorder; for others, they may play little to no role. In either case, the large literature on risk factors for EDs indicates that many individual and environmental factors affect these disorders and must be addressed in treatment. Therefore, efforts to address the spiritual needs of adolescents as part of their personhood should proceed alongside empirically based treatments such as FBT or AFT.

Viewing children as agents. EDs present unique questions about how to help youth express their agency appropriately when they are enacting behaviors, such as severe calorie restriction, that could ultimately be fatal. Anorexia in particular is unique in its commonly ego-syntonic nature, meaning that it is consistent with an individual's sense of self and values and, therefore, viewed as desirable or even an inherent part of one's identity. Studies assessing the themes of letters written by adult patients to their anorexia suggest that anorexia serves positive purposes or functions for many individuals, including helping with the management of negative emotions and contributing to their sense of security or control, confidence, identity, company/ belonging, being special, and feeling attractive. However, the view of anorexia is not entirely positive, as these individuals also describe more negative effects, such as being controlled by the disorder, experiencing intrusive thoughts about food, losing friends, and feeling betrayed by a disorder that wastes their lives (Marzola et al., 2015; Serpell et al., 1999). Therefore, many individuals with anorexia may experience a sense of ambivalence toward the disorder and its effects. On the one hand, it serves a number of important functions for them; on the other hand, its effects can be detrimental and damaging. Clients' attitudes toward treatment, then, may range from a full desire for recovery to full resistance, with many youth falling somewhere in between these extremes (and attitudes toward treatment varying even within the same youth over the course of therapy). As clinicians, we have to understand this dynamic and the potential for ambivalence and to make proverbial space in therapy for clients to express their true thoughts and feelings and to have their perspectives validated, not

because we agree with them or think they represent objective reality but because they reflect the client's actual experiences and views. When youth feel genuinely heard, which they may not experience within their families, we help set the stage for effective therapy in which we can join with youth and address their individual thoughts, feelings, and experiences within the context of treatment. If we fail to hear or dismiss these youths' thoughts and emotions, including their positive experience of the disorder or their ambivalence toward therapy, they will be less willing participants in treatment, which is, in turn, less likely to be effective.

One of the ethical issues in treating EDs, particularly in adults, revolves around balancing the client's self-determination and autonomy with "forced" or more coercive treatment (e.g., involuntary hospitalization, tube feeding, close surveillance during meals, exercise restriction, removal of privileges with treatment noncompliance; Matusek & O'Dougherty Wright, 2010). If a dangerously underweight client does not want to eat, should she be required to do so? Who gets to choose the client's behavior and outcomes: the client (to whom the body belongs but who may have severe cognitive distortions) or significant others, such as parents or professionals (who may have a more accurate understanding of the client's health)? Although there are ethical questions about autonomy in the treatment of any severe psychopathology, these questions are particularly relevant for individuals with EDs, which may be ego-syntonic and result in more treatment resistance. Furthermore, they are especially complex when the client is a child or adolescent, who has less autonomy in general. Because their cognitive and physical capacities are still developing, significant adults make many decisions for youth and place restrictions on their behavior, particularly when they are younger. However, ED symptoms are sometimes conceptualized as an expression of a need for control or a pushing back against an overly controlling environment (Dalgleish et al., 2001; Froreich et al., 2017; Williams et al., 1990). There is particular concern, then, about forcing a client with an ED, who may already feel she has little control over her life, to eat or not to engage in other disordered behaviors. Are we taking away the only means of directing her life that the client currently feels she has? If so, how does this approach affect her overall well-being, and what does it imply about our understanding of autonomy and agency?

Although treatment planning needs to individualize treatment based on an understanding of the particular factors and dynamics of the adolescent and family, in general, the best approach aims to promote both objective health and safety and developmentally appropriate autonomy. If a youth with an ED is medically unstable or in physical danger as the result of her symptoms, it is unethical to fail to take drastic, adult-initiated, evidence-based action to treat her symptoms, which may include hospitalization and/or refeeding. However, clinicians cannot neglect issues of control and agency. Treatment procedures and their rationale should be clearly explained to youth, in recognition of their agency as well as the long-term goal of the development of adaptive exertion of control over their lives. In addition, when it is appropriate for youth to have control or choice in certain aspects of treatment, opportunities should be provided for their active partici-

pation and self-direction (e.g., choosing which of two high-calorie foods they would rather eat, choosing when in the day they would like to engage in their permitted one hour of exercise). The FBT approach emphasizes increasing autonomy and agency on the client's part as treatment progresses; at the beginning of therapy, parents closely direct and supervise the adolescent's eating, but closer to the end of treatment, the client is allowed more freedom and choice. Even as intensive, other-determined treatment may be crucial early on, the movement toward adolescent self-direction is developmentally important. EDs are unique because their symptoms revolve around topics and stimuli— food and the body—which must be faced and addressed by every person on every day of life. Significant loss, frightening situations, and traumatic events do not happen every day for youth with depression, anxiety disorders, or PTSD, but individuals with EDs face their relationship with food on a daily basis. Therefore, preparing these youth for long-term positive functioning involves not only reducing current symptoms but also helping them develop the skills to manage their ongoing, unavoidable relationships with food and their bodies, particularly as they enter adulthood and are increasingly independent in their lives and choices.

One inventive prevention program called REbeL was designed to empower adolescents to challenge the thin-body ideal and create an environment that supports positive body image (Breithaupt et al., 2017b). Specially trained teachers facilitate voluntary group meetings and student-led education presentations for peers and parents on the topics of body image, eating disorders, mindful eating, exercise, self-esteem, bullying and weight bias, and media literacy. The REbeL program has been found to reduce adolescents' body checking behaviors (understood to reflect problematic cognitions) and internalization of the thin-body ideal, and to increase feelings of empowerment (Breithaupt et al., 2017a, 2019). This program is an example of a creative way to facilitate agency in a developmentally appropriate, adolescent-led but adult-supervised manner. Youth are given an opportunity not only to learn about disordered eating and related topics but also to take the ownership and initiative involved in presenting the information to significant others. Clinicians and parents might apply these ideas in work with individual youth, encouraging them to research and think critically about issues such as media messages and weight bias and to explore ways that they can make positive changes in their communities.

In addition to addressing food- and body-related issues, respecting adolescents' agency in treatment should involve helping clients and families identify other appropriate ways for youth to exert control and independence in their lives. An important foundation for this work involves psychoeducation about adolescent development, which is included as an element of FBT. Clinicians, youth, and families might discuss the processes of identity development and increasing autonomy that occur normatively in adolescence as well as how these issues may be apparent in an adolescents' thoughts, emotions, behaviors, and family dynamics. Parents should understand how and why their adolescents might need more freedom but also support as they discover who they are as independent people who will soon leave their families of origin. Youth should be aware of how various manifestations of identity exploration or the desire for autonomy can be adaptive or maladaptive. As these issues are explored in therapy, specific areas in which adolescents can have more autonomy and agency can be recognized. For example, in a given family, perhaps parents are overly controlling of what youth wear, who they spend time with, or how they manage their schoolwork. When youth are given developmentally appropriate outlets for exerting choice and control over their own lives, the role of these influences on disordered eating may decrease, and youth may become better prepared to explore the world in healthy ways as they become adults.

CASE STUDY

Pertinent history. Elizabeth "Lizzy" LeClair is referred for outpatient therapy following a brief inpatient hospitalization for anorexia nervosa. She is fifteen years old and will be entering the tenth grade. Lizzy displays an abnormal approach to food and eating (restricts the types of food she ate, keeps track of a very low daily calorie count), and engages in excessive exercise to keep from gaining weight. At the time of her hospitalization, Lizzy was at a very low weight, was tired and not sleeping well, experienced intestinal problems and anemia, had withdrawn from friends and family, and had ended her ninth-grade year with poor grades due to her difficulty concentrating. Inpatient treatment was effective in increasing her body weight and iron level though it remains low for her age and height, and she still has some physical symptoms linked to an eating disorder (loss of period, thin hair, sensitivity to cold). She continues to express a fear of gaining weight and has a distorted view of her body.

In addition to the eating disorder, Lizzy is experiencing significant emotional distress, including anxiety and sadness. She is often sad and expresses low self-esteem, a sense of inadequacy, and feelings of being unloved and worthless (e.g., "I shouldn't have good things," "Why would anyone like me?"). She evaluates her abilities and her interpersonal relationships negatively. She also has frequent and abrupt mood swings with difficulty managing her anger; Mrs. LeClair wonders if Lizzy becomes irritable because she is hungry. She displays physical symptoms, including fatigue and sleep disturbance, tenseness, and indecisiveness. Further, Lizzy worries about her friendships, rejection and embarrassment in front of others, and something bad happening to her mother. Lizzy has maintained friendships with the same group of peers throughout middle school and high school, though she is described as "quiet and shy." Lizzy often spends time with her friends, but Mrs. LeClair notes there seems to be "lots of drama" among the girls. In the past, Lizzy has expressed a passive desire to die and end all her problems. She does not have current suicidal ideation and has not engaged in self-injurious behavior. While hospitalized, Lizzy was also diagnosed with other specified depressive disorder not meeting full criteria for a depressive episode with anxious distress. Her discharge note described Lizzy as temperamentally an emotionally sensitive adolescent who has not yet developed strategies to appropriately manage the feelings she experiences.

Lizzy's symptoms are related to her desire to exert a sense of control over her environment. During the intake session (see below), the therapist learns Lizzy has experienced familial discord and multiple changes in family structure. Lizzy lives with her biological parents and two older brothers (ages eighteen and sixteen) in a rural Midwest town. Her eldest brother is currently away at college. Mr. and Mrs. LeClair have separated twice over the past four years (Mr. LeClair moved out of the house for three to five months), but they are currently back together and in marital therapy. They describe "good periods" as well as "stressful periods" in the past in which they argued frequently. They acknowledge that even when they were not fighting, it felt stressful in the home because "you never knew how long it would last." Currently, they describe an improved marital relationship. Lizzy worries about getting in trouble with both her parents and explains her parents yell at her for the "silliest things" (e.g., not putting her bathroom towel away). The LeClairs are a prominent family in their small, rural town. Mr. LeClair is an ER physician, and Mrs. LeClair works part-time as a school librarian in the local school district. They both came from a poor background and are proud of their achievements. They feel strongly that their children should work hard and excel in their endeavors. The family does not affiliate with any religion and have never attended religious services. They know the clinical psychologist to whom they were referred is Christian and check that religious content would not be brought up in the therapy process.

Discharge paperwork from Lizzy's hospitalization included recommendations for her parents to validate her feelings while refraining from rigid or critical parenting of Lizzy and to promote her independence and emotion regulation, as she has few coping skills to manage her emotions. It was strongly recommended Lizzy and her family first participate in family therapy to address family beliefs, attitudes, values, and processes that underlie Lizzy's maladaptive eating behavior and body image. Family therapy also was recommended to improve their relationships with one another by helping them better understand each other's perspectives, learn more effective communication, identify effective emotion expression and regulation within the home, and encourage Lizzy's sense of control within the family system as she progresses through adolescence. She was referred to a clinical psychologist who partners with a pediatrician and behavioral health consultant in the treatment of eating disorders. Therapy appointments are coordinated with medical appointments so Lizzy's weight can be monitored and psychoeducation about a healthy lifestyle (nutrition, physical activity) can be provided to the family as follow-up care to services provided during her hospitalization.

Course of treatment.

Phase I. In the first session, the clinician meets with Lizzy, her parents, and her sixteen-year-old brother, Matt. The therapist has received discharge paperwork from Lizzy's inpatient hospitalization and met with staff from a pediatrics department who will also be working with Lizzy. This session as well as the following session is scheduled for ninety minutes to allow time for information gathering and activities. The therapist begins the session by describing the typical course of therapy, explaining that this first session is meant for the family and the therapist to get to know each other and that the role of the therapist is to serve as a consultant to the

family. In order to get to know the family, the therapist first asks them to engage in an interactive task, planning a dream vacation together. The therapist observes that Mr. and Mrs. LeClair often negate Lizzy's and her brother's suggestions, sometimes with open ridicule. Lizzy tends to withdraw and display flat affect immediately afterwards, whereas her brother justifies his suggestions and argues the superiority of his suggestions even if they are not chosen. The therapist pays attention to her own increasing frustration while watching this interaction and with the lack of agency given to Lizzy; however, she also recognizes the positive affect expressed among family members and their effective use of humor that seems to help them enjoy the interaction. These strengths can be used in therapy. The family indicates this is a typical interaction for them.

The therapist's goal for this initial session, in addition to building rapport, is to start to gather information about the family's history and the history of eating disorder symptoms, and help the family externalize the eating disorder. Thus, the therapist opens discussion about the eating disorder by asking each family member to identify what they see as the effects of "the eating disorder" and one thing they would change about the eating disorder and their family if they had a magic wand. Lizzy's brother Matt describes Lizzy as a "health freak," and expresses annoyance that he has to attend these sessions. His feelings are reflected, though the therapist also notes the effect of his words on Lizzy (her face turned red, she sank into the couch). When asked how she feels, Lizzy states "embarrassed." The therapist explains the importance of recognizing the eating disorder and its power in the family without blaming Lizzy; everyone is on the same LeClair team to fight against the eating disorder and help each other. Matt is encouraged to describe the family prior to the eating disorder and now. He appears defensive and simply states the family was "fine but then was stressful." He would like the family to not have to worry as much and for his sister to eat so his parents don't argue with her. The therapist again gently points out that therapy will address the unhealthy behaviors surrounding food with the goal of improved eating behaviors and decreased stress for everyone.

Lizzy describes her concern about dieting, body weight, and problematic eating behaviors (e.g., "I am absolutely terrified about being overweight," "I feel guilty when I eat, even when I feel hungry"). Lizzy is unable to describe things she likes about her appearance. Her parents jump in to state she is not fat and ask how she possibly could be overweight since she does exercises (jumping jacks, burpees, leg lifts, long runs) after every time she eats. The therapist again takes note that though her parents were trying to counter Lizzy's negative self-view, the focus of their comment was on her weight and what she does to control it. The therapist redirects the conversation to Lizzy's hopes for the family's future. Lizzy states she would like the family to argue less and for herself to not think about food so much. The therapist takes this opportunity to ask Lizzy and her parents to explain what they learned during Lizzy's inpatient hospitalization about how eating disorders can affect a person's thinking and perceptions. The therapist reflects that both Lizzy and her brother would like the arguing to decrease in the family. Mr. and Mrs. LeClair are asked

what their goals for therapy are, and they agree that more positive interactions would be a "good start," and that they also want their daughter to be healthy.

Regarding the course of the eating disorder, the LeClair family agree that Lizzy started focusing on her appearance in eighth grade and had difficulty leaving the house some mornings because she would "be fretting" over how she looked. Lizzy reports that at first she tried to eat healthy so she would not gain weight, but she later started researching calories and nutritional values and keeping a food log. She challenged herself to decrease her caloric intake each week and started weighing herself twice a day to ensure she had not gained weight. When she got into ninth grade, Lizzy joined cross-country with some close friends. They would discuss the calories they burned each day and compare their body size (e.g., their "thigh gap," sides of their stomachs). She started getting positive comments from boys when she walked by, and her peers told her she was lucky to be so thin. As with most runners, her running also improved with her weight loss. After the season ended, Lizzy was not engaged in an extracurricular activity.

Her parents report noticing her engagement in various exercise routines throughout the day even when watching television (squats, leg lifts) and her increasing withdrawal from friends over the winter and spring. Lizzy begins to cry when describing the loneliness she felt and identifies her "obsessive" fear of numbers going up on the bathroom scale and her guilt for eating food as the main factors leading to continued weight loss. Her parents state they thought Lizzy was being healthy and that she looked healthy. They noticed a problem when they could not go out to eat together as a family without food selection being such a big deal and when their friends asked them if Lizzy had dropped too much weight. The therapist observes that Matt listens intently to his family talk about the course of the eating disorder. She asks for his thoughts and he states that he has not heard this before and did not realize everything that Lizzy went through. The therapist provides psychoeducation about the development of eating disorders and how insidious it can be. The therapist then concludes the session with a review of the collaboration with pediatrics staff and sharing of information about Lizzy's weekly weight check. The family has already removed the bathroom scale based on recommendations from her inpatient therapist. The therapist schedules the next session and explains it will be a family meal in order to help them counter the eating disorder during the important task of eating together.

The second session is conducted at the family's house during their dinnertime in order for the therapist to see mealtime in a naturalistic setting. Mr. and Mrs. LeClair have met with the behavioral health consultant and a nutritionist at the pediatrics office to identify meal options that will help Lizzy gain weight and include foods Lizzy likes. Of note, though parents are typically encouraged to use their own knowledge of healthy eating, this external support is important for the LeClairs because they do not have healthy eating habits themselves. The therapist explains she will be helping Mr. and Mrs. LeClair verbally encourage Lizzy to eat more than she wants to so she can restore her weight. The role of Lizzy's parents to plan, make, and supervise all Lizzy's meals is emphasized, as is the need

for Mr. and Mrs. LeClair to provide support and empathy for Lizzy. In order to continue externalizing the eating disorder, the therapist reminds the family that the eating disorder interferes with Lizzy's ability to make good decisions about eating and her activity level, thus requiring the direct intervention and support of her family. The therapist emphasizes to Lizzy that once they have defeated the eating disorder's power, she will regain control over these decisions.

As the meal begins, the therapist observes that Mr. and Mrs. LeClair quickly become frustrated and use a harsher tone with Lizzy. Matt is observed to withdraw during this time. The therapist first reinforces Matt's lack of criticism or complaint, and encourages him to offer praise to his sister when he notices her overcoming the eating disorder in her engagement in the family meal or with a bite of food. The therapist then asks what he would like to talk about, and as the meal progresses, Matt begins telling funny stories about his day. This brings levity to the family, and the atmosphere becomes more upbeat. The therapist then turns attention to encouragement of Mr. and Mrs. LeClair in their role of directly intervening to encourage Lizzy's eating. Her parents' cajoling her to eat and providing rationales for how the food would make her healthier seemed to result in Lizzy's annoyance and pushing of food around her plate. The difficult balance between being supportive and noncritical during meals and snacks even as they challenge Lizzy to increase consumption beyond her comfort level is normalized. Mr. and Mrs. LeClair are coached to use direct prompts in a warm, encouraging tone (e.g., "You need to eat three bites of the pasta," "Put some butter on the corn on the cob now"). During the meal, Lizzy frequently makes negative comments about the food, and her parents and brother are encouraged to ignore these comments. Lizzy's distress after eating is visible, and with the therapist's support, she is able to identify her discomfort with eating. The family engages in problem solving about how to provide a distraction after meals so the eating disorder does not "discount" or undermine Lizzy's progress. They report that they all typically "go do their own thing" after dinner. In order to help Lizzy's anxiety decrease after mealtime, they decide to engage in family board game nights and choose television shows to watch together for the first hour after eating dinner. This also serves to increase their positive interactions as a family.

Given that the family expressed their desire to exclude spiritual or religious content from therapy, the therapist carefully considers her own process of implicit integration throughout therapy. Her self-reflection challenges her to view and interact with the family in helpful ways that are consistent with her theological views of children and effective child treatment. The therapist loves working with youth because she is able to affect their developing brain, regulation, and values. She also enjoys working with families as they support their child's development. However, she personally finds it more difficult to work with some families, and thus has learned she must approach therapy with these families in a reflective manner. When engaged in family therapy, the therapist facilitates sessions with the goal of treating each member with the kindness, respect, and dignity they deserve as being made in the image of God. Each person in the LeClair family has dignity and worth

and a special place in his creation. She also sees her role in sessions as helping the family's relationships reflect characteristics of compassion and submission. Within the first couple of sessions, the therapist recognizes her unhelpful ways of thinking about Lizzy's parents. She challenges herself to think about the steps the family is taking to overcome their susceptibility to engage Lizzy in harmful ways and their love for her that can overcome the many risk factors the therapist can identify in this family system. She prays prior to each session to be filled with empathy for all the difficult things each family member is dealing with, and with patience to meet the family where they are at.

Typically, when the therapist engages in this treatment with Christian families, she introduces therapy from the foundational belief that God will be walking alongside them in recovery from the eating disorder; he will help them even with the struggle and pain that is part of the recovery process. This foundational principle opens up discussion about the difficult aspects of recovery and builds natural, genuine bonds between individuals involved in therapy. The therapist also typically addresses aspects of the client's mind, body, and spirit; with the LeClair family, she explicitly acknowledges the important connection between the body and the mind due to the physiological effects of the eating disorder. She also seeks to instill hope in the family for healing from their pain and suffering, though her own hope for the family is provided in Christ. The therapist witnesses God's kindness and redemption in the treatment of the family by other professionals on the team, and the acknowledgment that God is constantly at work maintains her own hope and awareness that God wants Lizzy and this family to flourish and have abundant lives.

Following the meal observation, the next five sessions have the goal of restoring Lizzy's weight and healthy eating patterns and preventing her past patterns of excessive exercise. Lizzy and her parents first go to the pediatrician's office for a weight check. The focus for Mr. and Mrs. LeClair is to gain control of Lizzy's eating behavior and reduce her eating disorder symptoms. Thus, Mr. and Mrs. LeClair must monitor Lizzy's meals, to ensure she is eating a healthy amount of nutritional foods, and also monitor her activity level. Because it is summer, the family is able to change their schedules so someone is with Lizzy for meals and snacks throughout the day. They have planned high caloric snacks that Lizzy likes throughout the day, though they need the therapist's coaching to determine the most effective way to ensure Lizzy's compliance and promote her weight gain. Mr. and Mrs. LeClair also determine a reasonable exercise routine for Lizzy in consultation with pediatric staff, as they are prone to permit more exercise than would promote appropriate weight gain for Lizzy at this point in her treatment.

Matt continues to attend these sessions, though he is often quiet. The therapist explores his relationship with Lizzy, and learns they used to be close and do many activities together until Matt went to high school. Lizzy feels that Matt began to make fun of her around his friends when he entered ninth grade and she was in eighth, including comments about her appearance. They are asked to share memories about what they used to do together and what their relationship was like. Matt explains it has been hard for him to watch his sister's health decline, hear negative

comments about her at school, and be worried about her. The therapist emphasizes that Matt can still be comforting and supportive, and refrain from criticism, as they battle this eating disorder together. Mr. and Mrs. LeClair also express negative views of the eating disorder and describe how it has affected the family, which is an encouraging display of their externalization of the disorder. The family together discusses how the eating disorder has contributed to stress within the family through conflict (e.g., fighting about food, about withdrawal from the family) and their worries about Lizzy's well-being.

The therapist also addresses each family member's approach toward body weight and health to help them monitor the messages Lizzy is exposed to. Mrs. LeClair reports not talking about food or body image in front of Lizzy and focusing on giving compliments to Lizzy about her appearance when Lizzy makes negative comments. Yet, Lizzy and her brother point out that Mrs. LeClair frequently makes comments about her own "heavy" size and is on a constant diet or new eating regimen (e.g., protein-only or gluten-free or Mediterranean diet). She also worries about the physical health of all family members. Prior to Lizzy's hospitalization, Mr. LeClair mainly drank protein shakes for sustenance during the day until dinner. He expresses that he has learned a lot about nutrition and recognizes he was not modeling healthy eating patterns. However, he continues to work out for several hours a day.

In working with clients with eating disorders, the therapist has considered theological implications of her work. She appreciates that the body is important because it is made by God but seeks to help families recognize the "goodness" of the body that is not based on body size or fitness; rather, it can be related to the body's capabilities, health, and engagement in activities they love. The therapist helps the family make a list of the strengths of their own bodies as well as other important individual characteristics, such as creativity, intelligence, responsibility, work ethic, and compassion. In general, Lizzy experiences self-loathing and feels love and acceptance is conditional (that what is accepted in her family is "thin" and "excellence"). When working with Christian clients, the therapist is able to explore the knowledge that God created the client and loves her. The therapist knows God delights in Lizzy as well as the family in general (Zephaniah 3:17) and that God offers them a place of honor. The therapist understands she cannot talk explicitly about God's love but she can help Lizzy *experience* unconditional love through the nonspecific factors of therapy and through facilitation of healthy family relationships without it being explicitly spiritual.

Through discussions in session, the therapist helps the family recognize that Lizzy has heightened sensitivity to criticism or negative comments about her appearance as well as any focus in the environment on eating and appearance in general. In a nonjudgmental manner, the therapist encourages the family to evaluate their own self- and other-directed comments around eating, appearance, and weight first; however, the family also begins to recognize other comments that indicate a general tendency toward "good-bad" and judgmental thinking in their home. As an exercise for each session, Mr. and Mrs. LeClair and Matt identify positive characteristics Lizzy possesses. Their competitiveness is channeled into a contest to see how many

judging comments each other makes that they can catch and reframe during the week.

The therapist feels an underlying annoyance at Mr. and Mrs. LeClair being controlling about odd things during therapy and with Lizzy's significant anxiety and resultant avoidant behaviors. The therapist also experiences frustration because the LeClairs do not start from the premise that Lizzy has inherent worth; within their family system, she earns her worth through achievement. The therapist seeks consultation with a colleague because she knows her role is to provide support for this family and that it is not helpful when blame is placed on parents or Lizzy's choices are judged. Her colleague gently reminds her of the power of empathy to encourage the parents to help Lizzy expose herself to eating and coach her through disordered behaviors. In discussion with her colleague, the therapist also articulates how treatment is a tremendous challenge for this family (and any family), but the LeClairs are committed and showing up, which is amazing. The therapist recognizes that their commitment to therapy leads to greater effectiveness of the treatment. She also bears in mind that Mr. and Mrs. LeClair do see Lizzy and her brother as gifts: there is much love within the family that can help overcome the criticism and "conditional" nature of their love. She recommits herself to helping the parents to be direct agents of love, grace, instruction, and discipline (consistent with Scripture). She mindfully observes and experiences joy in the family during sessions, including their use of humor, kind words spoken to each other, and recognition that the parents' high standards are born out of love for their children.

The focus within this family has been on physical and social aspects of functioning, with high standards placed on both. The therapist ultimately seeks to bring all aspects of functioning together for Lizzy's well-being and healthy development over the course of treatment, consistent with her theological understanding of personhood. The therapist first recognizes her own strong desire for change in this family and focuses on facilitating patience in therapy with treatment goals for Lizzy's biological and behavioral functioning. The therapist is careful to acknowledge Lizzy's agency in this first phase of treatment. By explaining the treatment program and the purpose of treatment objectives to combat ED symptoms, the therapist builds Lizzy's trust and openness to therapy so Lizzy can accept and "sign onto" even Phase I of treatment, in which her parents exert more control than she feels comfortable with. She finds ways to help Lizzy have a voice in this part of the treatment, even if not around eating behavior.

Through active listening, the therapist helps Mr. and Mrs. LeClair and Matt listen to Lizzy's experiences, thoughts, and feelings so she feels genuinely heard and active in writing her own life. Thus, during this phase of treatment, Lizzy's expression of her emotions is encouraged. She describes feeling out of control around food ("like it is driving me and clouding my head"), though this experience has decreased following inpatient treatment and increased exposure to more food items. Lizzy explains that she tries to fight her preoccupation to be thinner through distraction and by challenging her own thoughts. Her parents and Matt describe Lizzy's apparent anxiety at meal times, and Lizzy agrees that she feels heightened anxiety just before eating and immediately after meals. The therapist emphasizes the need for behavioral change as

crucial to treatment (exposure to anxiety-provoking situations will decrease anxiety over time) as well as the benefits of healthy eating behaviors. By having Lizzy monitor and report on her anxiety levels after every meal, she recognizes that with each exposure she feels slightly more comfortable. For example, the eating disorder pushed a discomfort with eating foods that were on her "bad food" list or having a full stomach, which now has less control over her. Lizzy and her parents report less conflict at meals, and Lizzy willingly follows her parents' lead regarding her eating. Mr. and Mrs. LeClair report feeling more confident in their ability to help Lizzy.

Phase II. After the first seven sessions of treatment, the therapist schedules sessions every other week over the next ten weeks. Goals for therapy turn to handing responsibility of healthy behavior from Mr. and Mrs. LeClair over to Lizzy, and the therapist continues to function as a coach for the family. Lizzy continues to track her weight at the pediatrician's office. With the start of a new school year, the family brings many topics and situations to therapy for discussion. Lizzy prepares the menu for several of the family's dinners using nutritional information she has gained about healthy eating and incorporating a wider range of foods she is willing to eat. As she had always liked cooking, this responsibility increases her confidence and sense of empowerment. However, Lizzy expresses her frustration that her family made a few negative comments about the meals. Her parents are coached to explore her perceptions without defensiveness. They then explain to Lizzy that their comments were not meant to be critical, and though it is clearly difficult for them, they acknowledge how she could have interpreted their comments this way. As her brother does not attend the first two sessions of this phase, the therapist enforces the need for Matt to attend in order to continue to involve all members of the family system in the treatment. At the third session, Matt begins coming again, and Lizzy is coached in assertive communication to express herself to her brother. Mr. and Mrs. LeClair and the therapist encourage his continued support of Lizzy fighting the eating disorder.

Over the course of these sessions, Mr. and Mrs. LeClair first provide decreasing direction to Lizzy about the number of snacks she eats at home independently. Lizzy plans to eat lunch at school by herself, about which her mother particularly expresses fear. Her feelings are explored and evaluated in the context of appropriately giving control to Lizzy over aspects of her life, including her eating. In recognition of Lizzy's history of feeling that things generally happen to her (rather than being able to control her environment), the family is encouraged to express confidence in Lizzy's ability to make responsible decisions. They permit her to spend an increasing amount of time with friends outside of the home, and eventually she is permitted to eat out with her friends. The therapist coaches the family in collaborative problem solving around other decisions that arise, such as attending birthday parties and spending the night at a friend's house, in order to continue to shift more control to Lizzy.

This phase of treatment with the LeClairs naturally leads to work on developmental tasks that were affected by the eating disorder, which is an aspect of this treatment approach. As Lizzy reenters school, her low self-esteem becomes apparent in the context of her peer relationships. She often feels left out and "not as good" as her friends. Looking at social media accounts and her friends' "stories" leads to negative thoughts about her body and her relationships. Matt confesses he sometimes feels the same way, and Mrs. LeClair acknowledges her own "obsession" with her social media accounts. The family decides together to help each other limit their time spent on social media and to have daily check-ins about the negative feelings they may experience to facilitate monitoring and discussion.

Lizzy wants to return to cross-country but seems hesitant to do so. After supportive reflection by her parents facilitated by the therapist, Lizzy describes the pressure she feels to perform as well as she did the previous year. Her parents' statements about this extracurricular (e.g., "If you don't try hard, then how will you get better?" "You can cut at least a minute off of last year's times") are evaluated in terms of how they may impact Lizzy. She also expresses the belief that her parents should not love her because of her inherent flaws. The therapist and Lizzy identify the ways Mr. and Mrs. LeClair could communicate support and how Lizzy could communicate when she feels pressure or a lack of acceptance from her parents. The lies the eating disorder will try to tell her (e.g., that she can feel better if she just lost weight, that others like her more when she is thin) are identified. The therapist helps Lizzy and her parents identify healthy coping strategies for when she feels lonely or overwhelmed and "catch" the negative thoughts and strong emotions.

The therapist is concerned that part of Lizzy's desire to rejoin the cross-country team may be for the wrong reasons (e.g., the attention on body and performance). However, Lizzy also needs to be given agency in her own life. The therapist endeavors to guide the family to focus on what is important to them outside of body image and accomplishments. Given their pre-occupation with status in general, the therapist reflects on how she can talk with them about "where their treasure is" without a spiritual focus and decides on a values-based discussion linked to actions they then can take within their family. The therapist asks questions about what values are leading to the decision to rejoin cross-country and listens for values focused on body image and performance. As she listens to the family's discussion, the therapist reflects internally that idolatry of perfection, excellence, and striving is prominent in the family. She recognizes the negative impact of pride, control, and a desire for human acceptance within the family, which guides her scaffolding of family discussions toward mindfulness of the motivations behind their decisions.

Phase III. Over the course of these sessions, Lizzy has reached a healthy weight for her height and build and is no longer engaging in disordered eating behavior (e.g., restriction of her eating, counting calories, excessive exercise). She also has successfully taken back control of her eating behavior from her parents. She no longer needs to be seen by pediatrics staff prior to sessions. Thus, the therapist moves into the third phase of treatment. Lizzy, her parents, and the therapist decide together to meet monthly over the next four months with a focus on strengthening the parent-adolescent relationship, problem solving around developmental challenges that arise in Lizzy's life, and providing continued monitoring of Lizzy's progress in healthy eating behavior. For example, Lizzy and her parents notice some of

the rules she still has about eating (eating in a certain order, avoiding categories of foods that are "bad") for which they then set goals for exposure and anxiety management. The therapist also continues to provide psychoeducation about adolescent development as well as recovery from anorexia in order to normalize the family's experiences.

Therapy sessions mainly focus on continued facilitation of effective communication, adaptive emotion expression and regulation within the home, and encouragement of Lizzy's sense of control within the family system to help them navigate adolescence. For example, regarding interpersonal relations, Lizzy reports ongoing feelings of stress and tension in her personal relationships, a feeling of being excluded from social activities, and a negative perception of her social relationships and friendships with peers (e.g., "I get left out of things"; "I always feel lonely"). Lizzy's attitude toward school and teachers is generally positive, but she feels immense pressure to perform well and "get perfect grades." She also reports problems in her relationship with her parents, such as feeling not esteemed by them (e.g., "My parents are hard to please"). Lizzy feels confused about her parents' relationship and the negative interactions she observes between them despite her parents' affirmation that they are not separating. The therapist helps Mr. and Mrs. LeClair explain in an appropriate manner to Lizzy their engagement in marital therapy and their desire to strengthen their relationship. They are encouraged to remain open to questions from Lizzy when she experiences confusion and worry about her parents' marriage, which will in turn help her to have a greater sense of control in her life rather than resorting to seeking control through eating behaviors. Family discussions lead to their decision to engage in more family activities together and to create more opportunities for conversations. Lizzy appreciates her parents' reflective listening about her peer relationships and their sharing of different perspectives about friendships. The therapist helps Lizzy identify peers who help her feel good about herself and who focus on things outside of appearance and performance with whom she could develop stronger friendships.

The eating disorder has not only made Lizzy feel lonely over the last year but also led to difficulty focusing on the activities she really wanted to put energy into. For example, Lizzy would like to join the photography club at her school. This activity initially is discounted by Lizzy's parents, as it does not contribute much to strengthening her application for college. Rather than withdrawing and experiencing both resentment and a lack of control, Lizzy is helped to explain what she likes about the activity and how she benefits from it. Her parents are assisted in actively listening to Lizzy, challenging their own assumptions, and identifying their values while letting Lizzy develop her own values and appropriately make her own choices.

As the therapist seeks to help the family communicate and navigate normal issues of adolescent development in healthy ways, she challenges them to develop a broader and less dualistic perspective. In the case of peer relationships, it is important for the therapist to facilitate discussion and "call out" the family's tendency to blame Lizzy's peer group for excluding her and making her feel lonely, as this forecloses discussion and fits into the family's tendency toward judgment and a good-bad mentality. Other individuals in Lizzy's life are complex, and it is important for everyone in the family to practice nonjudgment and openness while also making choices for Lizzy's health. These discussions can serve as a foundation for spiritual growth even if not explicitly spiritual or religious in nature. Regarding normative adolescent issues, such as selection of photography as an extracurricular (an aspect of identity development), the therapist seeks to help Lizzy select adaptive paths for herself (agency) in communication with her parents in order to increase her sense of control and to limit Mr. and Mrs. LeClair's overinvolvement and promote their acceptance of Lizzy no matter what she chooses. These seemingly minor decisions can help Lizzy develop a sense of purpose, identity, and meaning that is missing from her life.

The therapist appreciates her privilege of connecting with this family and journeying through life with them in both joy and pain. She rests in her hope that the family experienced her as trustworthy, consistent, and loving, which can make an imprint on their spiritual development. In the final session, during which the family's progress is celebrated, the therapist also reviews specific skills she observed the family learning and using with the goal of relapse prevention. The family identifies the healthy coping skills they have found most helpful and how they can apply them to possible future difficulties. The family reviews how to engage in collaborative problem solving when disagreements arise between Lizzy and her parents regarding rules and expectations. The strategies Lizzy used to disagree with the eating disorder are reinforced so she can continue to have agency in her ongoing recovery.

Additional considerations from a developmental psychopathology framework. At first, Mr. and Mrs. LeClair are overwhelmed by the intensity of treatment and the requirements on them to provide monitoring of Lizzy's eating and well-being. They abruptly decide to pull out of commitments they had made (i.e., serving on the board of a community organization, attending book club) and to stop their own therapy. The therapist encourages Lizzy's parents to continue their participation in marital therapy. They are helped to identify sources of support for themselves outside of the family. During the second phase of treatment, Mrs. LeClair also begins individual therapy for herself, attributing the self-awareness she began to have through family discussions and observing Lizzy's progress in therapy. This is a difficult decision for Mrs. LeClair as it involves recognition of her own weaknesses, and the therapist praises the strength Mrs. LeClair displays in beginning the hard work of therapy herself and reinforces her willingness to change.

With recognition that the family is achievement oriented and motivated to become experts, they are encouraged to develop their understanding of eating disorders. The therapist recommends relevant and appropriate websites for additional information, such as feast-ed.org, eatingwithyouranorexic.com, and the website for the Academy for Eating Disorders. By directing the family to resources they can access on their own, the therapist encourages the family's sense agency as well as their ability to address future questions and challenges that arise without necessarily needing to return to family therapy.

At the conclusion of therapy, Lizzy is referred for individual therapy to continue to address her tendency toward negative perceptions of relationships (e.g., loneliness and disconnection), and symptoms of depression and anxiety. She is also encouraged to continue to openly discuss the eating disorder and ways to fight it throughout the rest of high school. The LeClairs should continue to monitor her weight and healthy eating behaviors in consultation with the pediatrics team. It is recommended that Lizzy's parents engage in parent consultation sessions to help identify effective parenting strategies to create a consistent, supportive home environment (e.g., clear house rules and expectations, coordinated parenting, provision of positive messages).

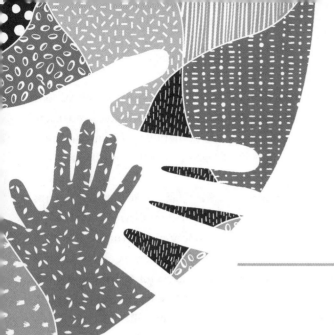

Chapter Ten

Going Beyond
the Literature:
Gender Dysphoria

I N THE PREVIOUS CHAPTERS of this book, we have introduced you to the field of developmental psychopathology and its implications for treatment, discussed the concept of evidence-based practice in psychology, explored Christian biblical and theological ideas that can shape the integrative treatment of psychopathology in youth, and applied these ideas to seven types of disorders commonly seen in youth. For each of the disorders we have discussed in detail so far, high-quality research has at least begun to identify effective psychological treatments, and for the most part, significant research exists on the risk factors and developmental processes that occur within each disorder. Furthermore, theological writing about some of these disorders can be found in other sources (though it is sometimes more focused on adults than youth), and we imagine that our integrative thinking is not particularly controversial for most Christians. Therefore, from an empirically based and theologically informed per-

spective that complements your professional training, we hope you are well-prepared to work with youth who experience disorders such as depression, anxiety, disruptive behavior disorders, and ADHD. However, we recognize that youth experience many other disorders as well, including disorders with a weaker treatment research base and more theological complexity. One such disorder is gender dysphoria (GD), which involves experiencing a sense of gender identity that is different from one's natal gender, the gender assigned at birth due to one's biological characteristics. We chose GD because it has received a significant amount of attention lately from both secular and Christian psychological communities, and although the research base is growing quickly, GD is still not well understood in youth, and little research exists on psychosocial treatments. In this chapter, after a brief literature review, we will use GD as a case example for how one might approach a topic within child clinical psychology that (1) does not have clear research support for effective psychological treatment and/or (2) is theologically complex or controversial.

GENDER DYSPHORIA

GD (formerly "gender identity disorder") is characterized by "a marked incongruence between one's experienced/expressed gender and assigned gender" (American Psychiatric Association, 2013, p. 452). The DSM-5 contains two sets of GD criteria, one for children and one for adolescents and adults, accounting for the developmental changes in how gender identity is likely to be expressed across the lifespan. Children must display at least six of the following symptoms, including the first symptom listed, in order to be diagnosed with GD: (1) strong desire to be the other gender (or consistently asserting that one actually is the other gender), (2) strong preference for other-gender clothing, (3) strong preference for other-gender roles in play, (4) strong preference for stereotypically other-gender toys/games/activities, (5) strong preference for playing with peers of the other gender, (6) strong rejection of toys/games/activities stereotypically preferred by children of one's assigned gender, (7) a strong dislike of own sexual organs, and (8) a strong desire to possess other-gender sex characteristics. The adolescent/adult criteria, of which one must exhibit only two symptoms for diagnosis, include: (1) strong incongruence between one's expressed/experienced gender and one's sex characteristics, (2) strong desire to be rid of one's sex characteristics because of this incongruence, (3) strong desire to possess other-gender sex characteristics, (4) strong desire to be the other gender/an alternative gender, (5)

strong desire to have others see and treat one as the other gender/an alternative gender, and (6) strong sense that one's feelings and reactions are those of the other gender/an alternative gender. For individuals of any age, symptoms must last for at least six months and cause significant distress and/or impairment in functioning (American Psychiatric Association, 2013). Sexual attraction is not part of the criteria for GD, as gender dysphoric youth may experience same-sex, opposite-sex, or bisexual attraction or orientation (Drummond et al., 2008; Steensma, McGuire, et al., 2013).

Youth with GD are at heightened risk for other psychological problems, including both internalizing and externalizing disorders (Cohen-Kettenis & van Goozen, 2002; Chen, Hidalgo, & Garofalo, 2017). Suicidal ideation and behavior also occur frequently in these youth and increase with age (Aitken et al., 2016; Fox et al., 2020). However, as with any disorder, there is significant individual variation. Some gender dysphoric youth do not have emotional or behavioral problems (de Vries, Doreleijers, et al., 2011), and in those who do, they often appear to be related to interpersonal stressors, such as family conflict, poor relationships with peers, or being bullied (Cohen-Kettenis & van Goozen, 2002; de Vries, Steensma, et al., 2016; Shiffman et al., 2016). Social support appears to have a particularly significant impact on mental health outcomes in youth with GD (Parr & Howe, 2019; Puckett et al., 2019). However, it has also been argued that the experience of incongruence between one's gender identity and one's assigned gender is in and of itself distressing, regardless of social support, which may also contribute to psychological comorbidity (Zucker et al., 2014). Finally, it is not uncommon for gender dysphoric youth to have symptoms of an autism spectrum disorder (de Vries et al., 2010; Nabbijohn et al., 2018; Skagerberg et al., 2015), which preliminary work suggests may be due to abnormal brain growth in utero that has been linked to both conditions (VanderLaan et al., 2015).

It is estimated that between .17% and 1.3% of youth experience gender dysphoria (Connolly et al., 2016). Research on the course of GD suggests that many youth who experience gender dysphoria in childhood—likely well over 50%—are considered "desisters," no longer reporting symptoms as they age, with a smaller number of "persisters" continuing to experience symptoms into adolescence (Drummond et al., 2008; Steensma et al., 2010 Steensma, McGuire, et al., 2013; Wallien & Cohen-Kettenis, 2008). Children with more intense symptoms, such as body dissatisfaction or stereotypically other-sex behavior, and natal females are more likely to experience persistent GD, whereas there are no links between GD persistence and social factors or psychological problems. Some children whose symptoms desist may not have been truly gender dysphoric (disliking or feeling disconnected to their natal gender) but rather found the idea of being the other gender appealing until they became more comfortable with their own bodies over time (Steensma et al., 2010). In contrast, more intense early symptoms may be signs of more persistent discomfort with one's assigned gender. However, due to societal expectations that individuals should behave in ways that are perceived to be consistent with their assigned genders, and the resulting pressure on gender-nonconforming individuals, it may be

difficult to accurately assess the rate of true GD desistence (Steensma & Cohen-Kettenis, 2015). In addition, there is heated debate in the professional literature about how to best assess desistence and persistence and how clinicians should consider the implications of varying patterns of continuity as they develop individual treatment plans (Steensma & Cohen-Kettenis, 2018; Temple Newhook et al., 2018; Winters et al., 2018; Zucker, 2018).

Though causes are still not well understood, GD is thought to result from the interaction of biological and environmental factors (de Vries, Kreukels, et al., 2014; Steensma, Kreukels, et al., 2013). Biological risk factors include genetic predisposition, abnormal prenatal sex hormone exposure, and structural and/or functional differences in certain brain regions (Bakker, 2014; Hoekzema et al., 2015; Klink & Den Heijer, 2014). Although nonbiological factors also play a role in the development of GD (Sasaki et al., 2016), there is more limited support for specific environmental factors, including family dynamics (such as limit setting around cross-gender behavior; Cohen-Kettenis & Arrindell, 1990; Zucker & Bradley, 1995) and gender assignment (in the case of individuals with disorders of sex development whose natal gender is not clearly male or female; Callens et al., 2016). These factors likely interact dynamically with one another as well as other aspects of development to predict risk toward GD. For example, it has been suggested that gender-related behaviors may shape the developing brain over time, and biologically influenced aspects of gender identity may elicit certain responses from the environment (de Vries, Kreukels, et al., 2014; Steensma, Kreukels, et al., 2013). In addition, the relative strength of different types of risk factors for GD varies by gender; environmental factors appear to influence cross-gender behavior and identity more in males than in females, whereas genetic factors are stronger in females than in males (Knafoet al., 2005; Sasaki et al., 2016; van Beijsterveldt et al., 2006).

Research on the treatment of GD in youth is still in its infancy compared to empirical support for treatments of many other childhood disorders (Spivey & Edwards-Leeper, 2019). There are three main views on how to best treat GD in children (American Psychological Association, 2015; Drescher, 2014). Given the percentage of children whose cross-gender identification desists, one view encourages clinicians to help children conform to their assigned gender. Clinicians may embrace this view because they believe that it is more beneficial for a child to change her gender identity to match her assigned gender, either for moral/religious reasons or because of the challenges associated with undergoing medical procedures to change her assigned gender as well as living in a society in which she will likely face prejudice and discrimination. The second view, sometimes called "watchful waiting" (Yarhouse, 2015) or "delayed transition" (Human Rights Campaign, 2016), is a sort of middle ground approach in which the child's symptoms and gender identity persistence are monitored, but little action is taken toward increasing conformity between assigned and expressed gender; rather, the child is permitted to express his or her gender identity in any way without either discouragement or affirmation. Perspectives on this view range from the belief that it is the most responsible course of action for youth with GD, which may desist over time (Royal College of Psychiatrists, 2018), to the view that it is effectively a method of withholding treatment from a child whose distress is likely to continue without intervention (HRC, 2016; Telfer et al., 2020). The third view encourages clinicians to help children and families embrace a nonconforming youth's sense of gender identity and, as is developmentally appropriate, to support the child in transitioning to life as a different gender. With children, such affirming approaches are generally psychosocial in nature, including education and support, though they may include nonmedical interventions to help the child live as their experienced gender (e.g., dressing and grooming as that gender). There has historically been disagreement in the psychological community as to whether encouraging children to change their gender identity is beneficial or harmful. However, the emphasis in the literature has more recently shifted toward an emphasis on affirming interventions as most beneficial (Chen et al., 2018; Spivey & Edwards-Leeper, 2019), with some critiques of even the watchful waiting approach as harmful due to its lack of action or affirmation (HRC, 2016).

For adolescents, as well as adults, changing natal gender to match gender identity is commonly accepted as the standard of treatment (American Psychological Association, 2015; World Professional Association for Transgender Health, 2012). The psychosocial interventions that are often considered most appropriate with gender dysphoric adolescents include long-term treatment to address distress, body image, and self-esteem issues; social difficulties; and comorbid symptoms as well as support for families and youth during the process of medical treatment

(Cousino et al., 2014; de Vries & Cohen-Kettenis, 2012, 2016; Vanderburgh, 2009; WPATH, 2012). In addition, mental health professionals play an important role in the process of assessing youths' GD symptoms, comorbid conditions, and individual and family readiness for medical interventions such as hormone therapy or surgery.

There are three categories of medical interventions to change the physical aspects of one's gender (Hembree, 2011; Hembree et al., 2009). Fully reversible interventions involve the use of hormones and steroids to suppress (delay) puberty or to promote the development of physical characteristics that are consistent with gender identity; the latter is sometimes referred to as gender-affirming cross-sex hormone (CSH) therapy (Mahfouda et al., 2019). Limited research suggests that adolescents' psychological responses to puberty suppression are generally positive (de Vries, Steensma, et al., 2011) and that the use of CSH can lead to improved quality of life and mental health outcomes (Mahfouda et al., 2019; Salas-Humara et al., 2019). Partially reversible interventions include the use of hormones to create other physical changes, such as the growth of larger breasts or the deepening of the voice. Surgery to change primary or secondary sex characteristics and other aspects of facial and body structure is an irreversible intervention. Detailed recommendations exist for assessing the appropriateness of each of these interventions, which generally occur in a stepwise fashion in the order listed above, with the age of the youth also being considered (WPATH, 2012). Sex reassignment surgery is not generally recommended during adolescence but may follow reversible interventions when youth become

adults (Hembree, 2011). Research has found variability in adolescents' well-being following surgery (de Vries, McGuire, et al., 2014; Smith, Van Goozen, & Cohen-Kettenis, 2001; Smith et al., 2005). Given the potential for harm following either a lack of treatment or irreversible treatment, the ethics of medical interventions for youth with GD are complex, including issues such as informed consent, stability and change in gender identity over time, and effects of treatment on future fertility and other aspects of brain and body development (Giordano, 2014; Holman & Goldberg, 2006).

Furthermore, there are some unique ethical and legal complexities to consider in the treatment of individuals with GD. The choice between different approaches to treatment —affirming versus change-oriented—has increasingly become seen in the professional realm as having a universally right and wrong direction rather than being based on clinician and client values and preferences. For example, a number of professional organizations have taken official stances that endorse only affirming treatments and oppose gender identity change efforts or even the endorsement of a binary view of gender (American Psychological Association, Task Force on Appropriate Therapeutic Responses to Sexual Orientation, 2009; National Association of Social Workers, 2015; WPATH, 2012). Furthermore, a number of nations and states have enacted laws banning the use of therapeutic efforts to change the gender identity (as well as the sexual orientation) of individuals under eighteen (Fitzsimons, 2020). Some clinicians who have concerns about utilizing an affirming approach with a particular client, for whatever reason, may find themselves in an ethical bind. The latest version of the American Counseling Association's code of ethics (2014) explicitly prohibits counselors from "referring prospective and current clients based solely on the counselor's personally held values, attitudes, beliefs . . . especially when the counselor's values are inconsistent with the client's goals or are discriminatory in nature" (p. 8), creating a situation in which clinicians may be legally barred from engaging in gender identity change efforts and ethically prohibited from referring a client to a different treatment provider. Therefore, it is extremely important for clinicians to be thoughtful and careful about how they approach their work with clients with GD, understanding as best they can the current treatment literature as well as how their theology informs their view of this work.

APPROACHING A CHALLENGING TOPIC

From a psychological perspective: When treatment research is lacking. It is part of a clinician's ethical responsibility to consider treatment research when selecting the best course of intervention for a client. However, not all presenting problems and diagnoses have a strong treatment research base. How, then, might a conscientious clinician proceed in exploring the literature to inform treatment choices when this is the case? We outline below some steps that can be helpful and use GD as an illustration of how to implement them.

Begin with summary sources. One helpful type of resource that can be useful in addressing the question of whether empirically supported treatments exist for a particular disorder are summary websites, standards of care documents, and review articles and

chapters. APA Division 53, the Society of Clinical Child and Adolescent Psychology, maintains the site effectivechildtherapy.org, which provides information on the state of research on evidence-based practice in psychology (EBPP) for specific psychological disorders in youth. This site is a great starting point for identifying whether research points to effective treatments for a disorder, the level of support for a treatment (e.g., well-established, probably efficacious), and literature review articles that cite primary research studies and treatment manuals. Standards of care documents that are published by various professional and advocacy organizations to outline principles for best practices with a particular population and/or presenting problem are often easily found online when they exist. For GD, both the American Psychological Association (2015) and the World Professional Association for Transgender Health (2012) have published standards of care documents for working with transgender and gender-nonconforming individuals, which includes those who may meet the criteria for GD. Though primarily concerned with recommendations for adult clients, both of these documents include material for clinicians working with children and adolescents. Therefore, some recommendations may be more easily applied with youth, whereas others may need to be evaluated in light of developmental considerations. As with any website, keep in mind that the content may or may not reflect the latest research, especially if it is not updated frequently. However, high-quality, reliable online resources like these can be a helpful starting point. Finally, published peer-reviewed summary sources such as literature reviews, meta-analyses, and book chapters on a particular disorder or presenting problem may provide a synopsis of the treatment literature and both an overview of the consensus in the empirical literature and references for individual studies.

Consider related research and theory that can inform treatment planning. For some disorders, such as GD, no empirically supported treatments for youth currently exist. When this is the case, clinicians may want to explore three categories of research on related treatments or conditions. First, there may be existing work that addresses treatment of a disorder of interest but which is limited for some reason, including theoretical ideas rather than empirical results, research that has not been replicated, case studies or studies with a small sample size, and investigations of the effects of a treatment on a population other than the one with whom a clinician is working (e.g., different in age, race/ethnicity/nationality, or other characteristics). Such studies may provide limited evidence of a treatment that has the potential to be effective. However, this type of related research should be used as one piece of a treatment plan that is informed in other ways, including the other methods discussed in this chapter. For clinicians working with gender dysphoric youth, a small number of articles describe psychological intervention programs for youth with GD and their families (Di Ceglie & Thümmel, 2006; Malpas, 2011; Meyer-Bahlburg, 2002; Rosenberg, 2002; Tishelman et al., 2015; Zucker et al., 2012). However, this work is descriptive rather than evaluative, and there are no systematic studies of the effects of specific psychosocial treatments on GD symptoms in youth. Therefore, clinicians are limited to drawing from these unassessed program models as well as from

articles or chapters that provide general theoretical principles for best mental health practices in treating gender dysphoric youth (Bernal & Coolhart, 2012; Cousino et al., 2014; de Vries & Cohen-Kettenis, 2012, 2016; Vanderburgh, 2009; WPATH, 2012). Youth-focused clinicians might also consider the adult literature when research on treatment of children and adolescents is insufficient for any reason. Unfortunately, as the professional consensus on appropriate treatment for adults with GD focuses on medical interventions (American Psychological Association, 2015; WPATH, 2012), this literature is not likely to be helpful for clinicians searching for information about psychosocial treatments for gender dysphoric youth.

Second, empirical studies of effective treatments for similar conditions may inform treatment planning. For example, if a clinician is treating an anxiety or impulse-control disorder for which treatment research is lacking, evidence-based interventions for other disorders of the same type can be a useful resource. Of course, one must be cautious about applying treatments for one disorder to a different set of symptoms, as even disorders that share features are unique in their presentation and causes. Significant alterations may be necessary to create a treatment program that is appropriate for the disorder being treated, but interventions that are supported for similar conditions can at least serve as an informative starting point. Again, unfortunately for clinicians seeking GD treatment resources, this direction is not likely to be fruitful. GD is a unique disorder that shares so little with other diagnoses in form and function that it is categorized by itself in the DSM (American Psychiatric Association, 2013).

Third, given the high level of psychological comorbidity in youth seeking treatment (Angold et al., 1999), addressing co-occurring disorders may be an important component of treatment. Therefore, informed by careful assessment, clinicians should identify any symptoms or disorders that are distinct from the main presenting problem but which need to be addressed clinically. Such issues may include symptoms that present a danger to the client or others (suicidality, severe aggression, or psychosis), cause significant distress and/or impairment, and worsen the presenting problem. If comorbid disorders that would benefit from treatment are identified, clinicians should draw from the treatment literature that addresses these comorbid problems. As reviewed earlier, comorbid symptomatology for gender dysphoric youth likely include depression, anxiety, externalizing symptoms, and suicidality (Aitken et al., 2016; Cohen-Kettenis & van Goozen, 2002), all of which have a richer treatment research literature than GD.

Be informed by developmental psychopathology. Developmental psychopathology is a valuable tool for informing individualized treatment planning, regardless of the amount of treatment research that exists for a particular disorder. As we have previously discussed (chapter one), developmental psychopathology considers disorder to be the result of the dynamic interaction of individual and environmental risk factors over the course of development. The beauty of this approach is that it emphasizes identifiable and often changeable factors that have directed the course of a child's unique development toward a particular disorder or disorders. Therefore, clinicians who take a developmental psychopathology–informed approach will begin

with a thorough assessment of the factors that are likely to have contributed to a child's current symptoms; these include biological variables, emotional and psychological child characteristics, family dynamics and features, and other peer and environmental influences on the child's well-being and development. Furthermore, this approach considers how these factors have interacted over time and the ways in which the child's behavior or symptoms may represent an adaptation to his environment. Treatment planning then includes the identification of risk factors that can be targeted. For example, effective treatment of anxiety in children generally needs to include addressing the ways in which anxiety may be modeled or inadvertently reinforced by parents. Furthermore, identifying and promoting protective factors within and around youth can also help redirect their pathways toward health and better functioning. An adolescent with depression might be helped to explore the ways she can best benefit from a strong social network within her family and her church community. Both the use of developmentally appropriate methods of assessment and a working knowledge of the research about risk and protective factors for a disorder are extremely helpful in facilitating this process.

GD is thought to develop as the result of the interaction between biological and environmental risk factors, but the details of what the specific factors are and how they operate and interact to create GD are still unclear, especially with regard to environmental influences on the disorder. Unfortunately, this lack of understanding of clear risk factors means that clinicians may not be able to aim to change the developmental pathways that have led to GD. The current research suggests that the biological factors that influence GD have genetic or poorly understood prenatal underpinnings, which eliminates them as psychotherapeutic targets. However, there is more evidence that the environmental and interpersonal risk factors that youth with GD experience may lead to comorbid emotional and behavioral symptoms. Therefore, identification of such stressors may be helpful in reducing other sources of distress and dysfunction even if they do not target GD symptoms themselves.

From a Christian perspective: Applying integrative resources. Integrating psychological approaches to the treatment of disorder with a Christian perspective is a process that is both communal and personal. It is communal in the sense that one is wise to draw from Christian thinking that others have done and to understand the intersection of faith and treatment in interaction with others; it is personal in that each Christian's experience of and understanding of both God and the process of treatment have unique elements, such that thoughtful integration may look different for every believer. In chapter two, we discussed some general frameworks and resources for integrating biblical and theological material with the treatment of childhood disorders. In this section, we will explore how these ideas might be applied to GD. Due to the theological complexity and controversy of this topic, rather than present theologically based conclusions, we will describe a variety of approaches in order to encourage readers to engage thoughtfully in their own integrative process. In this discussion, we will present three frameworks from which people commonly understand

gender dysphoria: the integrity framework, the disability framework, and the diversity framework (Yarhouse, 2015). We will revisit the idea that the three parts of the biblical story—creation, fall, and redemption—have implications for understanding and treating mental illness. We will also discuss the unique theological considerations for working with youth with GD stemming from the ideas that children are gifts, full persons, and agents (Miller-McLemore, 2003).

Theology of creation and human nature. We are created by God, in his image, as gendered beings (Genesis 1:27). However, Christians disagree about how to best understand God's intentions for gender. According to the *integrity framework*, clear distinctions between biological maleness and femaleness are sacred and embedded in our created nature. Therefore, GD (or any inconsistency between one's biological sex and one's experience of one's own gender) is a violation of God's intention for human nature. This is a common view within evangelical churches, and a number of conservative evangelical groups have put forth statements affirming the integrity framework (Coalition for Biblical Sexuality, 2017; Southern Baptist Convention, 2014). Furthermore, it has been suggested that the relatively rare occurrence of both gender dysphoria and intersex conditions (in which biological gender is not clear-cut) are actually evidence of the validity of a binary conceptualization of gender, as the physical characteristics and gender identity align as male or female for the vast majority of individuals (Looy & Bouma, 2005; Yarhouse, 2015).

Other Christian writers challenge this view as having the potential to overly simplify complex issues around gender. For example, some theologians focus on the meaning of our being created male and female as a reflection primarily of our inherent relationality and incompleteness rather than the centrality of binary gender to identity (Looy, 2002; Looy & Bouma, 2005). The difference between men and women—and the creation of woman as man's companion—highlights the incompleteness of each lone human (Grenz, 1998). Indeed, the *imago Dei* is argued to be only fully manifest when we are in relationship with one another. The incompleteness of each person on his own also highlights our need for a relationship with God. In addition, the joining of man and woman in marriage is used throughout Scripture as a reflection of the relationship between God and his people (Hosea 2; Ephesians 5:22-27). In this view, the creation of Adam and Eve primarily reflects each person's need for relationships to complete their imaging of God and the functioning for which they were created; the nature of creation as gendered, then, is not meant to create a rigid template for understanding gender norms. Though this view still affirms God's design for people as male or female, it also reminds us to guard against using the creation narrative to defend an overly rigid view of the male-female dichotomy that can risk excluding individuals who have more trouble fitting into these neat categories (Yarhouse, 2015).

Theology of the fall and suffering. The introduction of sin into the world has affected every aspect of our being, including our gendered nature. The *disability framework* understands gender dysphoria in terms of disorder; it reflects a biologically based abnormality in the normally congruent connection between biological sex and experienced gender. From a Christian perspective, this incongruence is the result of a fallen world in which creation does not function as God intended it. In contrast with the integrity framework, however, the disability framework does not view gender incongruence as a moral issue; rather, it is better conceptualized as a disorder that occurs as a result of the fall and the effects of sin but not as the result of individual sin or even choice. This view is parallel to a common theological approach to understanding other disabilities or disorders, ranging from hearing impairments to depression, which are seen as imperfections in the created order (specifically, people) that are the result of the fall.

It is because of the fall that pain and suffering, including the suffering that individuals with GD experience, exist in the world. However, God can—and does—use suffering to accomplish his purposes (Romans 5:3-5; 8:17-18). The difficulty of experiencing a gender identity that is incongruent with one's biological sex (and/or the expectations of one's culture) can create unique opportunities for self-exploration and meaning making (Yarhouse & Carr, 2012). Youth with gender dysphoria may be faced more imminently than their peers with questions such as: How do I see myself? How do I understand God's intentions for creation and gender? How do I discern God's will for my life? What does true community look like? Wrestling with these questions can produce deeper understandings of oneself, God, and the world, as well as develop characteristics such as strength, perseverance, and steadfastness. Therefore, as parents and clinicians, we want to be careful not to focus so heavily on ameliorating dysphoria that we dismiss the experience of struggling and suffering as wholly negative;

rather, we need to make space in our interactions with youth with GD for them to wrestle with difficult questions as we support them and trust God's ability to work all things for good as he makes these youth more like himself (Romans 8:28-29) without presuming we know God's specific plan for them. At the same time, we recognize that God does not desire for us to wallow in our misery, and that he does offer us joy even in our temporary time in this fallen world. The suffering experienced by many individuals with gender dysphoria—such as depression, autism, or cancer—is probably not part of God's original design for people. So, how does Christian theology help us understand the implications of redemption and healing for individuals with GD?

Theology of redemption and healing. The story of Scripture does not end with Adam and Eve's expulsion from the Garden of Eden, of course, but finds its continuation in the death and resurrection of Christ. We are offered rebirth, life, healing, and hope through Jesus (Isaiah 53:5; John 3:16; Titus 3:4-7). One of the pressing questions for Christians seeking to understand GD revolves around how we define healing and redemption for these individuals. The integrity framework recommends rejection of an incongruent gender identity and the embracing of one's biological sex as the only desirable option. The disability framework emphasizes management of dysphoria in the most effective manner, with no particular treatment direction being inherently morally superior to any other. The *diversity framework*, increasingly emphasized in Western cultures (though not commonly within the evangelical church), views diversity in gendered experiences and identifications as positive and praiseworthy.

At the extreme end of this view, binary conceptualizations of gender are inaccurate and repressive, and all forms of gender identification (including less common varieties such as pangender or gender-fluid) should be encouraged and celebrated. Therefore, within a diversity framework, healing is likely to take the form of accepting one's experienced gender identity, changing one's external presentation (sometimes including physical features) to match gender identity, rejecting cultural pressures to conform to traditional binary presentations of gender, and surrounding oneself with a community who supports and celebrates gender identity diversity. Therefore, clinicians need to discern which framework they think offers the best approach to understanding GD—as informed by psychological research as well as theological understandings of the nature of creation and sin—in order to develop a thoughtful, coherent approach to treatment.

Some authors have emphasized the value of integrating components of each of the three views into understandings of healing and treatment (Yarhouse, 2015). The integrity framework holds the distinctiveness of male and female in high regard; the disability framework encourages compassion and empathy; the diversity framework encourages meaning making and supportive community. Examining each framework for its potential to inform how we respond wisely and compassionately to youth with GD is more helpful than closing our ears to them if we disagree with their main principles; we can listen to and learn from a variety of perspectives without compromising on our own beliefs and values. A more nuanced or integrated view might also help us consider more flexible approaches to treatment. For example, it has been suggested that understandings of "healthy" gender identity that focus solely on taking steps to ensure a match between biological and experienced gender (either by changing gender identity or by altering physical manifestations of sex and gender, such as with hormones or surgery) are too limited (Looy & Bouma, 2005; Yarhouse, 2015). Rather, such perspectives note that we might do well to widen our understanding of healing to include gender dysphoria that is managed in less dramatic ways that allow individuals to live productive and contented lives despite their dysphoria. That is, "rather than reject the person facing such [gender identity] conflicts, the Christian community would do well to recognize the conflict and try to work with the person to find the least invasive ways to manage the gender identity concerns" (Yarhouse, 2015, p. 25).

We might also do well to consider how our understanding of the nature and role of gender shapes inclusion within the church and in particular roles (Looy & Bouma, 2005). For example, in many churches, particular roles may be either informally or formally limited to one gender or the other (e.g., women leading children's ministry, men serving as elders). What is the rationale behind these distinctions? Are they due to an understanding that only one gender is truly suited for particular roles, perhaps due to scriptural interpretations? Or are they in place because certain roles require certain characteristics that are more likely to be present in one gender or the other but are not truly confined to only men or women? In both cases, what are the implications for individuals who experience gender dysphoria

(as well as those who are intersex)? Are there instances when the gendered nature of particular roles within the church excludes these individuals from participation, and how do we respond to these limits? In what ways do they help or hinder the spiritual development of individuals as well as the work of the church?

Finally, as we have discussed earlier (chapter two), sin still affects the world, and Christ's work on the cross will not be consummated until his second coming and the establishment of the new heaven and the new earth. This truth means that while we can experience some freedom and healing in this life, suffering still exists, significantly for some individuals. Unfortunately, for those with GD, the centrality of gender to identity, combined with varying cultural and societal expectations and pressures, means that they may continue to experience some form or source of distress or impairment as the result of their gender incongruence. Individuals who choose to manage their dysphoria in less drastic ways, often in ways that are consistent with their biological sex, may still experience distress in situations that trigger their dysphoria (e.g., when a natal female with GD attends a formal event in which she is expected to dress in a highly feminine manner; Yarhouse, 2015). Those who as adults pursue more invasive treatments, such as hormone therapy and/or sex reassignment surgery, may experience distress as the result of either regret about an irreversible decision or from the side effects of biologically based interventions whose long-term effects are not well studied. In any case, we must remember that our hope does not lie in our experiences in this life but in the eternal life to come and in the completion of Christ's work that will "wipe every tear from [our] eyes" (Revelation 21:4). This eternal focus should not be used to dismiss the very real here-and-now concerns and struggles of youth with GD but provides encouragement and hope that full healing and freedom can ultimately occur by God's grace.

Children as gifts. In addition to the broader theological ideas of creation, sin, and redemption, as clinicians desiring to work well with youth with gender dysphoria, we also need to consider how theological ideas about childhood inform this work. One implication of the view that children are gifts is that we must do our best to care well for those who are suffering. For youth with disorders whose treatment has been more thoroughly researched, this responsibility may be somewhat easier. However, it is equally important for us to care well for youth with GD, for whom the most effective treatment is much less clear, as their suffering is as valid and important as that of their peers with anxiety or disruptive behavior disorders. Therefore, we must be discerning stewards of the treatment research that does exist as well as any other sources of information that can help us craft a responsible treatment plan, including research on the causes of GD, research on treating adults with GD, research into effective treatments for comorbid conditions, theologically based perspectives on gender, and the voices of these youth themselves as they speak about their experiences, thoughts, and feelings. It will take more time, effort, and perhaps creativity on the part of the clinician working with a child or adolescent with GD to craft and implement a treatment plan than it generally takes to follow a manualized intervention, but if we value these children as gifts,

these are important investments to make. The energy we pour into these youth as caregivers not only honors God, the giver of the gift, but also communicates to the youths themselves that they are loved, valuable, and worthy of care. These messages are especially important for youth with GD who may have faced criticism, condemnation, and a lack of support from other significant adults, particularly in the context of the church (Yarhouse & Carr, 2012; Yarhouse, 2015).

An important task for clinicians working with youth with GD is to assess their context and support systems. In the context of understanding children as gifts, this task may lead clinicians to ask specific questions, including: How do their families view their GD? What messages of acceptance (conditional or unconditional) or rejection have they received from their parents or broader communities? In what ways have their families encouraged stronger identification for either their biological sex or their experienced gender? Do they have peers and/or adults with whom they can be completely open and honest? If they are involved in a religious community, in what ways have members of that community been supportive or unsupportive of their thoughts, feelings, experiences, and desires? Within that community (as well as the youth's family), is gender incongruence viewed as a moral or a nonmoral issue? What do youths' families and communities understand as the causes of GD (e.g., individual sinfulness, environmental factors, biological influences)? Which framework—integrity, disability, or diversity—is most heavily emphasized in the contexts in which the youth lives? We need to understand these messages and contexts in order to assess youths' social support as well as the messages they may have internalized, their views of themselves as valued and valuable, risk for comorbid disorders, and the range of treatments that is likely to be considered acceptable and helpful. Since clinicians who work with youth are almost always interacting with their clients' families as well, it is important to explore parents' views of gender and their child and work with family members to explore how they can best support and care for their transgender family member with GD; this conversation may take more time and nuance if members of the same family endorse different frameworks for understanding GD (e.g., one family member embraces the diversity framework and encourages nonbinary gender expression, while another family member takes the integrity perspective and believes that gender expression should conform to natal or assigned gender).

Another important role of the therapeutic context, larger than just the content of the intervention itself, is the support provided by the therapist. Common factors research suggests that the therapeutic alliance, the trust-based, positive working relationship between a clinician and a client, is an extremely important component of whether a treatment will be effective (Wampold, 2015). In addition, the hope for change that therapy provides is also predictive of improvement, even apart from the substance of the treatment itself. Therefore, clinicians working with youth with GD may play an important supportive and caring role, even when they do not have a manualized, highly empirically supported intervention to implement. Given the degree of alienation they often experience within families and broader communities, these youth

especially may benefit from a trusting relationship with a clinician who listens empathically to their experiences and concerns and communicates to them that change is possible. Therapists who work with youth who are struggling to understand how God views them may also focus on helping clients understand that God loves them as he loves all of his creation and that they are fearfully and wonderfully made.

Children as persons. If youth are fully human, then our theologically based views of human nature, the fall, and redemption apply equally to them. Youth are created as gendered beings, in the image of God, with an incompleteness that can only be rectified through relationships with God and other people. God can use their suffering to shape them and their faith. In addition, part of their humanity is their ongoing development. Development occurs through all of life, of course, but the rapid and significant changes that characterize childhood and adolescence demand attention to developmental sensitivity in considering GD in youth. As we work with youth with GD, we should be aware that their understandings of gender and gender roles—both their own and those of others—are affected by their developmental stage (Martin & Ruble, 2010). As these understandings change over time, gender identification may fluctuate as well. Indeed, this pattern may be a significant contributor to the high rates of desistance of gender dysphoria from childhood into adolescence and adulthood. We should be appropriately cautious, then, about implementing interventions that may be inappropriate for a developmentally temporary experience or even harmful in the long run (e.g., starting a child on hormone therapy to suppress puberty when it is unclear whether her dysphoria will persist and this treatment could negatively impact bone density or future fertility). Similarly, even with help and support, children (and perhaps also adolescents) are unlikely to have the cognitive and social maturity to make decisions that have a lifelong impact, such as sex reassignment surgery. However, we also need to be sensitive to a child's experiences of their own gendered nature and their dysphoria and walk closely with them, truly considering their experiences and perspectives in the ongoing processes of assessment and treatment. Recognizing the full humanity of youth includes supporting their development both now and into the future; for youth with GD, this entails coming alongside them and their families as they consider the short- and long-term impacts of various treatment options, helping them manage their dysphoria in the present in a way that also enables healthy long-term growth and development.

We also want to guard against reducing identity to issues of gender (DeFranza, 2015). One's gender, and the degree of conformity to culturally based expectations about gender, is a significant component of how we see others and ourselves. When a couple is expecting a baby, one of the first questions others ask them is often about the child's gender, and a perusal of the baby gear department of any large store makes it apparent that norms and expectations about gender differences are in place well before a child is born. However, as Christians, we recognize that our identity is much broader than being male or female; we are created in God's image, foreknown, chosen, loved, redeemed, and saved by God.

Indeed, our status as believers in Christ is so unifying that the importance of earthly differences—including in gender—is eliminated by our entry into his family (Galatians 3:28; Colossians 3:11). These truths do not mean that these differences cease to exist; indeed, the diversity of the great multitude that will praise God at the end of time is purposeful and praiseworthy (Revelation 5:9; 7:9-10). We would do well to encourage individuals who struggle with issues of gender identity that gender is not their only defining feature, even as we are careful not to dismiss or minimize their concerns (i.e., "Since your identity is rooted in Christ, you shouldn't be bothered by your experience of gender incongruence"). Given the fact that complex and dialectical thought is still developing in children and adolescents (Santrock, 2017), we should be especially purposeful in encouraging them to develop a multifaceted sense of their own identities, defined by a wide variety of appropriate characteristics and features and, for youth who are believers, being rooted in Christ as the central feature through which all other components of identity are filtered.

Children as agents. As full persons, children have the potential to be agents in both their own development and in the world around them. Youth receive a barrage of input about gender roles and norms from a variety of sources beginning early in life. Given the relative infrequency of gender dysphoria and intersex conditions in the population, these voices and pressures are likely to come primarily from others who experience consistency between their biological sex and their gender identity. Therefore, there is a high risk that the unique perspectives of youth who experience GD will be overshadowed by the voices of those whose experiences of gender are more normative. We have a special responsibility, then, to make space in both therapy and society more broadly for these youth to have their voices heard. Regardless of the framework on gender dysphoria (integrity, disability, or diversity) that one finds most appealing, there is value in listening to the thoughts, feelings, and experiences of all people, including youth with GD. For example, individuals with GD may be in a position to speak into spiritual issues in unique ways. For example, Yarhouse (2015) describes his experience with transgender Christians who report that they experience the masculine and feminine aspects of God's character more richly because of their gender identity concerns. Individuals with GD, particularly those who are Christians, may also be in special positions to speak into how the church can show kindness and compassion to the suffering and marginalized (Yarhouse & Carr, 2012). As we listen, we can gain a better sense of the variety of human experiences, and that helps us build empathy and connection with even those who are very different from us.

Giving these youth the space to be heard is beneficial to them, providing support and care for those at high risk for depression and anxiety as well as enhancing their own sense of agency. The message that their perspectives are valued by others can be empowering for a group of youth who frequently feel powerless. Depending on the framework they embrace, families might consider how to maximize these children's ability to make choices in their own lives (e.g., in terms of the types of toys they play with or the clothes they wear, at least in certain settings). It is important to remember that identity exploration is an important developmental process, and we want to allow youth with GD the same appropriate freedom to explore who they are that their peers are given. Within the context of treatment, we want to be intentional about giving these youth, especially older children and adolescents, a meaningful role in determining the direction of their own treatment (Temple Newhook et al., 2018; WPATH, 2012). We need to listen carefully to their experiences and desires in order to understand the nature of their dysphoria, what tools and resources have been most helpful for managing it, what experiences are most challenging or distressing, and when and how their dysphoria manifests most strongly (which may help us discern its likelihood to persist as well as the degree to which it interferes with functioning and well-being). It may also be helpful to work with youth to identify—and help them understand—the framework by which they understand their experiences. Do they see their dysphoria as a distortion in the clear line between male and female intended by God (integrity framework), as a disorder that they did not choose and which is a nonmoral issue (disability framework), as an experience to be celebrated (diversity framework), or as some combination of these? What frameworks are being emphasized by significant others in their lives (e.g., family members, peers, school personnel, church community), and how does the consistency or conflict between their views and those of others impact their well-being? Finally, when we help these youth do the hard work of understanding their own experiences and how these may be consistent or inconsistent with the expectations of the culture, we are supporting the development of skills that will serve them well as they mature into adulthood. Rather than characterizing their experiences for them or making one-sided decisions about determining treatment direction and defining positive outcomes in a particular way, we want youth to be as involved in this process as possible so that they may be able to navigate any ongoing gender identity issues in a way that is thoughtful, adaptive, and faithful to their own informed understanding of a life well lived.

CONCLUSIONS

The work of wrestling through these difficult questions and issues both for one's own understanding and for the benefit of one's client is important work for God's kingdom. All youth and families need and deserve the best possible clinical care, and the provision of such care is generally more challenging when treatment cannot be guided by a detailed manual or when presenting problems are theologically complex. We hope that the guidance we offer above—including drawing on relevant clinical material and utilizing a theological understanding of creation, suffering, and redemption—will help you approach your young clients and their treatment in a way that is beneficial to them and honoring to God.

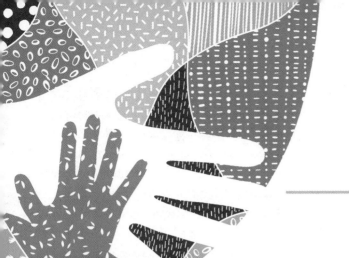

Conclusion

A T THE TIME OF THIS WRITING, it is week seven of the coronavirus pandemic, and we are quarantined in our homes with our children who range from age three to age seventeen. We are observing children's health and adjustment through our roles as child clinicians, educators, neighbors, and mothers. Challenging and traumatic events can lead to strong feelings of grief and helplessness and can interfere with typical development. Yet they can also highlight the protective factors that help us thrive here on God's earth and alter developmental trajectories. One critical protective factor is supportive relationships. Now more than ever, it is clear how important it is for youth to have adults who support them. Children need adults who listen to and validate their experiences, who provide acceptance and a sense of security, are predictable and convey warmth, are flexible in problem solving and responding to their needs, display patience with their development, are self-reflective and make changes or amends when needed, and maintain hope and faith even when it seems difficult. We are so excited

that you have the opportunity to be one of these adults to the youth you work with in your clinical practice as they face the stressors associated with psychopathology.

We hope this book has enlightened you, encouraged you, challenged you, and uplifted you in your work. Ideally, we hope it has inspired your practice to be more science-based, theologically informed, creative, and Spirit-led. To fully value and respect children and their agency, we must set an intention throughout life to better understand and care for them. As lifelong learners and developing individuals yourselves, we encourage you to invest in continued professional and spiritual development in order to strengthen your ability to provide effective treatments to youth and families and to thrive in this important work you are undertaking. We cannot emphasize enough the value of supervision and consultation with other people. These people may include more experienced professionals, clinicians who are peers, researchers or instructors, and spiritual mentors. Scripture is clear that we are not meant to function alone, and input from and reflection with trusted individuals is crucial in the process of discerning theological truths and treatment planning with clients whose presenting problems and their treatment are particularly challenging for whatever reason. We hope that this book will continue to be one of many resources that you draw from as you design and implement treatment plans for your young clients as you value them as gifts, respect them as fully human, and work to promote their agency.

We pray that you receive this work as encouraging and energizing for the crucial work that you do with children and their families. As you go forward . . .

Trust that God has prepared you for this good work. Your personal characteristics, your life experiences, your faith, and your training have led you to this work. God is with you and for you as he places children in your care.

Trust in the importance of your work. You are helping to develop skills children need now and in the future to overcome difficulties. When therapy does not go as planned, remember that your role right now may be to plant a seed for future growth. You may be providing the safe place a child needs to experience. Even if therapy is short-lived, you may be preparing a child and their caregivers to engage in future treatment by giving them a positive experience, communi-

cating the expectations of therapy, and encouraging them to be open to and seek out support.

Trust in the compassion and love God has given you. Through your compassionate desire to fully understand a child's experience, you are helping that child glimpse who he or she truly is—a gift created and loved by a gracious God. This is a holy space and enterprise.

Trust in your role as a blessing. You are serving the least of these and God will guide you in this opportunity to enrich the lives of the children and families you care for. Be playful with them, allow yourself to feel their joys and their sorrows, generously give of your knowledge and skills, and shower God's affection on them.

And at the end of the day, *trust that God is with these youth and will provide peace and hope and grace to them over the course of their lives.*

> We live in a world in which we need to share responsibility. It's easy to say, "It's not my child, not my community, not my world, not my problem." Then there are those who see the need and respond. I consider those people my heroes.
>
> FRED ROGERS

> Have courage for the great sorrows of life and patience for the small ones; and when you have laboriously accomplished your daily task, go to sleep in peace. God is awake.
>
> VICTOR HUGO

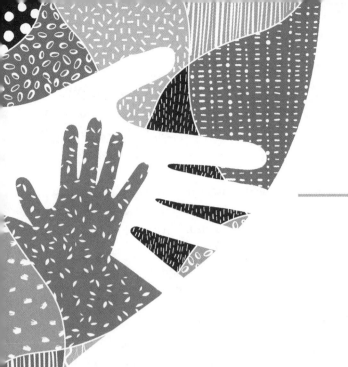

References

Abela, J. R. Z., Brozina, K., & Haigh, E. P. (2002). An examination of the response styles theory of depression in third- and seventh-grade children: A short-term longitudinal study. *Journal of Abnormal Child Psychology, 30*(5), 515-27.

Abikoff, H., Gallagher, R., Wells, K. C., Murray, D. W., Huang, L., Lu, F., & Petkova, E. (2013). Remediating organizational functioning in children with ADHD: Immediate and long-term effects from a randomized controlled trial. *Journal of Consulting and Clinical Psychology, 81*(1), 113-28. https://doi.org/10.1037/a0029648

Abikoff, H., Hechtman, L., Klein, R. G., Gallagher, R., Fleiss, K., Etcovitch, J., Cousins, L., Greenfield, B., Martin, D., & Pollack, S. (2004a). Social functioning in children with ADHD treated with long-term methylphenidate and multimodal psychosocial treatment. *Journal of the American Academy of Child & Adolescent Psychiatry, 43*(7), 820-29. https://doi.org/10.1097/01.chi.0000128797.91601.1a

Abikoff, H., Hechtman, L., Klein, R. G., Weiss, G., Fleiss, K., Etcovitch, J., Cousins, L., Greenfield, B., Martin, D., & Pollack, S. (2004b). Symptomatic improvement in children with ADHD treated with long-term methylphenidate and multimodal psychosocial treatment. *Journal of the American Academy of Child & Adolescent Psychiatry, 43*(7), 802-11. https://doi.org/10.1097/01.chi.0000128791.10014.ac

Abikoff, H. B., Thompson, M., Laver-Bradbury, C., Long, N., Forehand, R. L., Brotman, L. M., Klein, R. G., Reiss, P., Huo, L., & Sonuga-Barke, E. (2015). Parent training for preschool ADHD: A randomized controlled trial of specialized and generic programs. *Journal of Child Psychology and Psychiatry, 56*(6), 618-31. https://doi.org/10.1111/jcpp.12346

Achenbach, T. M. (1991a). *Manual for the child behavior checklist and 1991 profile*. University of Vermont Department of Psychiatry.

Achenbach, T. M. (1991b). *Manual for the youth self-report and 1991 profile*. University of Vermont Department of Psychiatry.

Achenbach, T. M., Howell, C. T., Quay, H. C., Conners, C. K. (1991). National survey of problems and competencies among four to sixteen-year-olds: Parents' reports for normative and clinical samples. *Monographs of the Society for Research in Child Development, 56*(3, Serial No. 225).

Adams, Z. W., Sumner, J. A., Danielson, C. K., McCauley, J. L., Resnick, H. S., Grös, K., Paul, L. A., Welsh, K. E., & Ruggiero, K. J. (2014). Prevalence and predictors of PTSD and depression among adolescent victims of the Spring 2011 tornado outbreak. *Journal of Child Psychology and Psychiatry, 55*(9), 1047-55. https://doi.org/10.1111/jcpp.12220

Affrunti, N. W., & Ginsburg, G. S. (2012). Exploring parental predictors of child anxiety: The mediating role of child interpretation bias. *Child & Youth Care Forum, 41*(6), 517-27.

Affrunti, N. W., & Woodruff-Borden, J. (2015). The effect of maternal psychopathology on parent-child agreement of child anxiety symptoms: A hierarchical linear modeling approach. *Journal of Anxiety Disorders, 32*, 56-65. https://doi.org/10.1016/j.janxdis.2015.03.010

Agha, S. S., Zammit, S., Thapar, A., & Langley, K. (2017). Maternal psychopathology and offspring clinical outcome: A four-year follow-up of boys with ADHD. *European Child & Adolescent Psychiatry, 26*(2), 253-62. https://doi.org/10.1007/s00787-016-0873-y

Agras, W. S., Bryson, S., Hammer, L. D., & Kraemer, H. C. (2007). Childhood risk factors for thin body preoccupation and social pressure to be thin. *Journal of the American Academy of Child & Adolescent Psychiatry, 46*(2), 171-78. https://doi.org/10.1097/chi.0b013e31802bd997

Ahmadzadeh, Y. I., Eley, T. C., Leve, L. D., Shaw, D. S., Natsuaki, M. N., Reiss, D., Neiderhiser, J. M., & McAdams, T. A. (2019). Anxiety in the family: A genetically informed analysis of transactional associations between mother, father and child anxiety symptoms. *Journal of Child Psychology and Psychiatry, 60*(12), 1269-77. https://doi.org/10.1111/jcpp.13068

Ainsworth, M. D. S. (1979). Infant-mother attachment. *American Psychologist, 34*(10), 932-37.

Aitken, M., VanderLaan, D. P., Wasserman, L., Stojanovski, S., & Zucker, K. J. (2016). Self-harm and suicidality in children referred for gender dysphoria. *Journal of the American Academy of Child & Adolescent Psychiatry, 55*(6), 513-20. https://doi.org/10.1016/j.jaac.2016.04.001

Aktar, E., Majdandžić, M., de Vente, W., & Bögels, S. M. (2014). Parental social anxiety disorder prospectively predicts toddlers' fear/avoidance in a social referencing paradigm. *Journal of Child Psychology and Psychiatry, 55*(1), 77-87.

Albrecht, B., Brandeis, D., Uebel-von Sandersleben, H., Valko, L., Heinrich, H., Xu, X., Drechsler, R., Heise, A., Kuntsi, J., Müller, U. C., Asherson, P., Steinhausen, H. C., Rothenberger, A., & Banaschewski, T. (2014). Genetics of preparation and response control in ADHD: the role of DRD4 and DAT1. *Journal of Child Psychology and Psychiatry, and Allied Disciplines, 55*(8), 914–923. https://doi.org/10.1111/jcpp.12212

Alderson, R., Rapport, M., & Kofler, M. (2007). Attention-deficit/hyperactivity disorder and behavioral inhibition: A meta-analytic review of the stop-signal paradigm. *Journal of Abnormal Child Psychology, 35*(5), 745-58. https://doi.org/10.1007/s10802-007-9131-6

Alink, L. A., Cicchetti, D., Kim, J., & Rogosch, F. A. (2009). Mediating & moderating processes in the relation between maltreatment and psychopathology: Mother-child relationship quality & emotion regulation. *Journal of Abnormal Child Psychology, 37*(6), 831-43.

Allen, K. L., Byrne, S. M., & Crosby, R. D. (2015). Distinguishing between risk factors for bulimia nervosa, binge eating disorder, and purging disorder. *Journal of Youth and Adolescence, 44*(8), 1580-91. https://doi.org/10.1007/s10964-014-0186-8

Allen, K. L., Byrne, S. M., Forbes, D., & Oddy, W. H. (2009). Risk factors for full- and partial-syndrome early adolescent eating disorders: A population-based pregnancy cohort study. *Journal of the American Academy of Child & Adolescent Psychiatry, 48*(8), 800-809. https://doi.org/10.1097/CHI.0b013e3181a8136d

Alloy, L. B., Abramson, L. Y., Walshaw, P. D., Cogswell, A., Grandin, L. D., Hughes, M. E., Iacoviello, B. M., Whitehouse, W. G., Urošević, S., Nusslock, R., & Hogan, M. E. (2008). Behavioral approach system and behavioral inhibition system sensitivities and bipolar spectrum disorders: Prospective prediction of bipolar mood episodes. *Bipolar Disorders, 10*(2), 310-22.

Alloy, L. B., Black, S. K., Young, M. E., Goldstein, K. E., Shapero, B. G., Stange, J. P., Boccia, A. S., Matt, L. M., Boland, E. M., Moore, L. C., & Abramson, L. Y. (2012). Cognitive vulnerabilities and depression versus other psychopathology symptoms and diagnoses in early adolescence. *Journal of Clinical Child and Adolescent Psychology, 41*(5), 539-60.

Alloy, L. B., Urošević, S., Abramson, L. Y., Jager-Hyman, S., Nusslock, R., Whitehouse, W. G., & Hogan, M. (2012). Progression along the bipolar spectrum: A longitudinal study of predictors of conversion from bipolar spectrum conditions to bipolar I and II disorders. *Journal of Abnormal Psychology, 121*(1), 16-27.

Amado, L., Jarque, S., & Ceccato, R. (2016). Differential impact of a multimodal versus pharmacological therapy on the core symptoms of attention deficit/hyperactivity disorder in childhood. *Research in Developmental Disabilities, 59*, 93-104. https://doi.org/10.1016/j.ridd.2016.08.004

American Academy of Pediatrics. (2011). ADHD: Clinical practice guideline for the diagnosis, evaluation, and treatment of attention-deficit/hyperactivity disorder in children and adoles-cents. *Pediatrics, 128*(5), 1007-22. https://doi.org/10.1542/peds.2011-2654

American Counseling Association (2014). *2014 ACA Code of Ethics.* Retrieved from https://www.counseling.org/knowledge-center/ethics

American Psychiatric Association. (1980). *Diagnostic and statistical manual of mental disorders* (3rd ed.). American Psychiatric Publishing.

American Psychiatric Association. (1994). *Diagnostic and statistical manual of mental disorders* (4th ed., text revision). American Psychiatric Publishing.

American Psychiatric Association. (2013). *Diagnostic and statistical manual of mental disorders* (5th ed.). American Psychiatric Publishing.

American Psychological Association. (2002). Criteria for evaluating treatment guidelines. *American Psychologist, 57*(12), 1052-59. https://doi.org/10.1037/0003-066X.57.12.1052

American Psychological Association. (2015). Guidelines for psychological practice with transgender and gender nonconforming people. *American Psychologist, 70*(9), 832-64.

American Psychological Association. (2017). *Ethical principles of psychologists and code of conduct* (2002, amended effective June 1, 2010, and January 1, 2017). http://www.apa.org/ethics/code/index.aspx

American Psychological Association, Task Force on Appropriate Therapeutic Responses to Sexual Orientation. (2009). *Report of the American Psychological Association Task Force on Appropriate Therapeutic Responses to Sexual Orientation.* Retrieved from https://www.apa.org/pi/lgbt/resources/sexual-orientation

Amorim, W. N., & Marques, S. C. (2018). Inhibitory control and cognitive flexibility in children with attention-deficit/hyperactivity disorder. *Psychology & Neuroscience, 11*(4), 364-74. https://doi.org/10.1037/pne0000156

An, J. Y., Lin, K., Zhu, L., Werling, D. M., Dong, S., Brand, H., Wang, H. Z., Zhao, X., Schwartz,

G. B., Collins, R. L., Currall, B. B., Dastmalchi, C., Dea, J., Duhn, C., Gilson, M. C., Klei, L., Liang, L., Markenscoff-Papadimitriou, E., Pochareddy, S., Ahituv, N., . . . Sanders, S. J. (2018). Genome-wide de novo risk score implicates promoter variation in autism spectrum disorder. *Science, 362*(6420), 1-8.

Angold, A., Costello, E. J., & Erkanli, A. (1999). Comorbidity. *Journal of Child Psychology and Psychiatry, 40*(1), 57-88.

Anixt, J. S., Vaughn, A. J., Powe, N. R., & Lipkin, P. H. (2016). Adolescent perceptions of outgrowing childhood attention-deficit hyperactivity disorder: Relationship to symptoms and quality of life. *Journal of Developmental and Behavioral Pediatrics, 37*(3), 196–204. https://doi.org/10.1097/DBP.0000000000000279

APA Presidential Task Force on Evidence-Based Practice. (2006). Evidence-based practice in psychology. *American Psychologist, 61*(4), 271-85.

Armstrong, T. D., & Costello, E. J. (2002). Community studies on adolescent substance use, abuse, or dependence and psychiatric comorbidity. *Journal of Consulting and Clinical Psychology, 70*, 1224-39.

Arnett, A. B., Macdonald, B., & Pennington, B. F. (2013). Cognitive and behavioral indicators of ADHD symptoms prior to school age. *Journal of Child Psychology and Psychiatry and Allied Disciplines, 54*(12), 1284–1294. https://doi.org/10.1111/jcpp.12104

Arnett, J. J., & Jensen, L. A. (2019). *Human development: A cultural approach* (3rd ed.). Pearson.

Arnold, L. E., Abikoff, H. B., Cantwell, D. P., Conners, C. K., Elliott, G. R., Greenhill, L. L., Hechtman, L., Hinshaw, S. P., Hoza, B., Jensen, P. S., Kraemer, H. C., March, J. S., Newcorn, J. H., Pelham, W. E., Richters, J. E., Schiller, E., Severe, J. B., Swanson, J. M., Vereen, D., & Wells, K. C. (1997). NIMH collaborative multimodal treatment study of children with ADHD (MTA): Design, methodology, and protocol evolution.

Journal of Attention Disorders, 2(3), 141-58. https://doi.org/10.1177/108705479700200301

Arnsten, A., & Pliszka, S. (2011). Catecholamine influences on prefrontal cortical function: Relevance to treatment of attention deficit/hyperactivity disorder and related disorders. *Pharmacology, Biochemistry and Behavior, 99*(2), 211-16. https://doi.org/10.1016/j.pbb.2011.01.020

Atherton, O. E., Ferrer, E., & Robins, R. W. (2018). The development of externalizing symptoms from late childhood through adolescence: A longitudinal study of Mexican-origin youth [Supplemental material]. *Developmental Psychology, 54*(6), 1135-47. https://doi.org/10.1037/dev0000489.supp

Atherton, O. E., Lawson, K. M., Ferrer, E., & Robins, R. W. (2019). The role of effortful control in the development of ADHD, ODD, and CD symptoms [Supplemental material]. *Journal of Personality and Social Psychology, 118*(6), 1226-46. https://doi.org/10.1037/pspp0000243.supp

Atkin, T., Nuñez, N., & Gobbi, G. (2017). Practitioner review: The effects of atypical antipsychotics and mood stabilisers in the treatment of depressive symptoms in paediatric bipolar disorder. *Journal of Child Psychology and Psychiatry, 58*(8), 865-79. https://doi.org/10.1111/jcpp.12735

Atkinson, L., Beitchman, J., Gonzalez, A., Young, A., Wilson, B., Escobar, M., Chisholm, V., Brownlie, E., Khoury, J. E., Ludmer, J., & Villani, V. (2015). Cumulative risk, cumulative outcome: A 20-year longitudinal study. *PLOS ONE, 10*(6), e0127650. https://doi.org/10.1371/journal.pone.0127650

Auerbach, J. G., Berger, A., Atzaba-Poria, N., Arbelle, S., Cypin, N., Friedman, A., & Landau, R. (2008). Temperament at 7, 12, and 25 months in children at familial risk for ADHD. *Infant and Child Development, 17*(4), 321-38. https://doi.org/10.1002/icd.579

Augustine. (1986). *The confessions of St. Augustine* (H. M. Helms, Trans.). Paraclete. (Original work published 398)

Axelson, D. A., & Birmaher, B. (2001). Relation between anxiety and depressive disorders in childhood and adolescence. *Depression & Anxiety, 14,* 67-78.

Bagwell, C. L., Molina, B. G., Kashdan, T. B., Pelham, W. J., & Hoza, B. (2006). Anxiety and mood disorders in adolescents with childhood attention-deficit/hyperactivity disorder. *Journal of Emotional and Behavioral Disorders, 14*(3), 178-87. https://doi.org/10.1177/10634266060140030501

Bai, D., Yip, B. H. K., Windham, G. C., Sourander, A., Francis, R., Yoffe, R., Glasson, E., Mahjani, B., Suominen, A., Leonard, H., Gissler, M., Buxbaum, J. D., Wong, K., Schendel, D., Kodesh, A., Breshnahan, M., Levine, S. Z., Parner, E. T., Hansen, S. N., . . . Sandin, S. (2019). Association of genetic and environmental factors with autism in a 5-country cohort. *JAMA Psychiatry, 76*(10), 1035-43. https://doi.org/10.1001/jamapsychiatry.2019.1411

Bailey, A., Le Couteur, A., Gottesman, I., & Bolton, P. (1995). Autism as a strongly genetic disorder: Evidence from a British twin study. *Psychological Medicine, 25*(1), 63-77. https://doi.org/10.1017/S0033291700028099

Bakeman, R., & Adamson, L. B. (1984). Coordinating attention to people and objects in mother-infant and peer-infant interaction. *Child Development, 55*(4), 1278-89. https://doi.org/10.2307/1129997

Baker, C., & Kuhn, L. (2018). Mediated pathways from maternal depression and early parenting to children's executive function and externalizing behaviour problems. *Infant and Child Development, 27*(1), e2052. https://doi.org/10.1002/icd.2052

Baker, J. H., Higgins Neyland, M. K., Thornton, L. M., Runfola, C. D., Larsson, H., Lichtenstein, P., & Bulik, C. (2019). Body dissatisfaction in adolescent boys [Supplemental material]. *Developmental Psychology, 55*(7), 1566-78. https://doi.org/10.1037/dev0000724.supp

Baker, J. H., Maes, H. H., Lissner, L., Aggen, S. H., Lichtenstein, P., & Kendler, K. S. (2009). Genetic risk factors for disordered eating in adolescent males and females. *Journal of Abnormal Psychology, 118*(3), 576-86. https://doi.org/10.1037/a0016314

Baker-Ericzén, M. J., Brookman-Frazee, L., & Stahmer, A. (2005). Stress levels and adaptability in parents of toddlers with and without autism spectrum disorders. *Research and Practice for Persons with Severe Disabilities, 30*(4), 194-204. https://doi.org/10.2511/rpsd.30.4.194

Bakker, J. (2014). Sex differentiation: Organizing effects of sex hormones. In B. P. C. Kreukels, T. D. Steensma, & A. L. C. de Vries (Eds.), *Gender dysphoria and disorders of sex development: Progress in care and knowledge* (pp. 3-23). Springer.

Balaban, V. (2009). Assessment of children. In E. B. Foa, T. M. Keane, M. J. Friedman, & J. A. Cohen (Eds.), *Effective treatments for PTSD: Practice guidelines from the International Society for Traumatic Stress Studies., 2nd ed.* (pp. 62–80). The Guilford Press.

Ballaban-Gil, K., & Tuchman, R. (2000). Epilepsy and epileptiform EEG: Association with autism and language disorders. *Mental Retardation and Developmental Disabilities Research Reviews, 6*(4), 300-308. https://doi.org/10.1002/1098-2779(2000)6:4<300::AID-MRDD9>3.0.CO;2-R

Balswick, J. O., & Balswick, J. K. (2014). *The family: A Christian perspective on the contemporary home* (4th ed.). Baker Academic.

Bandura, A. (1977). *Social learning theory.* Prentice Hall.

Banerjee, T. D., Middleton, F., & Faraone, S. V. (2007). Environmental risk factors for attention-deficit hyperactivity disorder. *Acta*

Paediatrica, *96*(9), 1269–1274. https://doi.org/10.1111/j.1651-2227.2007.00430.x

Banks, D. M., & Weems, C. F. (2014). Family and peer social support and their links to psychological distress among hurricane-exposed minority youth. *The American Journal of Orthopsychiatry*, *84*(4), 341–352. https://doi.org/10.1037/ort0000006

Banny, A. M., Cicchetti, D., Rogosch, F. A., Oshri, A., & Crick, N. R. (2013). Vulnerability to depression: A moderated mediation model of the roles of child maltreatment, peer victimization, and serotonin transporter linked polymorphic region genetic variation among children from low socioeconomic status backgrounds. *Development and Psychopathology*, *25*, 599-614.

Barbaresi, W. J., Katusic, S. K., Colligan, R. C., Weaver, A. L., Leibson, C. L., & Jacobsen, S. J. (2014). Long-term stimulant medication treatment of attention-deficit/hyperactivity disorder: results from a population-based study. *Journal of Developmental and Behavioral Pediatrics*, *35*(7), 448–457. https://doi.org/10.1097/DBP.0000000000000099

Bardone-Cone, A. M., & Cass, K. M. (2007). What does viewing a pro-anorexia website do? An experimental examination of website exposure and moderating effects. *International Journal of Eating Disorders*, *40*(6), 537-48. https://doi.org/10.1002/eat.20396

Barger, B. D., Campbell, J. M., & McDonough, J. D. (2013). Prevalence and onset of regression within autism spectrum disorders: A meta-analytic review. *Journal of Autism and Developmental Disorders*, *43*(4), 817-28. https://doi.org/10.1007/s10803-012-1621-x

Bar-Haim, Y., Lamy, D., Pergamin, L., Bakermans-Kranenburg, M. J., & van IJzendoorn, M. H. (2007). Threat-related attentional bias in anxious and nonanxious individuals: A meta-analytic study. *Psychological Bulletin*, *133*(1), 1-24.

Barkley, R. (1997). *ADHD and the nature of self-control*. Guilford Press.

Barkley, R. A. (2013). *Defiant children: A clinician's manual for assessment and parent training* (3rd ed.). Guilford.

Barkley, R. A., Fischer, M., Smallish, L., & Fletcher, K. (2002). The persistence of attention-deficit/hyperactivity disorder into young adulthood as a function of reporting source and definition of disorder. *Journal of Abnormal Psychology*, *111*(2), 279-89. https://doi.org/10.1037/0021-843X.111.2.279

Barrett, P. M. (2000). *FRIENDS program for children: Group leaders manual*. Australian Academic Press.

Barrett, P. M. (2004a). *FRIENDS for Life program for children—Group leader's workbook for children* (4th ed.). Australian Academic Press.

Barrett, P. M. (2004b). *FRIENDS for Life program for children—Group leader's workbook for youth* (4th ed.). Australian Academic Press.

Barrett, P. M., Dadds, M. R., & Rapee, R. M. (1996). Family treatment of childhood anxiety: A controlled trial. *Journal of Consulting and Clinical Psychology*, *64*(2), 333-42.

Barrett, P. M., Rapee, R. M., Dadds, M. M., & Ryan, S. M. (1996). Family enhancement of cognitive style in anxious and aggressive children. *Journal of Abnormal Child Psychology*, *24*(2), 187-203.

Bartels, M., van Beijsterveldt, C. E. M., Derks, E. M., Stroet, T. M., Polderman, T. J. C., Hudziak, J. J., & Boomsma, D. I. (2007). Young Netherlands Twin Register (Y-NTR): A longitudinal multiple informant study of problem behavior. *Twin Research and Human Genetics*, *10*(1), 3-11.

Barth, K. (2009). *Church dogmatics* (Vol. 3, Part 1) (G. W. Bromley & T. F. Torrence, Eds.) (J. W. Edwards, O. Bussey, & H. Knight, Trans.). T & T Clark. (Original work published 1945)

Bastiani, A. M., Rao, R., Weltzin, T., & Kaye, W. H. (1995). Perfectionism in anorexia nervosa.

International Journal of Eating Disorders, 17(2), 147-52. https://doi.org/10.1002/1098-108X (199503)17:2<147::AID-EAT2260170207 >3.0.CO;2-X

Battaglia, M., Touchette, É., Garon-Carrier, G., Dionne, G., Côté, S. M., Vitaro, F., Tremblay, R. E., & Boivin, M. (2016). Distinct trajectories of separation anxiety in the preschool years: Persistence at school entry and early-life associated factors. *Journal of Child Psychology and Psychiatry, 57*(1), 39-46.

Bauermeister, J. J., Shrout, P. E., Ramírez, R., Bravo, M., Alegría, M., Martínez-Taboas, A., Chávez, L., Rubio-Stipec, M., García, P., Ribera, J., & Canino, G. (2007). ADHD correlates, comorbidity, and impairment in community and treated samples of children and adolescents. *Journal of Abnormal Child Psychology, 35*(6), 883-98. https://doi.org/10.1007/s10802-007-9141-4

Baumrind, D. (1966). Effects of authoritative parental control on child behavior. *Child Development, 37*(4), 887-907.

Bayley, N. (2006). *Bayley Scales of Infant and Toddler Development—Third Edition (Bayley-III)*. Harcourt Assessment.

Ben-Sasson, A., & Gill, S. V. (2014). Motor and language abilities from early to late toddlerhood: Using formalized assessments to capture continuity and discontinuity in development. *Research in Developmental Disabilities, 35*(7), 1425-32. https://doi.org/10.1016/j.ridd.2014.03.036

Beauchaine, T. P., Hinshaw, S. P., & Pang, K. L. (2010). Comorbidity of attention-deficit/hyperactivity disorder and early-onset conduct disorder: Biological, environmental, and developmental mechanisms. *Clinical Psychology: Science and Practice, 17*(4), 327-36. https://doi.org/10.1111/j.1468-2850.2010.01224.x

Beauchaine, T. P., Webster-Stratton, C., & Reid, M. J. (2005). Mediators, moderators, and predictors of 1-year outcomes among children treated for early-onset conduct problems: A latent growth curve analysis. *Journal of Consulting and Clinical Psychology, 73*(3), 371-88.

Beck, A. T., & Steer, R. (1993). *Beck Depression Inventory*. Psychological Corporation.

Becker, A. E., Burwell, R. A., Herzog, D. B., Hamburg, P., & Gilman, S. E. (2002). Eating behaviours and attitudes following prolonged exposure to television among ethnic Fijian adolescent girls. *The British Journal of Psychiatry, 180*(6), 509-14. https://doi.org/10.1192/bjp.180.6.509

Becker, E., Jensen-Doss, A., Kendall, P., Birmaher, B., & Ginsburg, G. (2016). All anxiety is not created equal: Correlates of parent/youth agreement vary across subtypes of anxiety. *Journal of Psychopathology and Behavioral Assessment, 38*(4), 528-37. https://doi.org/10.1007/s10862-016-9544-z

Becker, S. P., Langberg, J. M., Eadeh, H., Isaacson, P. A., & Bourchtein, E. (2019). Sleep and daytime sleepiness in adolescents with and without ADHD: Differences across ratings, daily diary, and actigraphy. *Journal of Child Psychology and Psychiatry, 60*(9), 1021-31.

Beesdo, K., Bittner, A., Pine, D. S., Stein, M. B., Höfler, M., Lieb, R., & Wittchen, H. U. (2007). Incidence of social anxiety disorder and the consistent risk for secondary depression in the first three decades of life. *Archivs of General Psychiatry, 64*(8), 903-12.

Beesdo, K., Knappe, S., & Pine, D. S. (2009). Anxiety and anxiety disorders in children and adolescents: Developmental issues and implications for DSM-V. *Psychiatric Clinics of North America, 32*(3), 483-524.

Behnken, M. P., Abraham, W. T., Cutrona, C. E., Russell, D. W., Simons, R. L., & Gibbons, F. X. (2014). Linking early ADHD to adolescent and early adult outcomes among African Americans. *Journal of Criminal Justice, 42*(2), 95–103. https://doi.org/10.1016/j.jcrimjus.2013.12.005

Beidas, R. S., Benjamin, C. L., Puleo, C. M., Edmunds, J. M., & Kendall, P. C. (2010). Flexible applications of the coping cat program for anxious youth. *Cognitive and Behavioral Practice, 17*(2), 142-153. https://doi.org/10.1016/j.cbpra.2009.11.002

Beidel, D. C., & Roberson-Nay, R. (2005). Treating childhood social phobia: Social Effectiveness Therapy for Children. In E. D. Hibbs & P. S. Jensen (Eds.), *Psychosocial treatments for child and adolescent disorders* (2nd ed., pp. 75-96). American Psychological Association.

Beidel, D. C., Turner, S. M., & Morris, T. L. (2000). Behavioral treatment of childhood social phobia. *Journal of Consulting and Clinical Psychology, 68*(6), 1072-80.

Beidel, D. C., Turner, S. M., Young, B., & Paulson, A. (2005). Social Effectiveness Therapy for Children: Three-year follow-up. *Journal of Consulting and Clinical Psychology, 73*(4), 721-25.

Beidel, D. C., Turner, S. M., & Young, B. J. (2006). Social Effectiveness Therapy for Children: Five years later. *Behavior Therapy, 37*(4), 416-25.

Bender, P. K., Pons, F., Harris, P. L., Esbjørn, B. H., & Reinholdt-Dunne, M. L. (2015). Emotion understanding in clinically anxious children: A preliminary investigation. *Frontiers in Psychology, 6,* 1916.

Bender, P. K., Reinholdt-Dunne, M. L., Esbjørn, B. H., & Pons, F. (2012). Emotion dysregulation and anxiety in children and adolescents: Gender differences. *Personality and Individual Differences, 53*(3), 284-88.

Bender, P. K., Sømhovd, M., Pons, F., Reinholdt-Dunne, M. L., & Esbjørn, B. H. (2015). The impact of attachment security and emotion dysregulation on anxiety in children and adolescents. *Emotional & Behavioural Difficulties, 20*(2), 189-204.

Bennett, D. C., Modrowski, C. A., Chaplo, S. D., & Kerig, P. K. (2016). Facets of emotion dysregulation as mediators of the association between trauma exposure and posttraumatic stress symptoms in justice-involved adolescents. *Traumatology, 22*(3), 174-83. https://doi.org/10.1037/trm0000085

Bennett, D. C., Modrowski, C. A., Kerig, P. K., & Chaplo, S. D. (2015). Investigating the dissociative subtype of posttraumatic stress disorder in a sample of traumatized detained youth. *Psychological Trauma: Theory, Research, Practice, and Policy, 7*(5), 465-72. https://doi.org/10.1037/tra0000057

Berge, J. M., Wall, M., Larson, N., Eisenberg, M. E., Loth, K. A., & Neumark-Sztainer, D. (2014). The unique and additive associations of family functioning and parenting practices with disordered eating behaviors in diverse adolescents. *Journal of Behavioral Medicine, 37*(2), 205-17. https://doi.org/10.1007/s10865-012-9478-1

Berg-Nielsen, T. S., Vikan, A., & Dahl, A. A. (2002). Parenting related to child and parental psychopathology: A descriptive review of the literature. *Clinical Child Psychology and Psychiatry, 7*(4), 529-52. https://doi.org/10.1177/1359104502007004006

Bernal, A. T., & Coolhart, D. (2012). Treatment and ethical considerations with transgender children and youth in family therapy. *Journal of Family Psychotherapy, 23*(4), 287-303. https://doi.org/10.1080/08975353.2012.735594

Berner, L. A., & Kaye, W. H. (2017). Disturbances of the central nervous system in anorexia nervosa and bulimia nervosa. In K. D. Brownell & B. T. Walsh (Eds.), *Eating disorders and obesity: A comprehensive handbook* (pp. 265-70). Guilford.

Berner, L. A., & Marsh, R. (2014). Frontostriatal circuits and the development of bulimia nervosa. *Frontiers in Behavioral Neuroscience, 8,* 395.

Bert, F., Gualano, M. R., Camussi, E., & Siliquini, R. (2016). Risks and threats of social media websites: Twitter and the proana movement. *Cyberpsychology, Behavior, and Social Net-*

working, 19(4), 233-38. https://doi.org/10.1089/cyber.2015.0553

Bethge, E. (2000). *Dietrich Bonhoeffer: A biography; theologian, Christian, man for his times.* Fortress Press.

Bhide, S., Sciberras, E., Anderson, V., Hazell, P., & Nicholson, J. M. (2017). Association between parenting style and social outcomes in children with and without attention-deficit/hyperactivity disorder: An 18-month longitudinal study. *Journal of Developmental and Behavioral Pediatrics, 38*(6), 369-77. https://doi.org/10.1097/DBP.0000000000000453

Biederman, J., Faraone, S., Mick, E., Wozniak, J., Chen, L., Ouellette, C., Marrs, A., Moore, P., Garcia, J., Mennin, D., & Lelon, E. (1996). Attention-deficit hyperactivity disorder and juvenile mania: An overlooked comorbidity? *Journal of the American Academy of Child and Adolescent Psychiatry, 35*(8), 997-1008.

Biederman, J., Faraone, S. V., & Monuteaux, M. C. (2002a). Differential effect of environmental adversity by gender: Rutter's index of adversity in a group of boys and girls with and without ADHD. *The American Journal of Psychiatry, 159*(9), 1556-62. https://doi.org/10.1176/appi.ajp.159.9.1556

Biederman, J., Faraone, S. V., & Monuteaux, M. C. (2002b). Impact of exposure to parental attention-deficit hyperactivity disorder on clinical features and dysfunction in the offspring. *Psychological Medicine, 32*(5), 817-27. https://doi.org/10.1017/S0033291702005652

Biederman, J., Melmed, R. D., Patel, A., McBurnett, K., Konow, J., Lyne, A., & Scherer, N. (2008). A randomized, double-blind, placebo-controlled study of guanfacine extended release in children and adolescents with attention-deficit/hyperactivity disorder. *Pediatrics, 121*(1), 73-84. https://doi.org/10.1542/peds.2006-3695

Biederman, J., Mick, E., & Faraone, S. V. (2000). Age-dependent decline of symptoms of attention deficit hyperactivity disorder: Impact of remission definition and symptom type. *The American Journal of Psychiatry, 157*(5), 816-18. https://doi.org/10.1176/appi.ajp.157.5.816

Biederman, J., Milberger, S., Faraone, S. V., Kiely, K., Guite, J., Mick, E., Ablon, S., Warburton, R., & Reed, E. (1995). Family-environment risk factors for attention-deficit hyperactivity disorder: A test of Rutter's indicators of adversity. *Archives of General Psychiatry, 52*(6), 464-70. https://doi.org/10.1001/archpsyc.1995.03950180050007

Biederman, J., Petty, C. R., Dolan, C., Hughes, S., Mick, E., Monuteaux, M. C., & Faraone, S. V. (2008). The long-term longitudinal course of oppositional defiant disorder and conduct disorder in ADHD boys: Findings from a controlled 10-year prospective longitudinal follow-up. *Psychological Medicine, 38*(7), 1027-36.

Biederman, J., Petty, C. R., Fried, R., Woodworth, K. Y., & Faraone, S. V. (2014). Is the diagnosis of ADHD influenced by time of entry to school? An examination of clinical, familial, and functional correlates in children at early and late entry points. *Journal of Attention Disorders, 18*(3), 179–185. https://doi.org/10.1177/1087054712445061

Biederman, J., Petty, C. R., Hirshfeld-Becker, D. R., Henin, A., Faraone, S. V., Fraire, M., Henry, B., McQuade, J., & Rosenbaum, J. F. (2007). Developmental trajectories of anxiety disorders in offspring at high risk for panic disorder and major depression. *Psychiatry Research, 153*(3), 245–252. https://doi.org/10.1016/j.psychres.2007.02.016

BigFoot, D. S., & Schmidt, S. R. (2012). American Indian and Alaska Native children: Honoring children—Mending the circle. In J. A. Cohen, A. P. Mannarino, & E. Deblinger (Eds.), *Trauma-focused CBT for children and adolescents: Treatment applications* (pp. 280-300). Guilford Press.

Billstedt, E., Gillberg, I. C., & Gillberg, C. (2007). Autism in adults: Symptom patterns and early childhood predictors. Use of the DISCO in a community sample followed from childhood. *Journal of Child Psychology and Psychiatry, 48*(11), 1102-10. https://doi.org/10.1111/j.1469-7610.2007.01774.x

Binder, E. B., Bradley, R. G., Liu, W., Epstein, M. P., Deveau, T. C., Mercer, K. B., Tang, Y., Gillespie, C. F., Heim, C. M., Nemeroff, C. B., Schwartz, A. C., Cubells, J. F., & Ressler, K. J. (2008). Association of FKBP5 polymorphisms and childhood abuse with risk of posttraumatic stress disorder symptoms in adults. *JAMA, 299*(11), 1291–1305. https://doi.org/10.1001/jama.299.11.1291

Birmaher, B. (2013). Bipolar disorder in children and adolescents. *Child and Adolescent Mental Health, 18*(3), 140-48.

Birmaher, B., Brent, D. A., Chiappetta, L., Bridge, J., Monga, S., & Baugher, M. (1999). Psychometric properties of the Screen for Child Anxiety Related Emotional Disorders (SCARED): A replication study. *Journal of the American Academy of Child and Adolescent Psychiatry, 38*(10), 1230-36.

Birmaher, B., & Sakolsky, D. (2013). Pharmacological treatment of anxiety disorders in children and adolescents. In C. A. Essau & T. H. Ollendick (Eds.), *The Wiley-Blackwell handbook of the treatment of childhood and adolescent anxiety* (pp. 229-48). Wiley-Blackwell.

Birmaher, B., Williamson, D. E., Dahl, R. E., Axelson, D. A., Kaufman, J., Dorn, L. D., & Ryan, N. D. (2004). Clinical presentation and course of depression in youth: Does onset in childhood differ from onset in adolescence? *Journal of the American Academy of Child & Adolescent Psychiatry, 43*(1), 63-70.

Bitsko, R., Holbrook, J., Ghandour, R., Blumberg, S., Visser, S., Perou, R., & Walkup, J. (2018). Epidemiology and impact of health care provider–diagnosed anxiety and depression among us children. *Journal of Developmental & Behavioral Pediatrics, 39*(5), 395-403. https://doi.org/10.1097/DBP.0000000000000571

Black, B. T., Soden, S. E., Kearns, G. L., & Jones, B. L. (2016). Clinical and pharmacologic considerations for guanfacine use in very young children. *Journal of Child and Adolescent Psychopharmacology, 26*(6), 498-504. https://doi.org/10.1089/cap.2014.0159

Black, P. J., Woodworth, M., Tremblay, M., & Carpenter, T. (2012). A review of trauma-informed treatment for adolescents. *Canadian Psychology/Psychologie Canadienne, 53*(3), 192-203. https://doi.org/10.1037/a0028441

Blain-Arcaro, C., & Vaillancourt, T. (2019). Longitudinal associations between externalizing problems and symptoms of depression in children and adolescents. *Journal of Clinical Child and Adolescent Psychology, 48*(1), 108-19. https://doi.org/10.1080/15374416.2016.1270830

Blastland, M. (2006) *The only boy in the world: A father explores the mysteries of autism.* Marlowe and Company.

Blumberg, H. P., Fredericks, C., Wang, F., Kalmar, J. H., Spencer, L., Papademetris, X., Pittman, B., Martin, A., Peterson, B. S., Fulbright, R. K., & Krystal, J. H. (2005). Preliminary evidence for persistent abnormalities in amygdala volumes in adolescents and young adults with bipolar disorder. *Bipolar Disorders, 7*(6), 570-76.

Boase, E. (2014). The traumatized body: Communal trauma and somatization in lamentations. In E. M. Becker, J. Dochhorn, & E. K. Holt (Eds.), *Trauma and traumatization in individual and collective dimensions: Insights from biblical studies and beyond* (pp. 193-209). Vandenhoeck & Ruprecht.

Boden, J. M., Fergusson, D. M., & Horwood, L. J. (2010). Risk factors for conduct disorder and oppositional/defiant disorder: evidence from a New Zealand birth cohort. *Journal of the*

American Academy of Child and Adolescent Psychiatry, 49(11), 1125–1133. https://doi.org/10.1016/j.jaac.2010.08.005

Boggs, S. R., Eyberg, S. M., Edwards, D., Rayfield, A., Jacobs, J., Bagner, D., & Hood, K. (2004). Outcomes of parent-child interaction therapy: A comparison of dropouts and treatment completers one to three years after treatment. *Child and Family Behavior Therapy, 26*, 1-22.

Bolton, D., Hill, J., O'Ryan, D., Udwin, O., Boyle, S., & Yule, W. (2004). Long-term effects of psychological trauma on psychosocial functioning. *Journal of Child Psychology and Psychiatry, 45*(5), 1007-14. https://doi.org/10.1111/j.1469-7610.2004.t01-1-00292.x

Bonander, C., Beckman, L., Janson, S., & Jernbro, C. (2016). Injury risks in schoolchildren with attention-deficit/hyperactivity or autism spectrum disorder: Results from two school-based health surveys of 6- to 17-year-old children in Sweden. *Journal of Safety Research, 58,* 49-56. https://doi.org/10.1016/j.jsr.2016.06.004

Bonhoeffer, D. (1954). *Life together.* Harper & Row.

Bonhoeffer, D. (2012). Overcoming fear. In I. Best (Ed)., *The collected sermons of Dietrich Bonhoeffer* (pp. 59-66). Fortress Press.

Boone, L., Soenens, B., Braet, C., & Goossens, L. (2010). An empirical typology of perfectionism in early-to-mid adolescents and its relation with eating disorder symptoms. *Behaviour Research and Therapy, 48*(7), 686-91. https://doi.org/10.1016/j.brat.2010.03.022

Borduin, C. M., Mann, B. J., Cone, L. T., Henggeler, S. W., Fucci, B. R., Blaske, D. M., & Williams, R. A. (1995). Multisystemic treatment of serious juvenile offenders: Long-term prevention of criminality and violence. *Journal of Consulting and Clinical Psychology, 63*(4), 569-78. https://doi.org/10.1037/0022-006X.63.4.569

Borquist-Conlon, D., Maynard, B., Brendel, K., & Farina, A. (2019). Mindfulness-based interventions for youth with anxiety: A systematic review and meta-analysis. *Research on Social Work Practice, 29*(2), 195-205.

Borzekowski, D. G., Schenk, S., Wilson, J. L., & Peebles, R. (2010). e-Ana and e-Mia: A content analysis of pro–eating disorder web sites. *American Journal of Public Health, 100*(8), 1526-34. https://doi.org/10.2105/AJPH.2009.172700

Bosquet, M., & Egeland, B. (2006). The development and maintenance of anxiety symptoms from infancy through adolescence in a longitudinal sample. *Development and Psychopathology, 18*(2), 517-50.

Bowlby, J. (1989). The role of attachment in personality development and psychopathology. In S. Greenspan & G. Pollock (Eds.), *The course of life* (Vol. 1, pp. 229-70). International Universities Press.

Boyatzis, C. J., & McConnell, K. M. (2006). Quest orientation in young women: age trends during emerging adulthood and relations to body image and disordered eating. *The International Journal for the Psychology of Religion, 16*(3), 197-207.

Boyle, C. A., Boulet, S., Schieve, L. A., Cohen, R. A., Blumberg, S. J., Yeargin-Allsopp, M., Visser, S., & Kogan, M. D. (2011). Trends in the prevalence of developmental disabilities in US children, 1997–2008. *Pediatrics, 127*(6), 1034-42. https://doi.org/10.1542/peds.2010-2989

Bralten, J., Franke, B., Waldman, I., Rommelse, N., Hartman, C., Asherson, P., Banaschewski, T., Ebstein, R. P., Gill, M., Miranda, A., Oades, R. D., Roeyers, H., Rothenberger, A., Sergeant, J. A., Oosterlaan, J., Sonuga-Barke, E., Steinhausen, H.-C., Faraone, S. V., Buitelaar, J. K., & Arias-Vasquez, A. (2013). Candidate genetic pathways for attention-deficit/hyperactivity disorder (ADHD) show association to hyperactive/impulsive symptoms in children with ADHD. *Journal of the American Academy of Child and Adolescent Psychiatry, 52*(11), 1204-12.

Brand, S., Wilhelm, F. H., Kossowsky, J., Holsboer-Trachsler, E., & Schneider, S. (2011). Children suffering from separation anxiety disorder (SAD) show increased HPA axis activity compared to healthy controls. *Journal of Psychiatric Research, 45*(4), 452-59.

Brazelton, T. (2013). *Learning to listen: A life caring for children.* Da Capo Press.

Breaux, R. P., & Harvey, E. A. (2019). A longitudinal study of the relation between family functioning and preschool ADHD symptoms. *Journal of Clinical Child and Adolescent Psychology, 48*(5), 749-64. https://doi.org/10.1080/15374416.2018.1437737

Breaux, R. P., Harvey, E. A., & Lugo-Candelas, C. I. (2014). The role of parent psychopathology in the development of preschool children with behavior problems. *Journal of Clinical Child and Adolescent Psychology, 43*(5), 777-90.

Breithaupt, L., Eickman, L., Byrne, C. E., & Fischer, S. (2017a). Enhancing empowerment in eating disorder prevention: Another examination of the REbeL peer education model. *Eating Behaviors, 25,* 38-41. https://doi.org/10.1016/j.eatbeh.2016.05.003

Breithaupt, L., Eickman, L., Byrne, C. E., & Fischer, S. (2017b). REbeL Peer Education: A model of a voluntary, after-school program for eating disorder prevention. *Eating Behaviors, 25,* 32-37. https://doi.org/10.1016/j.eatbeh.2016.08.003

Breithaupt, L., Eickman, L., Byrne, C. E., & Fischer, S. (2019). REbeL Peer Education: A model of a voluntary, after-school program for eating disorder prevention. *Eating Behaviors, 32,* 111-16. https://doi.org/10.1016/j.eatbeh.2016.10.010

Bremner, J. D. (2006). Stress and brain atrophy. *CNS & Neurological Disorders—Drug Targets, 5*(5), 503-12.

Briere, J., Johnson, K., Bissada, A., Damon, L., Crouch, J., Gil, E., Hanson, R., & Ernst, V. (2001). The trauma symptom checklist for young children (TSCYC): Reliability and association with abuse exposure in a multi-site study. *Child Abuse & Neglect, 25*(8), 1001-14. https://doi.org/10.1016/S0145-2134(01)00253-8

Brion, M., Victora, C., Matijasevich, A., Horta, B., Anselmi, L., Steer, C., Menezes, A. M. B., Lawlor, D. A., & Smith, G. D. (2010). Maternal smoking and child psychological problems: Disentangling causal and noncausal effects. *Pediatrics, 126*(1), e57-e65. https://doi.org/10.1542/peds.2009-2754

Broderick, P. C., & Korteland, C. (2002). Coping style and depression in early adolescence: Relationships to gender, gender role, and implicit beliefs. *Sex Roles, 46*(7-8), 201-13.

Broeren, S., Muris, P., Diamantopoulou, S., & Baker, J. R. (2013). The course of childhood anxiety symptoms: Developmental trajectories and child-related factors in normal children. *Journal of Abnormal Child Psychology, 41*(1), 81-95.

Bronfenbrenner, U. (1979). *The ecology of human development: Experiments by nature and design.* Harvard University Press.

Brookings, J. B., & Wilson, J. F. (1994). Personality and family-environment predictors of self-reported eating attitudes and behaviors. *Journal of Personality Assessment, 63*(2), 313-26. https://doi.org/10.1207/s15327752jpa6302_10

Brouillard, C., Brendgen, M., Vitaro, F., Dionne, G., & Boivin, M. (2018). Links between the mother–adolescent and father–adolescent relationships and adolescent depression: A genetically informed study. *Journal of Clinical Child and Adolescent Psychology, 47*(Suppl 1), S397–S408. https://doi.org/10.1080/15374416.2017.1350964

Brown, A. D., Becker-Weidman, E., & Saxe, G. N. (2014). A developmental perspective on childhood traumatic stress. In M. J. Friedman,

T. M. Keane, & P. A. Resick (Eds.), *Handbook of PTSD: Science and practice* (2nd ed., pp. 331-50). Guilford Press.

Brumariu, L. E., Kerns, K. A., & Seibert, A. (2012). Mother–child attachment, emotion regulation, and anxiety symptoms in middle childhood. *Personal Relationships, 19*(3), 569-85.

Bryant-Waugh, R. J., Cooper, P. J., Taylor, C. L., & Lask, B. D. (1996). The use of the eating disorder examination with children: A pilot study. *International Journal of Eating Disorders, 19*(4), 391-97. https://doi.org/10.1002/(SICI)1098-108X(199605)19:4<391::AID-EAT6>3.0.CO;2-G

Buckingham-Howes, S., Armstrong, B., Pejsa-Reitz, M. C., Wang, Y., Witherspoon, D. O., Hager, E. R., & Black, M. M. (2018). BMI and disordered eating in urban, African American, adolescent girls: The mediating role of body dissatisfaction. *Eating Behaviors, 29,* 59-63. https://doi.org/10.1016/j.eatbeh.2018.02.006

Bufferd, S. J., Dougherty, L. R., Carlson, G. A., Rose, S., & Klein, D. N. (2012). Psychiatric disorders in preschoolers: Continuity from ages 3 to 6. *The American Journal of Psychiatry, 169*(11), 1157-64.

Bufferd, S. J., Dougherty, L. R., Olino, T. M., Dyson, M. W., Carlson, G. A., & Klein, D. N. (2018). Temperament distinguishes persistent/recurrent from remitting anxiety disorders across early childhood. *Journal of Clinical Child and Adolescent Psychology, 47*(6), 1004-13. https://doi.org/10.1080/15374416.2016.1212362

Buie, T., Campbell, D. B., Fuchs, G. I., Furuta, G. T., Levy, J., VandeWater, J., Whitaker, A. H., Atkins, D., Bauman, M. L., Beaudet, A. L., Carr, E. G., Gershon, M. D., Hyman, S. L., Jirapinyo, P., Jyonouchi, H., Kooros, K., Kushak, R., Levitt, P., Levy, S., . . . Winter, H. (2010). Evaluation, diagnosis, and treatment of gastrointestinal disorders in individuals with ASDs: A consensus report. *Pediatrics, 125*(Suppl 1), s1-s18. https://doi.org/10.1542/peds.2009-1878C

Bulik, C. M. (2002). Eating disorders in adolescents and young adults. *Child and Adolescent Psychiatric Clinics of North America, 11*(2), 201-18. https://doi.org/10.1016/S1056-4993(01)00004-9

Bulik, C. M., Sullivan, P. F., & Kendler, K. S. (1998). Heritability of binge-eating and broadly defined bulimia nervosa. *Biological Psychiatry, 44*(12), 1210-18. https://doi.org/10.1016/S0006-3223(98)00280-7

Bulik, C. M., Sullivan, P. F., Tozzi, F., Furberg, H., Lichtenstein, P., & Pedersen, N. L. (2006). Prevalence, heritability, and prospective risk factors for anorexia nervosa. *Archives of General Psychiatry, 63*(3), 305-12. https://doi.org/10.1001/archpsyc.63.3.305

Bullitt-Jonas, M. (1999). *Holy hunger: A memoir of desire.* A. A. Knopf.

Bunte, T. L., Laschen, S., Schoemaker, K., Hessen, D. J., van der Heijden, P. M., & Matthys, W. (2013). Clinical usefulness of observational assessment in the diagnosis of DBD and ADHD in preschoolers. *Journal of Clinical Child and Adolescent Psychology, 42*(6), 749-61. https://doi.org/10.1080/15374416.2013.773516

Bunte, T. L., Schoemaker, K., Hessen, D. J., van der Heijden, P. M., & Matthys, W. (2014). Stability and change of ODD, CD and ADHD diagnosis in referred preschool children. *Journal of Abnormal Child Psychology, 42*(7), 1213-24. https://doi.org/10.1007/s10802-014-9869-6

Burke, J. D., Pardini, D. A., & Loeber, R. (2008). Reciprocal relationships between parenting behavior and disruptive psychopathology from childhood through adolescence. *Journal of Abnormal Child Psychology, 36*(5), 679-92. https://doi.org/10.1007/s10802-008-9219-7

Buss, K. A., & Kiel, E. J. (2011). Do maternal protective behaviors alleviate toddlers' fearful distress? *International Journal of Behavioral Development, 35*(2), 136-43.

Busso, D. S., McLaughlin, K. A., & Sheridan, M. A. (2014). Media exposure and sympathetic nervous system reactivity predict PTSD symptoms after the Boston Marathon bombings. *Depression and Anxiety, 31*(7), 551-58. https://doi.org/10.1002/da.22282

Butcher, F., Galanek, J. D., Kretschmar, J. M., & Flannery, D. J. (2015). The impact of neighborhood disorganization on neighborhood exposure to violence, trauma symptoms, and social relationships among at-risk youth. *Social Science & Medicine, 146*, 300-306.

Butler, L. D., & Nolen-Hoeksema, S. (1994). Gender differences in responses to depressed mood in a college sample. *Sex Roles, 30*(5-6), 331-46.

Button, E. J., Chadalavada, B., & Palmer, R. L. (2010). Mortality and predictors of death in a cohort of patients presenting to an eating disorders service. *International Journal of Eating Disorders, 43*(5), 387-92.

Butzlaff, R. L., & Hooley, J. M. (1998). Expressed emotion and psychiatric relapse: a meta-analysis. *Archives of General Psychiatry, 55*(6), 547-52.

Cadman, T., Findon, J., Eklund, H., Hayward, H., Howley, D., Cheung, C., Kuntsi, J., Glaser, K., Murphy, D., & Asherson, P. (2016). Six-year follow-up study of combined type ADHD from childhood to young adulthood: Predictors of functional impairment and comorbid symptoms. *European Psychiatry, 35,* 47-54. https://doi.org/10.1016/j.eurpsy.2015.08.007

Caglayan, A. O. (2010). Genetic causes of syndromic and non-syndromic autism. *Developmental Medicine and Child Neurology, 52*(2), 130–138. https://doi.org/10.1111/j.1469-8749.2009.03523.x

Calati, R., Pedrini, L., Alighieri, S., Alvarez, M. I., Desideri, L., Durante, D., Favero, F., Lero, L., Magnani, G., Pericoli, V., Polmonari, A., Raggini, R., Raimondi, E., Riboni, V., Scaduto, M. C., Serretti, A., & De Girolamo, G. (2011). Is cognitive behavioural therapy an effective complement to antidepressants in adolescents? A meta-analysis. *Acta Neuropsychiatrica, 23*(6), 263-71.

Calhoun, B. H., Ridenour, T. A., & Fishbein, D. H. (2019). Associations between child maltreatment, harsh parenting, and sleep with adolescent mental health. *Journal of Child and Family Studies, 28*(1), 116-30. https://doi.org/10.1007/s10826-018-1261-7

Callens, N., Van Kuyk, M., van Kuppenveld, J. H., Drop, S. S., Cohen-Kettenis, P. T., & Dessens, A. B. (2016). Recalled and current gender role behavior, gender identity and sexual orientation in adults with Disorders/Differences of Sex Development. *Hormones and Behavior, 86*, 8-20. https://doi.org/10.1016/j.yhbeh.2016.08.008

Calvin, J. (1847–1850). *Calvin's Commentaries, Vol. 8: Psalms, Part I* (John King, Trans.). Retrieved from http://www.sacred-texts.com/chr/calvin/cc08/cc08013.htm

Campbell, J. M., Ruble, L. A., & Hammond, R. K. (2014). Comprehensive developmental assessment model. In L. A. Wilkinson (Ed.), *Autism spectrum disorder in children and adolescents: Evidence-based assessment and intervention in schools* (pp. 51-73). American Psychological Association. https://doi.org/10.1037/14338-004

Campbell, K., & Peebles, R. (2014). Eating disorders in children and adolescents: State of the art review. *Pediatrics, 134*(3), 582-92. https://doi.org/10.1542/peds.2014-0194

Campbell, S. B., Leezenbaum, N. B., Mahoney, A. S., Day, T. N., & Schmidt, E. N. (2015). Social engagement with parents in 11-month-old siblings at high and low genetic risk for autism spectrum disorder. *Autism, 19*(8), 915-24. https://doi.org/10.1177/1362361314555146

Canals, J., Sancho, C., & Arija, M. V. (2009). Influence of parent's eating attitudes on eating disorders in school adolescents. *European Child & Adolescent Psychiatry, 18*(6), 353-59. https://doi.org/10.1007/s00787-009-0737-9

Cannon, M. F., & Weems, C. F. (2010). Cognitive biases in childhood anxiety disorders: Do interpretive and judgment biases distinguish anxious youth from their non-anxious peers? *Journal of Anxiety Disorders, 24*(7), 751-58.

Capaldi, D. M., & Patterson, G. R. (1994). Interrelated influences of contextual factors on antisocial behavior in childhood and adolescence for males. *Progress in Experimental Personality & Psychopathology Research*, 165-98.

Carlson, E. A., Jacobvitz, D., & Sroufe, L. A. (1995). A developmental investigation of inattentiveness and hyperactivity. *Child Development, 66*(1), 37-54. https://doi.org/10.2307/1131189

Carr, D. M. (2014). *Holy resilience: The Bible's traumatic origins*. Yale University Press.

Carter, A. S., Godoy, L., Wagmiller, R. L., Veliz, P., Marakovitz, S., & Briggs-Gowan, M. J. (2010). Internalizing trajectories in young boys and girls: The whole is not a simple sum of its parts. *Journal of Abnormal Child Psychology, 38*(1), 19-31.

Carter, J. S., & Garber, J. (2011). Predictors of the first onset of a major depressive episode and changes in depressive symptoms across adolescence: Stress and negative cognitions. *Journal of Abnormal Psychology, 120*(4), 779-96.

Carthy, T., Horesh, N., Apter, A., & Gross, J. J. (2010). Patterns of emotional reactivity and regulation in children with anxiety disorders. *Journal of Psychopathology and Behavioral Assessment, 32*(1), 23-36.

Castellanos, F. X., Lee, P. P., Sharp, W., Jeffries, N. O., Greenstein, D. K., Clasen, L. S., Blumenthal, J., D., James, R. S., Ebens, C. L., Walter, J. M.,

Zijdenbos, A., Evans, A. C., Giedd, J. N., & Rapoport, J. L. (2002). Developmental trajectories of brain volume abnormalities in children and adolescents with attention-deficit/hyperactivity disorder. *Journal of the American Medical Association, 288*(14), 1740-48.

Castro, J., Gila, A., Gual, P., Lahortiga, F., Saura, B., & Toro, J. (2004). Perfectionism dimensions in children and adolescents with anorexia nervosa. *Journal of Adolescent Health, 35*(5), 392-98. https://doi.org/10.1016/j.jadohealth.2003.11.094

Castro-Fornieles, J., Gual, P., Lahortiga, F., Gila, A., Casulà, V., Fuhrmann, C., Imirizaldu, M., Saura, B., Martínez, E., & Toro, J. (2007). Self-oriented perfectionism in eating disorders. *International Journal of Eating Disorders, 40*(6), 562-68. https://doi.org/10.1002/eat.20393

Cautela, J. R., & Kearney, A. J. (1986). *The covert conditioning handbook*. Springer.

Cénat, J. M., & Derivois, D. (2015). Long-term outcomes among child and adolescent survivors of the 2010 Haitian earthquake. *Depression and Anxiety, 32*(1), 57-63. https://doi.org/10.1002/da.22275

Cervera, S., Lahortiga, F., Martínez-González, M. A., Gual, P., Irala-Estévez, J. D., & Alonso, Y. (2003). Neuroticism and low self-esteem as risk factors for incident eating disorders in a prospective cohort study. *International Journal of Eating Disorders, 33*(3), 271-80. https://doi.org/10.1002/eat.10147

Chacko, A., Wymbs, B. T., Wymbs, F. A., Pelham, W. E., Swanger-Gagne, M. S., Girio, E., Pirvics, L., Herbst, L., Guzzo, J., Phillips, C., & O'Connor, B. (2009). Enhancing traditional behavioral parent training for single mothers of children with ADHD. *Journal of Clinical Child and Adolescent Psychology, 38*(2), 206-18. https://doi.org/10.1080/15374410802698388

Chamberlain, P., Reid, J. B., Ray, J., Capaldi, D., & Fisher, P. (1997). Parent inadequate discipline.

In T. A. Widiger, A. J. Frances, H. A. Pincus, R. Ross, M. B. First, & W. Davis (Eds.), *DSM-IV source book* (Vol. 3, pp. 560-629). American Psychiatric Association.

Chambless, D. L., & Hollon, S. D. (1998). Defining empirically supported therapies. *Journal of Consulting and Clinical Psychology, 66*(1), 7-18. https://doi.org/10.1037/0022-006X.66.1.7

Chan, E., Fogler, J. M., & Hammerness, P. G. (2016). Treatment of attention-deficit/hyperactivity disorder in adolescents: A systematic review. *JAMA: Journal of the American Medical Association, 315*(18), 1997-2008. https://doi.org/10.1001/jama.2016.5453

Chang, C., Kaczkurkin, A. N., McLean, C. P., & Foa, E. B. (2018). Emotion regulation is associated with PTSD and depression among female adolescent survivors of childhood sexual abuse. *Psychological Trauma: Theory, Research, Practice, and Policy, 10*(3), 319-26. https://doi.org/10.1037/tra0000306

Chang, Z., Lichtenstein, P., Asherson, P. J., & Larsson, H. (2013). Developmental twin study of attention problems: High heritabilities throughout development. *Jama Psychiatry, 70*(3), 311-18. https://doi.org/10.1001/jamapsychiatry.2013.287

Chaplo, S. D., Kerig, P. K., Bennett, D. C., & Modrowski, C. A. (2015). The roles of emotion dysregulation and dissociation in the association between sexual abuse and self-injury among juvenile justice–involved youth. *Journal of Trauma & Dissociation, 16*(3), 272.

Chen, D., Edwards-Leeper, L., Stancin, T., & Tishelman, A. (2018). Advancing the practice of pediatric psychology with transgender youth: State of the science, ongoing controversies, and future directions. *Clinical Practice in Pediatric Psychology, 6*(1), 73-83. https://doi.org/10.1037/cpp0000229

Chen, D., Hidalgo, M. A., & Garofalo, R. (2017). Parental perceptions of emotional and behavioral difficulties among prepubertal gender-nonconforming children [Supplemental material]. *Clinical Practice in Pediatric Psychology, 5*(4), 342-52. https://doi.org/10.1037/cpp0000217.supp

Chen, J., Li, X., Natsuaki, M. N., Leve, L. D., & Harold, G. T. (2014). Genetic and environmental influences on depressive symptoms in Chinese adolescents. *Behavior Genetics, 44*, 36-44.

Chen, Q., Brikell, I., Lichtenstein, P., Serlachius, E., Kuja-Halkola, R., Sandin, S., & Larsson, H. (2017). Familial aggregation of attention-deficit/hyperactivity disorder. *Journal of Child Psychology and Psychiatry, 58*(3), 231-39. https://doi.org/10.1111/jcpp.12616

Chen, X., Fu, R., & Leng, L. (2014). Culture and developmental psychopathology. In M. Lewis & K. D. Rudolph (Eds.), *Handbook of developmental psychopathology* (3rd ed., pp. 225-41). Springer. https://doi.org/10.1007/978-1-4614-9608-3

Cherkasova, M., Sulla, E. M., Dalena, K. L., Pondé, M. P., & Hechtman, L. (2013). Developmental course of attention deficit hyperactivity disorder and its predictors. *Journal of the Canadian Academy of Child and Adolescent Psychiatry, 22*(1), 47–54.

Cheung, C. M., Rijdijk, F., McLoughlin, G., Faraone, S. V., Asherson, P., & Kuntsi, J. (2015). Childhood predictors of adolescent and young adult outcome in ADHD. *Journal of Psychiatric Research, 62,* 92-100. https://doi.org/10.1016/j.jpsychires.2015.01.011

Cheung, K., & Theule, J. (2016). Parental psychopathology in families of children with ADHD: A meta-analysis. *Journal of Child and Family Studies, 25*(12), 3451-61. https://doi.org/10.1007/s10826-016-0499-1

Chien, H., Gau, S. S., Hsu, Y., Chen, Y., Lo, Y., Shih, Y., & Tseng, W. I. (2015). Altered cortical thickness and tract integrity of the mirror neuron system and associated social communication in autism spectrum disorder. *Autism*

Research, 8(6), 694-708. https://doi.org/10.1002/aur.1484

Child Anxiety Network. (2007). *I Can Relax! A Relaxation CD for Children* [Album]. http://www.childanxiety.net/I_Can_Relax!_CD_for_Children.htm

Childress, A. C., Brewerton, T. D., Hodges, E. L., & Jarrell, M. P. (1993). The Kids' Eating Disorders Survey (KEDS): A study of middle school students. *Journal of the American Academy of Child & Adolescent Psychiatry, 32*(4), 843-50. https://doi.org/10.1097/00004583-199307000-00021

Chiodo, L. M., Jacobson, S. W., & Jacobson, J. L. (2004). Neurodevelopmental effects of postnatal lead exposure at very low levels. *Neurotoxicology and Teratology, 26*(3), 359-71. https://doi.org/10.1016/j.ntt.2004.01.010

Chorpita, B. F. (2007). *Modular cognitive-behavioral therapy for childhood anxiety disorders.* Guilford.

Chow, C. M., & Tan, C. C. (2018). The role of fat talk in eating pathology and depressive symptoms among mother-daughter dyads. *Body Image, 24,* 36-43. https://doi.org/10.1016/j.bodyim.2017.11.003

Christensen, D. L., Baio, J., Braun, K. V. N., Bilder, D., Charles, J., Constantino, J. N., Daniels, J., Durkin, M. S., Fitzgerald, R. T., Kurzius-Spencer, M., Lee, L., Pettygrove, S., Robinson, C., Schulz, E., Wells, C., Wingate, M. S., Zahorodny, W., & Yeargin-Allsopp, M. (2016). Prevalence and characteristics of autism spectrum disorder among children aged 8 years—Autism and Developmental Disabilities Monitoring Network, 11 Sites, United States, 2012. *Morbidity and Mortality Weekly Report Surveillance Summaries, 65*(SS-3), 1-23. https://doi.org/10.15585/mmwr.ss6503a1

Christensen, J., Grønborg, T. K., Sørensen, M. J., Schendel, D., Parner, E. T., Pedersen, L. H., & Vestergaard, M. (2013). Prenatal valproate exposure and risk of autism spectrum disorders and childhood autism. *JAMA: Journal of the American Medical Association, 309*(16), 1696-1703. https://doi.org/10.1001/jama.2013.2270

Chronis, A. M., Lahey, B. B., Pelham, W. J., Williams, S. H., Baumann, B. L., Kipp, H., Jones, H. A., & Rathouz, P. J. (2007). Maternal depression and early positive parenting predict future conduct problems in young children with attention-deficit/hyperactivity disorder. *Developmental Psychology, 43*(1), 70-82. https://doi.org/10.1037/0012-1649.43.1.70

Chronis-Tuscano, A., Molina, B. S. G., Pelham, W. E., Applegate, B., Dahlke, A., Overmyer, M., & Lahey, B. B. (2010). Very early predictors of adolescent depression and suicide attempts in children with attention-deficit/hyperactivity disorder. *Archives of General Psychiatry, 67*(10), 1044–1051. https://doi.org/10.1001/archgen-psychiatry.2010.127

Cicchetti, D. (2006). Development and psychopathology. In D. Cicchetti & D. J. Cohen (Eds.), *Developmental psychopathology: Vol. 1. Theory and method* (2nd ed., pp. 1-23). Wiley & Sons.

Cicchetti, D., & Rogosch, F. A. (1996). Equifinality and multifinality in developmental psychopathology. *Development and Psychopathology, 8*(4), 597-600.

Cicchetti, D., & Rogosch, F. A. (2014). Genetic moderation of child maltreatment effects on depression and internalizing symptoms by serotonin transporter linked polymorphic region (5-HTTLPR), brain-derived neurotrophic factor (BDNF), norepinephrine transporter (NET), and corticotropin releasing hormone receptor 1 (CRHR1) genes in African American children. *Development and Psychopathology, 26,* 1219-39.

Cicero, D. C., Epler, A. J., & Sher, K. J. (2009). Are there developmentally limited forms of bipolar disorder? *Journal of Abnormal Psychology, 118*(3), 431-47.

Cisler, J. M., Sigel, B. A., Kramer, T. L., Smith-erman, S., Vanderzee, K., Pemberton, J., & Kilts, C. D. (2015). Amygdala response predicts trajectory of symptom reduction during Trauma-Focused Cognitive-Behavioral Therapy among adolescent girls with PTSD. *Journal of Psychiatric Research, 71,* 33-40.

Clark, D. B., Cornelius, J., Wood, D. S., & Vanyukov, M. (2004). Psychopathology risk transmission in children of parents with substance use disorders. *American Journal of Psychiatry, 161*(4), 685-91.

Clayborne, Z. M., Varin, M., & Colman, I. (2019). Systematic review and meta-analysis: Adolescent depression and long-term psychosocial outcomes. *Journal of the American Academy of Child & Adolescent Psychiatry, 58*(1), 72-79. https://doi.org/10.1016/j.jaac.2018.07.896

Cloitre, M., Stolbach, B. C., Herman, J. L., van der Kolk, B., Pynoos, R., Wang, J., & Petkova, E. (2009). A developmental approach to complex PTSD: childhood and adult cumulative trauma as predictors of symptom complexity. *Journal of Traumatic Stress, 22*(5), 399-408.

Coalition for Biblical Sexuality. (2017). Nashville statement. Retrieved from https://cbmw.org/nashville-statement/

Cobb, G. (2017). "This is *not* pro-ana": Denial and disguise in pro-anorexia online spaces. *Fat Studies: An Interdisciplinary Journal of Body Weight and Society, 6*(2), 189-205. http://doi.org/10.1080/21604851.2017.1244801

Cockcroft, K. (2011). Working memory functioning in children with attention-deficit/hyperactivity disorder (ADHD): A comparison between subtypes and normal controls. *Journal of Child and Adolescent Mental Health, 23*(2), 107–118. https://doi.org/10.2989/17280583.2011.634545

Cohen, H., Amerine-Dickens, M., & Smith, T. (2006). Early intensive behavioral treatment: Replication of the UCLA model in a community setting. *Journal of Developmental and Behavioral Pediatrics, 27*(Suppl2), S145-S155. https://doi.org/10.1097/00004703-200604002-00013

Cohen, J. A., Bukstein, O., Walter, H., Benson, S. R., Chrisman, A., Farchione, T. R., Hamilton, J., Keable, H., Kinlan, J., Schoettle, U., Siegel, M., Stock, S., & Medicus, J. (2010). Practice parameter for the assessment and treatment of children and adolescents with posttraumatic stress disorder. *Journal of the American Academy of Child & Adolescent Psychiatry, 49*(4), 414-30. https://doi.org/10.1097/00004583-201004000-00021

Cohen, J. A., Deblinger, E., Mannarino, A. P., & Steer, R. A. (2004). A multisite, randomized controlled trial for children with sexual abuse-related PTSD symptoms. *Journal of the American Academy of Child & Adolescent Psychiatry, 43*(4), 393-402.

Cohen, J. A., & Mannarino, A. P. (1996). A treatment study for sexually abused preschool children: Initial treatment and outcome findings. *Journal of the American Academy of Child and Adolescent Psychiatry, 35*(1), 42-50.

Cohen, J. A., Mannarino, A. P., & Deblinger, E. (2006). *Treating trauma and traumatic grief in children and adolescents.* Guilford.

Cohen, J. A., Mannarino, A. P., & Deblinger, E. (2017). Trauma-focused cognitive-behavioral therapy for traumatized children. In J. R. Weisz & A. E. Kazdin (Eds.), *Evidence-based psychotherapies for children and adolescents* (3rd ed., pp. 253-71). Guilford.

Cohen-Kettenis, P. T., & Arrindell, W. A. (1990). Perceived parental rearing style, parental divorce and transsexualism: A controlled study. *Psychological Medicine, 20*(3), 613-20.

Cohen-Kettenis, P. T., & van Goozen, S. M. (2002). Adolescents who are eligible for sex reassignment surgery: Parental reports of emotional and behavioural problems. *Clinical Child Psychology and Psychiatry, 7*(3), 412-22. https://doi.org/10.1177/1359104502007003008

Cole, D. A., Nolen-Hoeksema, S., Girgus, J. S., & Paul, G. (2006). Stressexposure and stress generation in child and adolescent depression: Alatent trait-state-error approach to longitudinal analysis. *Journal of Abnormal Psychology, 115*, 40–51.

Cole, P. M., Hall, S. E., & Radzioch, A. M. (2009). Emotional dysregulation and the development of serious misconduct. In S. Olson & A. Sameroff (Eds.), *Biopsychosocial regulatory processes in the development of childhood behavior problems* (pp. 186-211). Cambridge University Press.

Cole, P. M., Zahn-Waxler, C., Fox, N. A., Usher, B. A., & Welsh, J. D. (1996). Individual differences in emotion regulation and behavior problems in preschool children. *Journal of Abnormal Psychology, 105*(4), 518-29.

Cole, P. M., Zahn-Waxler, C., & Smith, K. D. (1994). Expressive control during a disappointment: Variations related to preschoolers' behavior problems. *Developmental Psychology, 30*(6), 835-46.

Colonnesi, C., Draijer, E. M., Stams, G. J., Van der Bruggen, C. O., Bögels, S. M., & Noom, M. J. (2011). The relation between insecure attachment and child anxiety: A meta-analytic review. *Journal of Clinical Child and Adolescent Psychology, 40*(4), 630-45.

Comas-Díaz, L. (2006). Cultural variation in the therapeutic relationship. In *Evidence-based psychotherapy: Where practice and research meet* (pp. 81-105). American Psychological Association. https://doi.org/10.1037/11423-004

Comer, J. S., Hong, N., Poznanski, B., Silva, K., & Wilson, M. (2019). Evidence base update on the treatment of early childhood anxiety and related problems. *Journal of Clinical Child and Adolescent Psychology, 48*(1), 1-15. https://doi.org/10.1080/15374416.2018.1534208

Comer, R. J., & Comer, J. S. (2018). *Abnormal psychology* (10th ed.). Worth.

Compas, B. E., Connor-Smith, J., & Jaser, S. S. (2004). Temperament, stress reactivity, and coping: Implications for depression in childhood and adolescence. *Journal of Clinical Child and Adolescent Psychology, 33*(1), 21-31.

Compton, S. N., Kratochvil, C. J., & March, J. S. (2007). Pharmacotherapy for anxiety disorders in children and adolescents: An evidence-based medicine review. *Psychiatric Annals, 37*, 504-17.

Conduct Problems Prevention Research Group. (2011). The effects of the Fast Track preventive intervention on the development of conduct disorder across childhood. *Child Development, 82*(1), 331-45. https://doi.org/10.1111/j.1467-8624.2010.01558.x

Conners, C. K. (2008). *Conners 3rd edition manual*. Multi-Health Systems.

Conners, C. K., Epstein, J. N., March, J. S., Angold, A., Wells, K. C., Klaric, J., Swanson, J., Arnold, L. E., Abikoff, H. B., Elliott, G. R., Greenhill, L. L., Hechtman, L., Hinshaw, S. P., Hoza, B., Jensen, P. S., Kraemer, H. C., Newcorn, J. H., Pelham, W. E., Severe, J. B., . . . Wigal, T. (2001). Multimodal treatment of ADHD in the MTA: An alternative outcome analysis. *Journal of the American Academy of Child & Adolescent Psychiatry, 40*(2), 159-67. https://doi.org/10.1097/00004583-200102000-00010

Connolly, M., Zervos, M., Barone, C., Johnson, C., & Joseph, C. (2016). The mental health of transgender youth: Advances in understanding. *Journal of Adolescent Health, 59*(5), 489-95. https://doi.org/10.1016/j.jadohealth.2016.06.012

Conrad, P., & Bergey, M. R. (2014). The impending globalization of ADHD: Notes on the expansion and growth of a medicalized disorder. *Social Science & Medicine, 122*, 31-43. https://doi.org/10.1016/j.socscimed.2014.10.019

Contractor, A. A., Layne, C. M., Steinberg, A. M., Ostrowski, S. A., Ford, J. D., & Elhai, J. D. (2013). Do gender and age moderate the symptom structure of PTSD? Findings from a national clinical sample of children and adolescents. *Psychiatry Research, 210*(3), 1056-64. https://doi.org/10.1016/j.psychres.2013.09.012

Cook, A., Blaustein, M., Spinazzola, J., & van der Kolk, B. A. (Eds.). (2003). *Complex trauma in children and adolescents*. National Child Traumatic Stress Network. Retrieved from http://www.NCTSNet.org

Cook, A., Spinazzola, J., Ford, J., Lanktree, C., Blaustein, M., Cloitre, M., DeRosa, R., Hubbard, R., Kagan, R., Liautaud, J., Mallah, K., Olafson, E., & van der Kolk, B. (2005). Complex trauma in children and adolescents. *Psychiatric Annals, 35*(5), 390-98.

Cooley, E., Toray, T., Wang, M. C., & Valdez, N. N. (2008). Maternal effects on daughters' eating pathology and body image. *Eating Behaviors, 9*(1), 52-61. https://doi.org/10.1016/j.eatbeh.2007.03.001

Cooper, M., Martin, J., Langley, K., Hamshere, M., & Thapar, A. (2014). Autistic traits in children with ADHD index clinical and cognitive problems. *European Child & Adolescent Psychiatry, 23*(1), 23-34. https://doi.org/10.1007/s00787-013-0398-6

Copeland, W. E., Keeler, G., Angold, A., & Costello, E. J. (2007). Traumatic events and posttraumatic stress in childhood. *Archives of General Psychiatry, 64*(5), 577-84.

Cortese, S., Faraone, S. V., Konofal, E., & Lecendreux, M. (2009). Sleep in children with attention-deficit/hyperactivity disorder: Meta-analysis of subjective and objective studies. *Journal of the American Academy of Child & Adolescent Psychiatry, 48*(9), 894-908. https://doi.org/10.1097/CHI.0b013e3181ae09c9

Costello, E. J., Angold, A., Burns, B. J., Stangl, D. K., Tweed, D. L., Erkanli, A., & Worthman, C. M. (1996). The Great Smoky Mountains Study of Youth. Goals, design, methods, and the prevalence of DSM-III-R disorders. *Archives of General Psychiatry, 53*(12), 1129–1136. https://doi.org/10.1001/archpsyc.1996.01830120067012

Costello, E. J., Erkanli, A., & Angold, A. (2006). Is there an epidemic of child or adolescent depression? *Journal of Child Psychology and Psychiatry, 47*(12), 1263-71.

Costello, E. J., Mustillo, S., Erkanli, A., Keeler, G., & Angold, A. (2003). Prevalence and development of psychiatric disorders in childhood and adolescence. *Archives of General Psychiatry, 60*(8), 837-44.

Côté, S., Vaillancourt, T., LeBlanc, J. C., Nagin, D. S., & Tremblay, R. E. (2006). The development of physical aggression from toddlerhood to pre-adolescence: A nation wide longitudinal study of Canadian children. *Journal of Abnormal Child Psychology, 34*(1), 71-85.

Counts, C. A., Nigg, J. T., Stawicki, J. A., Rappley, M. D., & von Eye, A. (2005). Family adversity in DSM-IV ADHD combined and inattentive subtypes and associated disruptive behavior problems. *Journal of the American Academy of Child and Adolescent Psychiatry, 44*(7), 690–698. https://doi.org/10.1097/01.chi.0000162582.87710.66

Cousino, M. K., Davis, A., Ng, H., & Stancin, T. (2014). An emerging opportunity for pediatric psychologists: Our role in a multidisciplinary clinic for youth with gender dysphoria. *Clinical Practice in Pediatric Psychology, 2*(4), 400-411. https://doi.org/10.1037/cpp0000077

Couturier, J., Kimber, M., & Szatmari, P. (2013). Efficacy of family-based treatment for adolescents with eating disorders: A systematic review and meta-analysis. *International Journal of Eating Disorders, 46*(1), 3-11. https://doi.org/10.1002/eat.22042

Couturier, J., Lock, J., Forsberg, S., Vanderheyden, D., & Lee, H. Y. (2007). The addition of parent and clinician component to the eating disorder examination for children and adolescents. *International Journal of Eating Disorders, 40*(5), 472-75. https://doi.org/10.1002/eat.20379

Craske, M. G., Rauch, S. L., Ursano, R., Prenoveau, J., Pine, D. S., & Zinbarg, R. E. (2009). What is an anxiety disorder? *Depression and Anxiety, 26*(12), 1066-85.

Craske, M. G., Waters, A. M., Lindsey, B. R., Naliboff, B., Lipp, O. V., Negoro, H., & Ornitz, E. M. (2008). Is aversive learning a marker of risk for anxiety disorders in children? *Behaviour Research and Therapy, 46*(8), 954-67.

Crea, T. M., Chan, K., & Barth, R. P. (2014). Family environment and attention-deficit/hyperactivity disorder in adopted children: Associations with family cohesion and adaptability. *Child: Care, Health and Development, 40*(6), 853-62. https://doi.org/10.1111/cch.12112

Creswell, C., & O'Connor, T. G. (2011). Interpretation bias and anxiety in childhood: Stability, specificity and longitudinal associations. *Behavioural and Cognitive Psychotherapy, 39*(2), 191-204.

Crick, N. R., & Dodge, K. A. (1994). A review and reformulation of social information-processing mechanisms in children's social adjustment. *Psychological Bulletin, 115*(1), 74-101.

Croen, L. A., Grether, J. K., Yoshida, C. K., Odouli, R., & Hendrick, V. (2011). Antidepressant use during pregnancy and childhood autism spectrum disorders. *Archives of General Psychiatry, 68*(11), 1104-12. https://doi.org/10.1001/archgenpsychiatry.2011.73

Culbert, K. M., Burt, S. A., McGue, M., Iacono, W. G., & Klump, K. L. (2009). Puberty and the genetic diathesis of disordered eating attitudes and behaviors. *Journal of Abnormal Psychology, 118*(4), 788-96. https://doi.org/10.1037/a0017207

Culpin, I., Stapinski, L., Miles, Ö. B., Araya, R., & Joinson, C. (2015). Exposure to socioeconomic adversity in early life and risk of depression at 18 years: The mediating role of locus of control. *Journal of Affective Disorders, 183*(1), 269-78. https://doi.org/10.1016/j.jad.2015.05.030

Curchack-Lichtin, J. T., Chacko, A., & Halperin, J. M. (2014). Changes in ADHD symptom endorsement: preschool to school age. *Journal of Abnormal Child Psychology, 42*(6), 993–1004. https://doi.org/10.1007/s10802-013-9834-9

Curry, J., Rohde, P., Simons, A., Silva, S., Vitiello, B., Kratochvil, C., Reinecke, M., Feeny, N., Wells, K., Pathak, S., Weller, E., Rosenberg, D., Kennard, B., Robins, M., Ginsburg, G., March, J., & TADS Team (2006). Predictors and moderators of acute outcome in the Treatment for Adolescents with Depression Study (TADS). *Journal of the American Academy of Child and Adolescent Psychiatry, 45*(12), 1427–1439. https://doi.org/10.1097/01.chi.0000240838.78984.e2Curtis, D. F. (2010). ADHD symptom severity following participation in a pilot, 10-week, manualized family-based behavioral intervention. *Child and Family Behavior Therapy, 32*(3), 231-41.

Curtis, N. M., Ronan, K. R., & Borduin, C. M. (2004). Multisystemic treatment: A meta-analysis of outcome studies. *Journal of Family Psychology, 18*(3), 411-19. https://doi.org/10.1037/0893-3200.18.3.411

Daleiden, E. L., & Vasey, M. W. (1997). An information-processing perspective on childhood anxiety. *Clinical Psychology Review, 17*(4), 407-29.

Dalgleish, T., Tchanturia, K., Serpell, L., Hems, S., de Silva, P., & Treasure, J. (2001). Perceived control over events in the world in patients with eating disorders: A preliminary study. *Personality and Individual Differences, 31*, 453-60.

Dalsgaard, S., Kvist, A. P., Leckman, J. F., Nielsen, H. S., & Simonsen, M. (2014). Cardiovascular safety of stimulants in children with attention-deficit/hyperactivity disorder: A nationwide prospective cohort study. *Journal of Child and Adolescent Psychopharmacology*, *24*(6), 302-10. https://doi.org/10.1089/cap.2014.0020

Dalsgaard, S., Østergaard, S. D., Leckman, J. F., Mortensen, P. B., & Pedersen, M. G. (2015). Mortality in children, adolescents, and adults with attention deficit hyperactivity disorder: A nationwide cohort study. *The Lancet*, *385*(9983), 2190-96. https://doi.org/10.1016/S0140-6736(14)61684-6

D'Andrea, W., Ford, J., Stolbach, B., Spinazzola, J., & van der Kolk, B. A. (2012). Understanding interpersonal trauma in children: Why we need a developmentally appropriate trauma diagnosis. *American Journal of Orthopsychiatry*, *82*(2), 187-200. https://doi.org/10.1111/j.1939-0025.2012.01154.x

Danforth, J. S., Harvey, E., Ulaszek, W. R., & McKee, T. E. (2006). The outcome of group parent training for families with attention-deficit hyperactivity disorder and defiant/aggressive behavior. *Journal of Behavior Therapy and Experimental Psychiatry*, *37*(3), 188-205.

Daniels, A. M., Halladay, A. K., Shih, A., Elder, L. M., & Dawson, G. (2014). Approaches to enhancing the early detection of autism spectrum disorders: A systematic review of the literature. *Journal of the American Academy of Child & Adolescent Psychiatry*, *53*(2), 141-52. https://doi.org/10.1016/j.jaac.2013.11.002

Daniels, A. M., & Mandell, D. S. (2014). Explaining differences in age at autism spectrum disorder diagnosis: A critical review. *Autism*, *18*(5), 583-97. https://doi.org/10.1177/1362361313480277

Daniels, J. K., Lamke, J., Gaebler, M., Walter, H., & Scheel, M. (2013). White matter integrity and its relationship to PTSD and childhood trauma—A systematic review and meta-analysis. *Depression and Anxiety*, *30*(3), 207-16. https://doi.org/10.1002/da.22044

Dapretto, M., Davies, M. S., Pfeifer, J. H., Scott, A. A., Sigman, M., Bookheimer, S. Y., & Iacoboni, M. (2006). Understanding emotions in others: Mirror neuron dysfunction in children with autism spectrum disorders. *Nature Neuroscience*, *9*(1), 28-30. https://doi.org/10.1038/nn1611

Davis, M. M., Miernicki, M. E., Telzer, E. H., & Rudolph, K. D. (2019). The contribution of childhood negative emotionality and cognitive control to anxiety-linked neural dysregulation of emotion in adolescence. *Journal of Abnormal Child Psychology*, *47*(3), 515-27. https://doi.org/10.1007/s10802-018-0456-0

Davis, N. O., & Carter, A. S. (2008). Parenting stress in mothers and fathers of toddlers with autism spectrum disorders: Associations with child characteristics. *Journal of Autism and Developmental Disorders*, *38*(7), 1278-91. https://doi.org/10.1007/s10803-007-0512-z

Dawson, G., Jones, E. H., Merkle, K., Venema, K., Lowy, R., Faja, S., Kamara, D., Murias, M., Greenson, J., Winter, J., Smith, M., Rogers, S. J., & Webb, S. J. (2012). Early behavioral intervention is associated with normalized brain activity in young children with autism. *Journal of the American Academy of Child & Adolescent Psychiatry*, *51*(11), 1150-59. https://doi.org/10.1016/j.jaac.2012.08.018

Dawson, G., Rogers, S., Munson, J., Smith, M., Winter, J., Greenson, J., Donaldson, A., & Varley, J. (2010). Randomized, controlled trial of an intervention for toddlers with autism: The Early Start Denver Model. *Pediatrics*, *125*(1), e17-e23. https://doi.org/10.1542/peds.2009-0958

Dawson, G., Toth, K., Abbott, R., Osterling, J., Munson, J., Estes, A., & Liaw, J. (2004). Early social attention impairments in autism: Social orienting, joint attention, and attention to distress. *Developmental Psychology*, *40*(2), 271-83. https://doi.org/10.1037/0012-1649.40.2.271

Dawson, G., Webb, S. J., & McPartland, J. (2005). Understanding the nature of face processing impairment in autism: Insights from behavioral and electrophysiological studies. *Developmental Neuropsychology, 27*(3), 403-24. https://doi.org/10.1207/s15326942dn2703_6

Dawson, K. S., Joscelyne, A., Meijer, C., Tampubolon, A., Steel, Z., & Bryant, R. A. (2014). Predictors of chronic posttraumatic response in Muslim children following natural disaster. *Psychological Trauma: Theory, Research, Practice, and Policy, 6*(5), 580–587. https://doi.org/10.1037/a0037140

de Albuquerque, P. P., & de Albuquerque Williams, L. C. (2015). Predictor variables of PTSD symptoms in school victimization: A retrospective study with college students. *Journal of Aggression, Maltreatment & Trauma, 24*(10), 1067-85. https://doi.org/10.1080/10926771.2015.1079281

de Arellano, M. A., Danielson, C. K., & Felton, J. W. (2012). Children of Latino descent: Culturally modified TF-CBT. In J. A. Cohen, A. P. Mannarino, & E. Deblinger (Eds.), *Trauma-focused CBT for children and adolescents: Treatment applications* (pp. 253-79). Guilford Press.

De Bellis, M. D., Casey, B. J., Dahl, R. E., Birmaher, B., Williamson, D. E., Thomas, K. M., Axelson, D. A., Frustaci, K., Boring, A. M., Hall, J., & Ryan, N. D. (2000). A pilot study of amygdala volumes in pediatric generalized anxiety disorder. *Biological Psychiatry, 48*(1), 51–57. https://doi.org/10.1016/s0006-3223(00)00835-0

Dearey, P. (2009). Do the autistic have a prayer? *Journal of Religion, Disability, and Health, 13*, 40-50.

Deater-Deckard, K., & Plomin, R. (1999). An adoption study of the etiology of teacher and parent reports of externalizing behavior problems in middle childhood. *Child Development, 70*(1), 144-54.

Deault, L. C. (2010). A systematic review of parenting in relation to the development of comorbidities and functional impairments in children with attention-deficit/hyperactivity disorder (ADHD). *Child Psychiatry and Human Development, 41*(2), 168-92. https://doi.org/10.1007/s10578-009-0159-4

De Bellis, M. D. (2001). Developmental traumatology: The psychobiological development of maltreated children and its implications for research, treatment, and policy. *Development and Psychopathology, 13*(3), 539-64.

Deblinger, E., Lippmann, J., & Steer, R. A. (1996). Sexually abused children suffering posttraumatic stress symptoms: Initial treatment outcome findings. *Child Maltreatment, 1*(4), 310-21.

Deeba, F., & Rapee, R. M. (2015). Prevalence of traumatic events and risk for psychological symptoms among community and at-risk children and adolescents from Bangladesh. *Child and Adolescent Mental Health, 20*(4), 218-24. https://doi.org/10.1111/camh.12093

DeFranza, M. K. (2015). *Sex differences in Christian theology: Male, female, and intersex in the image of God.*: Eerdmans

de Graaf, R., Bijl, R. V., Spijker, J., Beekman, A. F., & Vollebergh, W. M. (2003). Temporal sequencing of lifetime mood disorders in relation to comorbid anxiety and substance use disorders: Findings from the Netherlands Mental Health Survey and Incidence Study. *Social Psychiatry & Psychiatric Epidemiology, 38*(1), 1-11.

Del Giudice, M., Ellis, B. J., & Shirtcliff, E. A. (2011). The Adaptive Calibration Model of stress responsivity. *Neuroscience and Biobehavioral Reviews, 35*(7), 1562-92. https://doi.org/10.1016/j.neubiorev.2010.11.007

Demeter, C. A., Youngstrom, E. A., Carlson, G. A., Frazier, T. W., Rowles, B. M., Lingler, J., McNamara, N. K., Difrancesco, K. E., Calabrese, J. R., & Findling, R. L. (2013). Age differences in the phenomenology of pediatric bipolar disorder. *Journal of Affective Disorders,*

147(1-3), 295–303. https://doi.org/10.1016/j.jad.2012.11.021

den Houting, J. (2019). Neurodiversity: An insider's perspective. *Autism, 23,* 271-73. https://doi.org/10.1177/1362361318820762

Depue, R. A., Krauss, S., Spoont, M. R., & Arbisi, P. (1989). General Behavior Inventory identification of unipolar and bipolar affective conditions in a nonclinical university population. *Journal of Abnormal Psychology, 98*(2), 117-26.

Derenne, J. L., & Beresin, E. V. (2006). Body image, media, and eating disorders. *Academic Psychiatry, 30*(3), 257-61.

Desrosiers, A., & Miller, L. (2008). Substance use versus anxiety in adolescents: Are some disorders more spiritual than others? *Research in the Social Scientific Study of Religion, 19,* 237-53.

Devita-Raeburn, E. (2016, August 11). Is the most common therapy for autism cruel? *The Atlantic.* Retrieved from https://www.theatlantic.com/health/archive/2016/08/aba-autism-controversy/495272/

de Vries, A. C., & Cohen-Kettenis, P. T. (2012). Clinical management of gender dysphoria in children and adolescents: The Dutch approach. *Journal of Homosexuality, 59*(3), 301-20. https://doi.org/10.1080/00918369.2012.653300

de Vries, A. C., & Cohen-Kettenis, P. T. (2016). Gender dysphoria in children and adolescents. In R. Ettner, S. Monstrey, & E. Coleman (Eds.), *Principles of transgender medicine and surgery* (pp. 180-207). Routledge/Taylor & Francis Group.

de Vries, A. L. C., Doreleijers, T. H., Steensma, T. D., & Cohen-Kettenis, P. T. (2011). Psychiatric comorbidity in gender dysphoric adolescents. *Journal of Child Psychology and Psychiatry, 52*(11), 1195-1202. https://doi.org/10.1111/j.1469-7610.2011.02426.x

de Vries, A. L. C., Kreukels, B. P. C., Steensma, T. D., & McGuire, J. K. (2014). Gender identity development: A biopsychosocial perspective. In B. P. C. Kreukels, T. D. Steensma, & A. L. C. de Vries, *Gender dysphoria and disorders of sex development: Progress in care and knowledge* (pp. 53-80). Springer.

de Vries, A. L. C., McGuire, J. K., Steensma, T. D., Wagenaar, E. F., Doreleijers, T. H., & Cohen-Kettenis, P. T. (2014). Young adult psychological outcome after puberty suppression and gender reassignment. *Pediatrics, 134*(4), 696-704. https://doi.org/10.1542/peds.2013-2958

de Vries, A. L. C., Noens, I. J., Cohen-Kettenis, P. T., van Berckelaer-Onnes, I. A., & Doreleijers, T. A. (2010). Autism spectrum disorders in gender dysphoric children and adolescents. *Journal of Autism and Developmental Disorders, 40*(8), 930-36. https://doi.org/10.1007/s10803-010-0935-9

de Vries, A. L. C., Steensma, T. D., Cohen-Kettenis, P. T., VanderLaan, D. P., & Zucker, K. J. (2016). Poor peer relations predict parent- and self-reported behavioral and emotional problems of adolescents with gender dysphoria: A cross-national, cross-clinic comparative analysis. *European Child & Adolescent Psychiatry, 25*(6), 579-88. https://doi.org/10.1007/s00787-015-0764-7

de Vries, A. L., Steensma, T. D., Doreleijers, T. A., & Cohen-Kettenis, P. T. (2011). Puberty suppression in adolescents with gender identity disorder: a prospective follow-up study. *Journal of sexual Medicine, 8*(8), 2276–2283. https://doi.org/10.1111/j.1743-6109.2010.01943.x

De Young, A. C., Kenardy, J. A., & Cobham, V. E. (2011). Diagnosis of posttraumatic stress disorder in preschool children. *Journal of Clinical Child and Adolescent Psychology, 40*(3), 375-84. https://doi.org/10.1080/15374416.2011.563474

Di Ceglie, D., & Thümmel, E. C. (2006). An experience of group work with parents of children and adolescents with gender identity disorder. *Clinical Child Psychology and*

Psychiatry, 11(3), 387-96. https://doi.org/10.1177/1359104506064983

Dickstein, S., Bannon, K., Castellanos, F. X., & Milham, M. (2006). The neural correlates of attention deficit hyperactivity disorder: An ALE meta-analysis. *Journal of Child Psychology and Psychiatry, 47*(10), 1051-62. https://doi.org/10.1111/j.1469-7610.2006.01671.x

Dierckx, B., Dieleman, G., Tulen, J. H., Treffers, P. D., Utens, E. M., Verhulst, F. C., & Tiemeier, H. (2012). Persistence of anxiety disorders and concomitant changes in cortisol. *Journal of Anxiety Disorders, 26*(6), 635-41.

Di Giunta, L., Rothenberg, W. A., Lunetti, C., Lansford, J. E., Pastorelli, C., Eisenberg, N., Thartori, E., Basili, E., Favini, A., Yotanyama-neewong, S., Peña Alampay, L., Al-Hassan, S. M., Bacchini, D., Bornstein, M. H., Chang, L., Deater-Deckard, K., Dodge, K. A., Oburu, P., Skinner, A. T., . . . Uribe Tirado, L. M. (2020). Longitudinal associations between mothers' and fathers' anger/irritability expressiveness, harsh parenting, and adolescents' socioemotional functioning in nine countries [Supplemental material]. *Developmental Psychology, 56*(3), 458-74. https://doi.org/10.1037/dev0000849.supp

Dimoska, A., Johnstone, S., Barry, R., & Clarke, A. (2003). Inhibitory motor control in children with attention-deficit/hyperactivity disorder: Event-related potentials in the stop-signal paradigm. *Biological Psychiatry, 54*(12), 1345-54. https://doi.org/10.1016/S0006-3223(03)00703-0

Dishion, T. J., Spracklen, K. M., Andrews, D. W., & Patterson, G. R. (1996). Deviancy training in male adolescent friendships. *Behavior Therapy, 27*(3), 373-90.

Docherty, M., Kubik, J., Herrera, C. M., & Boxer, P. (2018). Early maltreatment is associated with greater risk of conduct problems and lack of guilt in adolescence. *Child Abuse & Neglect,*

79, 173-82. https://doi.org/10.1016/j.chiabu.2018.01.032

Dodge, K. A., Lansford, J. E., Burks, V. S., Beter, J. E., Pettit, G. S., Fontaine, R., & Price, J. M. (2003). Peer rejection and social information-processing factors in the development of aggressive behavior problems in children. *Child Development, 74*(2), 374-93.

Dodge, K. A., Price, J. M., Bachorowski, J., & Newman, J. P. (1990). Hostile attributional biases in severely aggressive adolescents. *Journal of Abnormal Psychology, 99*(4), 385-92.

Dogan-Ates, A. (2010). Developmental differences in children's and adolescents' post-disaster reactions. *Issues in Mental Health Nursing, 31*(7), 470-76. https://doi.org/10.3109/01612840903582528

Donnelly, C. L. (2009). Psychopharmacotherapy for children and adolescents. In E. B. Foa, T. M. Keane, M. J. Friedman, & J. A. Cohen (Eds.), *Effective treatments for PTSD* (pp. 269-78). Guilford.

Doshi-Velez, F., Ge, Y., & Kohane, I. (2014). Comorbidity clusters in autism spectrum disorders: An electronic health record time-series analysis. *Pediatrics, 133*(1), e54-e63. https://doi.org/10.1542/peds.2013-0819

Dougherty, L. R., Smith, V. C., Bufferd, S. J., Kessel, E. M., Carlson, G. A., & Klein, D. N. (2016). Disruptive mood dysregulation disorder at the age of 6 years and clinical and functional outcomes 3 years later. *Psychological Medicine, 46*(5), 1103-46.

Doyle, A. C., & Le Grange, D. (2015). Family-based treatment for anorexia nervosa in adolescents. In H. Thompson-Brenner (Ed.), *Casebook of evidence-based therapy for eating disorders* (pp. 43-70). Guilford.

Drescher, J. (2014). Controversies in gender diagnoses. *LGBT Health, 1*(1), 1-5.

Drieberg, H., McEvoy, P. M., Hoiles, K. J., Shu, C. Y., & Egan, S. J. (2019). An examination of direct, indirect and reciprocal relationships between perfectionism, eating disorder symptoms, anxiety, and depression in children and adolescents with eating disorders. *Eating Behaviors, 32,* 53-59. https://doi.org/10.1016/j.eatbeh.2018.12.002

Drummond, K. D., Bradley, S. J., Peterson-Badali, M., & Zucker, K. J. (2008). A follow-up study of girls with gender identity disorder. *Developmental Psychology, 44*(1), 34-45. https://doi.org/10.1037/0012-1649.44.1.34

Duncombe, M. E., Havighurst, S. S., Holland, K. A., & Frankling, E. J. (2012). The contribution of parenting practices and parent emotion factors in children at risk for disruptive behavior disorders. *Child Psychiatry & Human Development, 43,* 715-33.

Duncombe, M., Havighurst, S. S., Holland, K. A., & Frankling, E. J. (2013). Relations of emotional competence and effortful control to child disruptive behavior problems. *Early Education and Development, 24*(5), 599-615.

Dunsmore, J. C., Booker, J. A., & Ollendick, T. H. (2013). Parental emotion coaching and child emotion regulation as protective factors for children with oppositional defiant disorder. *Social Development, 22*(3), 444-66.

DuPaul, G. J., & Kern, L. (2011). *Young children with ADHD: Early identification and intervention.* American Psychological Association. https://doi.org/10.1037/12311-000

DuPaul, G. J., Morgan, P. L., Farkas, G., Hillemeier, M. M., & Maczuga, S. (2016). Academic and social functioning associated with attention-deficit/hyperactivity disorder: Latent class analyses of trajectories from kindergarten to fifth grade. *Journal of Abnormal Child Psychology, 44*(7), 1425-38. https://doi.org/10.1007/s10802-016-0126-z

DuPaul, G. J., & Stoner, G. (2014). *ADHD in the schools: Assessment and intervention strategies* (3rd ed). Guilford.

DuPaul, G. J., & Weyandt, L. L. (2006). School-based intervention for children with attention deficit hyperactivity disorder: Effects on academic, social, and behavioural functioning. *International Journal of Disability, Development and Education, 53*(2), 161-76. https://doi.org/10.1080/10349120600716141

Duric, N. S., Assmus, J., Gundersen, D., Golos, A. D., & Elgen, I. B. (2017). Multimodal treatment in children and adolescents with attention-deficit/hyperactivity disorder: A 6-month follow-up. *Nordic Journal of Psychiatry, 71*(5), 386-94. https://doi.org/10.1080/08039488.2017.1305446

Du Rietz, E., Cheung, C. M., McLoughlin, G., Brandeis, D., Banaschewski, T., Asherson, P., & Kuntsi, J. (2016). Self-report of ADHD shows limited agreement with objective markers of persistence and remittance. *Journal of Psychiatric Research, 82,* 91-99. https://doi.org/10.1016/j.jpsychires.2016.07.020

Dworzynski, K., Ronald, A., Bolton, P., & Happé, F. (2012). How different are girls and boys above and below the diagnostic threshold for autism spectrum disorders? *Journal of the American Academy of Child & Adolescent Psychiatry, 51*(8), 788-97. https://doi.org/10.1016/j.jaac.2012.05.018

Eamon, M. K. (2002). Influences and mediators of the effect of poverty on young adult depressive symptoms. *Journal of Youth and Adolescence, 31,* 231-42.

Eapen, V., Črnčec, R., & Walter, A. (2013). Clinical outcomes of an early intervention program for preschool children with autism spectrum disorder in a community group setting. *BMC Pediatrics, 13*(1), 1-9. https://doi.org/10.1186/1471-2431-13-3

Edmunds, H., & Hill, A. J. (1999). Dieting and the family context of eating in young adolescent children. *International Journal of Eating*

Disorders, 25(4), 435-40. https://doi.org/10.1002/(SICI)1098-108X(199905)25:4<435::AID-EAT8>3.0.CO;2-3

Efron, D., Bryson, H., Lycett, K., & Sciberras, E. (2016). Children referred for evaluation for ADHD: Comorbidity profiles and characteristics associated with a positive diagnosis. *Child: Care, Health and Development, 42*(5), 718-24. https://doi.org/10.1111/cch.12364

Egger, H., Kondo, D., & Angold, A. (2006). The epidemiology and diagnostic issues in preschool attention-deficit/hyperactivity disorder: A review. *Infants & Young Children, 19*(2), 109-22.

Egger, H. L., Erkanli, A., Keeler, G., Potts, E., Walter, B. K., & Angold, A. (2006). Test-retest reliability of the Preschool Age Psychiatric Assessment (PAPA). *Journal of the American Academy of Child & Adolescent Psychiatry, 45*(5), 538-49. https://doi.org/10.1097/01.chi.0000205705.71194.b8

Eikeseth, S. (2011). Intensive early intervention. In J. L. Matson & P. Sturmey (Eds.), *International handbook of autism and pervasive developmental disorders* (pp. 321-38). Springer. https://doi.org/10.1007/978-1-4419-8065-6_20

Eikeseth, S., Klintwall, L., Jahr, E., & Karlsson, P. (2012). Outcome for children with autism receiving early and intensive behavioral intervention in mainstream preschool and kindergarten settings. *Research in Autism Spectrum Disorders, 6*(2), 829-35. http://doi.org/10.1016/j.rasd.2011.09.002

Eikeseth, S., Smith, T., Jahr, E., & Eldevik, S. (2002). Intensive behavioral treatment at school for 4- to 7-year-old children with autism: A 1-year comparison controlled study. *Behavior Modification, 26*(1), 49-68. https://doi.org/10.1177/0145445502026001004

Eikeseth, S., Smith, T., Jahr, E., & Eldevik, S. (2007). Outcome for children with autism who began intensive behavioral treatment between ages 4 and 7: A comparison controlled study. *Behavior Modification, 31*(3), 264-78. https://doi.org/10.1177/0145445506291396

Eisen, A. R., & Schaefer, C. E. (2005). *Separation anxiety in children and adolescents.* Guilford.

Eisenberg, N., Cumberland, A., & Spinrad, T. L. (1998). Parental socialization of emotion. *Psychological Inquiry, 9*(4), 241-73.

Eisenberg, N., Guthrie, I. K., Fabes, R. A., Shepard, S., Losoya, S., Murphy, B. C., Jones, S., Poulin, R., & Reiser, M. (2000). Prediction of elementary school children's externalizing problem behaviors from attentional and behavioral regulation and negative emotionality. *Child Development, 71*(5), 1367–1382. https://doi.org/10.1111/1467-8624.00233

Eley, T. C., Bolton, D., O'Connor, T. G., Perrin, S., Smith, P., & Plomin, R. (2003). A twin study of anxiety-related behaviours in pre-school children. *Journal of Child Psychology and Psychiatry, 44*(7), 945-60.

Eley, T. C., Lichtenstein, P., & Moffitt, T. E. (2003). A longitudinal behavioral genetic analysis of the etiology of aggressive and nonaggressive antisocial behavior. *Development and Psychopathology, 15*(2), 383-402.

Elliott, M. A. (2006). *Faithful feelings: Rethinking emotion in the New Testament.* Kregel.

Elmore, A. L., Nigg, J. T., Friderici, K. H., Jernigan, K., & Nikolas, M. A. (2016). Does 5HTTLPR genotype moderate the association of family environment with child attention-deficit hyperactivity disorder symptomatology? *Journal of Clinical Child and Adolescent Psychology, 45*(3), 348-60. https://doi.org/10.1080/15374416.2014.979935

El-Sheikh, M., Hinnant, J. B., Kelly, R. J., & Erath, S. (2010). Maternal psychological control and child internalizing symptoms: Vulnerability and protective factors across bioregulatory and ecological domains. *Journal of Child Psychology and Psychiatry, 51*(2), 188-98.

Emslie, G. J. (2012). The psychopharmacology of adolescent depression. *Journal of Child and Adolescent Psychopharmacology, 22*(1), 2-4.

Enlow, M. B., Blood, E., & Egeland, B. (2013). Sociodemographic risk, developmental competence, and PTSD symptoms in young children exposed to interpersonal trauma in early life. *Journal of Traumatic Stress, 26*(6), 686–694. https://doi.org/10.1002/jts.21866

Enlow, M. B., Egeland, B., Carlson, E., Blood, E., & Wright, R. J. (2014). Mother-infant attachment and the intergenerational transmission of posttraumatic stress disorder. *Development and Psychopathology, 26*(1), 41–65. https://doi.org/10.1017/S0954579413000515

Entwistle, D. (2015). *Integrative approaches to psychology and Christianity* (3rd ed.). Cascade Books.

Ercan, E. S., Ardic, U. A., Kutlu, A., & Durak, S. (2012). No beneficial effects of adding parent training to methylphenidate treatment for ADHD + ODD/CD children: A 1-year prospective follow-up study. *Journal of Attention Disorders, 18*(2), 145-57. https://doi.org/10.1177/1087054711432884

Erickson, M. J. (2013). *Christian theology* (3rd ed.). Baker Academic.

Erikson, E. H. (1950). *Childhood and society*. W. W. Norton.

Erikson, E. H. (1985). *Children and society*. W. W. Norton.

Ernst, M., Moolchan, E. T., & Robinson, M. L. (2001). Behavioral and neural consequences of prenatal exposure to nicotine. *Journal of the American Academy of Child & Adolescent Psychiatry, 40*(6), 630-41. https://doi.org/10.1097/00004583-200106000-00007

Esbjørn, B. H., Bender, P. K., Reinholdt-Dunne, M. L., Munck, L. A., & Ollendick, T. H. (2012). The development of anxiety disorders: Considering the contributions of attachment and emotion regulation. *Clinical Child and Family Psychology Review, 15*(2), 129-43.

Espil, F. M., Viana, A. G., & Dixon, L. J. (2016). Post-traumatic stress disorder and depressive symptoms among inpatient adolescents: The underlying role of emotion regulation. *Residential Treatment for Children & Youth, 33*(1), 51-68. https://doi.org/10.1080/0886571X.2016.1159939

Essau, C. A. (2003). Comorbidity of anxiety disorders in adolescents. *Depression & Anxiety, 18*(1), 1-6.

Essau, C. A., & Ollendick, T. H. (2009). Diagnosis and assessment of adolescent depression. In S. Nolen-Hoeksema & L. M. Hilt (Eds.), *Handbook of depression in adolescents* (pp. 33-52). Routledge.

Estes, A., Munson, J., Dawson, G., Koehler, E., Zhou, X., & Abbott, R. (2009). Parenting stress and psychological functioning among mothers of preschool children with autism and developmental delay. *Autism, 13*(4), 375-87. https://doi.org/10.1177/1362361309105658

Estes, A., Munson, J., Rogers, S. J., Greenson, J., Winter, J., & Dawson, G. (2015). Long-term outcomes of early intervention in 6-year-old children with autism spectrum disorder. *Journal of the American Academy of Child & Adolescent Psychiatry, 54*(7), 580-87. https://doi.org/10.1016/j.jaac.2015.04.005

Estes, A., Zwaigenbaum, L., Gu, H., St John, T., Paterson, S., Elison, J. T., Hazlett, H., Botteron, K., Dager, S. R., Schultz, R. T., Kostopoulos, P., Evans, A., Dawson, G., Eliason, J., Alvarez, S., Piven, J., & IBIS network (2015). Behavioral, cognitive, and adaptive development in infants with autism spectrum disorder in the first 2 years of life. *Journal of Neurodevelopmental Disorders, 7*(1), 24. https://doi.org/10.1186/s11689-015-9117-6

Evans, A. S., Spirito, A., Celio, M., Dyl, J., & Hunt, J. (2007). The relation of substance use to trauma and conduct disorder in an adolescent psychiatric population. *Journal of Child &*

Adolescent Substance Abuse, 17(1), 29-49. https://doi.org/10.1300/J029v17n01_02

Evans, E. H., Adamson, A. J., Basterfield, L., Le Couteur, A., Reilly, J. K., Reilly, J. J., & Parkinson, K. N. (2017). Risk factors for eating disorder symptoms at 12 years of age: A 6-year longitudinal cohort study. *Appetite, 108*, 12–20. https://doi.org/10.1016/j.appet.2016.09.005

Evans, G.W., & Kim, P. (2007). Childhood poverty and health: Cumulative risk exposure and stress dysregulation. *Psychological Science, 18*(11), 953-957. https://doi.org/10.1111/j.1467-9280.2007.02008.x

Evans, G. W., Li, D., & Whipple, S. S. (2013). Cumulative risk and child development. *Psychological Bulletin, 139*(6), 1342-96. https://doi.org/10.1037/a0031808.supp

Evans, L. D., Kouros, C. D., Samanez-Larkin, S., & Garber, J. (2016). Concurrent and short-term prospective relations among neurocognitive functioning, coping, and depressive symptoms in youth. *Journal of Clinical Child & Adolescent Psychology, 45*(1), 6-20.

Evans, S. W., Owens, J. S., Wymbs, B. T., & Ray, A. R. (2018). Evidence-based psychosocial treatments for children and adolescents with attention deficit/hyperactivity disorder. *Journal of Clinical Child and Adolescent Psychology, 47*(2), 157-98. https://doi.org/10.1080/15374416.2017.1390757

Eyberg, S. M., Funderburk, B. W., Hembree-Kigin, T. L., McNeil, C. B., Querido, J. G., & Hood, K. (2001). Parent-child interaction therapy with behavior problem children: One and two year maintenance of treatment effects in the family. *Child and Family Behavior Therapy, 23*(4), 1-20.

Fabiano, G. A., Pelham, W. J., Coles, E. K., Gnagy, E. M., Chronis-Tuscano, A., & O'Connor, B. C. (2009). A meta-analysis of behavioral treatments for attention-deficit/hyperactivity disorder. *Clinical Psychology Review, 29*(2), 129-40. https://doi.org/10.1016/j.cpr.2008.11.001

Fabiano, G. A., Schatz, N. K., & Pelham, W. J. (2014). Summer treatment programs for youth with ADHD. *Child and Adolescent Psychiatric Clinics of North America, 23*(4), 757-73. https://doi.org/10.1016/j.chc.2014.05.012

Fabiano, G. A., Vujnovic, R. K., Pelham, W. E., Waschbusch, D. A., Massetti, G. M., Pariseau, M. E., Naylor, J., Yu, J., Robins, M., Carnefix., T., Greiner, A. R., & Volker, M. (2010). Enhancing the effectiveness of special education programming for children with attention deficit hyperactivity disorder using a daily report card. *School Psychology Review, 39*(2), 219-39.

Fahim, C., He, Y., Yoon, U., Chen, J., Evans, A., & Perusse, D. (2011). Neuroanatomy of childhood disruptive behavior disorders. *Aggressive Behavior, 37*(4), 326-37.

Fairburn, C. G., & Beglin, S. J. (1994). Assessment of eating disorders: Interview or self-report questionnaire? *International Journal of Eating Disorders, 16*(4), 363-70.

Fairburn, C. G., & Cooper, Z. (1993). The Eating Disorder Examination (12th edition). In C. G. Fairburn & G. T. Wilson (Eds.), *Binge eating: Nature, assessment, and treatment* (pp. 317–360). New York: Guilford Press.

Fairburn, C. G., Cooper, Z., Doll, H. A., & Welch, S. L. (1999). Risk factors for anorexia nervosa: Three integrated case-control comparisons. *Archives of General Psychiatry, 56*(5), 468-76. https://doi.org/10.1001/archpsyc.56.5.468

Fairburn, C. G., Doll, H. A., Welch, S. L., Hay, P. J., Davies, B. A., & O'Connor, M. E. (1998). Risk factors for binge eating disorder: A community-based, case-control study. *Archives of General Psychiatry, 55*(5), 425-32. https://doi.org/10.1001/archpsyc.55.5.425

Faja, S., & Dawson, G. (2017). Autism spectrum disorder. In T. P. Beauchaine & S. P. Hinshaw (Eds.), *Child and adolescent psychopathology* (3rd ed., pp. 745-82). Wiley.

Fantuzzo, J. W., & Fusco, R. A. (2007). Children's direct exposure to types of domestic violence crime: A population-based investigation. *Journal of Family Violence, 22*(7), 543-52. https://doi.org/10.1007/s10896-007-9105-z

Faraone, S., Perlis, R., Doyle, A., Smoller, J., Goralnick, J., Holmgren, M., & Sklar, P. (2005). Molecular genetics of attention-deficit/hyperactivity disorder. *Biological Psychiatry, 57*(11), 1313-23. https://doi.org/10.1016/j.biopsych.2004.11.024

Feeny, N. C., Silva, S. G., Reinecke, M. A., McNulty, S., Findling, R. L., Rohde, P., Curry, J. F., Ginsburg, G. S., Kratochvil, C. J., Pathak, S. M., May, D. E., Kennard, B. D., Simons, A. D., Wells, K. C., Robins, M., Rosenberg, D., & March, J. S. (2009). An exploratory analysis of the impact of family functioning on treatment for depression in adolescents. *Journal of Clinical Child and Adolescent Psychology, 38*(6), 814-25.

Feldman, R., Vengrober, A., Eidelman-Rothman, M., & Zagoory-Sharon, O. (2013). Stress reactivity in war-exposed young children with and without posttraumatic stress disorder: Relations to maternal stress hormones, parenting, and child emotionality and regulation. *Development and Psychopathology, 25*(4), 943-55. https://doi.org/10.1017/S0954579413000291

Feng, X., Keenan, K., Hipwell, A. E., Henneberger, A. K., Rischall, M. S., Butch, J., Coyne, C., Boeldt, D., Hinze, A. K., & Babinski, D. E. (2009). Longitudinal associations between emotion regulation and depression in preadolescent girls: Moderation by the caregiving environment. *Developmental Psychology, 45*(3), 798-808.

Feng, X., Shaw, D. S., Kovacs, M., Lane, T., O'Rourke, F. E., & Alarcon, J. H. (2008). Emotion regulation in preschoolers: The roles of behavioral inhibition, maternal affective behavior, and maternal depression. *Journal of Child Psychology and Psychiatry, 49*(2), 132-41.

Ferreira, J. E., de Souza, P. R., Jr, da Costa, R. S., Sichieri, R., & da Veiga, G. V. (2013). Disordered eating behaviors in adolescents and adults living in the same household in metropolitan area of Rio de Janeiro, Brazil. *Psychiatry Research, 210*(2), 612–617. https://doi.org/10.1016/j.psychres.2013.06.021

Ferreiro, F., Seoane, G., & Senra, C. (2012). Gender-related risk and protective factors for depressive symptoms and disordered eating in adolescence: A 4-year longitudinal study. *Journal of Youth and Adolescence, 41*(5), 607-22. https://doi.org/10.1007/s10964-011-9718-7

Ferreiro, F., Seoane, G., & Senra, C. (2014). Toward understanding the role of body dissatisfaction in the gender differences in depressive symptoms and disordered eating: A longitudinal study during adolescence. *Journal of Adolescence, 37*(1), 73-84. https://doi.org/10.1016/j.adolescence.2013.10.013

Ferreiro, F., Wichstrøm, L., Seoane, G., & Senra, C. (2014). Reciprocal associations between depressive symptoms and disordered eating among adolescent girls and boys: A multiwave, prospective study. *Journal of Abnormal Child Psychology, 42*(5), 803-12. https://doi.org/10.1007/s10802-013-9833-x

Festa, C. C., & Ginsburg, G. S. (2011). Parental and peer predictors of social anxiety in youth. *Child Psychiatry and Human Development, 42*(3), 291-306.

Fettig, A., & Fleury, V. P. (2017). Early intervention services for children with autism. In D. Zager, D. F. Cihak, & A. Stone-MacDonald (Eds.), *Autism spectrum disorders: Identification, education, and treatment.*, 4th ed. (pp. 124–141). Routledge/Taylor & Francis Group.

Findling, R. L., Gracious, B. L., McNamara, N. K., Youngstrom, E. A., Demeter, C. A., Branicky, L. A., & Calabrese, J. R. (2001).

Rapid, continuous cycling and psychiatric co-morbidity in pediatric bipolar I disorder. *Bipolar Disorders, 3*(4), 202-10.

Fisak, B., Jr., & Grills-Taquechel, A. E. (2007). Parental modeling, reinforcement, and information transfer: Risk factors in the development of child anxiety? *Clinical Child & Family Psychology Review, 10*(3), 213-31.

Fitzpatrick, K. K., Hoste, R. R., Lock, J., & Le Grange, D. (2015). Adolescent-focused therapy for anorexia nervosa. In H. Thompson-Brenner (Ed.), *Casebook of evidence-based therapy for eating disorders* (pp. 343-61). Guilford Press.

Fitzpatrick, K. K., Moye, A., Hoste, R., Lock, J., & Le Grange, D. (2010). Adolescent focused psychotherapy for adolescents with anorexia nervosa. *Journal of Contemporary Psychotherapy, 40*(1), 31-39. https://doi.org/10.1007/s10879-009-9123-7

Fitzsimons, T. (2020, May 8). *Germany is 5th country to ban conversion therapy for minors.* NBC News. https://www.nbcnews.com/feature/nbc-out/germany-5th-country-ban-conversion-therapy-minors-n1203166

Flanagan, J. E., Landa, R., Bhat, A., & Bauman, M. (2012). Head lag in infants at risk for autism: A preliminary study. *American Journal of Occupational Therapy, 66*(5), 577-85. https://doi.org/10.5014/ajot.2012.004192

Flanagan, K. S., & Hall, S. E. (2014). Overview of developmental psychopathology and integrative themes. In K. S. Flanagan & S. E. Hall (Eds.), *Christianity and developmental psychopathology: Foundations and approaches* (pp. 1-42). InterVarsity Press.

Fleming, J. E., & Offord, D. R. (1990). Epidemiology of childhood depressive disorders: A critical review. *Journal of the American Academy of Child & Adolescent Psychiatry, 29*, 571-80.

Fletcher, A. C., Steinberg, L., & Williams-Wheeler, M. (2004). Parental influences on adolescent problem behavior: Revisiting Stattin and Kerr. *Child Development, 75*(3), 781-96. https://doi.org/10.1111/j.1467-8624.2004.00706.x

Fletcher, K. E. (2007). Posttraumatic stress disorder. In E. J. Mash & R. A. Barkley (Eds.), *Assessment of childhood disorders* (4th ed., pp. 398-483). Guilford Press.

Flett, G. L., Druckman, T., Hewitt, P. L., & Wekerle, C. (2012). Perfectionism, coping, social support, and depression in maltreated adolescents. *Journal of Rational-Emotive & Cognitive-Behavior Therapy, 30*, 118-31.

Foa, E. B., Asnaani, A., Zang, Y., Capaldi, S., & Yeh, R. (2018). Psychometrics of the Child PTSD Symptom Scale for DSM-5 for trauma-exposed children and adolescents. *Journal of Clinical Child and Adolescent Psychology, 47*(1), 38-46. https://doi.org/10.1080/15374416.2017.1350962

Foa, E. B., Ehlers, A., Clark, D. M., Tolin, D. F., & Orsillo, S. M. (1999). The Posttraumatic Cognitions Inventory (PTCI): Development and validation. *Psychological Assessment, 11*(3), 303-14. https://doi.org/10.1037/1040-3590.11.3.303

Folk, J. B., Zeman, J. L., Poon, J. A., & Dallaire, D. H. (2014). A longitudinal examination of emotion regulation: Pathways to anxiety and depressive symptoms in urban minority youth. *Child and Adolescent Mental Health, 19*(4), 243-50.

Fonagy, P., Cottrell, D., Phillips, J., Bevington, D., Glaser, D., & Allison, E. (2015). *What works for whom?: A critical review of treatments for children and adolescents.* Guilford Press.

Ford, J. D. (2009). Neurobiological and developmental research: Clinical implications. In C. A. Courtois & J. D. Ford (Eds.), *Treating complex traumatic stress disorders: An evidence-based guide* (pp. 31-58). Guilford Press.

Forehand, R., & Kotchick, B. A. (2016). Cultural diversity: A wake-up call for parent training.

Behavior Therapy, 47(6), 981-92. https://doi.org/10.1016/j.beth.2016.11.010

Forgatch, M. S., & Patterson, G. R. (2010). Parent Management Training—Oregon Model: An intervention for antisocial behavior in children and adolescents. In J. R. Weisz & A. E. Kazdin (Eds.), *Evidence-based psychotherapies for children and adolescents* (2nd ed., pp. 159-78). Guilford.

Fout, J. A. (2015). What do I fear when I fear my God? A theological reexamination of a biblical theme. *Journal of Theological Interpretation, 9*(1), 23-38.

Fox, K. R., Choukas-Bradley, S., Salk, R. H., Marshal, M. P., & Thoma, B. C. (2020). Mental health among sexual and gender minority adolescents: Examining interactions with race and ethnicity [Supplemental material]. *Journal of Consulting and Clinical Psychology, 88*(5), 402-15. https://doi.org/10.1037/ccp0000486.supp

Fox, N. A., Nichols, K. E., Henderson, H. A., Rubin, K., Schmidt, L., Hamer, D., Ernst, M., & Pine, D. S. (2005). Evidence for a gene-environment interaction in predicting behavioral inhibition in middle childhood. *Psychological Science, 16*(12), 921-26.

France, R. T. (1994). Matthew. In G. J. Wenham, J. A. Motyer, D. A. Carson, & R. T. France (Eds.), *New Bible commentary* (21st century edition, pp. 904-45). Inter-Varsity Press.

Francis, L. A., & Birch, L. L. (2005). Maternal influences on daughters' restrained eating behavior. *Health Psychology, 24*(6), 548-54. https://doi.org/10.1037/0278-6133.24.6.548

Francisco, R., Espinoza, P., González, M. L., Penelo, E., Mora, M., Rosés, R., & Raich, R. M. (2015). Body dissatisfaction and disordered eating among Portuguese and Spanish adolescents: The role of individual characteristics and internalisation of sociocultural ideals. *Journal of Adolescence, 41*, 7-16. https://doi.org/10.1016/j.adolescence.2015.02.004

Franke, B., Neale, B., & Faraone, S. (2009). Genome-wide association studies in ADHD. *Human Genetics, 126*(1), 13-50.

Frankel, F., Myatt, R., Cantwell, D. P., & Feinberg, D. T. (1997). Parent-assisted transfer of children's social skills training: Effects on children with and without attention-deficit hyperactivity disorder. *Journal of the American Academy of Child & Adolescent Psychiatry, 36*(8), 1056-64. https://doi.org/10.1097/00004583-199708000-00013

Freeman, A. J., Youngstrom, E. A., Freeman, M. J., Youngstrom, J. K., & Findling, R. L. (2011). Is caregiver-adolescent disagreement due to differences in thresholds for reporting manic symptoms? *Journal of Child and Adolescent Psychopharmacology, 21*, 425-32.

Fried, R., Chan, J., Feinberg, L., Pope, A., Woodworth, K. Y., Faraone, S. V., & Biederman, J. (2016). Clinical correlates of working memory deficits in youth with and without ADHD: A controlled study. *Journal of Clinical and Experimental Neuropsychology, 38*(5), 487-96. https://doi.org/10.1080/13803395.2015.1127896

Friederich, H. C., Wu, M., Simon, J. J., & Herzog, W. (2013). Neurocircuit function in eating disorders. *International Journal of Eating Disorders, 46*(5), 425–432. https://doi.org/10.1002/eat.22099

Fristad, M. (2016). Evidence-based psychotherapies and nutritional interventions for children with bipolar spectrum disorders and their families. *The Journal of Clinical Psychiatry, 77*(Suppl E1), 04. https://doi.org/10.4088/JCP.15017su1c.04

Fristad, M. A., Gavazzi, S. M., & Mackinaw-Koons, B. (2003). Family psychoeducation: An adjunctive intervention for children with bipolar disorder. *Biological Psychiatry, 53*(11), 1000-1008.

Fristad, M. A., Goldberg-Arnold, J. S., & Gavazzi, S. M. (2003). Multi-family psychoeducation groups in the treatment of children with mood disorders. *Journal of Marital and Family Therapy, 29*(4), 491-504.

Fristad, M. A., & MacPherson, H. A. (2014). Evidence-based psychosocial treatments for child and adolescent bipolar spectrum disorders. *Journal of Clinical Child & Adolescent Psychology, 43*(3), 339-55.

Fristad, M. A., Verducci, J. S., Walters, K., & Young, M. E. (2009). Impact of multifamily psychoeducational psychotherapy in treating children aged 8 to 12 years with mood disorders. *Archives of General Psychiatry, 66*(9), 1013-20.

Froehlich-Santino, W., Londono Tobon, A., Cleveland, S., Torres, A., Phillips, J., Cohen, B., Torigoe, T., Miller, J., Fedele, A., Collins, J., Smith, K., Lotspeich, L., Croen, L. A., Ozonoff, S., Lajonchere, C., Grether, J. K., O'Hara, R., & Hallmayer, J. (2014). Prenatal and perinatal risk factors in a twin study of autism spectrum disorders. *Journal of Psychiatric Research, 54,* 100-108. https://doi.org/10.1016/j.jpsychires .2014.03.019

Froreich, F. V., Vartanian, L. R., Zawadzki, M. J., Grisham, J. R., & Touyz, S. W. (2017). Psychological need satisfaction, control, and disordered eating. *British Journal of Clinical Psychology, 56*(1), 53-68. https://doi.org/10.1111/ bjc.12120

Furr, J. M., Comer, J. S., Edmunds, J. M., & Kendall, P. C. (2010). Disasters and youth: A meta-analytic examination of posttraumatic stress. *Journal of Consulting and Clinical Psychology, 78*(6), 765-80. https://doi.org/10.1037/ a0021482

Fussner, L. M., Luebbe, A. M., Mancini, K. J., & Becker, S. P. (2018). Emotion dysregulation mediates the longitudinal relation between peer rejection and depression: Differential effects of gender and grade. *International Journal of Behavioral Development, 42*(2), 155-66. https://doi.org/10.1177/0165025416669062

Gaffrey, M. S., Tillman, R., Barch, D. M., & Luby, J. L. (2018). Continuity and stability of preschool depression from childhood through adolescence and following the onset of puberty. *Comprehensive Psychiatry, 86,* 39-46. https://doi. org/10.1016/j.comppsych.2018.07.010

Galambos, N. L., Leadbeater, B. J., & Barker, E. T. (2004). Gender differences in and risk factors for depression in adolescents: A 4-year longitudinal study. *International Journal of Behavior Development, 28,* 16-25.

Galano, M. M., Miller, L. E., & Graham-Bermann, S. A. (2014). Avoidance symptom presentation of preschoolers exposed to Intimate Partner Violence in a group therapy setting. *Child Care in Practice, 20*(4), 399-414.

Gale, L., Channon, S., Larner, M., & James, D. (2016). Experiences of using pro-eating disorder websites: A qualitative study with service users in NHS eating disorder services. *Eating and Weight Disorders, 21*(3), 427-34. https://doi.org/10.1007/s40519-015-0242-8

Galéra, C., Côté, S. M., Bouvard, M. P., Pingault, J., Melchior, M., Michel, G., Boivin, M., & Tremblay, R. E. (2011). Early risk factors for hyperactivity-impulsivity and inattention trajectories from age 17 months to 8 years. *Archives of General Psychiatry, 68*(12), 1267-75. https://doi .org/10.1001/archgenpsychiatry.2011.138

Gallagher, R., Abikoff, H. B., & Spira, E. G. (2014). *Organizational skills training for children with ADHD: An empirically supported treatment.* Guilford Press.

Garber, J., Braafladt, N., & Weiss, B. (1995). Affect regulation in depressed and nondepressed children & young adolescents. *Development and Psychopathology, 7*(1), 93-115.

Garcia, A. M., Medina, D., & Sibley, M. H. (2019). Conflict between parents and adolescents with ADHD: Situational triggers and the role of comorbidity. *Journal of Child and Family Studies, 28*(12), 3338-45. https://doi.org/10.1007/s10826 -019-01512-7

García, J., Grau, C., & Garcés, J. (2015). Learning and behaviour of three- to five-year-old children with ADHD. *Infancia y Aprendizaje/ Journal for the Study of Education and Development, 38*(4), 775-807. https://doi.org/10.108 0/02103702.2015.1076268

Gardener, H., Spiegelman, D., & Buka, S. L. (2011). Perinatal and neonatal risk factors for autism: A comprehensive meta-analysis. *Pediatrics, 128*(2), 344-55. https://doi.org/10.1542/ peds.2010-1036

Gardner, R. M., Stark, K., Friedman, B. N., & Jackson, N. A. (2000). Predictors of eating disorder scores in children ages 6 through 14: a longitudinal study. *Journal of Psychosomatic Research, 49*(3), 199–205. https://doi. org/10.1016/s0022-3999(00)00172-0

Garland, A. F., Hawley, K. M., Brookman-Frazee, L., & Hurlburt, M. S. (2008). Identifying common elements of evidence-based psychosocial treatments for children's disruptive behavior problems. *Journal of the American Academy of Child & Adolescent Psychiatry, 47*(5), 505-14. https://doi.org/10.1097/ CHI.0b013e31816765c2

Garner, D.M. (2004). *Eating Disorder Inventory-3 professional manual.* Lutz, FL: Psychological Assessment Resources.

Garrett, A. S., Reiss, A. L., Howe, M. E., Kelley, R. G., Singh, M. K., Adleman, N. E., Karchemskiy, A., & Chang, K. D. (2012). Abnormal amygdala and prefrontal cortex activation to facial expressions in pediatric bipolar disorder. *Journal of the American Academy of Child & Adolescent Psychiatry, 51*(8), 821-31.

Gaub, M., & Carlson, C. (1997). Gender differences in ADHD: A meta-analysis and critical review. *Journal of the American Academy of Child & Adolescent Psychiatry, 36*(8), 1036-45. https:// doi.org/10.1097/00004583-199708000-00011

Gavita, O. A., Capris, D., Bolno, J., & David, D. (2012). Anterior cingulate cortex findings in child disruptive behavior disorders. A meta-analysis. *Aggression and Violent Behavior, 17,* 507-13.

Ge, X., Lorenz, F. O., Conger, R. D., Elder, G. H., & Simons, R. L. (1994). Trajectories of stressful life events and depressive symptoms during adolescence. *Developmental Psychology, 30*(4), 467-83.

Ge, X., Natsuaki, M. N., & Conger, R. D. (2006). Trajectories of depressive symptoms and stressful life events among male and female adolescents in divorced and nondivorced families. *Development and Psychopathology, 18*(1), 253-73.

Gejman, P., Sanders, A., & Duan, J. (2010). The role of genetics in the etiology of schizophrenia. *The Psychiatric Clinics of North America, 33*(1), 35-66. https://doi.org/10.1016/j. psc.2009.12.003

Geller, B., Luby, J. L., Joshi, P., Wagner, K. D., Emslie, G., Walkup, J. T., Axelson, D. A., Bolhofner, K., Robb, A., Wolf, D. V., Riddle, M. A., Birmaher, B., Nusrat, N., Ryan, N. D., Vitiello, B., Tillman, R., & Lavori, P. (2012). A randomized controlled trial of risperidone, lithium, or divalproex sodium for initial treatment of bipolar I disorder, manic or mixed phase, in children and adolescents. *Archives of General Psychiatry, 69*(5), 515-28. https://doi. org/10.1001/archgenpsychiatry.2011.1508

Geller, B., Tillman, R., Bolhofner, K., & Zimerman, B. (2008). Child bipolar I disorder: Prospective continuity with adult bipolar I disorder; characteristics of second and third episodes; predictors of 8-year outcome. *Archives of General Psychiatry, 65*(10), 1125-33.

Geller, B., Williams, M., Zimerman, B., Frazier, J., Beringer, L., & Warner, K. L. (1998). Prepubertal and early adolescent bipolarity differentiate from ADHD by manic symptoms, grandiose delusions, ultra-rapid or ultradian cycling. *Journal of Affective Disorders, 51*(2), 81-91.

Geller, B., Zimerman, B., Williams, M., DelBello, M., Bolhofner, K., Craney, J., Frazier, J., Beringer, L., & Nickelsburg, M. (2002). DSM-IV mania symptoms in a prepubertal and early adolescent bipolar disorder phenotype compared to attention-deficit hyperactive and normal controls. *Journal of Child and Adolescent Psychopharmacology, 12*(1), 11-25.

George, M. W., Fairchild, A. J., Mark Cummings, E., & Davies, P. T. (2014). Marital conflict in early childhood and adolescent disordered eating: Emotional insecurity about the marital relationship as an explanatory mechanism. *Eating Behaviors, 15*(4), 532-39. https://doi.org/10.1016/j.eatbeh.2014.06.006

Ghandour, R., Sherman, L., Vladutiu, C., Ali, M., Lynch, S., Bitsko, R., & Blumberg, S. (2019). Prevalence and treatment of depression, anxiety, and conduct problems in US children. *The Journal of Pediatrics, 206*, 256-67. https://doi.org/10.1016/j.jpeds.2018.09.021

Giaconia, R. M., Reinherz, H. Z., Hauf, A. C., Paradis, A. D., Wasserman, M. S., & Langhammer, D. M. (2000). Comorbidity of substance use and post-traumatic stress disorders in a community sample of adolescents. *American Journal of Orthopsychiatry, 70*(2), 253-62. https://doi.org/10.1037/h0087634

Gibb, B. E., Alloy, L. B., Walshaw, P. D., Comer, J. S., Shen, G. C., & Villari, A. G. (2006). Predictors of attributional style change in children. *Journal of Abnormal Child Psychology, 34*(3), 425-39.

Gibb, B. E., Stone, L. B., & Crossett, S. E. (2012). Peer victimization and prospective changes in children's inferential styles. *Journal of Clinical Child & Adolescent Psychology, 41*(5), 561-69.

Gibbs, V., Aldridge, F., Chandler, F., Witzlsperger, E., & Smith, K. (2012). An exploratory study comparing diagnostic outcomes for autism spectrum disorders under DSM-IV-TR with the proposed DSM-5 revision. *Journal of Autism and Developmental Disorders, 42*(8), 1750-56. https://doi.org/10.1007/s10803-012-1560-6

Gidaya, N. B., Lee, B. K., Burstyn, I., Yudell, M., Mortensen, E. L., & Newschaffer, C. J. (2014). In utero exposure to selective serotonin reuptake inhibitors and risk for autism spectrum disorder. *Journal of Autism and Developmental Disorders, 44*(10), 2558-67. https://doi.org/10.1007/s10803-014-2128-4

Giedd, J., Blumenthal, J., Molloy, E., & Castellanos, F. (2001). Brain imaging of attention deficit/hyperactivity disorder. *Annals of the New York Academy of Sciences, 931*(1), 33-49. https://doi.org/10.1111/j.1749-6632.2001.tb05772.x

Gillberg, C., & Billstedt, E. (2000). Autism and Asperger syndrome: Coexistence with other clinical disorders. *Acta Psychiatrica Scandinavica, 102*(5), 321-30. https://doi.org/10.1034/j.1600-0447.2000.102005321.x

Gillespie, C. F., Phifer, J., Bradley, B., & Ressler, K. J. (2009). Risk and resilience: Genetic and environmental influences on development of the stress response. *Depression and Anxiety, 26*(11), 984-92. https://doi.org/10.1002/da.20605

Gilliam, J. E. (2014). *Gilliam Autism Rating Scale, Third Edition (GARS-3)*. Pro-Ed.

Gilliom, M., Shaw, D. S., Beck, J. E., Schonberg, M. A., & Lukon, J. L. (2002). Anger regulation in disadvantaged preschool boys: Strategies, antecedents, and the development of self-control. *Developmental Psychology, 38*(2), 222-35.

Gillogly, R. R. (1981). Spanking hurts everybody. *Theology Today, 37*(4), 415-24.

Giordano, S. (2014). Medical treatment for children with gender dysphoria: Conceptual and ethical issues. In B. P. C. Kreukels, T. D. Steensma, & A. L. C. de Vries, *Gender dysphoria and disorders of sex development: Progress in care and knowledge* (pp. 205-30). Springer.

Girirajan, S., Dennis, M. Y., Baker, C., Malig, M., Coe, B. P., Campbell, C. D., Mark, K., Vu, T. H., Alkan, C., Cheng, Z., Biesecker, L. G., Bernier, R., & Eichler, E.E. (2013). Refinement and discovery of new hotspots of copy-number variation associated with autism spectrum disorder. *American Journal of Human Genetics, 92*, 221-37. https://doi.org/10.1016/j.ajhg.2012.12.016

Gizer, I. R., Waldman, I. D., Abramowitz, A., Barr, C. L., Feng, Y., Wigg, K. G., Misener, V. L., & Rowe, D. C. (2008). Relations between multi-informant assessments of ADHD symptoms, DAT1, and DRD4. *Journal of Abnormal Psychology, 117*(4), 869-80. https://doi.org/10.1037/a0013297

Gladstone, T. G., & Kaslow, N. J. (1995). Depression and attributions in children and adolescents: A meta-analytic review. *Journal of Abnormal Child Psychology, 23*, 597-606.

Goenjian, A. K., Pynoos, R. S., Steinberg, A. M., Endres, D., Abraham, K., Geffner, M. E., & Fairbanks, L. A. (2003). Hypothalamic-pituitary-adrenal activity among Armenian adolescents with PTSD symptoms. *Journal of Traumatic Stress, 16*(4), 319-23. https://doi.org/10.1023/A:1024453632458

Goin-Kochel, R. P., Mire, S. S., & Dempsey, A. G. (2015). Emergence of autism spectrum disorder in children from simplex families: relations to parental perceptions of etiology. *Journal of Autism and Developmental Disorders, 45*(5), 1451–1463. https://doi.org/10.1007/s10803-014-2310-8

Goldberg, W. A., Osann, K., Filipek, P. A., Laulhere, T., Jarvis, K., Modahl, C., Flodman, P., & Spence, M. A. (2003). Language and other regression: Assessment and timing. *Journal of Autism and Developmental Disorders, 33*(6), 607-16. https://doi.org/10.1023/B:JADD.0000005998.47370.ef

Golden, N. H., & Ornstein, R. M. (2016). Eating problems in children and adolescents. In B. T. Walsh, E. Attia, D. R. Glasofer, & R. Sysko (Eds.), *Handbook of assessment and treatment of eating disorders* (pp. 45-63). American Psychiatric Association Publishing.

Goldschmidt, A. B., Doyle, A. C., & Wilfley, D. E. (2007). Assessment of binge eating in overweight youth using a questionnaire version of the child eating disorder examination with instructions. *International Journal of Eating Disorders, 40*(5), 460-67. https://doi.org/10.1002/eat.20387

Goldstein, B. I., Sassi, R., & Diler, R. S. (2012). Pharmacologic treatment of bipolar disorder in children and adolescents. *Child and Adolescent Psychiatric Clinics of North America, 21*(4), 911-39.

Goldstein, B. I., Strober, M., Axelson, D., Goldstein, T. R., Gill, M. K., Hower, H., Dickstein, D., Hunt, J., Yen, S., Kim, E., Ha, W., Liao, F., Fan, J., Iyengar, S., Ryan, N. D., Keller, M. B., & Birmaher, B. (2013). Predictors of first-onset substance use disorders during the prospective course of bipolar spectrum disorders in adolescents. *Journal of the American Academy of Child & Adolescent Psychiatry, 52*(10), 1026-37.

Goldstein, L. H., Harvey, E. A., & Friedman-Weieneth, J. L. (2007). Examining subtypes of behavior problems among 3-year-old children: Part III. Investigating differences in parenting practices and parenting stress. *Journal of Abnormal Child Psychology, 35*(1), 125-36.

Goldstein, P., & Ault, M. (2015). Including individuals with disabilities in a faith community: A framework and example. *Journal of Disability & Religion, 19*(1), 1-14. https://doi.org/10.1080/23312521.2015.992601

Goldstein, T. R., Axelson, D. A., Birmaher, B., & Brent, D. A. (2007). Dialectical behavior therapy for adolescents with bipolar disorder: A 1-year open trial. *Journal of the American Academy of Child & Adolescent Psychiatry,*

46(7), 820-30. https://doi.org/10.1097/chi.0b013 e31805c1613

Goldstein, T. R., Birmaher, B., Axelson, D., Goldstein, B. I., Gill, M. K., Esposito-Smythers, C., Ryan, N. D., Strober, M. A., Hunt, J., & Keller, M. (2009). Family environment and suicidal ideation among bipolar youth. *Archives of Suicide Research, 13*(4), 378-88.

Goldstein, T. R., Fersch-Podrat, R. K., Rivera, M., Axelson, D. A., Merranko, J., Yu, H., Brent, D., & Birmaher, B. (2015). Dialectical behavior therapy for adolescents with bipolar disorder: Results from a pilot randomized trial. *Journal of Child and Adolescent Psychopharmacology, 25*(2), 140-49. https://doi.org/10.1089/cap.2013.0145

Gonzalez, A., Peris, T. S., Vreeland, A., Kiff, C. J., Kendall, P. C., Compton, S. N., Albano, A. M., Birmaher, B., Ginsburg, G. S., Keeton, C. P., March, J., McCracken, J., Sherrill, R. M., Walkup, J. T., & Piacentini, J. (2015). Parental anxiety as a predictor of medication and CBT response for anxious youth. *Child Psychiatry and Human Development, 46*(1), 84-93.

Goodheart, C. D. (2006). Evidence, endeavor, and expertise in psychology practice. In C. D. Goodheart, A. E. Kazdin, & R. J. Sternberg (Eds.), *Evidence-based psychotherapy: Where practice and research meet* (pp. 37-61). American Psychological Association. https://doi.org/10.1037/11423-002

Goodkind, J. R., Lanoue, M. D., & Milford, J. (2010). Adaptation and implementation of cognitive behavioral intervention for trauma in schools with American Indian youth. *Journal of Clinical Child and Adolescent Psychology, 39*(6), 858–872. https://doi.org/10.1080/15374416.2010.517166

Goodman, S. H., & Brand, S. R. (2009). Infants of depressed mothers. In C. H. Zeanah (Ed.), *Handbook of infant mental health* (3rd ed., pp. 153-70). Guilford.

Goodyer, I., Dubicka, B., Wilkinson, P., Kelvin, R., Roberts, C., Byford, S., Breen, S., Ford, C., Barrett, B., Leech, A., Rothwell, J., White, L., & Harrington, R. (2007). Selective serotonin reuptake inhibitors (SSRIs) and routine specialist care with and without cognitive behaviour therapy in adolescents with major depression: Randomised controlled trial. *BMJ: British Medical Journal, 335*(7611), 142.

Goodyer, I. M., Herbert, J., Tamplin, A., Secher, S. M., & Pearson, J. (1997). Short-term outcome of major depression: II. Life events, family dysfunction, and friendship difficulties as predictors of persistent disorder. *Journal of the American Academy of Child and Adolescent Psychiatry, 36*(4), 474–480. https://doi.org/10.1097/00004583-199704000-00009

Gorman-Smith, D., Henry, D. B., & Tolan, P. H. (2004). Exposure to community violence and violence perpetration: The protective effects of family functioning. *Journal of Clinical Child and Adolescent Psychology, 33*(3), 439-49. https://doi.org/10.1207/s15374424jccp3303_2

Gorrell, S., & Le Grange, D. (2019). Update on treatments for adolescent bulimia nervosa. *Child and Adolescent Psychiatric Clinics of North America, 28*(4), 537-47. https://doi.org/10.1016/j.chc.2019.05.002

Grabe, S., Ward, L. M., & Hyde, J. S. (2008). The role of the media in body image concerns among women: A meta-analysis of experimental and correlational studies. *Psychological Bulletin, 134*(3), 460-76.

Gracious, B. L., Youngstrom, E. A., Findling, R. L., & Calabrese, J. R. (2002). Discriminative validity of a parent version of the Young Mania Rating Scale. *Journal of the American Academy of Child & Adolescent Psychiatry, 41*(11), 1350-59.

Grandin, T. (2006). *Thinking in pictures.* Vintage Books.

Grandin, T., & Barron, S. (2017). *Unwritten rules of social relationships: Decoding social mysteries through the unique perspectives of autism* (2nd ed.). Future Horizons.

Granpeesheh, D., & Tarbox, J. (2014). Philosophy and mores. In D. Granpeesheh, J. Tarbox, A. C. Najdowski, & J. Kornack (Eds.), *Evidence-based treatment for children with autism: The CARD Model* (pp. 7-17). Academic Press.

Grant, K. E., Compas, B. E., Stuhlmacher, A. F., Thurm, A. E., McMahon, S. D., & Halpert, J. A. (2003). Stressors and child and adolescent psychopathology: Moving from markers to mechanisms of risk. *Psychological Bulletin, 129*(3), 447-66. https://doi.org/10.1037/0033-2909.129.3.447

Grasso, D., Greene, C., & Ford, J. D. (2013). Cumulative trauma in childhood. In J. D. Ford & C. A. Courtois (Eds.), *Treating complex traumatic stress disorders in children and adolescents: Scientific foundations and therapeutic models* (pp. 79-99). Guilford Press.

Graziano, P. A., & Garcia, A. (2016). Attention-deficit hyperactivity disorder and children's emotion dysregulation: A meta-analysis. *Clinical Psychology Review, 46,* 106-23. https://doi.org/10.1016/j.cpr.2016.04.011

Green, G., Brennan, L. C., & Fein, D. (2002). Intensive behavioral treatment for a toddler at high risk for autism. *Behavior Modification, 26*(1), 69–102. https://doi.org/10.1177/0145445502026001005

Greene, C. A., Grasso, D. J., & Ford, J. D. (2014). Emotion regulation in the wake of complex childhood trauma. In R. Pat-Horenczyk, D. Brom, & J. M. Vogel (Eds.), *Helping children cope with trauma: Individual, family and community perspectives* (pp. 19-40). Routledge/Taylor & Francis Group.

Greenhill, L., Kollins, S., Abikoff, H., McCracken, J., Riddle, M., Swanson, J., McGough, J., Wigal, S., Wigal, T., Vitiello, B., Skrobala, A., Posner, K., Ghuman, J., Cunningham, C., Davis, M., Chuang, S., & Cooper, T. (2006). Efficacy and safety of immediate-release methylphenidate treatment for preschoolers with ADHD. *Journal of the American Academy of Child & Adolescent Psychiatry, 45*(11), 1284-93. https://doi.org/10.1097/01.chi.0000235077.32661.61

Grenz, S. J. (1998). Theological foundations for male-female relationships. *Journal of the Evangelical Theological Society, 41*(4), 615-30.

Grenz, S. J. (2000). *Renewing the center: Evangelical theology in a post-theological era.* Baker Academic.

Gressier, F., Calati, R., Balestri, M., Marsano, A., Alberti, S., Antypa, N., & Serretti, A. (2013). The 5-HTTLPR polymorphism and posttraumatic stress disorder: A meta-analysis. *Journal of Traumatic Stress, 26*(6), 645-53. https://doi.org/10.1002/jts.21855

Griffith, S. F., Arnold, D. H., Rolon-Arroyo, B., & Harvey, E. A. (2019). Neuropsychological predictors of ODD symptom dimensions in young children. *Journal of Clinical Child and Adolescent Psychology, 48*(1), 80-92. https://doi.org/10.1080/15374416.2016.1266643

Groh, A.M., Fearon, R.P., Bakermans-Kranenburg, M.J., van Ijzendoorn, M.H., Steele, R.D., & Roisman, G.I. (2014). The significance of attachment security for children's social competences with peers: A meta-analytic study. *Attachment and Human Development, 16*(2), 103-136. https://doi.10.1080/14616734.2014.883636

Gruber, J., Gilbert, K. E., Youngstrom, E., Youngstrom, J. K., Feeny, N. C., & Findling, R. L. (2013). Reward dysregulation and mood symptoms in an adolescent outpatient sample. *Journal of Abnormal Child Psychology, 41,* 1053-65.

Guarneri-White, M. E., Jensen-Campbell, L. A., & Knack, J. M. (2015). Is co-ruminating with friends related to health problems in victimized adolescents? *Journal of Adolescence,*

39, 15–26. https://doi.org/10.1016/j.adoles cence.2014.11.004

Guedeney, A. (2007). Withdrawal behavior and depression in infancy. *Infant Mental Health Journal, 28*(4), 393-408.

Guerra, C., Farkas, C., & Moncada, L. (2018). Depression, anxiety and PTSD in sexually abused adolescents: Association with self-efficacy, coping and family support. *Child Abuse & Neglect, 76*, 310-20. https://doi.org/10.1016/j. chiabu.2017.11.013

Guerry, J. D., & Hastings, P. D. (2011). In search of HPA axis dysregulation in child and adolescent depression. *Clinical Child and Family Psychology Review, 14*(2), 135-60.

Gullone, E. (2000). The development of normal fear. *Clinical Psychology Review, 20*(4), 429-51.

Gunlick, M. L., & Mufson, L. (2009). Interpersonal psychotherapy for depressed adolescents. In S. Nolen-Hoeksema & L. M. Hilt (Eds.), *Handbook of depression in adolescents* (pp. 511-29). Routledge.

Gunnar, M. R., & Vazquez, D. M. (2001). Low cortisol and a flattening of expected daytime rhythm: Potential indices of risk in human development. *Development and Psychopathology, 13*(3), 515-38. https://doi.org/10.1017/ S0954579401003066

Gurevitz, M., Geva, R., Varon, M., & Leitner, Y. (2014). Early markers in infants and toddlers for development of ADHD. *Journal of Attention Disorders, 18*(1), 14-22. https://doi. org/10.1177/1087054712447858

Hadwin, J. A., Garner, M., & Perez-Olivas, G. (2006). The development of information processing biases in childhood anxiety: A review and exploration of its origins in parenting. *Clinical Psychology Review, 26*(7), 876-94.

Hails, K. A., Reuben, J. D., Shaw, D. S., Dishion, T. J., & Wilson, M. N. (2018). Transactional associations among maternal depression, parent–child coercion, and child conduct problems during early childhood. *Journal of Clinical Child and Adolescent Psychology, 47*(Suppl 1), S291-S305. https://doi.org/10.1080 /15374416.2017.1280803

Halevi, G., Djalovski, A., Vengrober, A., & Feldman, R. (2016). Risk and resilience trajectories in war-exposed children across the first decade of life. *Journal of Child Psychology and Psychiatry, 57*(10), 1183-93. https://doi. org/10.1111/jcpp.12622

Halmi, K. A., Bellace, D., Berthod, S., Ghosh, S., Berrettini, W., Brandt, H. A., Bulik, C. M., Crawford, S., Fichter, M. M., Johnson, C. L., Kaplan, A., Kaye, W. H., Thornton, L., Treasure, J., Blake Woodside, D., & Strober, M. (2012). An examination of early childhood perfectionism across anorexia nervosa subtypes. *International Journal of Eating Disorders, 45*(6), 800–807. https://doi.org/10.1002/eat.22019

Hall, S. E. (2014). Emotion regulation. In K. S. Flanagan & S. E. Hall (Eds.), *Christianity and developmental psychopathology: Theory and application for working with youth* (pp. 63-97). InterVarsity Press.

Hall, S. E., Watson, T. E., Kellums, M., & Kimmel, J. (2016). Mental health needs and resources in Nepal. *International Journal of Culture and Mental Health, 9*, 278-84.

Hallett, V., Ronald, A., Rijsdijk, F., & Eley, T. C. (2009). Phenotypic and genetic differentiation of anxiety-related behaviors in middle childhood. *Depression and Anxiety, 26*(4), 316-24.

Halligan, S., Cooper, P., Fearon, P., Wheeler, S., Crosby, M., & Murray, L. (2013). The longitudinal development of emotion regulation capacities in children at risk for externalizing disorders. *Development and Psychopathology, 25*(2), 391-406. https://doi.org/10.1017/ S0954579412001137

Halligan, S. L., & Philips, K. J. (2010). Are you thinking what I'm thinking? Peer group similarities in adolescent hostile attribution tendencies. *Developmental Psychology, 46*(5), 1385-88.

Hallmayer, J., Cleveland, S., Torres, A., Phillips, J., Cohen, B., Torigoe, T., Miller, J., Fedele, A., Collins, J., Smith, K., Lotspeich, L., Croen, L. A., Ozonoff, S., Lajonchere, C., Grether, J. K., & Risch, N. (2011). Genetic heritability and shared environmental factors among twin pairs with autism. *Archives of General Psychiatry, 68*(11), 1095-1102. https://doi.org/10.1001/archgenpsychiatry.2011.76

Hambour, V. K., Zimmer-Gembeck, M. J., Clear, S., Rowe, S., & Avdagic, E. (2018). Emotion regulation and mindfulness in adolescents: Conceptual and empirical connection and associations with social anxiety symptoms. *Personality and Individual Differences, 134*, 7-12. https://doi.org/10.1016/j.paid.2018.05.037

Hammen, C., Rudolph, K., Weisz, J., Rao, U, & Burge, D. (1999). The context of depression in clinic-referred youth: Neglected areas in treatment. *Journal of the American Academy of Child & Adolescent Psychiatry, 38*, 64-71.

Handford, C. M., Rapee, R. M., & Fardouly, J. (2018). The influence of maternal modeling on body image concerns and eating disturbances in preadolescent girls. *Behaviour Research and Therapy, 100*, 17-23. https://doi.org/10.1016/j.brat.2017.11.001

Hankin, B. L. (2008). Rumination and depression in adolescence: Investigating symptom specificity in a multiwave prospective study. *Journal of Clinical Child and Adolescent Psychology, 37*(4), 701-13.

Hankin, B. L., Young, J. F., Gallop, R., & Garber, J. (2018). Cognitive and interpersonal vulnerability to adolescent depression: Classification of risk profiles for a personalized prevention approach. *Journal of Abnormal Child Psychology, 46*(7), 1521-1533. https://doi.org/10.1007/s10802-018-0401-2

Hanley, G. P. (2012). Functional assessment of problem behavior: Dispelling myths, over-coming implementation obstacles, and developing new lore. *Behavior Analysis in Practice, 5*(1), 54-72.

Hardman, R. K., Berrett, M. E., & Richards, P. S. (2003). Spirituality and ten false beliefs and pursuits of women with eating disorders: implications for counselors. *Counseling and Values, 48*(1), 67-78.

Harpold, T. L., Wozniak, J., Kwon, A., Gilbert, J., Wood, J., Smith, L., & Biederman, J. (2005). Examining the association between pediatric bipolar disorder and anxiety disorders in psychiatrically referred children and adolescents. *Journal of Affective Disorders, 88*(1), 19-26.

Harrison, P., & Oakland, T. (2015). *Adaptive Behavior Assessment System, Third Edition (ABAS-3)*. Western Psychological Services.

Harstad, E., Weaver, A. L., Katusic, S. K., Colligan, R. C., Kumar, S., Chan, E., Voigt, R. G., & Barbaresi, W. J. (2014). ADHD, stimulant treatment, and growth: A longitudinal study. *Pediatrics, 134*(4), 935-44. https://doi.org/10.1542/peds.2014-0428

Harvey, E. A., Lugo-Candelas, C. I., & Breaux, R. P. (2015). Longitudinal changes in individual symptoms across the preschool years in children with ADHD. *Journal of Clinical Child and Adolescent Psychology, 44*(4), 580–594. https://doi.org/10.1080/15374416.2014.886253

Harvey, E. A., Metcalfe, L. A., Herbert, S. D., & Fanton, J. H. (2011). The role of family experiences and ADHD in the early development of oppositional defiant disorder. *Journal of Clinical Child and Adolescent Psychology, 41*, 784-95.

Hatch, B., Healey, D. M., & Halperin, J. M. (2014). Associations between birth weight and attention-deficit/hyperactivity disorder symptom severity: Indirect effects via primary neuropsychological functions. *Journal of Child Psychology and Psychiatry, 55*(4), 384-92. https://doi.org/10.1111/jcpp.12168

Havens, J. F., Gudiño, O. G., Biggs, E. A., Diamond, U. N., Weis, J. R., & Cloitre, M. (2012). Identification of trauma exposure and PTSD in adolescent psychiatric inpatients: An exploratory study. *Journal of Traumatic Stress, 25*(2), 171-78. https://doi.org/10.1002/jts.21683

Hawker, D. S. J., & Boulton, M. J. (2000). Twenty years' research on peer victimization and psychosocial maladjustment: A meta-analytic review of cross-sectional studies. *Journal of Child Psychology and Psychiatry, 41*(4), 441-55.

Hawkins, J., Catalano, R., Kosterman, R., Abbott, R., & Hill, K. (1999). Preventing adolescent health-risk behaviors by strengthening protection during childhood. *Archives of Pediatrics & Adolescent Medicine, 153*(3), 226-34.

Hayden, E. P., Seeds, P. M., & Dozois, D. J. A. (2009). Risk and vulnerability in adolescent depression. In C. A. Essau (Ed.), *Treatments for adolescent depression* (pp. 27-56). Guilford.

Haynos, A. F., Watts, A. W., Loth, K. A., Pearson, C. M., & Neumark-Stzainer, D. (2016). Factors predicting an escalation of restrictive eating during adolescence. *Journal of Adolescent Health, 59*(4), 391-96. https://doi.org/10.1016/j.jadohealth.2016.03.011

Hayward, D., Eikeseth, S., Gale, C., & Morgan, S. (2009). Assessing progress during treatment for young children with autism receiving intensive behavioural interventions. *Autism, 13*(6), 613-33. https://doi.org/10.1177/136236 1309340029

Healy, S. J., Murray, L., Cooper, P. J., Hughes, C., & Halligan, S. L. (2015). A longitudinal investigation of maternal influences on the development of child hostile attributions and aggression. *Journal of Clinical Child and Adolescent Psychology, 44*(1), 80-92.

Hechtman, L., Swanson, J. M., Sibley, M. H., Stehli, A., Owens, E. B., Mitchell, J. T., Arnold, L. E., Molina, B. S. G., Hinshaw, S. P., Jensen, P. S., Abikoff, H. B., Algorta, G. P., Howard, A. L.,

Hoza, B., Etcovitch, J., Houssais, S., Lakes, K. D., & Nichols, J. Q. (2016). Functional adult outcomes 16 years after childhood diagnosis of attention-deficit/hyperactivity disorder: MTA results. *Journal of the American Academy of Child & Adolescent Psychiatry, 55*(11), 945-52. https://doi.org/10.1016/j.jaac.2016.07.774

Heim, C., Newport, D. J., Mletzko, T., Miller, A. H., & Nemeroff, C. B. (2008). The link between childhood trauma and depression: insights from HPA axis studies in humans. *Psychoneuroendocrinology, 33*(6), 693-710.

Hembree, W. C. (2011). Guidelines for pubertal suspension and gender reassignment for transgender adolescents. *Child and Adolescent Psychiatric Clinics of North America, 20*(4), 725-32. https://doi.org/10.1016/j.chc.2011.08.004

Hembree, W. C., Cohen-Kettenis, P., Delemarre-van de Waal, H. A., Gooren, L. J., Meyer, W. J., III, Spack, N. P., Tangpricha, V., & Montori, V. M. (2009). Endocrine treatment of transsexual persons: An Endocrine Society clinical practice guideline. *Journal of Clinical Endocrinology & Metabolism, 94*(9), 3132-54.

Henggeler, S. W., & Schaeffer, C. M. (2017). Treating serious antisocial behavior using multisystemic therapy. In J. R. Weisz & A. E. Kazdin (Eds.), *Evidence-based psychotherapies for children and adolescents* (2nd ed., pp. 197-214). Guilford.

Henggeler, S. W., Schoenwald, S. K., Borduin, C. M., Rowland, M. D., & Cunningham, P. B. (2009). *Multisystemic therapy for antisocial behavior in children and adolescents* (2nd ed.). Guilford.

Henggeler, S. W., Schoenwald, S. K., Rowland, M. D., & Cunningham, P. B. (2002). *Serious emotional disturbance in children and adolescents: Multisystemic therapy.* Guilford.

Henry, B., Caspi, A., Moffitt, T. E., & Silva, P. A. (1996). Temperamental and familial predictors of violent and nonviolent criminal convictions: Age 3 to age 18. *Developmental Psychology, 32*(4), 614-23.

Herrmann, S. (2016). Counting sheep: Sleep disorders in children With autism spectrum disorders. *Journal of Pediatric Health Care, 30*(2), 143–154. https://doi.org/10.1016/j.pedhc.2015.07.003

Herpertz-Dahlmann, B. (2009). Adolescent eating disorders: definitions, symptomatology, epidemiology and comorbidity. *Child and Adolescent Psychiatric Clinics of North America, 18*(1), 31–47. https://doi.org/10.1016/j.chc.2008.07.005

Herts, K. L., McLaughlin, K. A., & Hatzenbuehler, M. L. (2012). Emotion dysregulation as a mechanism linking stress exposure to adolescent aggressive behavior. *Journal of Abnormal Child Psychology, 40*(7), 1111-22.

Hewitt, P. L., & Flett, G. L. (1991). Perfectionism in the self and social contexts: Conceptualization, assessment, and association with psychopathology. *Journal of Personality and Social Psychology, 60*(3), 456-70. https://doi.org/10.1037/0022-3514.60.3.456

Hicks, T. A., Bountress, K. E., Resnick, H. S., Ruggiero, K. J., & Amstadter, A. B. (2020). Caregiver support buffers posttraumatic stress disorder symptoms following a natural disaster in relation to binge drinking. *Psychological Trauma: Theory, Research, Practice, and Policy*. Advance online publication. https://doi.org/10.1037/tra0000553

Higa, C. K., & Daleiden, E. L. (2008). Social anxiety and cognitive biases in non-referred children: The interaction of self-focused attention and threat interpretation biases. Journal of Anxiety Disorders, 22(3), 441-52.

Higa-McMillan, C. K., Francis, S. E., & Chorpita, B. F. (2014). Anxiety disorders. In E. J. Mash & R. A. Barkley (Eds.), *Child psychopathology* (3rd ed., pp. 345-28). Guilford.

Higa-McMillan, C. K., Francis, S. E., Rith-Najarian, L., & Chorpita, B. F. (2016). Evidence base update: 50 years of research on treatment for child and adolescent anxiety. *Journal of Clinical Child and Adolescent Psychology, 45*(2), 91-113.

Hildebrandt, T., Alfano, L., Tricamo, M., & Pfaff, D. W. (2010). Conceptualizing the role of estrogens and serotonin in the development and maintenance of bulimia nervosa. *Clinical Psychology Review, 30*(6), 655-68. https://doi.org/10.1016/j.cpr.2010.04.011

Hilt, L. M., & Nolen-Hoeksema S. (2006). The emergence of gender differences in depression in adolescence. In S. Nolen-Hoeksema & L. M. Hilt (Eds.), *Handbook of depression in adolescents* (pp. 111-35). Routledge.

Hinshaw, S. P. (2005). Enhancing social competence in children with attention-deficit/hyperactivity disorder: Challenges for the new millennium. In E. D. Hibbs & P. S. Jensen (Eds.), *Psychosocial treatments for child and adolescent disorders: Empirically based strategies for clinical practice* (2nd ed., pp. 351-376). American Psychological Association.

Hinshaw, S. P. (2017). Developmental psychopathology as a scientific discipline. In T. P. Beauchaine & S. P. Hinshaw (Eds.), *Child and adolescent psychopathology* (3rd ed., pp. 3-32). John Wiley & Sons.

Hinshaw, S. P., & Arnold, L. E. (2015). Attention-deficit hyperactivity disorder, multimodal treatment, and longitudinal outcome: Evidence, paradox, and challenge. *Wires Cognitive Science, 6*(1), 39-52. https://doi.org/10.1002/wcs.1324

Hirshfeld-Becker, D. R., Biederman, J., & Rosenbaum, J. F. (2004). Behavioral inhibition. In T. L. Morris & J. S. March (Eds.), *Anxiety disorders in children and adolescents* (2nd ed., pp. 27-58). Guilford.

Hitchcock, C., Ellis, A. A., Williamson, P., & Nixon, R. V. (2015). The prospective role of cognitive appraisals and social support in predicting children's posttraumatic stress. *Journal of Abnormal Child Psychology, 43*(8), 1485-92. https://doi.org/10.1007/s10802-015-0034-7

Hoek, H. W., & van Hoeken, D. (2003). Review of the prevalence and incidence of eating disorders. *International Journal of Eating Disorders, 34*(4), 383-96. https://doi.org/10.1002/eat.10222

Hoekzema, E., Schagen, S. E., Kreukels, B. C., Veltman, D. J., Cohen-Kettenis, P. T., Delemarre-van de Waal, H., & Bakker, J. (2015). Regional volumes and spatial volumetric distribution of gray matter in the gender dysphoric brain. *Psychoneuroendocrinology, 55,* 59-71. https://doi.org/10.1016/j.psyneuen.2015.01.016

Holman, C. W., & Goldberg, J. M. (2006). Ethical, legal, and psychosocial issues in care of transgender adolescents. *International Journal of Transgenderism, 9*(3-4), 95-110. https://doi.org/10.1300/J485v09n03_05

Holmes, M. M. (2000). A terrible thing happened: A story for children who have witnessed violence or trauma. Magination Press.

Hong, J. S., Tillman, R., & Luby, J. L. (2015). Disruptive behavior in preschool children: Distinguishing normal misbehavior from markers of current and later childhood conduct disorder. *The Journal of Pediatrics, 166*(3), 723-30.

Howard, K.A.S., Budge, S.L., & McKay, K.M. (2010). Youth exposed to violence: The role of protective factors. *Journal of Community Psychology, 38,* 63-79. https://doi.org/10.1002/JCOP.20352

Howlin, P., Goode, S., Hutton, J., & Rutter, M. (2004). Adult outcome for children with autism. *Journal of Child Psychology and Psychiatry, 45*(2), 212-29. https://doi.org/10.1111/j.1469-7610.2004.00215.x

Hoza, B. (2007). Peer functioning in children with ADHD. *Journal of Pediatric Psychology, 32*(6), 655-63. https://doi.org/10.1093/jpepsy/jsm024

Huberty, T. J. (2012). *Anxiety and depression in children and adolescents: Assessment, intervention, and prevention.* Springer.

Hudec, K. L., Alderson, R. M., Patros, C. G., Lea, S. E., Tarle, S. J., & Kasper, L. J. (2015). Hyperactivity in boys with attention-deficit/hyperactivity disorder (ADHD): The role of executive and non-executive functions. *Research in Developmental Disabilities, 45-46,* 103-9. https://doi.org/10.1016/j.ridd.2015.07.012

Hudson, J. L., Dodd, H. F., & Bovopoulos, N. (2011). Temperament, family environment and anxiety in preschool children. *Journal of Abnormal Child Psychology, 39*(7), 939-51.

Huey, S. J., & Polo, A. J. (2018). Evidence-based psychotherapies with ethnic minority children and adolescents. In J. R. Weisz & A. E. Kazdin (Eds.), *Evidence-based psychotherapies for children and adolescents* (3rd ed., pp. 361-78). Guilford Press.

Hughes, C., White, A., Sharpen, J., & Dunn, J. (2000). Antisocial, angry, and unsympathetic: "Hard-to-manage" preschoolers' peer problems and possible cognitive influences. *Journal of Child Psychology and Psychiatry, 41*(2), 169-79.

Hughes, E. K., Goldschmidt, A. B., Labuschagne, Z., Loeb, K. L., Sawyer, S. M., & Grange, D. L. (2013). Eating disorders with and without comorbid depression and anxiety: Similarities and differences in a clinical sample of children and adolescents. *European Eating Disorders Review, 21,* 386-94.

Hughes, E. K., Gullone, E., & Watson, S. D. (2011). Emotional functioning in children and adolescents with elevated depressive symptoms. *Journal of Psychopathology and Behavior Assessment, 33,* 335-45.

Hulme, P. A. (2011). Childhood sexual abuse, HPA axis regulation, and mental health: An integrative review. *Western Journal of Nursing Research*, *33*(8), 1069-97. https://doi.org/10.1177/0193945910388949

Hultman, C., Sandin, S., Levine, S., Lichtenstein, P., & Reichenberg, A. (2011). Advancing paternal age and risk of autism: New evidence from a population-based study and a meta-analysis of epidemiological studies. *Molecular Psychiatry, 16*(12), 1203-12.

Hultman, C. M., Sparén, P., & Cnattingius, S. (2002). Perinatal risk factors for infantile autism. *Epidemiology, 13*(4), 417-23.

Hulvershorn, L. A., Cullen, K., & Anand, A. (2011). Toward dysfunctional connectivity: A review of neuroimaging findings in pediatric major depressive disorder. *Brain Imaging and Behavior, 5*(4), 307-28.

Human Rights Campaign. (2016). *Supporting & caring for transgender children*. Retrieved September 9, 2020, from https://www.hrc.org/resources/supporting-caring-for-transgender-children

Hummel, R. M., & Gross, A. M. (2001). Socially anxious children: An observational study of parent-child interaction. *Child & Family Behavior Therapy, 23*(3), 19-41.

Hummer, T. A., Wang, Y., Kronenberger, W. G., Dunn, D. W., & Mathews, V. P. (2015). The relationship of brain structure to age and executive functioning in adolescent disruptive behavior disorder. *Psychiatry Research: Neuroimaging, 231*(3), 210-17.

Hurrell, K. E., Hudson, J. L., & Schniering, C. A. (2015). Parental reactions to children's negative emotions: Relationships with emotion regulation in children with an anxiety disorder. *Journal of Anxiety Disorders, 29*, 72-82.

Hutchison, L., Feder, M., Abar, B., & Winsler, A. (2016). Relations between parenting stress, parenting style, and child executive functioning for children with ADHD or autism. *Journal of Child and Family Studies, 25*(12), 3644-56. https://doi.org/10.1007/s10826-016-0518-2

Ingersoll, B., Dvortcsak, A., Whalen, C., & Sikora, D. (2005). The effects of a developmental, social-pragmatic language intervention on rate of expressive language production in young children with autistic spectrum disorders. *Focus on Autism and Other Developmental Disabilities, 20*(4), 213-22. https://doi.org/10.1177/10883576050200040301

Ipser, J. C., Stein, D. J., Hawkridge, S., & Hoppe, L. (2009). Pharmacotherapy for anxiety disorders in children and adolescents. *Cochrane Database of Systematic Reviews, 3*, 1-24.

Ivey, A., D'Andrea, M., & Ivey, M. (2011). *Theories of counseling and psychotherapy: A multicultural perspective* (7th ed.). Sage Publications.

Jacobson, L. A., Crocetti, D., Dirlikov, B., Slifer, K., Denckla, M. B., Mostofsky, S. H., & Mahone, E. M. (2018). Anomalous brain development is evident in preschoolers with attention deficit hyperactive disorder. *Journal of the International Neuropsychology Society, 24*(6), 531-39. https://doi.org/10.1017/S1355617718000103

Jaffe, S. R. (2017). Child maltreatment and risk for psychopathology. In T. P. Beauchaine & S. P. Hinshaw (Eds.), *Child and adolescent psychopathology* (3rd ed., pp. 144-77). Wiley.

Jaffee, S. R., Caspi, A., Moffitt, T. E., & Taylor, A. (2004). Physical maltreatment victim to antisocial child: Evidence of an environmentally mediated process. *Journal of Abnormal Psychology, 113*(1), 44-55.

Jalbrzikowski, M., Larsen, B., Hallquist, M. N., Foran, W., Calabro, F., & Luna, B. (2017). Development of white matter microstructure and intrinsic functional connectivity between the amygdala and ventromedial prefrontal cortex: Associations with anxiety and depression. *Biological Psychiatry, 82*(7), 511-21. https://doi.org/10.1016/j.biopsych.2017.01.008

Jameson, N. D., Sheppard, B. K., Lateef, T. M., Vande Voort, J. L., He, J., & Merikangas, K. R. (2016). Medical comorbidity of attention-deficit/hyperactivity disorder in US adolescents. *Journal of Child Neurology, 31*(11), 1282-89. https://doi.org/10.1177/08830738166 53782

Janssen, T. W., Heslenfeld, D. J., van Mourik, R., Logan, G. D., & Oosterlaan, J. (2015). Neural correlates of response inhibition in children with attention-deficit/hyperactivity disorder: A controlled version of the stop-signal task. *Psychiatry Research, 233*(2), 278–284. https://doi.org/10.1016/j.pscychresns.2015.07.007

Javaras, K. N., Laird, N. M., Reichborn-Kjennerud, T., Bulik, C. M., Pope, H. J., & Hudson, J. I. (2008). Familiality and heritability of binge eating disorder: Results of a case-control family study and a twin study. *International Journal of Eating Disorders, 41*(2), 174-79. https://doi.org/10.1002/eat.20484

Jaycox, L. (2004). *Cognitive-Behavioral Intervention for Trauma in Schools*. Sopris West.

Jaycox, L. H., Cohen, J. A., Mannarino, A. P., Walker, D. W., Langley, A. K., Gegenheimer, K. L., Scott, M., & Schonlau, M. (2010). Children's mental health care following Hurricane Katrina: A field trial of trauma-focused psychotherapies. *Journal of Traumatic Stress, 23*(2), 223-31.

Jensen, D. H. (2005). *Graced vulnerability: A theology of childhood*. Pilgrim Press.

Jett, S., LaPorte, D. J., & Wanchisn, J. (2010). Impact of exposure to pro-eating disorder websites on eating behaviour in college women. *European Eating Disorders Review, 18*(5), 410-16. https://doi.org/10.1002/erv.1009

Johnson, C., & Myers, S. (2007). Identification and evaluation of children with autism spectrum disorders. *Pediatrics, 120*(5), 1183-215.

Johnson, E. L. (1987). Sin, weakness, and psychopathology. *Journal of Psychology and Theology, 15*, 218-26.

Johnson, S., Kochhar, P., Hennessy, E., Marlow, N., Wolke, D., & Hollis, C. (2016). Antecedents of attention-deficit/hyperactivity disorder symptoms in children born extremely preterm. *Journal of Developmental and Behavioral Pediatrics, 37*(4), 285-97. https://doi.org/10.1097/DBP.0000000000000298

Johnson, W. G., Grieve, F. G., Adams, C. D., & Sandy, J. (1999). Measuring binge eating in adolescents: Adolescent and parent versions of the Questionnaire of Eating and Weight Patterns. *International Journal of Eating Disorders, 26*(3), 301-14. https://doi.org/10.1002/(SICI)1098-108X(199911)26:3<301::AID-EAT8>3.0.CO;2-M

Johnston, C., & Mash, E. J. (2001). Families of children with attention-deficit/hyperactivity disorder: Review and recommendations for future research. *Clinical Child and Family Psychology Review, 4*(3), 183-207. https://doi.org/10.1023/A:1017592030434

Joiner, T. E., Catanzaro, S. J., & Laurent, J. (1996). Tripartite structure of positive and negative affect, depression, and anxiety in child and adolescent psychiatric inpatients. *Journal of Abnormal Psychology, 105*(3), 401-9.

Jones, D. C., Vigfusdottir, T. H., & Lee, Y. (2004). Body image and the appearance culture among adolescent girls and boys: An examination of friend conversations, peer criticism, appearance magazines, and the internalization of appearance ideals. *Journal of Adolescent Research, 19*(3), 323-39. https://doi.org/10.1177/0743558403258847

Jones, E. J., Gliga, T., Bedford, R., Charman, T., & Johnson, M. H. (2014). Developmental pathways to autism: a review of prospective studies of infants at risk. *Neuroscience and Biobehavioral Reviews, 39*(100), 1–33. https://doi.org/10.1016/j.neubiorev.2013.12.001

Jones, J. M., Bennett, S., Olmsted, M. P., Lawson, M. L., & Rodin, G. (2001). Disordered eating attitudes and behaviours in teenaged girls: A school-based study. *Canadian Medical Association Journal, 165*(5), 547-52.

Jones, S. L. (2010). An integration view. In E. L. Johnson (Ed.), *Psychology and Christianity: Five views* (2nd ed., pp. 101-28). InterVarsity Press.

Jones, S. L., Flanagan, K. F., & Butman, R. E. (2011). Behavior therapy. In S. L. Jones & R. E. Butman (Eds.), *Modern psychotherapies: A comprehensive Christian appraisal* (2nd ed., pp. 166-200). InterVarsity Press.

Jones, W., & Klin, A. (2013). Attention to eyes is present but in decline in 2-6-month-old infants later diagnosed with autism. *Nature, 504*(7480), 427-31. https://doi.org/10.1038/nature12715

Josephson, A. M., & Dell, M. L. (2004). Religion and spirituality in child and adolescent psychiatry: A new frontier. *Child and Adolescent Psychiatric Clinics of North America, 13*(1), 1-15. https://doi.org/10.1016/S1056-4993(03)00099-3

Jung, V., Short, R., Letourneau, N., & Andrews, D. (2007). Interventions with depressed mothers and their infants: Modifying interactive behaviours. *Journal of Affective Disorders, 98*(3), 199-205.

Juranek, J., Filipek, P. A., Berenji, G. R., Modahl, C., Osann, K., & Spence, M. A. (2006). Association between amygdala volume and anxiety level: Magnetic resonance imaging (MRI) study in autistic children. *Journal of Child Neurology, 21*(12), 1051-68. https://doi.org/10.1177/7010.2006.00237

Kagan, J., Reznick, J. S., Snidman, N., Gibbons, J., & Johnson, M. O. (1988). Childhood derivatives of inhibition and lack of inhibition to the unfamiliar. *Child Development, 59*(6), 1580-89.

Kalkbrenner, A. E., Schmidt, R. J., & Penlesky, A. C. (2014). Environmental chemical exposures and autism spectrum disorders: A review of the epidemiological evidence. *Current Problems in Pediatric and Adolescent Health Care, 44*(10), 277-318. https://doi.org/10.1016/j.cppeds.2014.06.001

Kaminski, J., & Claussen, A. (2017). Evidence base update for psychosocial treatments for disruptive behaviors in children. *Journal of Clinical Child and Adolescent Psychology, 46*(4), 477-99. https://doi.org/10.1080/15374416.2017.1310044

Kaplan, A. S., & Garfinkel, P. E. (1999). Difficulties in treating patients with eating disorders: A review of patient and clinician variables. *The Canadian Journal of Psychiatry, 44*(7), 665-70.

Kaplow, J. B., Rolon-Arroyo, B., Layne, C. M., Rooney, E., Oosterhoff, B., Hill, R., Steinberg, A. M., Lotterman, J., Gallagher, K. A. S., & Pynoos, R. S. (2020). Validation of the UCLA PTSD Reaction Index for DSM-5: A developmentally informed assessment tool for youth. *Journal of the American Academy of Child & Adolescent Psychiatry, 59*(1), 186-94. https://doi.org/10.1016/j.jaac.2018.10.019

Kassam-Adams, N. (2006). The acute stress checklist for children (ASC-Kids): Development of a child self-report measure. *Journal of Traumatic Stress, 19*(1), 129-39.

Kataoka, S. H., Santiago, C. D., Jaycox, L. H., Langley, A. K., Stein, B. D., & Vona, P. (2014). Cognitive behavioral intervention for trauma in schools: Dissemination and implementation of a school-based intervention. In R. S. Beidas & P. C. Kendall (Eds.), *Dissemination and implementation of evidence-based practices in child and adolescent mental health* (pp. 294-310). Oxford University Press.

Kataoka, S. H., Stein, B. D., Jaycox, L. H., Wong, M., Escudero, P., Tu, W., Zaragoza, C., & Fink, A. (2003). A school-based mental health program for traumatized Latino immigrant children. *Journal of the American Academy of Child & Adolescent Psychiatry, 42*(3), 311-18. https://doi.org/10.1097/00004583-200303000-00011

Kaufman, J., Birmaher, B., Axelson, D., Pereplet-chikova, F., Brent, D., & Ryan, N. (2016). *Kiddie Schedule for Affective Disorders and Schizophrenia for School Aged Children—Lifetime Version—DSM-5*. Retrieved from https://www.pediatricbipolar.pitt.edu/sites/default/files/KSADS_DSM_5_SCREEN_Final.pdf

Kaufman, J., Birmaher, B., Brent, D., Rao, U., Flynn, C., Moreci, P., Williamson, D., & Ryan, N. (1997). Schedule for Affective Disorders and Schizophrenia for School-Age Children—Present and Lifetime Version (K-SADS-PL): Initial reliability and validity data. *Journal of the American Academy of Child & Adolescent Psychiatry, 36*(7), 980-88.

Kaur, H., & Kearney, C. A. (2015). An examination of posttraumatic stress symptoms among maltreated multiracial youth. *Journal of Aggression, Maltreatment & Trauma, 24*(5), 487-500. https://doi.org/10.1080/10926771.2015.1029181

Kazdin, A. E. (2005). *Parent management training*. Oxford University Press.

Kazdin, A. E. (2008). Evidence-based treatment and practice: New opportunities to bridge clinical research and practice, enhance the knowledge base, and improve patient care. *American Psychologist, 63*(3), 146-59. https://doi.org/10.1037/0003-066X.63.3.146

Kazdin, A. E. (2010). Problem-solving skills training and parent management training for Oppositional Defiant Disorder and Conduct Disorder. In J.R. Weisz & A.E. Kazdin (Eds.). *Evidence-based psychotherapies for children and adolescents* (2nd ed., pp. 211-226). New York: Guilford Press.

Kazdin, A. E. (2018). Parent management training and problem-solving skills training for child and adolescent conduct problems. In J. R. Weisz & A. E. Kazdin (Eds.), *Evidence-based psychotherapies for children and adolescents* (3rd ed., pp. 142-58). Guilford Press.

Kearney, A. J. (2008). *Understanding applied behavior analysis*. Jessica Kingsley Publishers.

Keding, T. J., & Herringa, R. J. (2015). Abnormal structure of fear circuitry in pediatric posttraumatic stress disorder. *Neuropsychopharmacology, 40*(3), 537-45. https://doi.org/10.1038/npp.2014.239

Keel, P. K., Dorer, D. J., Eddy, K. T., Franko, D., Charatan, D. L., & Herzog, D. B. (2003). Predictors of mortality in eating disorders. *Archives of General Psychiatry, 60*(2), 179-83. https://doi.org/10.1001/archpsyc.60.2.179

Keel, P. K., Klump, K. L., Leon, G. R., & Fulkerson, J. A. (1998). Disordered eating in adolescent males from a school-based sample. *International Journal of Eating Disorders, 23*(2), 125-32. https://doi.org/10.1002/(SICI)1098-108X(199803)23:2<125::AID-EAT2>3.0.CO;2-M

Keenan, K., Shaw, D., Delliquadri, E., Giovannelli, J., & Walsh, B. (1999). Evidence for the continuity of early problem behaviors: Application of a developmental model. *Journal of Abnormal Child Psychology, 26*(6), 443-54.

Keenan, K., & Wakschlag, L. S. (2000). More than the terrible twos: The nature and severity of behavior problems in clinic-referred preschool children. *Journal of Abnormal Child Psychology, 28*(1), 33-46.

Keenan, K., & Wakschlag, L. S. (2002). Can a valid diagnosis of disruptive behavior disorders be made in preschool children? *American Journal of Psychiatry, 159*(3), 351-58.

Keenan, K., & Wakschlag, L. S. (2004). Are oppositional defiant disorder and conduct disorder symptoms normative behaviors in preschoolers? A comparison of referred and nonreferred children. *American Journal of Psychiatry, 161*(2), 356-58.

Keery, H., van den Berg, P., & Thompson, J. K. (2004). An evaluation of the Tripartite Influence Model of body dissatisfaction and eating disturbance with adolescent girls. *Body Image, 1*(3), 237-51. https://doi.org/10.1016/j.bodyim.2004.03.001

Keeshin, B. R., & Strawn, J. R. (2014). Psychological and pharmacologic treatment of youth with posttraumatic stress disorder: An evidence-based review. *Child and Adolescent Psychiatric Clinics of North America, 23*(2), 399-411. https://doi.org/10.1016/j.chc.2013.12.002

Keeshin, B. R., Strawn, J. R., Out, D., Granger, D. A., & Putnam, F. W. (2013). Cortisol awakening response in adolescents with acute sexual abuse related posttraumatic stress disorder. *Depression and Anxiety, 31*(2), 107-14. https://doi.org/10.1002/da.22154

Keil, V., Asbrand, J., Tuschen-Caffier, B., & Schmitz, J. (2017). Children with social anxiety and other anxiety disorders show similar deficits in habitual emotional regulation: Evidence for a transdiagnostic phenomenon. *European Child & Adolescent Psychiatry, 26*(7), 749-57. https://doi.org/10.1007/s00787-017-0942-x

Keller, M. B., Lavori, P. W., Wunder, J., Beardslee, W. R., Schwartz, C. E., & Roth, J. (1992). Chronic course of anxiety disorders in children and sdolescents. *Journal of the American Academy of Child & Adolescent Psychiatry, 31*(4), 595-99.

Kendall, P. C. (1994). Treating anxiety disorders in children: Results of a randomized clinical trial. *Journal of Consulting and Clinical Psychology, 62*(1), 100-10.

Kendall, P. C., Choudhury, M., Hudson, J., & Webb, A. (2002). *The C.A.T. Project manual.* Workbook Publishing.

Kendall, P. C., Crawford, E. A., Kagan, E. R., Furr, J. M. & Podell, J. L. (2017). Child-focused treatment of anxiety. In J. R. Weisz & A. E. Kazdin (Eds.), *Evidence-based psychotherapies for children and adolescents* (3rd. ed., pp. 17-34). Guilford.

Kendall, P. C., Cummings, C. M., Villabø, M. A., Narayanan, M. K., Treadwell, K., Birmaher, B., Compton, S., Piacentini, J., Sherrill, J., Walkup, J., Gosch, E., Keeton, C., Ginsburg, G., Suveg, C., & Albano, A. M. (2016). Mediators of change in the Child/Adolescent Anxiety Multimodal Treatment Study. *Journal of Consulting and Clinical Psychology, 84*(1), 1-14.

Kendall, P. C., Flannery-Schroeder, E., Panichelli-Mindel, S. M., Southam-Gerow, M., Henin, A., & Warman, M. (1997). Therapy for youths with anxiety disorders: A second randomized clinical trial. *Journal of Consulting and Clinical Psychology, 65*(3), 366-80.

Kendall, P. C., Furr, J. M., & Podell, J. L. (2010). Child-focused treatment of anxiety. In J. R. Weisz & A. E. Kazdin (Eds.), *Evidence-based psychotherapies for children and adolescents* (2nd ed., pp. 45-60). Guilford.

Kendall, P. C., Gosch, E., Furr, J., & Sood, E. (2008). Flexibility within fidelity. *Journal of the American Academy of Child & Adolescent Psychiatry, 47*(9), 987-87.

Kendall, P. C., & Hedtke, K. A. (2006). *Cognitive-behavioral therapy for anxious children: Therapist manual.* Workbook Publishing.

Kendall, P. C., Robin, J. A., Hedtke, K. A., Suveg, C., Flannery-Schroeder, E., & Gosch, E. (2005). Considering CBT with anxious youth? Think exposures. *Cognitive and Behavioral Practice, 12*(1), 136-48.

Kendler, K. S., MacLean, C., Neale, M. C., Kessler, R. C., Heath, A. C., & Eaves, L. J. (1991). The genetic epidemiology of bulimia nervosa. *American Journal of Psychiatry, 148*(12), 1627-37.

Kennard, B. D., Emslie, G. J., Mayes, T. L., Nakonezny, P. A., Jones, J. M., Foxwell, A. A., & King, J. (2014). Sequential treatment with fluoxetine and relapse-prevention CBT to improve outcomes in pediatric depression. *American Journal of Psychiatry, 171*(10), 1083-90.

Kerns, C. M., Kendall, P. C., Zickgraf, H., Franklin, M. E., Miller, J., Herrington, J. (2015). Not to be overshadowed or overlooked: Functional impairments associated with comorbid anxiety disorders in youth with ASD. *Behavior Therapy*, 46(1), 29-39. https://doi.org/10.1016/j.beth.2014.03.005

Kerns, K. A., Siener, S., & Brumariu, L. E. (2011). Mother–child relationships, family context, and child characteristics as predictors of anxiety symptoms in middle childhood. *Development and Psychopathology*, 23(2), 593-604.

Kessler, R. C., Adler, L., Barkley, R., Biederman, J., Conners, C. K., Demler, O., Faraone, S. V., Greenhill, L. L., Howes, M. J., Secnik, K., Spencer, T., Ustun, B., Walters, E. E., & Zaslavsky, A. M. (2006). The prevalence and correlates of adult ADHD in the United States: Results from the National Comorbidity Survey replication. *The American Journal of Psychiatry*, 163(4), 716-23. https://doi.org/10.1176/appi.ajp.163.4.716

Kessler, R. C., Avenevoli, S., Costello, E. J., Georgiades, K., Green, J. G., Gruber, M. J., He, J.-P., Koretz, D., McLaughlin, K. A., Petukhova, M., Sampson, N., Zaslavsky, A. M., & Merikangas, K. R. (2012). Prevalence, persistence, and sociodemographic correlates of *DSM-IV* disorders in the National Comorbidity Survey Replication Adolescent Supplement. *Archives of General Psychiatry*, 69(4), 372-80.

Kessler, R. C., Berglund, P., Demler, O., Jin, R., Merikangas, K. R., & Walters, E. E. (2005). Lifetime prevalence and age-of-onset distributions of DSM-IV disorders in the National Comorbidity Survey Replication. *Archives of General Psychiatry*, 62(6), 593-602.

Khamis, V. (2015). Coping with war trauma and psychological distress among school-age Palestinian children. *American Journal of Orthopsychiatry*, 85(1), 72-79. https://doi.org/10.1037/ort0000039

Kiliç, E. Z., Özgüven, H. D., & Sayil, I. (2003). The psychological effects of parental mental health on children experiencing disaster: The experience of Bolu earthquake in Turkey. *Family Process*, 42(4), 485-95. https://doi.org/10.1111/j.1545-5300.2003.00485.x

Kim, E. Y., Miklowitz, D. J., Biuckians, A., & Mullen, K. (2007). Life stress and the course of early-onset bipolar disorder. *Journal of Affective Disorders*, 99(1-3), 37-44.

Kim, J., & Cicchetti, D. (2010). Longitudinal pathways linking child maltreatment, emotion regulation, peer relations, and psychopathology. *Journal of Child Psychology and Psychiatry*, 51(6), 706-16.

Kim-Cohen, J., Arseneault, L., Caspi, A., Tomás, M. P., Taylor, A., & Moffitt, T. E. (2005). Validity of DSM-IV conduct disorder in 41/2-5-year-old children: a longitudinal epidemiological study. *The American Journal of Psychiatry*, 162(6), 1108-17.

Kimberlin, S., & Berrick, J.D. (2015). Poor for how long? Chronic vs. transient child poverty in the United States. In E. Fernandez, A. Zeira, T. Vecchiato, & C. Canali (Eds.). *Theoretical and empirical insights into child and family poverty: Cross national perspectives.* Springer Publisher.

Kimonis, E. R., Frick, P. J., & McMahon, R. J. (2014). Conduct and oppositional defiant disorders. In E. J. Mash & R. A. Barkley (Eds.), *Child psychopathology* (3rd ed., pp. 145-79). Guilford.

Klasen, F., Reissmann, S., Voss, C., & Okello, J. (2015). The guiltless guilty: Trauma-related guilt and psychopathology in former Ugandan child soldiers. *Child Psychiatry and Human Development*, 46(2), 180-93. https://doi.org/10.1007/s10578-014-0470-6

Kleim, B., Grey, N., Wild, J., Nussbeck, F. W., Stott, R., Hackmann, A., Clark, D. M., & Ehlers, A. (2013). Cognitive change predicts symptom reduction with cognitive therapy for posttraumatic stress disorder. *Journal of*

Consulting and Clinical Psychology, *81*(3), 383-93. https://doi.org/10.1037/a0031290

Klein, D. N., Dougherty, L. R., & Olino, T. M. (2005). Toward guidelines for evidence-based assessment of depression in children and adolescents. *Journal of Clinical Child and Adolescent Psychology, 34*(3), 412-32.

Kliethermes, M., Nanney, R. W., Cohen, J. A., & Mannarino, A. P. (2013). Trauma-focused cognitive-behavioral therapy. In J. D. Ford & C. A. Courtois (Eds.), *Treating complex traumatic stress disorders in children and adolescents: Scientific foundations and therapeutic models* (pp. 184-202). Guilford Press.

Kliewer, W., Murrelle, L., Mejia, R., Torres de G., Y., & Angold, A. (2001). Exposure to violence against a family member and internalizing symptoms in Colombian adolescents: The protective effects of family support. *Journal of Consulting and Clinical Psychology, 69*(6), 971-82. https://doi.org/10.1037/0022-006X.69.6.971

Klink, D., & Den Heijer, M. (2014). Genetic aspects of gender identity development and gender dysphoria. In B. C. Kreukels, T. D. Steensma, A. C. de Vries, (Eds.), *Gender dysphoria and disorders of sex development: Progress in care and knowledge* (pp. 25-51). Springer Science + Business Media. https://doi.org/10.1007/978-1-4614-7441-8_2

Klump, K. L., Culbert, K. M., O'Connor, S., Fowler, N., & Burt, S. A. (2017). The significant effects of puberty on the genetic diathesis of binge eating in girls. *International Journal of Eating Disorders, 50*(8), 984-89. https://doi.org/10.1002/eat.22727

Klump, K. L., Culbert, K. M., Slane, J. D., Burt, S. A., Sisk, C. L., & Nigg, J. T. (2012). The effects of puberty on genetic risk for disordered eating: Evidence for a sex difference. *Psychological Medicine, 42*(3), 627-37. https://doi.org/10.1017/S0033291711001541

Klump, K. L., Keel, P. K., Sisk, C., & Burt, S. A. (2010). Preliminary evidence that estradiol moderates genetic influences on disordered eating attitudes and behaviors during puberty. *Psychological Medicine, 40*(10), 1745-53. https://doi.org/10.1017/S0033291709992236

Klump, K. L., McGue, M., & Iacono, W. G. (2003). Differential heritability of eating attitudes and behaviors in prepubertal versus pubertal twins. *International Journal of Eating Disorders, 33*(3), 287-92. https://doi.org/10.1002/eat.10151

Klump, K. L., Miller, K. B., Keel, P. K., McGue, M., & Iacono, W. G. (2001). Genetic and environmental influences on anorexia nervosa syndromes in a population-based twin sample. *Psychological Medicine, 31*(4), 737-40. https://doi.org/10.1017/S0033291701003725

Klump, K. L., Perkins, P. S., Burt, S. A., McGue, M., & Iacono, W. G. (2007). Puberty moderates genetic influences on disordered eating. *Psychological Medicine, 37*(5), 627-34. https://doi.org/10.1017/S0033291707000189

Knafo, A., Iervolino, A. C., & Plomin, R. (2005). Masculine girls and feminine boys: genetic and environmental contributions to atypical gender development in early childhood. *Journal of Personality and Social Psychology, 88*(2), 400-12.

Knopik, V. S., Marceau, K., Bidwell, L. C., Palmer, R. C., Smith, T. F., Todorov, A., Evans, A. S., & Heath, A. C. (2016). Smoking during pregnancy and ADHD risk: A genetically informed, multiple-rater approach. *American Journal of Medical Genetics Part B: Neuropsychiatric Genetics, 171*(7), 971-81. https://doi.org/10.1002/ajmg.b.32421

Knutson, J. F., DeGarmo, D., Koeppl, G., & Reid, J. B. (2005). Care neglect, supervisory neglect, and harsh parenting in the development of children's aggression: A replication and extension. *Child Maltreatment, 10*(2), 92-107.

Kodituwakku, P. W., Kalberg, W., & May, P. A. (2001). The effects of prenatal alcohol exposure on executive functioning. *Alcohol Research & Health, 25*(3), 192-98.

Koegel, L. K., Koegel, R. L., Harrower, J. K., & Carter, C. M. (1999). Pivotal response intervention I: Overview of approach. *Journal of the Association for Persons with Severe Handicaps, 24*(3), 174-85. https://doi.org/10.2511/rpsd.24.3.174

Kofler, M. J., Larsen, R., Sarver, D. E., & Tolan, P. H. (2015). Developmental trajectories of aggression, prosocial behavior, and social-cognitive problem solving in emerging adolescents with clinically elevated attention-deficit/hyperactivity disorder symptoms. *Journal of Abnormal Psychology, 124*(4), 1027–1042. https://doi.org/10.1037/abn0000103

Kolevzon, A., Gross, R., & Reichenberg, A. (2007). Prenatal and perinatal risk factors for autism: a review and integration of findings. *Archives of Pediatrics & Adolescent Medicine, 161*(4), 326–333. https://doi.org/10.1001/archpedi.161.4.326

Kopp, C. B. (1989). Regulation of distress and negative emotions. *Developmental Psychology, 25*(3), 343-54.

Korrel, H., Mueller, K. L., Silk, T., Anderson, V., & Sciberras, E. (2017). Research review: Language problems in children with attention-deficit hyperactivity disorder—A systematic meta-analytic review. *Journal of Child Psychology and Psychiatry, 58*(6), 640-54. https://doi.org/10.1111/jcpp.12688

Koshy, A. J., & Sisti, D. A. (2015). Assent as an ethical imperative in the treatment of ADHD. *Journal of Medical Ethics, 41*(12), 977-81. https://doi.org/10.1136/medethics-2014-102166

Koss, K. J., Cummings, E. M., Davies, P. T., Hetzel, S., & Cicchetti, D. (2018). Harsh parenting and serotonin transporter and BDNF Val66Met polymorphisms as predictors of adolescent depressive symptoms. *Journal of Clinical Child and Adolescent Psychology, 47*(Suppl 1), S205–S218. https://doi.org/10.1080/15374416.2016.1220311

Kouros, C. D., & Garber, J. (2014). Trajectories of individual depressive symptoms in adolescents: Gender and family relationships as predictors. *Developmental Psychology, 50*(12), 2633-43.

Kotler, L. A., Cohen, P., Davies, M., Pine, D. S., & Walsh, B. T. (2001). Longitudinal relationships between childhood, adolescent, and adult eating disorders. *Journal of the American Academy of Child & Adolescent Psychiatry, 40*(12), 1434-40. https://doi.org/10.1097/00004583-200112000-00014

Kovacs, M. (1992). *Children's Depression Inventory manual.* Multi-Health Systems.

Kovacs, M. (1996). Presentation and course of major depressive disorder during childhood and later years of the life span. *Journal of the American Academy of Child & Adolescent Psychiatry, 35,* 705-15.

Kowatch, R. A., Fristad, M., Birmaher, B., Wagner, K. D., Findling, R. L., & Hellander, M. (2005). Treatment guidelines for children and adolescents with bipolar disorder. *Journal of the American Academy of Child & Adolescent Psychiatry, 44*(3), 213-35.

Krahnstoever Davison, K., Markey, C. N., & Birch, L. L. (2003). A longitudinal examination of patterns in girls' weight concerns and body dissatisfaction from ages 5 to 9 years. *International Journal of Eating Disorders, 33*(3), 320-32. https://doi.org/10.1002/eat.10142

Krakowiak, P., Walker, C. K., Bremer, A. A., Baker, A. S., Ozonoff, S., Hansen, R. L., & Hertz-Picciotto, I. (2012). Maternal metabolic conditions and risk for autism and other neurodevelopmental disorders. *Pediatrics, 129*(5), e1121-e1128. https://doi.org/10.1542/peds.2011-2583

Kuckertz, J. M., Mitchell, C., & Wiggins, J. L. (2018). Parenting mediates the impact of maternal depression on child internalizing symptoms. *Depression and Anxiety, 35*(1), 89-97. https://doi.org/10.1002/da.22688

Kumar, U., Arya, A., & Agarwal, V. (2017). Neural alterations in ADHD children as indicated by voxel-based cortical thickness and morphometry analysis. *Brain & Development, 39*(5), 403-10. https://doi.org/10.1016/j.braindev.2016.12.002

Kurz, S., Van Dyck, Z., Dremmel, D., Munsch, S., & Hilbert, A. (2015). Early-onset restrictive eating disturbances in primary school boys and girls. *European Child & Adolescent Psychiatry, 24*(7), 779-85. https://doi.org/10.1007/s00787-014-0622-z

Kutuk, M. O., Tufan, A. E., Guler, G., Yalin, O. O., Altintas, E., Bag, H. G., Uluduz, D., Toros, F., Aytan, N., Kutuk, O., & Ozge, A. (2018). Migraine and associated comorbidities are three times more frequent in children with ADHD and their mothers. *Brain & Development, 40*(10), 857-64. https://doi.org/10.1016/j.braindev.2018.06.001

Lachs, N. (2002). Isaac: A psychological perspective. *Jewish Bible Quarterly, 30*(4), 266-71.

Ladouceur, C. D., Farchione, T., Diwadkar, V., Pruitt, P., Radwan, J., Axelson, D. A., Birmaher, B., & Phillips, M. L. (2011). Differential patterns of abnormal activity and connectivity in the amygdala-prefrontal circuitry in bipolar-I and bipolar-NOS youth. *Journal of the American Academy of Child & Adolescent Psychiatry, 50*(12), 1275-89.

La Greca, A. M., Silverman, W. K., Lai, B., & Jaccard, J. (2010). Hurricane-related exposure experiences and stressors, other life events, and social support: Concurrent and prospective impact on children's persistent posttraumatic stress symptoms. *Journal of Consulting and Clinical Psychology, 78*(6), 794-805. https://doi.org/10.1037/a0020775

Lahey, B. B., Pelham, W. E., Loney, J., Kipp, H., Ehrhardt, A., Lee, S. S., Willcut, E. G., Hartung, C. M., Chronis, A., & Massetti, G. (2004). Three-year predictive validity of DSM-IV attention deficit hyperactivity disorder in children diagnosed at 4-6 years of age. *The American Journal of Psychiatry, 161*(11), 2014-20. https://doi.org/10.1176/appi.ajp.161.11.2014

Lahey, B. B., Pelham, W. E., Loney, J., Lee, S. S., & Willcutt, E. (2005). Instability of the DSM-IV subtypes of ADHD from preschool through elementary school. *Archives of General Psychiatry, 62*(8), 896-902. https://doi.org/10.1001/archpsyc.62.8.896

Landa, R., & Garrett-Mayer, E. (2006). Development in infants with autism spectrum disorders: A prospective study. *Journal of Child Psychology and Psychiatry, 47*(6), 629-38. https://doi.org/10.1111/j.1469-7610.2006.01531.x

Landolt, M. A., Vollrath, M., Timm, K., Gnehm, H. E., & Sennhauser, F. H. (2005). Predicting posttraumatic stress symptoms in children after road traffic accidents. *Journal of the American Academy of Child & Adolescent Psychiatry, 44*(12), 1276-83. https://doi.org/10.1097/01.chi.0000181045.13960.67

Langberg, J. M., Arnold, L. E., Flowers, A. M., Epstein, J. N., Altaye, M., Hinshaw, S. P., Swanson, J. M., Kotkin, R., Simpson, S., Molina, B. S. G., Jensen, P. S., Abikoff, H., Pelham, W. E., Vitiello, B., Wells, K. C., & Hechtman, L. (2010). Parent-reported homework problems in the MTA study: Evidence for sustained improvement with behavioral treatment. *Journal of Clinical Child and Adolescent Psychology, 39*(2), 220-33. https://doi.org/10.1080/15374410903532700

Langberg, J. M., Epstein, J. N., Becker, S. P., Girio-Herrera, E., & Vaughn, A. J. (2012). Evaluation of the Homework, Organization, and Planning

Skills (HOPS) intervention for middle school students with attention deficit hyperactivity disorder as implemented by school mental health providers. *School Psychology Review, 41*(3), 342-64.

Langberg, J. M., Epstein, J. N., Urbanowicz, C. M., Simon, J. O., & Graham, A. J. (2008). Efficacy of an organization skills intervention to improve the academic functioning of students with attention-deficit/hyperactivity disorder. *School Psychology Quarterly, 23*(3), 407-17. https://doi.org/10.1037/1045-3830.23.3.407

Laor, N., Wolmer, L., & Cohen, D. J. (2001). Mothers' functioning and children's symptoms 5 years after a SCUD missile attack. *The American Journal of Psychiatry, 158*(7), 1020-26. https://doi.org/10.1176/appi .ajp.158.7.1020

La Roche, M., Christopher, M. S., & West, L. M. (2017). Toward a cultural evidence-based psychotherapy. In J. M. Casas, L. A. Suzuki, C. M. Alexander, & M. A. Jackson (Eds.), *Handbook of multicultural counseling* (4th ed., pp. 177-87). Sage.

Larson, J., & Lochman, J. E. (2011). *Helping school-children cope with anger* (2nd ed). Guilford.

Laska, K. M., Gurman, A. S., & Wampold, B. E. (2014). Expanding the lens of evidence-based practice in psychotherapy: A common factors perspective. *Psychotherapy, 51*(4), 467-81. https://doi.org/10.1037/a0034332

Lastoria, M. D. (1990). A family systems approach to adolescent depression. *Journal of Psychology and Christianity, 9*(4), 44-54.

Lau, J. F., & Eley, T. C. (2006). Changes in genetic and environmental influences on depressive symptoms across adolescence and young adulthood. *British Journal of Psychiatry, 189*, 422-27.

Lau, J. Y. F., Lissek, S., Nelson, E. E., Lee, Y., Roberson-Nay, R., Poeth, K., Jenness, J., Ernst, M., Grillon, C., & Pine, D. S. (2008). Fear conditioning in adolescents with anxiety disorders: Results from a novel experimental paradigm. *Journal of the American Academy of Child & Adolescent Psychiatry, 47*(1), 94-102.

Laurent, J., Catanzaro, S. J., Rudolph, K. D., Joiner, T. J., Potter, K. I., Lambert, S., Osborne, L., & Gathright, T. (1999). A measure of positive and negative affect for children: Scale development and preliminary validation. *Psychological Assessment, 11*(3), 326-38.

Lavigne, J. V, Arend, R., Rosenbaum, D., Binns, H. J., Christoffel, K. K., & Gubbons, R. D. (1998). Psychiatric disorders with onset in the preschool years: I. Stability of diagnoses. *Journal of the American Academy of Child & Adolescent Psychiatry, 37*(12), 1246-54.

Lavigne, J. V., Bryant, F. B., Hopkins, J., & Gouze, K. R. (2019). Age 4 predictors of oppositional defiant disorder in early grammar school. *Journal of Clinical Child and Adolescent Psychology, 48*(1), 93-107. https://doi.org/10.1080/15374416.2017.1280806

Lavigne, J. V., Gibbons, R. D., Christoffel, K. K., Arend, R., Rosenbaum, D., Binns, H., Dawson, N., Sobel, H., & Isaacs, C. (1996). Prevalence rates and correlates of psychiatric disorders among preschool children. *Journal of the American Academy of Child & Adolescent Psychiatry, 35*(2), 204-14.

Lavigne, J. V., LeBailly, S. A., Hopkins, J., Gouze, K. R., & Binns, H. J. (2009). The prevalence of ADHD, ODD, depression, and anxiety in a community sample of 4-year-olds. *Journal of Clinical Child and Adolescent Psychology, 38*(3), 315-28.

Law, E. C., Sideridis, G. D., Prock, L. A., & Sheridan, M. A. (2014). Attention-deficit/hyperactivity disorder in young children: Predictors of diagnostic stability. *Pediatrics, 133*(4), 569-667.

Lawrence, P. J., Murayama, K., & Creswell, C. (2019). Systematic review and meta-analysis:

Anxiety and depressive disorders in offspring of parents with anxiety disorders. *Journal of the American Academy of Child & Adolescent Psychiatry, 58*(1), 46-60. https://doi.org/10.1016/j.jaac.2018.07.898

Lazarus, R. S. (1999). *Stress and emotion: A new synthesis.* Springer.

Le, J., Feygin, Y., Creel, L., Lohr, W. D., Jones, V. F., Williams, P. G., Myers, J. A., Pasquenza, N., & Davis, D. W. (2020). Trends in diagnosis of bipolar and disruptive mood dysregulation disorders in children and youth. *Journal of Affective Disorders, 264*, 242-48. https://doi.org/10.1016/j.jad.2019.12.018

Leaf, R., & McEachin, J. (2016). "The Lovaas Model: Love it or hate it, but first understand it." In R. Romanczyk & J. McEachin (Eds.), *Comprehensive models of autism spectrum disorder treatment: Points of divergence and convergence* (pp. 7-43). Springer.

Leckman, J. F. (2013). The risks and benefits of antidepressants to treat pediatric-onset depression and anxiety disorders: A developmental perspective. *Psychotherapy and Psychosomatics, 82*, 129-31.

Lee, Y., & Lin, P. (2010). Association between serotonin transporter gene polymorphism and eating disorders: A meta-analytic study. *International Journal of Eating Disorders, 43*(6), 498-504. https://doi.org/10.1002/eat.20732

Leenarts, L. W., Diehle, J., Doreleijers, T. H., Jansma, E. P., & Lindauer, R. L. (2013). Evidence-based treatments for children with trauma-related psychopathology as a result of childhood maltreatment: A systematic review. *European Child & Adolescent Psychiatry, 22*(5), 269-83.

Lee-Winn, A. E., Townsend, L., Reinblatt, S. P., & Mendelson, T. (2016). Associations of neuroticism and impulsivity with binge eating in a nationally representative sample of adolescents in the United States. *Personality and Individual Differences, 90*, 66-72. https://doi.org/10.1016/j.paid.2015.10.042

Legerstee, J. S., Verhulst, F. C., Robbers, S. C., Ormel, J., Oldehinkel, A. J., & van Oort, F. A. (2013). Gender-specific developmental trajectories of anxiety during adolescence: Determinants and outcomes. The TRAILS study. *Journal of the Canadian Academy of Child and Adolescent Psychiatry, 22*(1), 26-34.

Le Grange, D., Accurso, E. C., Lock, J., Agras, S., & Bryson, S. W. (2014). Early weight gain predicts outcome in two treatments for adolescent anorexia nervosa. *International Journal of Eating Disorders, 47*(2), 124-29. https://doi.org/10.1002/eat.22221

Le Grange, D., Crosby, R. D., Rathouz, P. J., & Leventhal, B. L. (2007). A randomized controlled comparison of family-based treatment and supportive psychotherapy for adolescent bulimia nervosa. *Archives of General Psychiatry, 64*(9), 1049-56. https://doi.org/10.1001/archpsyc.64.9.1049

Le Grange, D., Lock, J., Accurso, E. C., Agras, W. S., Darcy, A., Forsberg, S., & Bryson, S. W. (2014). Relapse from remission at two- to four-year follow-up in two treatments for adolescent anorexia nervosa. *Journal of the American Academy of Child & Adolescent Psychiatry, 53*(11), 1162-67. https://doi.org/10.1016/j.jaac.2014.07.014

Le Grange, D., Lock, J., Agras, W. S., Moye, A., Bryson, S. W., Jo, B., & Kraemer, H. C. (2012). Moderators and mediators of remission in family-based treatment and adolescent focused therapy for anorexia nervosa. *Behaviour Research and Therapy, 50*(2), 85-92. https://doi.org/10.1016/j.brat.2011.11.003

Le Grange, D., & Robin, A. L. (2017). Family-based treatment and behavioral family systems therapy for adolescent eating disorders. In J. R. Weisz & A. E. Kazdin (Eds.), *Evidence-based psychotherapies for children and adolescents* (3rd ed., pp. 308-24). Guilford.

Leitch, S., Sciberras, E., Post, B., Gerner, B., Rinehart, N., Nicholson, J. M., & Evans, S. (2019). Experience of stress in parents of children with ADHD: A qualitative study. *International Journal of Qualitative Studies on Health and Well-Being, 14*(1). https://doi.org/10.1080/17482631.2019.1690091

Leitenberg, H., Yost, L. W., & Carroll-Wilson, M. (1986). Negative cognitive errors in children: Questionnaire development, normative data, and comparisons between children with and without self-reported symptoms of depression, low self-esteem, and evaluation anxiety. *Journal of Consulting and Clinical Psychology, 54*(4), 528-36.

Lelwica, M. (1999). *Staving for salvation: The spiritual dimenstions of eating problems among American girls and women.* New York: Oxford University Press.

Lengua, L. J. (2002). The contribution of emotionality and self-regulation to the understanding of children's response to multiple risk. *Child Development, 73*(1), 144. https://doi.org/10.1111/1467-8624.00397

Lengua, L. J., West, S. G., & Sandler, I. N. (1998). Temperament as a predictor of symptomatology in children: Addressing contamination of measures. *Child Development, 69*(1), 164-81.

Leshem, B., Haj-Yahia, M. M., & Guterman, N. B. (2016). The role of family and teacher support in post-traumatic stress symptoms among Palestinian adolescents exposed to community violence. *Journal of Child and Family Studies, 25*(2), 488-502. https://doi.org/10.1007/s10826-015-0226-3

Levendosky, A. A., Bogat, G. A., & Martinez-Torteya, C. (2013). PTSD symptoms in young children exposed to intimate partner violence. *Violence Against Women, 19*(2), 187-201. https://doi.org/10.1177/1077801213476458

Levey, E. J., Oppenheim, C. E., Lange, B. C. L., Plasky, N. S., Harris, B. L., Lekpeh, G. G., Kekulah, I., Henderson, D. C., & Borba, C. C. (2016). A qualitative analysis of factors impacting resilience among youth in post-conflict Liberia. *Child and Adolescent Psychiatry and Mental Health, 10,* 26.

Levy, D., Ronemus, M., Yamrom, B., Lee, Y. H., Leotta, A., Kendall, J., Marks, S., Lakshmi, B., Pai, D., Ye, K., Buja, A., Krieger, A., Yoon, S., Troge, J., Rodgers, L., Iossifoc, I., & Wigler, M. (2011). Rare de novo and transmitted copy-number variation in autistic spectrum disorders. *Neuron, 70*(5), 886-97.

Levy, F., Hay, D. A., Bennett, K. S., & McStephen, M. (2005). Gender differences in ADHD subtype vomorbidity. *Journal of the American Academy of Child & Adolescent Psychiatry, 44*(4), 368–376. https://doi.org/10.1097/01.chi.0000153232.64968.cl

Lewinsohn, P. M., Klein, D. N., & Seeley, J. R. (1995). Bipolar disorders in a community sample of older adolescents: Prevalence, phenomenology, comorbidity, and course. *Journal of the American Academy of Child & Adolescent Psychiatry, 34*(4), 454-63.

Lewinsohn, P. M., Striegel-Moore, R. H., & Seeley, J. H. (2000). Epidemiology and natural course of eating disorders in young women from adolescence to young adulthood. *Journal of the American Academy of Child & Adolescent Psychiatry, 39*(10), 1284-92. https://doi.org/10.1097/00004583-200010000-00016

Lewis, M. (2014). Toward the development of the science of developmental psychopathology. In M. Lewis & K. D. Rudolph (Eds.), *Handbook of developmental psychopathology* (3rd ed., pp. 3-23). Springer.

Liberman, L. C., Lipp, O. V., Spence, S. H., & March, S. (2006). Evidence for retarded extinction of aversive learning in anxious children. *Behaviour Research and Therapy, 44*(10), 1491-1502.

Linehan, M. (1993). *Cognitive-behavioral treatment of borderline personality disorder.* Guilford Press.

Linke, J., Kircanski, K., Brooks, J., Perhamus, G., Gold, A. L., & Brotman, M. A. (2020). Exposure-based cognitive-behavioral therapy for disruptive mood dysregulation disorder: An evidence-based case study. *Behavior Therapy, 51*(2), 320-33. https://doi.org/10.1016/j.beth.2019.05.007

Linnet, K. M., Dalsgaard, S., Obel, C., Wisborg, K., Henriksen, T. B., Rodriquez, A., Kotimaa, A., Moilanen, I., Thomsen, P. H., Olsen, J., & Jarvelin, M. (2003). Maternal lifestyle factors in pregnancy risk of attention deficit hyperactivity disorder and associated behaviors: Review of the current evidence. *The American Journal of Psychiatry, 160*(6), 1028-40. http://doi.org/10.1176/appi.ajp.160.6.1028

Lipschitz, D. S., Rasmusson, A. M., Anyan, W., Gueorguieva, R., Billingslea, E. M., Cromwell, P. F., & Southwick, S. M. (2003). Posttraumatic stress disorder and substance use in inner-city adolescent girls. *Journal of Nervous and Mental Disease, 191*(11), 714-21. https://doi.org/10.1097/01.nmd.0000095123.68088.da

Little, K., Olsson, C. A., Youssef, G. J., Whittle, S., Simmons, J. G., Yücel, M., Sheeber, L. B., Foley, D. L., & Allen, N. B. (2015). Linking the serotonin transporter gene, family environments, hippocampal volume and depression onset: A prospective imaging gene × environment analysis. *Journal of Abnormal Psychology, 124*(4), 834-49.

Lim, K. X., Liu, C. Y., Schoeler, T., Cecil, C., Barker, E. D., Viding, E., Greven, C. U., & Pingault, J. B. (2018). The role of birth weight on the causal pathway to child and adolescent ADHD symptomatology: a population-based twin differences longitudinal design. *Journal of Child Psychology and Psychiatry, and Allied Disciplines, 59*(10), 1036–1043. https://doi.org/10.1111/jcpp.12949

Liu, J., Yao, L., Zhang, W., Xiao, Y., Liu, L., Gao, X., Shah, C., Li, S., Tao, B., & Lui, S. (2017). Gray matter abnormalities in pediatric autism spectrum disorder: A meta-analysis with signed differential mapping. *European Child & Adolescent Psychiatry, 26*(8), 933-45. https://doi.org/10.1007/s00787-017-0964-4

Liu, S. T., & Chen, S. H. (2015). A Community Study on the Relationship of Posttraumatic Cognitions to Internalizing and Externalizing Psychopathology in Taiwanese Children and Adolescents. *Journal of Abnormal Child Psychology, 43*(8), 1475–1484. https://doi.org/10.1007/s10802-015-0030-y

Liu, X., Lin, X., Heath, M. A., Zhou, Q., Ding, W., & Qin, S. (2018). Longitudinal linkages between parenting stress and oppositional defiant disorder (ODD) symptoms among Chinese children with ODD. *Journal of Family Psychology, 32*(8), 1078-86. https://doi.org/10.1037/fam0000466

Liu, Y., & Merritt, D. H. (2018). Examining the association between parenting and childhood depression among Chinese children and adolescents: A systematic literature review. *Children and Youth Services Review, 88*, 316-32. https://doi.org/10.1016/j.childyouth.2018.03.019

Lochman, J. E., Boxmeyer, C. L., Powell, N. P., Barry, T. D., & Pardini, D. A. (2010). Anger control training for aggressive youths. In J. R. Weisz & A. E. Kazdin (Eds.), *Evidence-based psychotherapies for children and adolescents* (2nd ed., pp. 227-42). Guilford.

Lochman, J. E., Dunn, S. E., & Wagner, E. E. (1997). Anger. In G. Bear, K. Minke, & A. Thomas (Eds.), *Children's Needs* (Vol. 2, pp. 149-60). National Association of School Psychology.

Lochman, J. E., FitzGerald, D. P., & Whidby, J. M. (1999). Anger management with aggressive children. In C. E. Schafer (Ed.), *Short-term psychotherapy groups for children* (pp. 301-50). Jason Aronson.

Lock, J. (2015). An update on evidence-based psychosocial treatments for eating disorders in children and adolescents. *Journal of Clinical Child & Adolescent Psychology, 44*(5), 707-21.

Lock, J. (2019). Updates on treatments for adolescent anorexia nervosa. *Child and Adolescent Psychiatric Clinics of North America, 28*(4), 523-35. https://doi.org/10.1016/j.chc.2019.05.001

Lock, J., & Le Grange, D. (2013). *Treatment manual for anorexia nervosa: A family-based approach.* Guilford.

Lock, J., Le Grange, D., Agras, W. S., Moye, A., Bryson, S. W., & Jo, B. (2010). Randomized clinical trial comparing family-based treatment with adolescent-focused individual therapy for adolescents with anorexia nervosa. *Archives of General Psychiatry, 67*(10), 1025-32. https://doi.org/10.1001/archgenpsychiatry.2010.128

Locke, R. L., Davidson, R. J., Kalin, N. H., & Goldsmith, H. H. (2009). Children's context inappropriate anger and salivary cortisol. *Developmental Psychology, 45*(5), 1284-97.

Loeber, R., Green, S. M., Keenan, K., & Lahey, B. B. (1995). Which boys will fare worse? Early predictors of the onset of conduct disorder in a six-year longitudinal study. *Journal of the American Academy of Child and Adolescent Psychiatry, 34*(4), 499-509.

Lønfeldt, N. N., Esbjørn, B. H., Normann, N., Breinholst, S., & Francis, S. E. (2017). Do mother's metacognitions, beliefs, and behaviors predict child anxiety-related metacognitions? *Child & Youth Care Forum, 46*(4), 577-99. https://doi.org/10.1007/s10566-017-9396-z

Lonigan, C. J., Phillips, B. M., & Hooe, E. S. (2003). Relations of positive and negative affectivity to anxiety and depression in children: Evidence from a latent variable longitudinal study. *Journal of Consulting and Clinical Psychology, 71*(3), 465-81.

Looy, H. (2002). Male and female God created them: The challenge of intersexuality. *Journal of Psychology and Christianity, 21*(1), 10-20.

Looy, H., & Bouma, H. I. (2005). The nature of gender: gender identity in persons who are intersexed or transgendered. *Journal of Psychology & Theology, 33*(3), 166-78.

Lopez-Duran, N. L., Kovacs, M., & George, C. J. (2009). Hypothalamic-pituitary-adrenal axis dysregulation in depressed children and adolescents: A meta-analysis. *Psychoneuroendocrinology, 34*(9), 1272-83.

Lord, C., Luyster, R. J., Gotham, K., & Guthrie, W. (2012). *Autism Diagnostic Observation Schedule, Second Edition (ADOS-2) Manual (Part II): Toddler Module.* Western Psychological Services.

Lord, C., Pickles, A., McLennan, J., Rutter, M., Bregman, J., Folstein, S., Fombonne, E., Leboyer, M., & Minshew, N. (1997). Diagnosing autism: Analyses of data from the Autism Diagnostic Interview. *Journal of Autism and Developmental Disorders, 27*(5), 501-17. https://doi.org/10.1023/A:1025873925661

Lord, C., Risi, S., DiLavore, P. S., Shulman, C., Thurm, A., & Pickles, A. (2006). Autism from 2 to 9 years of age. *Archives of General Psychiatry, 63*(6), 694–701. https://doi.org/10.1001/archpsyc.63.6.694

Lord, C., Risi, S., Lambrecht, L., Cook, E. J., Leventhal, B. L., DiLavore, P. C., Pickles, A., & Rutter, M. (2000). The Autism Diagnostic Observation Schedule—Generic: A standard measure of social and communication deficits associated with the spectrum of autism. *Journal of Autism and Developmental Disorders, 30*(3), 205-23. https://doi.org/10.1023/A:1005592401947

Lord, C., Rutter, M., DiLavore, P. C., Risi, S., Gotham, K., & Bishop, S. (2012). *Autism Diagnostic Observation Schedule, Second Edition (ADOS-2) Manual.* Western Psychological Services.

Lord, C., Rutter, M., & Le Couteur, A. (1994). Autism Diagnostic Interview—Revised: A revised version of a diagnostic interview for caregivers of individuals with possible pervasive developmental disorders. *Journal of Autism and Developmental Disorders, 24*(5), 659-85. https://doi.org/10.1007/BF02172145

Lougheed, J. P., & Hollenstein, T. (2012). A limited repertoire of emotion regulation strategies is associated with internalizing problems in adolescence. *Social Development, 21*(4), 704-21.

Lovaas, O. I. (1987). Behavioral treatment and normal educational and intellectual functioning in young autistic children. *Journal of Consulting and Clinical Psychology, 55*(1), 3-9. https://doi.org/10.1037/0022-006X.55.1.3

Lowe, M. R., Marmorstein, N., Iacono, W., Rosenbaum, D., Espel-Huynh, H., Muratore, A. F., Lantz, E. L., & Zhang, F. (2019). Body concerns and BMI as predictors of disordered eating and body mass in girls: An 18-year longitudinal investigation. *Journal of Abnormal Psychology, 128*(1), 32-43. https://doi.org/10.1037/abn0000394

Luby, J. L. (2009). Depression. In C. H. Zeanah (Ed.), *Handbook of infant mental health* (3rd ed., pp. 409-20). Guilford.

Luby, J. L., Gaffrey, M., Tillman, R., April, L., & Belden, A. (2014). Trajectories of preschool disorders to full DSM depression at school age and early adolescence: Continuity of preschool depression. *The American Journal of Psychiatry, 171*(7), 768-76. https://doi.org/10.1176/appi.ajp.2014.13091198

Luby, J. L., Heffelfinger, A. K., Mrakotsky, C., Brown, K. M., Hessler, M. J., Wallis, J. M., & Spitznagel, E. L. (2003). The clinical picture of depression in preschool children. *Journal of the American Academy of Child & Adolescent Psychiatry, 42*(3), 340-48.

Luby, J. L., Heffelfinger, A. K., Mrakotsky, C., Hessler, M. J., Brown, K. M., & Hildebrand, T. (2002). Preschool major depressive disorder: Preliminary validation for developmentally modified DSM-IV criteria. *Journal of the American Academy of Child & Adolescent Psychiatry, 41*(8), 928-37.

Luby, J. L., Sullivan, J., Belden, A., Stalets, M., Blankenship, S., & Spitznagel, E. (2006). An observational analysis of behavior in depressed preschoolers: Further validation of early-onset depression. *Journal of the American Academy of Child & Adolescent Psychiatry, 45*(2), 203-12.

Luebbe, A. M., & Bell, D. J. (2014). Positive and negative family emotional climate differentially predict youth anxiety and depression via distinct affective pathways. *Journal of Abnormal Child Psychology, 42*(6), 897-911.

Lupien, S. J., McEwen, B. S., Gunnar, M. R., & Heim, C. (2009). Effects of stress throughout the lifespan on the brain, behaviour and cognition. *Nature Reviews. Neuroscience, 10*(6), 434-45.

Luthar, S. S., & Cicchetti, D. (2000). The construct of resilience: Implications for interventions and social policies. *Development and Psychopathology, 12*(4), 857-85. https://doi.org/10.1017/S0954579400004156

Luthar, S. S., Cicchetti, D., & Becker, B. (2000). The construct of resilience: A critical evaluation and guidelines for future work. *Child Development, 71*(3), 543-62. https://doi.org/10.1111/1467-8624.00164

Luther, M. (1958). Lectures on Genesis (G. V. Schick, Trans.). In J. Pelikan (Ed.), *Luther's works* (pp. 60-70). Concordia. (Originally published 1545.)

Luyster, R., Gotham, K., Guthrie, W., Coffing, M., Petrak, R., Pierce, K., Bishop, S., Esler, A., Hus, V., Oti, R., Richler, J., Risi, S., & Lord, C. (2009). The Autism Diagnostic Observation Schedule—Toddler Module: A new module of a standardized diagnostic measure for autism spectrum disorders. *Journal of Autism and Developmental Disorders, 39*(9), 1305-20. https://doi.org/10.1007/s10803-009-0746-z

Lyubomirsky, S., & Nolen-Hoeksema, S. (1993). Self-perpetuating properties of dysphoric rumination. *Journal of Personality & Social Psychology, 65*(2), 339-49.

Lyubomirsky, S., & Nolen-Hoeksema, S. (1995). Effects of self-focused rumination on negative thinking and interpersonal problem solving. *Journal of Personality & Social Psychology, 69*(1), 176-90.

Macaskill, G. (2017). Autism spectrum disorders and the New Testament: Preliminary reflections. *Journal of Disability and Religion, 22*(1), 15-41. http://doi.org/10.1080/23312521.2017.1373613

MacBrayer, E. K., Milich, R., & Hundley, M. (2003). Attributional biases in aggressive children and their mothers. *Journal of Abnormal Psychology, 112*(4), 698-708.

Maciejewski, D. F., van Lier, P. C., Neumann, A., Van der Giessen, D., Branje, S. T., Meeus, W. J., & Koot, H. M. (2014). The development of adolescent generalized anxiety and depressive symptoms in the context of adolescent mood variability and parent-adolescent negative interactions. *Journal of Abnormal Child Psychology, 42*(4), 515-26.

MacPherson, H. A., Algorta, G. P., Mendenhall, A. N., Fields, B. W., & Fristad, M. A. (2014). Predictors and moderators in the randomized trial of multifamily psychoeducational psychotherapy for childhood mood disorders. *Journal of Clinical Child and Adolescent Psychology, 43*(3), 459-72.

Maenner, M.J., Shaw, K.A., Baio, J., Washington, A., Patrick, M., DiRienzo, M., Christensen, D. L., Wiggins, L. D., Pettygrove, S., Andrews, J. G., Lopez, M., Hudson, A., Baroud, T., Schwenk, Y., White, T., Rosenbrg, C. R., Lee, L., Harrington, R. A., Huston, M., . . . Dietz, P. M. (2020). Prevalence of autism spectrum disorder among children aged 8 years—Autism and Developmental Disabilities Monitoring Network, 11 Sites, United States, 2016. *MMWR Surveillance Summaries, 69*(4), 1-12. https://doi.org/10.15585/mmwr.ss6904a1

Maganto, C., Garaigordobil, M., & Kortabarria, L. (2016). Eating problems in adolescents and youths: Explanatory variables. *The Spanish Journal of Psychology, 19*, e81. https://doi.org/10.1017/sjp.2016.74

Mahfouda, S., Moore, J. K., Siafarikas, A., Hewitt, T., Ganti, U., Lin, A., & Zepf, F. D. (2019). Gender-affirming hormones and surgery in transgender children and adolescents. *The Lancet Diabetes & Endocrinology, 7*(6), 484-98.

Makino, M., Tsuboi, K., & Dennerstein, L. (2004). Prevalence of eating disorders: A comparison of Western and non-Western countries. *Medscape General Medicine, 6*(3), 49.

Mallott, M. A., & Beidel, D. C. (2014). Anxiety disorders in adolescents. In C. A. Alfano & D. C. Beidel (Eds.), *Comprehensive evidence-based interventions for children and adolescents* (pp. 111-27). Wiley.

Malm, H., Brown, A. S., Gissler, M., Gyllenberg, D., Hinkka-Yli-Salomäki, S., McKeague, I. W., Weissman, M., Wickramaratne, P., Artama, M., Gingrich, J. A., & Sourander, A. (2016). Gestational exposure to selective serotonin reuptake inhibitors and offspring psychiatric disorders: A national register-based study. *Journal of the American Academy of Child & Adolescent Psychiatry, 55*(5), 359-66. https://doi.org/10.1016/j.jaac.2016.02.013

Maloney, M. J., McGuire, J. B., & Daniels, S. R. (1988). Reliability testing of a children's version of the Eating Attitude Test. *Journal of the American Academy of Child & Adolescent Psychiatry, 27*(5), 541-43. https://doi.org/10.1097/00004583-198809000-00004

Mandy, W., & Lai, M. (2016). Annual research review: The role of the environment in the developmental psychopathology of autism spectrum condition. *Journal of Child Psychology and Psychiatry, 57*(3), 271-92. https://doi.org/10.1111/jcpp.12501

Mannarino, A. P., Cohen, J. A., Deblinger, E., Runyon, M. K., & Steer, R. A. (2012). Trauma-focused Cognitive-Behavioral Therapy for children: Sustained impact of treatment 6 and 12 months later. *Child Maltreatment, 17*(3), 2 3 1 - 4 1 . h t t p s : / / d o i . org/10.1177/1077559512451787

March, J. S. (1997). *Multidimensional Anxiety Scale for Children.* Pearson Education.

Maresh, E. L., Beckes, L., & Coan, J. A. (2013). The social regulation of threat-related attentional disengagement in highly anxious individuals. *Frontiers in Human Neuroscience, 7.* https://doi.org/10.3389/fnhum.2013.00515

Marshall, A. D. (2016). Developmental timing of trauma exposure relative to puberty and the nature of psychopathology among adolescent girls. *Journal of the American Academy of Child & Adolescent Psychiatry, 55*(1), 25-32. https://doi.org/10.1016/j.jaac.2015.10.004

Marshall, C., Noor, A., Vincent, J., Lionel, A., Feuk, L., Skaug, J., Shago, M; Moessner, R; Pinto, D; Ren, Y; Thiruvahindrapduram, B; Fiebig, A; Schreiber, S; Friedman, J; Ketelaars, C. E. J.; Vos, Y J; Ficicioglu, C; Kirkpatrick, S; Nicolson, R;. . . Scherer, S. (2008). Structural variation of chromosomes in autism spectrum disorder. *American Journal of Human Genetics, 82*(2), 477-88.

Martel, M. M., Nikolas, M., Jernigan, K., Friderici, K., Waldman, I., & Nigg, J. T. (2011). The dopamine receptor D4 gene (DRD4) moderates family environmental effects on ADHD. *Journal of Abnormal Child Psychology, 39*(1), 1-10. https://doi.org/10.1007/s10802-010-9439-5

Marthoenis, M., Ilyas, A., Sofyan, H., & Schouler-Ocak, M. (2019). Prevalence, comorbidity and predictors of post-traumatic stress disorder, depression, and anxiety in adolescents following an earthquake. *Asian Journal of Psychiatry, 43,* 154-59. https://doi.org/10.1016/j.ajp.2019.05.030

Martin, A. J. (2014). The role of ADHD in academic adversity: Disentangling ADHD effects from other personal and contextual factors. *School Psychology Quarterly, 29*(4), 395-408. https://doi.org/10.1037/spq0000069

Martin, C. L., & Ruble, D. N. (2010). Patterns of gender development. *Annual Review of Psychology, 61,* 353-81. https://doi.org/10.1146/annurev.psych.093008.100511

Martinussen, R., Hayden, J., Hogg-Johnson, S., & Tannock, R. (2005). A meta-analysis of working memory impairments in children with attention-deficit/hyperactivity disorder. *Journal of the American Academy of Child & Adolescent Psychiatry, 44*(4), 377-84. https://doi.org/10.1097/01.chi.0000153228.72591.73

Marzola, E., Abbate-Daga, G., Gramaglia, C., Amianto, F., & Fassino, S. (2015). A qualitative investigation into anorexia nervosa: The inner perspective. *Cogent Psychology, 2*(1). https://doi.org/10.1080/23311908.2015.1032493

Masi, G., Berloffa, S., Mucci, M., Pfanner, C., D'Acunto, G., Lenzi, F., Liboni, F., Manfredi, A., & Milone, A. (2018). A naturalistic exploratory study of obsessive-compulsive bipolar comorbidity in youth. *Journal of Affective Disorders, 231,* 21-26. https://doi.org/10.1016/j.jad.2018.01.020

Masten, A. S. (2014). *Ordinary magic: Resilience in development.* Guilford.

Masten, A. S., & Coatsworth, J. (1995). Competence, resilience, and psychopathology. In D. Cicchetti & D. Cohen (Eds.), *Developmental psychopathology: Vol. 2. Risk, disorder, and adaptation* (pp. 715-52). Wiley.

Masten, A. S., & Coatsworth, J. (1998). The development of competence in favorable and unfavorable environments: Lessons from research on successful children. *American Psychologist, 53*(2), 205-20.

Mathews, B. L., Kerns, K. A., & Ciesla, J. A. (2014). Specificity of emotion regulation difficulties related to anxiety in early adolescence. *Journal of Adolescence, 37*(7), 1089-97.

Matusek, J. A., & O'Dougherty Wright, M. (2010). Ethical dilemmas in treating clients with eating disorders: A review and application of an integrative ethical decision-making model. *European Eating Disorders Review, 18*(6), 434-52. https://doi.org/10.1002/erv.1036

Maughan, A., & Cicchetti, D. (2002). Impact of child maltreatment and interadult violence on children's emotion regulation abilities and socioemotional adjustment. *Child Development, 73*(5), 1525-42.

Maughan, B., Rowe, R., Messer, J., Goodman, R., & Meltzer, H. (2004). Conduct disorder and oppositional defiant disorder in a national sample: Developmental epidemiology. *Journal of Child Psychology and Psychiatry, 45*(3), 609-21.

Mazurek, M. O., Dovgan, K., Neumeyer, A. M., & Malow, B. A. (2019). Course and predictors of sleep and co-occurring problems in children with autism spectrum disorder. *Journal of Autism and Developmental Disorders, 49*, 2101-15. https://doi.org/10.1007/s10803-019-03894-5

Mazza, J. R., Pingault, J. B., Booij, L., Boivin, M., Tremblay, R., Lambert, J., Zunzunegui, M. V., & Côté, S. (2017). Poverty and behavior problems during early childhood: The mediating role of maternal depression symptoms and parenting. *International Journal of Behavioral Development, 41*(6), 670-80. https://doi.org/10.1177/0165025416657615

Mazzeo, S. E., Mitchell, K. S., Bulik, C. M., Reichborn-Kjennerud, T., Kendler, K. S., & Neale, M. C. (2009). Assessing the heritability of anorexia nervosa symptoms using a marginal maximal likelihood approach. *Psychological Medicine, 39*(3), 463-73. https://doi.org/10.1017/S0033291708003310

McCart, M., & Sheidow, A. (2016). Evidence-based psychosocial treatments for adolescents with disruptive behavior. *Journal of Clinical Child & Adolescent Psychology, 45*(5), 529-63.

McCauley, E., Myers, K., Mitchell, J., Calderon, R., Schloredt, K., & Treder, R. (1993). Depression in young people: Initial presentation and clinical course. *Journal of the American Academy of Child & Adolescent Psychiatry, 32*, 714-22.

McCracken, J. T., McGough, J. J., Loo, S. K., Levitt, J., Del'Homme, M., Cowen, J., Sturm, A., Whelan, F., Hellemann, G., Sugar, C., & Bilder, R. M. (2016). Combined stimulant and guanfacine administration in attention-deficit/hyperactivity disorder: A controlled, comparative study. *Journal of the American Academy of Child & Adolescent Psychiatry, 55*(8), 657-66. https://doi.org/10.1016/j.jaac.2016.05.015

McCrimmon, A. W., Matchullis, R. L., Altomare, A. A., & Smith-Demers, A. D. (2016). Executive functions in autism spectrum disorder. In J. L. Matson (Ed.), *Handbook of assessment and diagnosis of autism spectrum disorder* (pp. 403-25). Springer International Publishing. https://doi.org/10.1007/978-3-319-27171-2

McEachin, J. J., Smith, T., & Lovaas, O. I. (1993). Long-term outcome for children with autism who received early intensive behavioral treatment. *American Journal on Mental Retardation, 97*(4), 359-72.

McEwen, B. S. (2002). The neurobiology and neuroendocrinology of stress: Implications for post-traumatic stress disorder from a basic science perspective. *Psychiatric Clinics of North America, 25*(2), 469–494. https://doi.org/10.1016/S0193-953X(01)00009-0

McGee, D. (2010). Widening the door of inclusion for children with autism through faith communities. *Journal of Religion, Disability, and Health, 14,* 279-92.

McGoey, K. E., DuPaul, G. J., Haley, E., & Shelton, T. L. (2007). Parent and teacher ratings of attention-deficit/hyperactivity disorder in preschool: The ADHD Rating Scale-IV Preschool Version. *Journal of Psychopathological and Behavioral Assessment, 29*(4), 269-76.

McGovern, C. W., & Sigman, M. (2005). Continuity and change from early childhood to adolescence in autism. *Journal of Child Psychology and Psychiatry, 46*(4), 401-8. https://doi.org/10.1111/j.1469-7610.2004.00361.x

McLaughlin, K. A., Busso, D. S., Duys, A., Green, J. G., Alves, S., Way, M., & Sheridan, M. A. (2014). Amygdala response to negative stimuli predicts PTSD symptom onset following a terrorist attack. *Depression and Anxiety, 31*(10), 834-42. https://doi.org/10.1002/da.22284

McLaughlin, K. A., Hatzenbuehler, M. L., Mennin, D. S., & Nolen-Hoeksema, S. (2011). Emotion dysregulation and adolescent psychopathology: A prospective study. *Behaviour Research and Therapy, 49*(9), 544-54.

McLaughlin, K. A., Koenen, K. C., Hill, E. D., Petukhova, M., Sampson, N. A., Zaslavsky, A. M., & Kessler, R. C. (2013). Trauma exposure and posttraumatic stress disorder in a national sample of adolescents. *Journal of the American Academy of Child & Adolescent Psychiatry, 52*(8), 815-30. https://doi.org/10.1016/j.jaac.2013.05.011

McLaughlin, K. A., & Nolen-Hoeksema, S. (2012). Interpersonal stress generation as a mechanism linking rumination to internalizing symptoms in early adolescents. *Journal of Clinical Child & Adolescent Psychology, 41*(5), 584-97.

McLean, C. P., Rosenbach, S. B., Capaldi, S., & Foa, E. B. (2013). Social and academic functioning in adolescents with child sexual abuse-related PTSD. *Child Abuse & Neglect, 37*(9), 675-78. https://doi.org/10.1016/j.chiabu.2013.03.010

McLean, C. P., Yeh, R., Rosenfield, D., & Foa, E. B. (2015). Changes in negative cognitions mediate PTSD symptom reductions during client-centered therapy and prolonged exposure for adolescents. *Behaviour Research and Therapy, 68,* 64-69. https://doi.org/10.1016/j.brat.2015.03.008

McLeod, B. D., Wood, J. J., & Weisz, J. R. (2007). Examining the association between parenting and childhood anxiety: A meta-analysis. *Clinical Psychology Review, 27*(2), 155-72.

McLoyd, V. C. (1998). Socioeconomic disadvantage and child development. *American Psychologist, 53*(2), 185-204.

McMahon, R. J., Estes, A. M. (1997). Conduct problems. In E. J. Mash & L. G. Terdal (Eds), *Assessment of childhood disorders, 3rd ed.,* (pp. 130-193). New York: Guilford.

McMahon, R. J., & Frick, P. J. (2005). Evidence-based assessment of conduct problems in children and adolescents. *Journal of Clinical Child and Adolescent Psychology, 34,* 477-505.

McMahon, R. J., & Frick, P. J. (2007). Conduct and oppositional disorders. In E. J. Mash & R. A. Barkley (Eds), *Assessment of childhood disorders* (4th ed., pp. 132-83). Guilford.

McMinn, M. (2004). *Why sin matters: The surprising relationship between our sin and God's grace.* Tyndale.

McMinn, M. R., & Campbell, C. D. (2007). *Integrative psychotherapy: Toward a comprehensive Christian approach.* InterVarsity Press.

McNeil, C. B., Capage, L. C., & Bennett, G. M. (2002). Cultural issues in the treatment of young African American children diagnosed with disruptive behavior disorders. *Journal of Pediatric Psychology, 27*(4), 339-50. https://doi.org/10.1093/jpepsy/27.4.339

McRay, B., Yarhouse, M., & Butman, R. (2016). *Modern psychopathologies: A comprehensive Christian appraisal* (2nd ed.). InterVarsity Press.

McStay, R. L., Trembath, D., & Dissanayake, C. (2014). Maternal stress and family quality of life in response to raising a child with autism: From preschool to adolescence. *Research in Developmental Disabilities, 35*(11), 3119-30. https://doi.org/10.1016/j.ridd.2014.07.043

Meeuwsen, M., Perra, O., van Goozen, S. H. M., & Hay, D. F. (2019). Informants' ratings of activity level in infancy predict ADHD symptoms and diagnoses in childhood. *Development and Psychopathology, 31*(4), 1255-69. https://doi.org/10.1017/S0954579418000597

Meiser-Stedman, R., Smith, P., Bryant, R., Salmon, K., Yule, W., Dalgleish, T., & Nixon, R. V. (2009). Development and validation of the Child Post-Traumatic Cognitions Inventory (CPTCI). *Journal of Child Psychology and Psychiatry, 50*(4), 432-40. https://doi.org/10.1111/j.1469-7610.2008.01995.x

Meiser-Stedman, R. A., Yule, W., Dalgleish, T., Smith, P., & Glucksman, E. (2006). The role of the family in child and adolescent posttraumatic stress following attendance at an emergency department. *Journal of Pediatric Psychology, 31*(4), 397-402. https://doi.org/10.1093/jpepsy/jsj005

Mercer, J. A. (2005). *Welcoming children: A practical theology of childhood*. Chalice Press.

Merikangas, A. K., Calkins, M. E., Bilker, W. B., Moore, T. M., Gur, R. C., & Gur, R. E. (2017). Parental age and offspring psychopathology in the Philadelphia neurodevelopmental cohort. *Journal of the American Academy of Child & Adolescent Psychiatry, 56*(5), 391-400. https://doi.org/10.1016/j.jaac.2017.02.004

Merikangas, K. R., Cui, L., Kattan, G., Carlson, G. A., Youngstrom, E. A., & Angst, J. (2012). Mania with and without depression in a community sample of US adolescents. *JAMA Psychiatry, 69*(9), 943-51.

Merikangas, K. R., He, J., Burstein, M., Swanson, S. A., Avenevoli, S., Cui, L., Benjet, C., Georgiades, K., & Swendsen, J. (2010). Lifetime prevalence of mental disorders in U.S. adolescents: Results from the National Comorbidity Survey Replication–Adolescent Supplement (NCS-A). *Journal of the American Academy of Child & Adolescent Psychiatry, 49*(10), 980-89. https://doi.org/10.1016/j.jaac.2010.05.017

Merikangas, K. R., Nakamura, E., & Kessler, R. (2009). Epidemiology of mental disorders in children and adolescents. *Dialogues in Clinical Neuroscience, 11*(1), 7-20.

Meyer, A., Carlton, C., Crisler, S., & Kallen, A. (2018). The development of the error-related negativity in large sample of adolescent females: Associations with anxiety symptoms. *Biological Psychology, 138*, 96-103. https://doi.org/10.1016/j.biopsycho.2018.09.003

Meyer, A., Nelson, B., Perlman, G., Klein, D. N., & Kotov, R. (2018). A neural biomarker, the error-related negativity, predicts the first onset of generalized anxiety disorder in a large sample of adolescent females. *Journal of Child Psychology and Psychiatry, 59*(11), 1162-70. https://doi.org/10.1111/jcpp.12922

Meyer-Bahlburg, H. L. (2002). Gender identity disorder in young boys: A parent- and peer-based treatment protocol. *Clinical Child Psychology and Psychiatry, 7*(3), 360-76. https://doi.org/10.1177/1359104502007003005

Micali, N., Solmi, F., Horton, N. J., Crosby, R. D., Eddy, K. T., Calzo, J. P., Sonneville, K. R., Swanson, S. A., & Field, A. E. (2015). Adolescent eating disorders predict psychiatric, high-risk behaviors and weight outcomes in young adulthood. *Journal of the American Academy of Child & Adolescent Psychiatry, 54*(8), 652-59. https://doi.org/10.1016/j.jaac.2015.05.009

Mick, E., Biederman, J., Prince, J., Fischer, M. J., & Faraone, S. V. (2002). Impact of low birth weight on attention-deficit hyperactivity disorder. *Journal of Developmental and Behavioral Pediatrics, 23*(1), 16-22. https://doi.org/10.1097/00004703-200202000-00004

Mick, E., & Faraone, S. V. (2009). Family and genetic association studies of bipolar disorder in children. *Child and Adolescent Psychiatric Clinics of North America, 18*(2), 441-53.

Mikami, A. Y. (2015). Social skills training for youth with ADHD. In R. A. Barkley (Ed.), *Attention-deficit hyperactivity disorder: A handbook for diagnosis and treatment* (pp. 569-95). Guilford Press.

Mikami, A. Y., Griggs, M. S., Lerner, M. D., Emeh, C. C., Reuland, M. M., Jack, A., & Anthony, M. R. (2013). A randomized trial of a classroom intervention to increase peers' social inclusion of children with attention-deficit/hyperactivity disorder. *Journal of Consulting and Clinical Psychology, 81*(1), 100-112. https://doi.org/10.1037/a0029654

Mikami, A. Y., Hinshaw, S. P., Arnold, L. E., Hoza, B., Hechtman, L., Newcorn, J. H., & Abikoff, H. B. (2010). Bulimia nervosa symptoms in the multimodal treatment study of children with ADHD. *International Journal of Eating Disorders, 43*(3), 248-59.

Mikami, A. Y., Lerner, M. D., Griggs, M. S., McGrath, A., & Calhoun, C. D. (2010). Parental influence on children with attention-deficit/hyperactivity disorder: II. Results of a pilot intervention training parents as friendship coaches for children. *Journal of Abnormal Child Psychology, 38*(6), 737-49. https://doi.org/10.1007/s10802-010-9403-4

Miklowitz, D. J., Axelson, D. A., George, E. L., Taylor, D. O., Schneck, C. D., Sullivan, A. E., Dickinson, L. M., & Birmaher, B. (2009). Expressed emotion moderates the effects of family-focused treatment for bipolar adolescents. *Journal of the American Academy of Child and Adolescent Psychiatry, 48*(6), 643-51.

Miklowitz, D. J., Biuckians, A., & Richards, J. A. (2006). Early-onset bipolar disorder: A family treatment perspective. *Development and Psychopathology, 18*(4), 1247-65.

Miklowitz, D. J., George, E. L., Axelson, D. A., Kim, E. Y., Birmaher, B., Schneck, C., Beresford, C., Craighead, W. E., & Brent, D. A. (2004). Family-focused treatment for adolescents with bipolar disorder. *Journal of Affective Disorders, 82*(Suppl 1), 113-28.

Miklowitz, D. J., & Goldstein, T. R. (2010). Family-based approaches to treating bipolar disorder in adolescence: Family-focused therapy and dialectical behavior therapy. In D. J. Miklowitz & D. Cicchetti (Eds.), *Understanding bipolar disorder: A developmental psychopathology perspective.* (pp. 466-93). Guilford.

Miklowitz, D. J., Goldstein, M. J., Nuechterlein, K. H., Snyder, K. S., & Mintz, J. (1988). Family factors and the course of bipolar affective disorder. *Archives of General Psychiatry, 45*(3), 225-31.

Miklowitz, D. J., Mullen, K. L., & Chang, K. D. (2008). Family-focused treatment for bipolar disorder in adolescence. In B. Gellder & M. P. DelBello (Eds.), *Treatment of bipolar disorder in children and adolescents* (pp. 166-83). Guilford.

Miklowitz, D. J., Schneck, C. D., George, E. L., Taylor, D. O., Sugar, C. A., Birmaher, B., Kowatch, R. A., DelBello, M. P., & Axelson, D. A. (2014). Pharmacotherapy and family-focused treatment for adolescents with bipolar I and II disorders: a 2-year randomized trial. *American Journal of Psychiatry, 171*(6), 658-67.

Milea, B., & Cozman, D. (2012). Comparative study of multimodal and pharmacological therapy in treating school aged children with ADHD. *Applied Medical Informatics, 31*(3), 55-63.

Miller, A. L., Rathus, J. H., & Linehan, M. M. (2006). *Dialectical behavior therapy with suicidal adolescents.* Guilford.

Miller, M., Musser, E., Young, G., Olson, B., Steiner, R., & Nigg, J. (2018). Sibling recurrence risk and cross-aggregation of attention-deficit/hyperactivity disorder and autism spectrum disorder. *JAMA Pediatrics, 173*(2), 147-52. https://doi.org/10.1001/jamapediatrics.2018.4076

Miller-Graff, L. E., & Campion, K. (2016). Interventions for posttraumatic stress with children exposed to violence: Factors associated with treatment success. *Journal of Clinical Psychology, 72*(3), 226–248. https://doi.org/10.1002/jclp.22238

Miller-McLemore, B. J. (2003). *Let the children come: Reimagining childhood from a Christian perspective.* Jossey-Bass.

Malpas, J. (2011). Between pink and blue: a multidimensional family approach to gender nonconforming children and their families. *Family Process, 50*(4), 453–470. https://doi.org/10.1111/j.1545-5300.2011.01371.x

Mitchell, K. S., Neale, M. C., Bulik, C. M., Aggen, S. H., Kendler, K. S., & Mazzeo, S. E. (2010). Binge eating disorder, a symptom-level investigation of genetic and environmental influences on liability. *Psychological Medicine, 40*(11), 1899-1906. https://doi.org/10.1017/S0033291710000139

Mitchison, G. M., Liber, J. M., Hannesdottir, D. K., & Njardvik, U. (2020). Emotion dysregulation, ODD and conduct problems in a sample of five and six-year-old children. *Child Psychiatry and Human Development, 51*(1), 71-79. https://doi.org/10.1007/s10578-019-00911-7

Modrowski, C. A., Bennett, D. C., Chaplo, S. D., & Kerig, P. K. (2017). Screening for PTSD among detained adolescents: Implications of the changes in the DSM–5. *Psychological Trauma: Theory, Research, Practice, and Policy, 9*(1), 10-17. http://doi.org/10.1037/tra0000156

Moffitt, T. E. (1990). Juvenile delinquency and attention-deficit disorder: Developmental trajectories from age 3 to 15. *Child Development, 61*(3), 893-910.

Moffitt, T. E. (1993). Adolescence-limited and life-course-persistent antisocial behavior: A developmental taxonomy. *Psychological Review, 100*(4), 674-701.

Moffitt, T. E., Caspi, A., Dickson, N., Silva, P., & Stanton, W. (1996). Childhood-onset versus adolescent-onset conduct problems in males: Natural history from ages 3 to 18 years. *Development and Psychopathology, 8*(2), 399-424.

Moffitt, T. E., Caspi, A., Rutter, M., & Silva, P. A. (2001). *Sex differences in antisocial behavior: Conduct disorder, delinquency, and violence in the Dunedin Longitudinal Study.* Cambridge University Press.

Mohamed, F. E., Kamal, T. M., Zahra, S. S., Khfagy, M. H., & Youssef, A. M. (2017). Dopamine D4 receptor gene polymorphism in a sample of Egyptian children with attention-deficit hyperactivity disorder (ADHD). *Journal of Child Neurology, 32*(2), 188-93. https://doi.org/10.1177/0883073816674091

Mohammad, E. T., Shapiro, E. R., Wainwright, L. D., & Carter, A. S. (2015). Impacts of family and community violence exposure on child coping and mental health. *Journal of Abnormal Child Psychology, 43*(2), 203-15. https://doi.org/10.1007/s10802-014-9889-2

Molina, B. G., Hinshaw, S. P., Swanson, J. M., Arnold, L. E., Vitiello, B., Jensen, P. S., Epstein, J. N., Hoza, B., Hechtman, L., Abikoff, H. B., Elliott, G. R., Greenhill, L. L., Newcorn, J. H., Wells, K. C., Wigal, T., Gibbons, R. D., Hur, K., & Houck, P. R. (2009). The MTA at 8 years: Prospective follow-up of children treated for combined-type ADHD in a multisite study. *Journal of the American Academy of Child & Adolescent Psychiatry, 48*(5), 484-500. https://doi.org/10.1097/CHI.0b013e31819c23d0

Monk, C. S., Nelson, E. E., McClure, E. B., Mogg, K., Bradley, B. P., Leibenluft, E., Blair, R. J., Chen, G., Charney, D. S., Ernst, M., & Pine, D. S. (2006). Ventrolateral prefrontal cortex activation and attentional bias in response to angry faces in adolescents with generalized anxiety disorder. *The American Journal of Psychiatry, 163*(6), 1091-97.

Monk, C. S., Telzer, E. H., Mogg, K., Bradley, B. P., Mai, X., Louro, H. M., Chen, G., McClure-Tone, E. B., Ernst, M., & Pine, D. S. (2008). Amygdala and ventrolateral prefrontal cortex activation to masked angry faces in children and adolescents with generalized anxiety disorder. *Archives of General Psychiatry, 65*(5), 568-76.

Moore, M. N., Salk, R. H., Van Hulle, C. A., Abramson, L. Y., Hyde, J. S., Lemery-Chalfant, K., & Goldsmith, H. H. (2013). Genetic and environmental influences on rumination, distraction, and depressed mood in adolescence. *Clinical Psychological Science, 1*(3), 316-22.

Moore, P. S., Whaley, S. E., & Sigman, M. (2004). Interactions between mothers and children: Impacts of maternal and child anxiety. *Journal of Abnormal Psychology, 113*(3), 471-76.

Moreno, C., Laje, G., Blanco, C., Jiang, H., Schmidt, A. B., & Olfson, M. (2007). National trends in the outpatient diagnosis and treatment of bipolar disorder in youth. *Archives of General Psychiatry, 64*(9), 1032-39.

Morey, R. A., Haswell, C. C., Hooper, S. R., & De Bellis, M. D. (2016). Amygdala, hippocampus, and ventral medial prefrontal cortex volumes differ in maltreated youth with and without chronic posttraumatic stress disorder. *Neuropsychopharmacology, 41*(3), 791-801. https://doi.org/10.1038/npp.2015.205

Morgan, J. E., Loo, S. K., & Lee, S. S. (2018). Neurocognitive functioning mediates the prospective association of birth weight with youth ADHD symptoms. *Journal of Clinical Child and Adolescent Psychology, 47*(5), 727-36. https://doi.org/10.1080/15374416.2016.1183498

Morina, N., Koerssen, R., & Pollet, T. V. (2016). Interventions for children and adolescents with posttraumatic stress disorder: A meta-analysis of comparative outcome studies. *Clinical Psychology Review, 47*, 41–54. https://doi.org/10.1016/j.cpr.2016.05.006

Morley, C. A., & Kohrt, B. A. (2013). Impact of peer support on PTSD, hope, and functional impairment: A mixed-methods study of child soldiers in Nepal. *Journal of Aggression, Maltreatment & Trauma, 22*(7), 714-34. https://doi.org/10.1080/10926771.2013.813882

Morris, A. S., Silk, J. S., Steinberg, L., Sessa, F. M., Avenevoli, S., & Essex, M. J. (2002). Temperamental vulnerability and negative parenting as interacting predictors of child adjustment. *Journal of Marriage and Family, 64*(2), 461-71.

Morris, S. S. J., Musser, E. D., Tenenbaum, R. B., Ward, A. R., Martinez, J., Raiker, J. S., Coles, E. K., & Riopelle, C. (2020). Emotion regulation via the autonomic nervous system in children with attention-deficit/hyperactivity disorder (ADHD): Replication and extension. *Journal of Abnormal Child Psychology, 48*(3), 361-73. https://doi.org/10.1007/s10802-019-00593-8

Morrow, J., & Nolen-Hoeksema, S. (1990). Effects of responses to depression on the remediation of depressive affect. *Journal of Personality and Social Psychology, 58*(3), 519-27.

Morsette, A., Swaney, G., Stolle, D., Schuldberg, D., van den Pol, R., & Young, M. (2009). Cognitive Behavioral Intervention for Trauma in Schools (CBITS): school-based treatment on a rural American Indian reservation. *Journal of Behavior Therapy and Experimental Psychiatry, 40*(1), 169–178. https://doi.org/10.1016/j.jbtep.2008.07.006

Moscardino, U., Scrimin, S., Capello, F., & Altoè, G. (2014). Brief report: Self-blame and PTSD symptoms in adolescents exposed to terrorism: is school connectedness a mediator? *Journal of Adolescence, 37*(1), 47–52. https://doi.org/10.1016/j.adolescence.2013.10.011

Moskowitz, A., & Heim, G. (2011). Eugen Bleuler's *Dementia Praecox or the Group of Schizo-*

phrenias (1911): A centenary appreciation and reconsideration. *Schizophrenia Bulletin, 37*(3), 471-79. https://doi.org/10.1093/schbul/sbr016

Moss, J., Magiati, I., Charman, T., & Howlin, P. (2008). Stability of the Autism Diagnostic Interview—Revised from pre-school to elementary school age in children with autism spectrum disorders. *Journal of Autism and Developmental Disorders, 38*(6), 1081-91. https://doi.org/10.1007/s10803-007-0487-9

MTA Cooperative Group. (1999a). A 14-month randomized clinical trial of treatment strategies for attention-deficit/hyperactivity disorder. *Archives of General Psychiatry, 56*(12), 1073-86. https://doi.org/10.1001/archpsyc.56.12.1073

MTA Cooperative Group. (1999b). Moderators and mediators of treatment response for children with attention-deficit/hyperactivity disorder: The multimodal treatment study of children with attention-deficit/hyperactivity disorder. *Archives of General Psychiatry, 56*(12), 1088-96. https://doi.org/10.1001/archpsyc.56.12.1088

MTA Cooperative Group. (2004a). National Institute of Mental Health Multimodal Treatment Study of ADHD follow-up: 24-Month outcomes of treatment strategies for attention-deficit/hyperactivity disorder. *Pediatrics, 113*(4), 754-61.

MTA Cooperative Group. (2004b). National Institute of Mental Health Multimodal Treatment Study of ADHD follow-up: Changes in effectiveness and growth after the end of treatment. *Pediatrics, 113*(4), 762-69.

Mufson, L., Dorta, K. P., Moreau, D., & Weissman, M. M. (2004). *Interpersonal psychotherapy for depressed adolescents* (2nd ed.). Guilford.

Müller, T. D., Föcker, M., Holtkamp, K., Herpertz-Dahlmann, B., & Hebebrand, J. (2009). Leptin-mediated neuroendocrine alterations in anorexia nervosa: Somatic and behavioral

implications. *Child and Adolescent Psychiatric Clinics of North America, 18*(1), 117-29. https://doi.org/10.1016/j.chc.2008.07.002

Mulqueen, J. M., Bartley, C. A., & Bloch, M. H. (2015). Meta-analysis: Parental interventions for preschool ADHD. *Journal of Attention Disorders, 19*(2), 118-24. https://doi.org/10.1177/1087054713504135

Mumper, E. E., Dyson, M. W., Finsaas, M. C., Olino, T. M., & Klein, D. N. (2020). Life stress moderates the effects of preschool behavioral inhibition on anxiety in early adolescence. *Journal of Child Psychology and Psychiatry, 61*(2), 167-74. https://doi.org/10.1111/jcpp.13121

Munkholm, A., Olsen, E. M., Rask, C. U., Clemmensen, L., Rimvall, M. K., Jeppesen, P., Micali, N., & Skovgaard, A. M. (2016). Early predictors of eating problems in preadolescence—A prospective birth cohort study. *Journal of Adolescent Health, 58*(5), 533-42. https://doi.org/10.1016/j.jadohealth.2016.01.006

Munson, J., Dawson, G., Abbott, R., Faja, S., Webb, S. J., Friedman, S. D., Shaw, D., Artru, A., & Dager, S. R. (2006). Amygdalar volume and behavioral development in autism. *Archives of General Psychiatry, 63*(6), 686-93. https://doi.org/10.1001/archpsyc.63.6.686

Muratori, P., Milone, A., Nocentini, A., Manfredi, A., Polidori, L., Ruglioni, L., Lambruschi, F., Masi, G., & Lochman, J. E. (2015). Maternal depression and parenting practices predict treatment outcome in Italian children with disruptive behavior disorder. *Journal of Child and Family Studies, 24*(9), 2805-16.

Muris, P., Merckelbach, H., Gadet, B., & Moulaert, V. (2000). Fears, worries, and scary dreams in 4- to 12-year-old children: Their content, developmental pattern, and origins. *Journal of Clinical Child Psychology, 29*, 43-52.

Muris, P., van Brakel, A. L., Arntz, A., & Schouten, E. (2011). Behavioral inhibition as a risk factor for the development of childhood anxiety disorders: A longitudinal study. *Journal of Child and Family Studies, 20*(2), 157-70.

Murray, L., Creswell, C., & Cooper, P. J. (2009). The development of anxiety disorders in childhood: An integrative review. *Psychological Medicine, 39*(9), 1413-23.

Murray, L. K., Dorsey, S., & Lewandowski, E. (2014). Global dissemination and implementation of child evidence-based practices in low resources countries. In R. S. Beidas & P. C. Kendall (Eds.), *Dissemination and implementation of evidence-based practices in child and adolescent mental health* (pp. 179–203). Oxford University Press.

Murray, L., Pella, J. E., De Pascalis, L., Arteche, A., Pass, L., Percy, R., Creswell, C., & Cooper, P. J. (2014). Socially anxious mothers' narratives to their children and their relation to child representations and adjustment. *Development and Psychopathology, 2*, 1531-46.

Nabbijohn, A. N., van der Miesen, A. I. R., Santarossa, A., Peragine, D., de Vries, A. L. C., Popma, A., Lai, M., & VanderLaan, D. P. (2018). Gender variance and the autism spectrum: An examination of children ages 6–12 years. *Journal of Autism and Developmental Disorders.* https://doi.org/10.1007/s10803-018-3843-z

Naber, F., Bakermans-Kranenburg, M., van Ijzendoorn, M., Dietz, C., Daalen, E., Swinkels, S. H. N., Buitelaar, J. K., & van Engeland, H. (2008). Joint attention development in toddlers with autism. *European Child & Adolescent Psychiatry, 17*, 143-52. https://doi.org/10.1007/s00787-007-0648-6

Nadeem E., Jaycox L.H., Langley A.K., Wong M., Kataoka S.H., Stein B.D. (2014) Effects of trauma on students: Early intervention through the Cognitive Behavioral Intervention for Trauma in Schools. In M. Weist, N. Lever, C. Bradshaw, & J. Owens (Eds),

Handbook of school mental health. Issues in cinical child psychology. Boston: Springer. https://doi.org/10.1007/978-1-4614-7624-5_11

Nader, K. (2008). *Understanding and assessing trauma in children and adolescents: Measures, methods, and youth in context.* Routledge.

Nader, K., & Fletcher, K. E. (2014). Childhood posttraumatic stress disorder. In E. J. Mash & R. A. Barkley (Eds.), *Child psychopathology* (3rd ed., pp. 476-528). Guilford.

Nanda, M. M., Kotchick, B. A., & Grover, R. L. (2012). Parental psychological control and childhood anxiety: The mediating role of perceived lack of control. *Journal of Child and Family Studies, 21*, 637-45.

Narad, M. E., Garner, A. A., Peugh, J. L., Tamm, L., Antonini, T. N., Kingery, K. M., Simon, J. O., & Epstein, J. N. (2015). Parent–teacher agreement on ADHD symptoms across development. *Psychological Assessment, 27*(1), 239-48. https://doi.org/10.1037/a0037864

National Association of Social Workers. (2015). *Sexual orientation change efforts (SOCE) and conversion therapy with lesbians, gay men, bisexuals, and transgender persons.* Retrieved from https://www.socialworkers.org/LinkClick.aspx?fileticket=yH3UsGQQmYI%3d&portalid=0

National Research Council (2001). *Educating children with autism.* National Academy Press.

Neal-Barnett, A. M., & Smith, J. M., Sr. (1996). African American children and behavior therapy: Considering the Afrocentric approach. *Cognitive and Behavioral Practice, 3*(2), 351-69. https://doi.org/10.1016/S1077-7229(96)80023-X

Neill, E. L., Weems, C. F., & Scheeringa, M. S. (2018). CBT for child PTSD is associated with reductions in maternal depression: Evidence for bidirectional effects. *Journal of Clinical Child and Adolescent Psychology, 47*(3), 410-20. https://doi.org/10.1080/15374416.2016.1212359

Nelemans, S. A., Hale, W. W., III, Branje, S. J. T., van Lier, P. A. C., Koot, H. M., & Meeus, W. H. J. (2017). The role of stress reactivity in the long-term persistence of adolescent social anxiety symptoms. *Biological Psychology, 125*, 91-104. https://doi.org/10.1016/j.biopsycho.2017.03.003

Neppl, T., Donnellan, M., Scaramella, L., Widaman, K., Spilman, S., Ontai, L., & Conger, R. (2010). Differential stability of temperament and personality from toddlerhood to middle childhood. *Journal of Research in Personality, 44*(3), 386-96. https://doi.org/10.1016/j.jrp.2010.04.004

Neugebauer, R., Turner, J. B., Fisher, P. W., Yamabe, S., Zhang, B., Neria, Y., Gameroff, M., Bolton, P., & Mack, R. (2014). Posttraumatic stress reactions among Rwandan youth in the second year after the genocide: Rising trajectory among girls. *Psychological Trauma: Theory, Research, Practice, and Policy, 6*(3), 269-79. https://doi.org/10.1037/a0035240

Neumann, A., van Lier, P. A. C., Gratz, K. L., & Koot, H. M. (2010). Multidimensional assessment of emotion regulation difficulties using the Difficulties in Emotion Regulation Scale. *Assessment, 17*(1), 138-49.

Neumark-Sztainer, D., Wall, M., Larson, N. I., Eisenberg, M. E., & Loth, K. (2011). Dieting and disordered eating behaviors from adolescence to young adulthood: findings from a 10-year longitudinal study. *Journal of the American Dietetic Association, 111*(7), 1004–1011. https://doi.org/10.1016/j.jada.2011.04.012

Newman, B. J. (2011). *Autism and your church: Nurturing the spiritual growth of people with autism spectrum disorder*. Friendship Ministries.

Ngo, V., Langley, A., Kataoka, S. H., Nadeem, E., Escudero, P., & Stein, B. D. (2008). Providing evidence-based practice to ethnically diverse youths: examples from the Cognitive Behavioral Intervention for Trauma in Schools (CBITS) program. *Journal of the American Academy of Child and Adolescent Psychiatry, 47*(8), 858–862. https://doi.org/10.1097/CHI.0b013e3181799f19

NICHD Early Child Care Research Network. (1998). Early child care and self-control, compliance, and problem behavior at twenty-four and thirty-six months. *Child Development, 69*(4), 1145-70.

Nicholls, D. E., Lynn, R., & Viner, R. M. (2011). Childhood eating disorders: British national surveillance study. *The British Journal of Psychiatry, 198*(4), 295-301. https://doi.org/10.1192/bjp.bp.110.081356

Nicholls, D., Statham, R., Costa, S., Micali, N., & Viner, R. M. (2016). Childhood risk factors for lifetime bulimic or compulsive eating by age 30 years in a British national birth cohort. *Appetite, 105*, 266–273. https://doi.org/10.1016/j.appet.2016.05.036

Nicholls, D. E., & Viner, R. M. (2009). Childhood risk factors for lifetime anorexia nervosa by age 30 years in a national birth cohort. *Journal of the American Academy of Child and Adolescent Psychiatry, 48*(8), 791–799. https://doi.org/10.1097/CHI.0b013e3181ab8b75

Nickel, L. R., Thatcher, A. R., Keller, F., Wozniak, R. H., & Iverson, J. M. (2013). Posture development in infants at heightened versus low risk for autism spectrum disorders. *Infancy, 18*(5), 639-61. https://doi.org/10.1111/infa.12025

Nickl-Jockschat, T., & Michel., T. M. (2011). The role of neurotrophic factors in autism. *Molecular Psychiatry, 16*(5), 478-90.

Nigg, J. (2017). Attention-deficit/hyperactivity disorder. In T. P. Beauchaine & S. P. Hinshaw (Eds.), *Child and adolescent psychopathology* (3rd ed., pp. 407-48). Wiley.

Nigg, J. T., & Barkley, R. A. (2014). Attention-deficit/hyperactivity disorder. In E. J. Mash & R. A. Barkley (Eds). *Child psychopathology* (3rd ed., pp. 75-144). Guilford.

Nigg, J., Nikolas, M., & Burt, S. A. (2010). Measured gene-by-environment interaction in relation to attention-deficit/hyperactivity disorder. *Journal of the American Academy of Child & Adolescent Psychiatry, 49*(9), 863-73. https://doi.org/10.1016/j.jaac.2010.01.025

Nigg, J. T., Nikolas, M., Knottnerus, G., Cavanagh, K., & Friderici, K. (2010). Confirmation and extension of association of blood lead with attention-deficit hyperactivity disorder (ADHD) and ADHD symptom domains at population-typical exposure levels. *Journal of Child Psychology and Psychiatry, 51*(1), 58-65. https://doi.org/10.1111/j.1469 -7610.2009.02135.x

Nishikawa, S., Fujisawa, T. X., Kojima, M., & Tomoda, A. (2018). Type and timing of negative life events are associated with adolescent depression. *Frontiers in Psychiatry, 9*(41). https://doi.org/10.3389/fpsyt.2018.00041

Nitschke, J. B., Sarinopoulos, I., Oathes, D. J., Johnstone, T., Whalen, P. J., Davidson, R. J., & Kalin, N. H. (2009). Anticipatory activation in the amygdala and anterior cingulate in generalized anxiety disorder and prediction of treatment response. *American Journal of Psychiatry, 166*(3), 302-10.

Nixon, R. V., Nehmy, T. J., Ellis, A. A., Ball, S., Menne, A., & McKinnon, A. C. (2010). Predictors of posttraumatic stress in children following injury: The influence of appraisals, heart rate, and morphine use. *Behaviour Research and Therapy, 48*(8), 810-15. https://doi.org/10.1016/j.brat.2010.05.002

Nolen-Hoeksema, S., Girgus, J. S., & Seligman, M. E. (1992). Predictors and consequences of childhood depressive symptoms: A 5-year longitudinal study. *Journal of Abnormal Psychology, 101*(3), 405-22.

Nordanger, D. Ø., Hysing, M., Posserud, M., Lundervold, A. J., Jakobsen, R., Olff, M., & Stormark, K. M. (2013). Posttraumatic responses to the July 22, 2011 Oslo terror among Norwegian high school students. *Journal of Traumatic Stress, 26*, 679-85. https://doi.org/10.1002/jts.21856

Norris, M. L., Boydell, K. M., Pinhas, L., & Katzman, D. K. (2006). Ana and the Internet: a review of pro-anorexia websites. *International Journal of Eating Disorders, 39*(6), 443–447. https://doi.org/10.1002/eat.20305

Nottelmann, E., & Jensen, P. S. (1995). Comorbidity of disorders in children and adolescents: Developmental perspectives. In T. H. Ollendick & R. J. Prinz (Eds.)., *Advances in clinical child perspectives* (Vol. 17, pp. 109-55). Plenum Press.

Nymberg, C., Jia, T., Lubbe, S., Ruggeri, B., Desrivieres, S., Barker, G., Büchel, C., Fauth-Buehler, M., Cattrell, A., Conrod, P., Flor, H., Gallinat, J., Garavan, H., Heinz, A., Ittermann, B., Lawrence, C., Mann, K., Nees, F., Salatino-Oliveira, A., . . . Schumann, G. (2013). Neural mechanisms of attention-deficit/hyperactivity disorder symptoms are stratified by *MAOA* genotype. *Biological Psychiatry, 74*(8), 607-14. https://doi.org/10.1016/j.biopsych.2013.03.027

Ochsner, K. N., & Gross, J. J. (2005). The cognitive control of emotion. *Trends in Cognitive Sciences, 9*(5), 242-49.

Oehrlein, E. M., Burcu, M., Safer, D. J., & Zito, J. M. (2016). National trends in ADHD diagnosis and treatment: Comparison of youth and adult office-based visits. *Psychiatric Services, 67*(9), 964-69. https://doi.org/10.1176/appi.ps.201500269

O'Hara, C. B., Campbell, I. C., & Schmidt, U. (2015). A reward-centred model of anorexia nervosa: A focussed narrative review of the neurological and psychophysiological literature. *Neuroscience and Biobehavioral Reviews, 52*, 131-52. https://doi.org/10.1016/j.neubiorev.2015.02.012

Ollendick, T. H., Davis, T. E., & Muris, P. (2004). Treatment of specific phobia in children and adolescents. In P. M. Barrett & T. H. Ollendick (Eds.), *Handbook of interventions that work with children and adolescents* (pp. 273-99). John Wiley & Sons.

Olson, L., Maclin, V., Moriarty, G., & Bermudez, H. (2013). God images. In D. F. Walker & W. L. Hathaway (Eds.), *Spiritual interventions in child and adolescent psychotherapy* (pp. 209-32). American Psychological Association. https://doi.org/10.1037/13947-010

Olson, S. L., Ip, K. I., Gonzalez, R., Beyers-Carlson, E. E. A., & Volling, B. L. (2020). Development of externalizing symptoms across the toddler period: The critical role of older siblings. *Journal of Family Psychology, 34*(2), 165-74. https://doi.org/10.1037/fam0000581

Oppenheimer, C. W., Hankin, B. L., & Young, J. (2018). Effect of parenting and peer stressors on cognitive vulnerability and risk for depression among youth. *Journal of Abnormal Child Psychology, 46*(3), 597-612. https://doi.org/10.1007/s10802-017-0315-4

Oransky, M., Hahn, H., & Stover, C. S. (2013). Caregiver and youth agreement regarding youths' trauma histories: Implications for youths' functioning after exposure to trauma. *Journal of Youth and Adolescence, 42*(10), 1528-42. https://doi.org/10.1007/s10964-013-9947-z

Orgilés, M., Penosa, P., Morales, A., Fernández-Martínez, I., & Espada, J. P. (2018). Maternal anxiety and separation anxiety in children aged between 3 and 6 years: The mediating role of parenting style. *Journal of Developmental and Behavioral Pediatrics, 39*(8), 621-28.

Orobio de Castro, B., Merk, W., Koops, W., Veerman, J. W., & Bosch, J. D. (2005). Emotions in social information processing and their relations with reactive and proactive aggression in referred aggressive boys. *Journal of Clinical Child and Adolescent Psychology, 34*(1), 105-16.

Orobio de Castro, B., Veerman, J. W., Koops, W., Bosch, J. D., & Monshouwer, H. J. (2002). Hostile attribution of intent and aggressive behavior: A meta-analysis. *Child Development, 73*(3), 916-34.

Osofsky, J. D., Osofsky, H. J., Weems, C. F., King, L. S., & Hansel, T. C. (2015). Trajectories of post-traumatic stress disorder symptoms among youth exposed to both natural and technological disasters. *Journal of Child Psychology and Psychiatry, 56*(12), 1347-55. https://doi.org/10.1111/jcpp.12420

Østergaard, S. D., Larsen, J. T., Dalsgaard, S., Wilens, T. E., Mortensen, P. B., Agerbo, E., Mors, O., & Petersen, L. (2016). Predicting ADHD by assessment of Rutter's indicators of adversity in infancy. *PLOS ONE, 11*(6), e0157352.

Osterling, J. A., Dawson, G., & Munson, J. A. (2002). Early recognition of 1-year-old infants with autism spectrum disorder versus mental retardation. *Development and Psychopathology, 14*(2), 239-51. https://doi.org/10.1017/S0954579402002031

Östlund, H., Keller, E., & Hurd, Y. (2003). Estrogen receptor gene expression in relation to neuropsychiatric disorders. *Annals of the New York Academy of Sciences, 1007*(1), 54-63. https://doi.org/10.1196/annals.1286.006

Otto, M. W., Henin, A., Hirshfeld-Becker, D. R., Pollack, M. H., Biederman, J., & Rosenbaum, J. F. (2007). Posttraumatic stress disorder symptoms following media exposure to tragic events: Impact of 9/11 on children at risk for anxiety disorders. *Journal of Anxiety Disorders, 21*(7), 888-902. https://doi.org/10.1016/j.janxdis.2006.10.008

Overton, W. F. (2013). A new paradigm for developmental science: Relationism and relational-developmental systems. *Applied Developmental Science, 17*(2), 94-107. https://doi.org/10.1080/10888691.2013.778717

Ozbay, F., Johnson, D. C., Dimoulas, E., Morgan, C. I., Charney, D., & Southwick, S. (2007). Social support and resilience to stress: From neurobiology to clinical practice. *Psychiatry*, *4*(5), 35-40.

Ozer, E. J., & Weinstein, R. S. (2004). Urban adolescents' exposure to community violence: The role of support, school safety, and social constraints in a school-based sample of boys and girls. *Journal of Clinical Child and Adolescent Psychology, 33*(3), 463-76. https://doi. org/10.1207/s15374424jccp3303_4

Ozonoff, S., Williams, B. J., & Landa, R. (2005). Parental report of the early development of children with regressive autism: The delays-plus-regression phenotype. *Autism, 9*(5), 461-86. https://doi.org/10.1177/1362361305057880

Ozonoff, S., Young, G. S., Carter, A., Messinger, D., Yirmiya, N., Zwaigenbaum, L., Bryson, S., Carver, L. J., Constantino, J. N., Dobkins, K., Hutman, T., Iverson, J. M., Landa, R., Rogers, S. J., Sigman, M., & Stone, W. L. (2011). Recurrence risk for autism spectrum disorders: A Baby Siblings Research Consortium study. *Pediatrics, 128*(3), e488-e495.

Pagani, L. S. (2014). Environmental tobacco smoke exposure and brain development: The case of attention deficit/hyperactivity disorder. *Neuroscience and Biobehavioral Reviews, 44*, 195-205. https://doi.org/10.1016/j.neubiorev.2013.03.008

Pagliaccio, D., Luby, J. L., Bogdan, R., Agrawal, A., Gaffrey, M. S., Belden, A. C., Botteron, K. N., Harms, M. P., & Barch, D. M. (2015). Amygdala functional connectivity, HPA axis genetic variation, and life stress in children and relations to anxiety and emotion regulation. *Journal of Abnormal Psychology, 124*(4), 817-33.

Palosaari, E., Punamäki, R. L., Peltonen, K., Diab, M., & Qouta, S. R. (2016). Negative social relationships predict posttraumatic stress symptoms among war-affected children via posttraumatic cognitions *Journal of Abnormal Child Psychology, 44*(5), 845–857. https://doi. org/10.1007/s10802-015-0070-3

Parens, E., & Johnston, J. (2010). Controversies concerning the diagnosis and treatment of bipolar disorder in children. *Child and Adolescent Psychiatry and Mental Health, 4*(9). http://capmh.biomedcentral.com/articles/10.1186/1753-2000-4-9

Park, S., Cho, S., Kim, J., Shin, M., Yoo, H., Oh, S. M., Han, D. H., Cheong, J. H., & Kim, B. (2014). Differential perinatal risk factors in children with attention-deficit/hyperactivity disorder by subtype. *Psychiatry Research, 219*(3), 609-16. https://doi.org/10.1016/j.psychres.2014.05.036

Parker, S. (2015, March 20). Autism: Does ABA therapy open society's doors to children, or impose conformity? *The Guardian*. Retrieved from https://www.theguardian.com/society/2015/mar/20/autism-does-aba-therapy-open-societys-doors-to-children-or-impose-conformity

Parkinson, K. N., Drewett, R. F., Le Couteur, A. S., & Adamson, A. J. (2012). Earlier predictors of eating disorder symptoms in 9-year-old children A longitudinal study. *Appetite, 59*(1), 161–167. https://doi.org/10.1016/j.appet.2012.03.022

Parr, N. J., & Howe, B. G. (2019). Heterogeneity of transgender identity nonaffirmation microaggressions and their association with depression symptoms and suicidality among transgender persons. *Psychology of Sexual Orientation and Gender Diversity, 6*(4), 461-74. https://doi.org/10.1037/sgd0000347

Patros, C., Alderson, R. M., Hudec, K. L., Tarle, S. J., & Lea, S. E. (2017). Hyperactivity in boys with attention-deficit/hyperactivity disorder: The influence of underlying visuospatial working memory and self-control processes.

Journal of Experimental Child Psychology, 154, 1–12. https://doi.org/10.1016/j.jecp.2016.09.008

Patterson, C. A., & Miles, B. S. (2015). *1-2-3 a calmer me: Helping children cope when emotions get out of control.* American Psychological Association.

Patterson, G. R. (1982). *Coercive family process.* Eugene, OR: Castalia.

Patterson, G. R., & Yoerger, K. (2002). A developmental model for early- and late-onset delinquency. In J. B. Reid, G. R. Patterson, & J. Snyder (Eds.), *Antisocial behavior in children and adolescents: A developmental analysis and model for intervention.* American Psychological Association.

Pavuluri, M. N., Graczyk, P. A., Henry, D. B., Carbray, J. A., Heidenreich, J., & Miklowitz, D. J. (2004). Child- and family-focused cognitive-behavioral therapy for pediatric bipolar disorder: Development and preliminary results. *Journal of the American Academy of Child and Adolescent Psychiatry, 43*(5), 528-37.

Pavuluri, M. N., Passarotti, A. M., Harral, E. M., & Sweeney, J. A. (2009). An fMRI study of the neural correlates of incidental versus directed emotion processing in pediatric bipolar disorder. *Journal of the American Academy of Child & Adolescent Psychiatry, 48*(3), 308-19.

Pavuluri, M. N., West, A., Hill, S. K., Jindal, K., & Sweeney, J. A. (2009). Neurocognitive function in pediatric bipolar disorder: 3-year follow-up shows cognitive development lagging behind healthy youths. *Journal of the American Academy of Child and Adolescent Psychiatry, 48*(3), 299–307. https://doi.org/10.1097/CHI.0b013e318196b907

Pearce, M. (2016). *Cognitive behavioral therapy for Christians with depression: A practical tool-based primer.* Templeton.

Pearson, C. M., Miller, J., Ackard, D. M., Loth, K. A., Wall, M. M., Haynos, A. F., & Neumark-Sztainer, D. (2017). Stability and change in patterns of eating disorder symptoms from adolescence to young adulthood. *International Journal of Eating Disorders, 50*(7), 748–757. https://doi.org/10.1002/eat.22692

Pelham, W. E., Burrows-MacLean, L., Gnagy, E. M., Fabiano, G. A., Coles, E. K., Tresco, K. E., Chacko, A., Wymbs, B. T., Wienke, A. L., Walker, K. S., & Hoffman, M. T. (2005). Transdermal methylphenidate, behavioral, and combined treatment for children with ADHD. *Experimental and Clinical Psychopharmacology, 13*(2), 111-26. https://doi.org/10.1037/1064-1297.13.2.111

Pelham, W. E., Jr, Fabiano, G. A., & Massetti, G. M. (2005). Evidence-based assessment of attention deficit hyperactivity disorder in children and adolescents. *Journal of Clinical Child and Adolescent Psychology, 34*(3), 449–476. https://doi.org/10.1207/s15374424jccp3403_5

Pelham, W. J., Gnagy, E. M., Greiner, A. R., Fabiano, G. A., Waschbusch, D. A., & Coles, E. K. (2017). Summer treatment programs for attention-deficit/hyperactivity disorder. In J. R. Weisz & A. E. Kazdin (Eds.), *Evidence-based psychotherapies for children and adolescents* (3rd ed., pp. 215-32). Guilford Press.

Pelham, W. J., Massetti, G. M., Wilson, T., Kipp, H., Myers, D., Newman Standley, B. B., Billheimer, S., & Waschbusch, D. A. (2005). Implementation of a comprehensive schoolwide behavioral intervention: The ABC Program. *Journal of Attention Disorders, 9*(1), 248-60. https://doi.org/10.1177/1087054705281596

Pelletier Brochu, J., Meilleur, D., DiMeglio, G., Taddeo, D., Lavoie, E., Erdstein, J., Pauzé, R., Pesant, C., Thibault, I., & Frappier, J.-Y. (2018). Adolescents' perceptions of the quality of interpersonal relationships and eating disorder symptom severity: The mediating role of low self-esteem and negative mood. *Eating Disorders: The Journal of Treatment & Prevention, 26*(4), 388-406. https://doi.org/10.1080/10640266.2018.1454806

Penela, E. C., Walker, O. L., Degnan, K. A., Fox, N. A., & Henderson, H. A. (2015). Early behavioral inhibition and emotion regulation: Pathways toward social competence in middle childhood. *Child Development, 86*(4), 1227-40.

Peng, C., Grant, J. D., Heath, A. C., Reiersen, A. M., Mulligan, R. C., & Anokhin, A. P. (2016). Familial influences on the full range of variability in attention and activity levels during adolescence: A longitudinal twin study. *Development and Psychopathology, 28*(2), 517-26. https://doi.org/10.1017/S0954579415001091

Pereira, A. I., Barros, L., Mendonça, D., & Muris, P. (2014). The relationships among parental anxiety, parenting, and children's anxiety: The mediating effects of children's cognitive vulnerabilities. *Journal of Child and Family Studies, 23*(2), 399-409.

Perez, M., Kroon Van Diest, A. M., Smith, H., & Sladek, M. R. (2018). Body dissatisfaction and its correlates in 5- to 7-year-old girls: A social learning experiment. *Journal of Clinical Child and Adolescent Psychology, 47*(5), 757-69. https://doi.org/10.1080/15374416.2016.1157758

Pérez-Edgar, K., Roberson-Nay, R., Hardin, M. G., Poeth, K., Guyer, A. E., Nelson, E. E., McClure, E. B., Henderson, H. A., Fox, N. A., Pine, D. S., & Ernst, M. (2007). Attention alters neural responses to evocative faces in behaviorally inhibited adolescents. *Neuroimage, 35*(4), 1538-46.

Perou, R., Bitsko, R. H., Blumberg, S. J., Pastor, P., Ghandour, R. M., Gfroerer, J. C., Hedden, S. L., Crosby, A. E., Visser, S. N., Schieve, L. A., Parks, S. E., Hall, J. E., Brody, D., Simile, C. M., Thompson, W. W., Baio, J., Avenevoli, S., Kogan, M. D., Huang, L. N., & Centers for Disease Control and Prevention (CDC) (2013). Mental health surveillance among children--United States, 2005-2011. *MMWR Supplements, 62*(2), 1–35.

Peters, A. T., Henry, D. B., & West, A. E. (2015). Caregiver characteristics and symptoms of pediatric bipolar disorder. *Journal of Child and Family Studies, 24*(5), 1469-80.

Petersen, I. T., Bates, J. E., Goodnight, J. A., Dodge, K. A., Lansford, J. E., Pettit, G. S., Latendresse, S. J., & Dick, D. M. (2012). Interaction between serotonin transporter polymorphism (5-HTTLPR) and stressful life events in adolescents' trajectories of anxious/depressed symptoms. *Developmental Psychology, 48*(5), 1463-75.

Pettersson, E., Sjölander, A., Almqvist, C., Anckarsäter, H., D'Onofrio, B. M., Lichtenstein, P., & Larsson, H. (2015). Birth weight as an independent predictor of ADHD symptoms: A within-twin pair analysis. *Journal of Child Psychology and Psychiatry, 56*(4), 453-59. https://doi.org/10.1111/jcpp.12299

Pfefferbaum, B., Tucker, P., & Nitiéma, P. (2015). Adolescent survivors of Hurricane Katrina: A pilot study of hypothalamic–pituitary–adrenal axis functioning. *Child & Youth Care Forum, 44*(4), 527-47. https://doi.org/10.1007/s10566-014-9297-3

Pheula, G., Rohde, L., & Schmitz, M. (2011). Are family variables associated with ADHD, inattentive type? A case-control study in schools. *European Child & Adolescent Psychiatry, 20*(3), 137-45. https://doi.org/10.1007/s00787-011-0158-4

Piacentini, J., Bennett, S., Compton, S. N., Kendall, P. C., Birmaher, B., Albano, A. M., March, J., Sherrill, J., Sakolsky, D., Ginsburg, G., Rynn, M., Bergman, R. L., Gosch, E., Waslick, B., Iyengar, S., McCracken, J., & Walkup, J. (2014). 24- and 36-week outcomes for the Child/Adolescent Anxiety Multimodal Study (CAMS). *Journal of the American Academy of Child & Adolescent Psychiatry, 53*(3), 297-310.

Pike, K. M., Hilbert, A., Wilfley, D. E., Fairburn, C. G., Dohm, F., Walsh, B. T., & Striegel-Moore, R. (2008). Toward an understanding of risk factors for anorexia nervosa: A case-control study. *Psychological Medicine, 38*(10), 1443-53. https://doi.org/10.1017/S0033291707002310

Pike, K. M., & Rodin, J. (1991). Mothers, daughters, and disordered eating. *Journal of Abnormal Psychology, 100*(2), 198-204. https://doi.org/10.1037/0021-843X.100.2.198

Pina, A. A., Polo, A. J., & Huey, S. J. (2019). Evidence-based psychosocial interventions for ethnic minority youth: The 10-year update. *Journal of Clinical Child and Adolescent Psychology, 48*(2), 179-202. https://doi.org/10.1080/15374416.2019.1567350

Pinhas, L., Morris, A., Crosby, R. D., & Katzman, D. K. (2011). Incidence and age-specific presentation of restrictive eating disorders in children: a Canadian Paediatric Surveillance Program study. *Archives of Pediatrics & adolescent Medicine, 165*(10), 895–899. https://doi.org/10.1001/archpediatrics.2011.145

Pinto, D., Delaby, E., Merico, D., Barbosa, M., Merikangas, A., Klei, L., Thiruvahindrapuram, B., Xu, X., Ziman, R., Wang, Z., Vorstman, J. A., Thompson, A., Regan, R., Pilorge, M., Pellecchia, G., Pagnamenta, A. T., Oliveira, B., Marshall, C. R., Magalhaes, T. R., Lowe, J. K., … Scherer, S. W. (2014). Convergence of genes and cellular pathways dysregulated in autism spectrum disorders. *American Journal of Human Genetics, 94*(5), 677–694. https://doi.org/10.1016/j.ajhg.2014.03.018

lana, M. T., Torres, T., Rodríguez, N., Boloc, D., Gassó, P., Moreno, E., Lafuente, A., Castro-Fornieles, J., Mas, S., & Lazaro, L. (2019). Genetic variability in the serotoninergic system and age of onset in anorexia nervosa and obsessive-compulsive disorder. *Psychiatry Research, 271*, 554-58. https://doi.org/10.1016/j.psychres.2018.12.019

Popma, A., Doreleijers, T. H., Jansen, L. C., Van Goozen, S. M., Van Engeland, H., & Ver-meiren, R. (2007). The diurnal cortisol cycle in delinquent male adolescents and normal controls. *Neuropsychopharmacology, 32*(7), 1622-28.

Post, R. M. (2007). Kindling and sensitization as models for affective episode recurrence, cyclicity, and tolerance phenomena. *Neuroscience and Biobehavioral Reviews, 31*(6), 858–873.

Post, R. M., Leverich, G. S., Xing, G., & Weiss, S. B. (2001). Developmental vulnerabilities to the onset and course of bipolar disorder. *Development and Psychopathology, 13*, 581-98.

Powell, S. G., Frydenberg, M., & Thomsen, P. H. (2015). The effects of long-term medication on growth in children and adolescents with ADHD: an observational study of a large cohort of real-life patients. *Child and Adolescent Psychiatry and Mental Health, 9*, 50. https://doi.org/10.1186/s13034-015-0082-3

Powers, A., Stevens, J. S., O'Banion, D., Stenson, A. F., Kaslow, N., Jovanovic, T., & Bradley, B. (2020). Intergenerational transmission of risk for PTSD symptoms in African American children: The roles of maternal and child emotion dysregulation. *Psychological Trauma: Theory, Research, Practice, and Policy.* Advance online publication. https://doi.org/10.1037/tra0000543

Priebe, S., Wildgrube, C., & Müller-Oerling-hausen, B. (1989). Lithium prophylaxis and expressed emotion. *British Journal of Psychiatry, 154*, 396-99.

Pringsheim, T., Hirsch, L., Gardner, D., & Gorman, D. A. (2015). The pharmacological management of oppositional behaviour, conduct problems, and aggression in children and adolescents with attention-deficit hyperactivity disorder, oppositional defiant disorder, and conduct disorder: A systematic review and meta-analysis. Part 1: Psychostimulants, alpha-2 agonists, and atomoxetine. *The Canadian Journal of Psychiatry, 60*(2), 42-51.

Prizant, B. M. (2016). *Uniquely human: A different way of seeing autism*. Simon & Schuster.

Prizant, B. M., Wetherby, A. M., & Rydell, P. J. (2000). Communication intervention issues for children with autism spectrum disorders. In A. M. Wetherby & B. M. Prizant (Eds.), *Autism spectrum disorders: A transactional developmental perspective* (pp. 193-224). Paul H. Brookes.

Puckett, J. A., Matsuno, E., Dyar, C., Mustanski, B., & Newcomb, M. E. (2019). Mental health and resilience in transgender individuals: What type of support makes a difference? [Supplemental material]. *Journal of Family Psychology, 33*(8), 954-64. https://doi.org/10.1037/fam0000561.supp

Punamäki, R., Palosaari, E., Diab, M., Peltonen, K., & Qouta, S. R. (2015). Trajectories of post-traumatic stress symptoms (PTSS) after major war among Palestinian children: Trauma, family- and child-related predictors. *Journal of Affective Disorders, 172,* 133-40. https://doi.org/10.1016/j.jad.2014.09.021

Pynoos, R. S., Weathers, F. W., Steinberg, A. M., Marx, B. P., Layne, C. M., Kaloupek, D. G., Schnurr, P. P., Keane, T. M., Blake, D. D., Newman, E., Nader, K. O., & Kriegler, J. A. (2015). *Clinician-Administered PTSD Scale for DSM-5 - Child/Adolescent Version*. Scale available from the National Center for PTSD at www.ptsd.va.gov.

Racco, A., & Vis, J. A. (2015). Evidence based trauma treatment for children and youth. *Child & Adolescent Social Work Journal, 32*(2), 121–129. https://doi.org/10.1007/s10560-014-0347-3

Ramsden, S. R., & Hubbard, J. A. (2002). Family expressiveness and parental emotion coaching: Their role in children's emotion regulation and aggression. *Journal of Abnormal Child Psychology, 30*(6), 657-67.

Rapport, M. D., Chung, K., Shore, G., & Isaacs, P. (2001). A conceptual model of child Psycho-pathology: implications for understanding attention deficit hyperactivity disorder and treatment efficacy. *Journal of Clinical Child Psychology, 30*(1), 48-58.

Rasmussen, C., & Bisanz, J. (2009). Executive functioning in children with fetal alcohol spectrum disorders: Profiles and age-related differences. *Child Neuropsychology, 15*(3), 201-15. https://doi.org/10.1080/09297040802385400

Rathus, J. H., & Miller, A. L. (2015). *DBT skills manual for adolescents*. Guilford.

Ready, C. B., Hayes, A. M., Yasinski, C. W., Webb, C., Gallop, R., Deblinger, E., & Laurenceau, J. (2015). Overgeneralized beliefs, accommodation, and treatment outcome in youth receiving trauma-focused cognitive behavioral therapy for childhood trauma. *Behavior Therapy, 46*(5), 671-88.

Reichborn-Kjennerud, T., Bulik, C. M., Tambs, K., & Harris, J. R. (2004). Genetic and environmental influences on binge eating in the absence of compensatory behaviors: A population-based twin study. *International Journal of Eating Disorders, 36*(3), 307-14. https://doi.org/10.1002/eat.20047

Reyno, S. M., & McGrath, P. J. (2006). Predictors of parent training efficacy for child externalizing behavior problems—A meta-analytic review. *Journal of Child Psychology and Psychiatry, 47*(1), 99-111.

Reynolds, C. R., & Kamphaus, R. W. (2015). *Behavior Assessment System for Children* (3rd ed.; BASC-3). NCS Pearson, Inc.

Reynolds, C. R., & Richmond, B. O. (2008). *Revised Children's Manifest Anxiety Scale—2*. Western Psychological Services.

Reynolds, W. M. (2002). *Reynolds Adolescent Depression Scale: Professional manual* (2nd ed.). Psychological Assessment Resources, Inc.

Reynolds, W. M. (2010). *Reynolds Child Depression Scale: Professional manual* (2nd ed.). Psychological Assessment Resources, Inc.

Rice, F., Riglin, L., Lomax, T., Souter, E., Potter, R., Smith, D. J., Thapar, A. K., & Thapar, A. (2019). Adolescent and adult differences in major depression symptom profiles. *Journal of Affective Disorders*, 243, 175-81. https://doi.org/10.1016/j.jad.2018.09.015

Richdale, A. L., & Schreck, K. A. (2009). Sleep problems in autism spectrum disorders: Prevalence, nature, & possible biopsychosocial aetiologies. *Sleep Medicine Reviews*, 13(6), 403-11. https://doi.org/10.1016/j.smrv.2009.02.003

Richler, J., Huerta, M., Bishop, S. L., & Lord, C. (2010). Developmental trajectories of restricted and repetitive behaviors and interests in children with autism spectrum disorders. *Development and Psychopathology*, 22(1), 55-69. https://doi.org/10.1017/S0954579409990265

Riddle, M. A., Yershova, K., Lazzaretto, D., Paykina, N., Yenokyan, G., Greenhill, L., Abikoff, H., Vitiello, B., Wigal, T., McCracken, J. T., Kollins, S. H., Murray, D. W., Wigal, S., Kastelic, E., McGough, J. J., dosReis, S., Bauzó-Rosario, A., Stehli, A., & Posner, K. (2013). The Preschool Attention-Deficit/Hyperactivity Disorder Treatment Study (PATS) 6-year follow-up. *Journal of the American Academy of Child & Adolescent Psychiatry*, 52(3), 264-78. https://doi.org/10.1016/j.jaac.2012.12.007

Riglin, L., Collishaw, S., Thapar, A. K., Dalsgaard, S., Langley, K., Smith, G. D., Stergiakouli, E., Maughan, B., O'Donovan, M. C., & Thapar, A. (2016). Association of genetic risk variants with attention-deficit/hyperactivity disorder trajectories in the general population. *JAMA Psychiatry*, 73(12), 1285-92. https://doi.org/10.1001/jamapsychiatry.2016.2817

Rinne-Albers, M. W., van der Wee, N. A., Lamers-Winkelman, F., & Vermeiren, R. M. (2013). Neuroimaging in children, adolescents and young adults with psychological trauma. *European Child & Adolescent Psychiatry*, 22(12), 745-55. https://doi.org/10.1007/s00787-013-0410-1

Rizzolatti, G., & Craighero, L. (2004). The mirror-neuron system. *Annual Review of Neuroscience*, 27, 169-92. https://doi.org/10.1146/annurev.neuro.27.070203.144230

Roberts, B. A., Martel, M. M., & Nigg, J. T. (2017). Are there executive dysfunction subtypes within ADHD? *Journal of Attention Disorders*, 21(4), 284-93. https://doi.org/10.1177/1087054713510349

Robin, A. L., Siegel, P. T., Koepke, T., Moye, A. W., & Tice, S. (1994). Family therapy versus individual therapy for adolescent females with anorexia nervosa. *Journal of Developmental and Behavioral Pediatrics*, 15(2), 111-16. https://doi.org/10.1097/00004703-199404000-00008

Robin, A. L., Siegel, P. T., & Moye, A. (1995). Family versus individual therapy for anorexia: Impact on family conflict. *International Journal of Eating Disorders*, 17(4), 313-22. https://doi.org/10.1002/1098-108X(199505)17:4<313::AID-EAT2260170402>3.0.CO;2-8

Robin, A. L., Siegel, P. T., Moye, A. W., Gilroy, M., Dennis, A. B., & Sikand, A. (1999). A controlled comparison of family versus individual therapy for adolescents with anorexia nervosa. *Journal of the American Academy of Child & Adolescent Psychiatry*, 38(12), 1482-89. https://doi.org/10.1097/00004583-199912000-00008

Robins, D. L., Fein, D., Barton, M. L., & Green, J. A. (2001). The Modified Checklist for Autism in Toddlers: An initial study investigating the early detection of autism and pervasive developmental disorders. *Journal of Autism and Developmental Disorders*, 31(2), 131-44. https://doi.org/10.1023/A:1010738829569

Robinson, N. S., Garber, J., & Hilsman, R. (1995). Cognitions and stress: Direct and moderating effects on depressive versus externalizing symptoms during the junior high school transition. *Journal of Abnormal Psychology*, 104(3), 453-63.

Robson, D. A., Allen, M. S., & Howard, S. J. (2020). Self-regulation in childhood as a predictor of future outcomes: A meta-analytic review [Supplemental material]. *Psychological Bulletin, 146*(4), 324-54. https://doi.org/10.1037/bul0000227.supp

Rodgers, R. F., Lowy, A. S., Halperin, D. M., & Franko, D. L. (2016). A meta-analysis examining the influence of pro-eating disorder websites on body image and eating pathology. *European Eating Disorders Review, 24*(1), 3–8. https://doi.org/10.1002/erv.2390

Rodgers, R. F., Slater, A., Gordon, C. S., McLean, S. A., Jarman, H. K., & Paxton, S. J. (2020). A biopsychosocial model of social media use and body image concerns, disordered eating, and muscle-building behaviors among adolescent girls and boys. *Journal of Youth and Adolescence, 49*(2), 399-409. https://doi.org/10.1007/s10964-019-01190-0

Rodriguez, C. M. (2003). Parental discipline and abuse potential affects on child depression, anxiety, and attributions. *Journal of Marriage and Family, 65*(4), 809-17.

Rogers, S. J., & Dawson, G. (2010). *Early Start Denver Model for young children with autism: Promoting language, learning, and engagement.* New York: Guilford Press.

Rogers, S. J., Vismara, L., Wagner, A. L., McCormick, C., Young, G., & Ozonoff, S. (2014). Autism treatment in the first year of life: A pilot study of infant start, a parent-implemented intervention for symptomatic infants. *Journal of Autism and Developmental Disorders, 44*(12), 2981-95. https://doi.org/10.1007/s10803-014-2202-y

Rohde, P. (2009). Comorbidities with adolescent depression. In S. Nolen-Hoeksema & L. M. Hilt (Eds.), *Handbook of depression in adolescents* (pp. 139-77). Routledge.

Roid, G. H. (2003). *Stanford-Binet Intelligence Scales, Fifth Edition (SB-5): Technical manual.* Riverside Publishing.

Rojas, D. C., Peterson, E., Winterrowd, E., Reite, M. L., Rogers, S. J., & Tregellas, J. R. (2006).

Regional gray matter volumetric changes in autism associated with social and repetitive behavior symptoms. *BMC Psychiatry, 6.* https://doi.org/10.1186/1471-244X-6-56

Rojo-Moreno, L., Arribas, P., Plumed, J., Gimeno, N., García-Blanco, A., Vaz-Leal, F., Vila, M. L., & Livianos, L. (2015). Prevalence and comorbidity of eating disorders among a community sample of adolescents: 2-year follow-up. *Psychiatry Research, 227*(1), 52-57. https://doi.org/10.1016/j.psychres.2015.02.015

Rolon-Arroyo, B., Arnold, D. H., Breaux, R. P., & Harvey, E. A. (2018). Reciprocal relations between parenting behaviors and conduct disorder symptoms in preschool children. *Child Psychiatry and Human Development, 49*(5), 786-99. https://doi.org/10.1007/s10578-018-0794-8

Ronald, A., Larsson, H., Anckarsäter, H., & Lichtenstein, P. (2014). Symptoms of autism and ADHD: A Swedish twin study examining their overlap. *Journal of Abnormal Psychology, 123*(2), 440-51. https://doi.org/10.1037/a0036088

Ronald, A., Simonoff, E., Kuntsi, J., Asherson, P., & Plomin, R. (2008). Evidence for overlapping genetic influences on autistic and ADHD behaviours in a community twin sample. *Journal of Child Psychology and Psychiatry, 49*(5), 535-42. https://doi.org/10.1111/j.1469-7610.2007.01857.x

Rondeau, H. (2003). Our lost children: Bipolar disorder and the church. *Journal of Psychology and Christianity, 22*(2), 123-30.

Rosenbaum Asarnow, J., Tompson, M., Woo, S., & Cantwell, D. P. (2001). Is expressed emotion a specific risk factor for depression or a nonspecific correlate of psychopathology? *Journal of Abnormal Child Psychology, 29*(6), 573-83. https://doi.org/10.1023/A:1012237411007

Rosenberg, M. (2002). Children with gender identity issues and their parents in individual and group treatment. *Journal of the American Academy of Child & Adolescent Psychiatry,*

41(5), 619-21. https://doi.org/10.1097/00004583-200205000-00020

Ross, E. H., & Kearney, C. A. (2015). Identifying heightened risk for posttraumatic symptoms among maltreated youth. *Journal of Child and Family Studies, 24*(12), 3767-73. https://doi.org/10.1007/s10826-015-0184-9

Rothbart, M. K., & Bates, J. E. (2006). Temperament. In N. Eisenberg, W. Damon, & R. M. Lerner (Eds.), *Handbook of child psychology: Social, emotional, and personality development., Vol. 3, 6th ed.* (pp. 99–166). John Wiley & Sons, Inc.

Rowland, A. S., Skipper, B. J., Umbach, D. M., Rabiner, D. L., Campbell, R. A., Naftel, A. J., & Sandler, D. P. (2015). The prevalence of ADHD in a population-based sample. *Journal of Attention Disorders, 19*(9), 741-54. https://doi.org/10.1177/1087054713513799

Roy, A. K., Lopes, V., & Klein, R. G. (2014). Disruptive mood dysregulation disorder: A new diagnostic approach to chronic irritability in youth. *American Journal of Psychiatry, 171*(9), 918-24.

Royal College of Psychiatrists. (2018). *Supporting transgender and gender-diverse people.* Retrieved from https://www.rcpsych.ac.uk/pdf/PS02_18.pdf

Rudolph, K. D., Flynn, M., Abaied, J. L., Groot, A., & Thompson, R. (2009). Why is past depression the best predictor of future depression? Stress generation as a mechanism of depression continuity in girls. *Journal of Clinical Child and Adolescent Psychology, 38*(4), 473-85.

Rudolph, K. D., & Lambert, S. F. (2007). Child and adolescent depression. In E. J. Mash & R. A. Barkley (Eds.), *Assessment of childhood disorders., 4th ed.* (pp. 213–252). The Guilford Press.

Rueger, S. Y., & Malecki, C. K. (2011). Effects of stress, attributional style and perceived parental support on depressive symptoms in early adolescence: A prospective analysis. *Journal of Clinical Child and Adolescent Psychology, 40*(3), 347-59.

Russell, A. E., Ford, T., Williams, R., & Russell, G. (2016). The association between socioeconomic disadvantage and attention deficit/hyperactivity disorder (ADHD): A systematic review. *Child Psychiatry and Human Development, 47*(3), 440-58. https://doi.org/10.1007/s10578-015-0578-3

Russell, G., Ford, T., Rosenberg, R., & Kelly, S. (2014). The association of attention deficit hyperactivity disorder with socioeconomic disadvantage: Alternative explanations and evidence. *Journal of Child Psychology and Psychiatry, 55*(5), 436-45. https://doi.org/10.1111/jcpp.12170

Russell, G. F., Szmukler, G. I., Dare, C., & Eisler, I. (1987). An evaluation of family therapy in anorexia nervosa and bulimia nervosa. *Archives of General Psychiatry, 44*(12), 1047–1056. https://doi.org/10.1001/archpsyc.1987.01800240021004

Rutter, M., Bailey, A., & Lord, C. (2008). *The Social Communication Questionnaire.* Western Psychological Services.

Rutter, M., & Garmezy, N. (1983). Developmental psychopathology. In E. M. Hetherington (Ed.), *Carmichael's manual of child psychology: Vol. 4. Social and personality development* (pp. 659-95). Wiley.

Rydell, A., Berlin, L., & Bohlin, G. (2003). Emotionality, emotion regulation, and adaptation among 5- to 8-year-old children. *Emotion, 3*(1), 30-47.

Sacco, R., Gabriele, S., & Persico, A. M. (2015). Head circumference and brain size in autism spectrum disorder: A systematic review and meta-analysis. *Psychiatry Research: Neuroimaging, 234*(2), 239-51. https://doi.org/10.1016/j.pscychresns.2015.08.016

Salas-Humara, C., Sequeira, G. M, Rossi, W., & Dhar, C. P. (2019). Gender affirming medical care of transgender youth. *Current Problems in Pediatric and Adolescent Health Care, 49*(9), 1-21.

Salbach-Andrae, H., Lenz, K., Simmendinger, N., Klinkowski, N., Lehmkuhl, U., & Pfeiffer, E. (2008). Psychiatric comorbidities among female adolescents with anorexia nervosa. *Child Psychiatry and Human Development, 39*(3), 261-72. https://doi.org/10.1007/s10578-007-0086-1

Sallee, F. R., McGough, J., Wigal, T., Donahue, J., Lyne, A., & Biederman, J. (2009). Guanfacine extended release in children and adolescents with attention-deficit/hyperactivity disorder: A placebo-controlled trial. *Journal of the American Academy of Child & Adolescent Psychiatry, 48*(2), 155-65. https://doi.org/10.1097/CHI.0b013e318191769e

Salloum, A., Stover, C. S., Swaidan, V. R., & Storch, E. A. (2015). Parent and child PTSD and parent depression in relation to parenting stress among trauma-exposed children. *Journal of Child and Family Studies, 24*(5), 1203-12. https://doi.org/10.1007/s10826-014-9928-1

Sallows, G., & Graupner, T. (2005). Intensive behavioral treatment for autism: Four-year outcomes and predictors. *American Journal on Mental Retardation, 110*(6), 417-38.

Samek, D. R., Wilson, S., McGue, M., & Iacono, W. G. (2018). Genetic and environmental influences on parent–child conflict and child depression through late adolescence. *Journal of Clinical Child and Adolescent Psychology, 47*(Suppl 1), S5–S20. https://doi.org/10.1080/15374416.2016.1141357

Sameroff, A. J. (2014). A dialectical integration of development for the study of psychopathology. In M. Lewis & K. D. Rudolph (Eds.), *Handbook of developmental psychopathology* (3rd ed., pp. 25-43). Springer.

Sameroff, A. J., Seifer, R., Baldwin, A., & Baldwin, C. (1993). Stability of intelligence from preschool to adolescence: The influence of social and family risk factors. *Child Development, 64*(1), 80-97. https://doi.org/10.2307/1131438

Sameroff, A. J., Seifer, R., Zax, M., & Barocas, R. (1987). Early indicators of developmental risk: Rochester Longitudinal Study. *Schizophrenia Bulletin, 13*(3), 383-94. https://doi.org/10.1093/schbul/13.3.383

Sandbank, M., Bottema-Beutel, K., Crowley, S., Cassidy, M., Dunham, K., Feldman, J. I., Crank, J., Albarran, S. A., Raj, S., Mahbub, P., & Woynaroski, T. G. (2020). Project AIM: Autism intervention meta-analysis for studies of young children. *Psychological Bulletin, 146*(1), 1-29. https://doi.org/10.1037/bul0000215

Sandin, S., Schendel, D., Magnusson, P., Hultman, C., Surén, P., Susser, E., Grønborg, T., Gissler, M., Gunnes, N., Gross, R., Henning, M., Bresnahan, M., Sourander, A., Hornig, M., Carter, K., Francis, R., Parner, E., Leonard, H., Rosanoff, M., Stoltenberg, C., … Reichenberg, A. (2016). Autism risk associated with parental age and with increasing difference in age between the parents. *Molecular Psychiatry, 21*(5), 693–700. https://doi.org/10.1038/mp.2015.70

Sandstrom, A., Uher, R., & Pavlova, B. (2020). Prospective association between childhood behavioral inhibition and anxiety: A meta-analysis. *Journal of Abnormal Child Psychology, 48*(1), 57-66. https://doi.org/10.1007/s10802-019-00588-5

Santrock, J. W. (2017). *Lifespan development* (16th ed.). McGraw-Hill.

Sartory, G., Heine, A., Müller, B. W., & Elvermann-Hallner, A. (2002). Event- and motor-related potentials during the continuous performance task in attention-deficit/hyperactivity disorder. *Journal of Psychophysiology, 16*(2), 97-106. https://doi.org/10.1027//0269-8803.16.2.97

Sasaki, S., Ozaki, K., Yamagata, S., Takahashi, Y., Shikishima, C., Kornacki, T., Nonaka, K. & Ando, J. (2016). Genetic and environmental influences on traits of gender identity disorder:

A study of Japanese twins across developmental stages. *Archives of Sexual Behavior, 45*(7), 1681-95. https://doi.org/10.1007/s10508-016-0821-4

Sasser, T. R., Kalvin, C. B., & Bierman, K. L. (2016). Developmental trajectories of clinically significant attention-deficit/hyperactivity disorder (ADHD) symptoms from grade 3 through 12 in a high-risk sample: Predictors and outcomes. *Journal of Abnormal Psychology, 125*(2), 207–219. https://doi.org/10.1037/abn0000112

Sawyer, A. M., & Borduin, C. M. (2011). Effects of multisystemic therapy through midlife: a 21.9-year follow-up to a randomized clinical trial with serious and violent juvenile offenders. *Journal of Consulting and Clinical Psychology, 79*(5), 643–652. https://doi.org/10.1037/a0024862

Say, G. N., Karabekiroglu, K., & Yuce, M. (2015). Factors related to methylphenidate response in children with attention deficit/hyperactivity disorder: A retrospective study. *Düşünen Adam: Journal of Psychiatry and Neurological Sciences, 28*(4), 319-27. https://doi.org/10.5350/DAJPN2015280403

Scheeringa, M. S., Myers, L., Putnam, F. W., & Zeanah, C. H. (2015). Maternal factors as moderators or mediators of PTSD symptoms in very young children: A two-year prospective study. *Journal of Family Violence, 30*(5), 633-42. https://doi.org/10.1007/s10896-015-9695-9

Scheeringa, M. S., Peebles, C. D., Cook, C. A., & Zeanah, C. H. (2001). Toward establishing procedural, criterion, and discriminant validity for PTSD in early childhood. *Journal of the American Academy of Child & Adolescent Psychiatry, 40*(1), 52-60. https://doi.org/10.1097/00004583-200101000-00016

Scheeringa, M. S., Weems, C. F., Cohen, J. A., Amaya-Jackson, L., & Guthrie, D. (2011). Trauma-focused cognitive-behavioral therapy for posttraumatic stress disorder in three-through six year-old children: A randomized clinical trial. *Journal of Child Psychology and Psychiatry, 52*(8), 853-60. https://doi.org/10.1111/j.1469-7610.2010.02354.x

Scheeringa, M. S., Wright, M. J., Hunt, J. P., & Zeanah, C. H. (2006). Factors affecting the diagnosis and prediction of PTSD symptomatology in children and adolescents. *American Journal of Psychiatry, 163*(4), 644-51. https://doi.org/10.1176/appi.ajp.163.4.644

Scheeringa, M. S., & Zeanah, C. H. (2008). Reconsideration of harm's way: Onsets and comorbidity patterns of disorders in preschool children and their caregivers following Hurricane Katrina. *Journal of Clinical Child and Adolescent Psychology, 37*(3), 508-18. https://doi.org/10.1080/15374410802148178

Scheeringa, M. S., Zeanah, C. H., Myers, L., & Putnam, F. W. (2003). New findings on alternative criteria for PTSD in preschool children. *Journal of the American Academy of Child & Adolescent Psychiatry, 42*(5), 561-70. https://doi.org/10.1097/01.CHI.0000046822.95464.14

Scheeringa, M. S., Zeanah, C. H., Myers, L., & Putnam, F. W. (2005). Predictive validity in a prospective follow-up of PTSD in preschool children. *Journal of the American Academy of Child & Adolescent Psychiatry, 44*(9), 899-906. https://doi.org/10.1097/01.chi.0000169013.81536.71

Schepman, K., Fombonne, E., Collishaw, S., & Taylor, E. (2014). Cognitive styles in depressed children with and without comorbid conduct disorder. *Journal of Adolescence, 37*(5), 622-31. https://doi.org/10.1016/j.adolescence.2014.04.004

Schmidt, U., Lee, S., Beecham, J., Perkins, S., Treasure, J., Yi, I., Winn, S., Robinson, P., Murphy, R., Keville, S., Johnson-Sabine, E., Jenkins, M., Frost, S., Dodge, L., Berelowitz, M.,

& Eisler, I. (2007). A randomized controlled trial of family therapy and cognitive behavior therapy guided self-care for adolescents with bulimia nervosa and related disorders. *American Journal of Psychiatry, 164*(4), 591–598. https://doi.org/10.1176/ajp.2007.164.4.591

Schmiedeler, S., Niklas, F., & Schneider, W. (2014). Symptoms of attention-deficit hyperactivity disorder (ADHD) and home learning environment (HLE): Findings from a longitudinal study. *European Journal of Psychology of Education, 29*(3), 467-82. https://doi.org/10.1007/s10212-013-0208-z

Schneider, R. L., Arch, J. J., Landy, L. N., & Hankin, B. L. (2018). The longitudinal effect of emotion regulation strategies on anxiety levels in children and adolescents. *Journal of Clinical Child and Adolescent Psychology, 47*(6), 978-91. https://doi.org/10.1080/15374416.2016.1157757

Schoon, I., Parsons, S., & Sacker, A. (2004). Socioeconomic adversity, educational resilience, and subsequent levels of adult adaptation. *Journal of Adolescent Research, 19*(4), 383-404. https://doi.org/10.1177/0743558403258856

Schopler, E., Van Bourgondien, M., Wellman, J., & Love, S. (2010). *Childhood Autism Rating Scale—Second edition (CARS2): Manual.* Western Psychological Services.

Schrobsdorff, S. (2016). The kids are not all right. *Time, 188*(19), 44-51.

Schroeder, C. S., & Gordon, B. N. (2002). *Assessment and treatment of childhood problems* (2nd ed). Guilford.

Schuck, K., Munsch, S., & Schneider, S. (2018). Body image perceptions and symptoms of disturbed eating behavior among children and adolescents in Germany. *Child and Adolescent Psychiatry and Mental Health, 12.* https://doi.org/10.1186/s13034-018-0216-5

Schuhmann, E. M., Foote, R., Eyberg, S. M., Boggs, S., & Algina, J. (1998). Parent-child interaction therapy: Interim report of a randomized trial with short-term maintenance. *Journal of Clinical Child Psychology, 27,* 1-7.

Schumann, C. M., Hamstra, J., Goodlin-Jones, B. I., Lotspeich, L. J., Kwon, H., Buonocore, M. H., Lammers, C. R., Reiss, A. L., & Amaral, D. G. (2004). The amygdala is enlarged in children but not adolescents with autism; the hippocampus is enlarged at all ages. *The Journal of Neuroscience, 24*(28), 6392-401.

Schwartz, C. E., Snidman, N., & Kagan, J. (1999). Adolescent social anxiety as an outcome of inhibited temperament in childhood. *Journal of the American Academy of Child & Adolescent Psychiatry, 38*(8), 1008-15.

Schwartz, D. J., Phares, V., Tantleff-Dunn, S., & Thompson, J. K. (1999). Body image, psychological functioning, and parental feedback regarding physical appearance. *International Journal of Eating Disorders, 25*(3), 339-43. https://doi.org/10.1002/(SICI)1098-108X(199904)25:3<339::AID-EAT13>3.0.CO;2-V

Schwartz, O. S., Byrne, M. L., Simmons, J. G., Whittle, S., Dudgeon, P., Yap, M. B. H., Sheeber, L., & Allen, N. B. (2014). Parenting during early adolescence and adolescent-onset major depression: A 6-year prospective longitudinal study. *Clinical Psychological Science, 2*(3), 272-86.

Schwartz, O. S., Dudgeon, P., Sheeber, L. B., Yap, M. B. H., Simmons, J. G., & Allen, N. B. (2012). Parental behaviors during family interactions predict changes in depression and anxiety symptoms during adolescence. *Journal of Abnormal Child Psychology, 40*(1), 59-71.

Schwartz, S., & Correll, C. U. (2014). Efficacy and safety of atomoxetine in children and adolescents with attention-deficit/hyperactivity disorder: results from a comprehensive meta-analysis and metaregression. *Journal of the American Academy of Child and Adolescent Psychiatry, 53*(2), 174–187. https://doi.org/10.1016/j.jaac.2013.11.005

Sciberras, E., Bisset, M., Hazell, P., Nicholson, J. M., Anderson, V., Lycett, K., Jongeling, B., & Efron, D. (2016). Health-related impairments in young children with ADHD: A community-based study. *Child: Care, Health and Development, 42*(5), 709-17. https://doi.org/10.1111/cch.12363

Segool, N. K., & Carlson, J. S. (2008). Efficacy of cognitive-behavioral and pharmacological treatments for children with social anxiety. *Depression and Anxiety, 25*(7), 620-31.

Sehm, M., & Warschburger, P. (2018). Prospective associations between binge eating and psychological risk factors in adolescence. *Journal of Clinical Child and Adolescent Psychology, 47*(5), 770-84. https://doi.org/10.1080/15374416.2016.1178124

Seidman, L., Valera, E., & Makris, N. (2005). Structural brain imaging of attention-deficit/hyperactivity disorder. *Biological Psychiatry, 57*(11), 1263-72. https://doi.org/10.1016/j.biopsych.2004.11.019

Seligman, L. S., Swedish, E. F., & Ollendick, T. H. (2014). Anxiety disorders in children. In C. A. Alfano & D. C. Beidel (Eds.), *Comprehensive evidence-based interventions for children and adolescents* (pp. 93-109). Wiley.

Seltzer, M. M., Shattuck, P., Abbeduto, L., & Greenberg, J. S. (2004). Trajectory of development in adolescents and adults with autism. *Mental Retardation and Developmental Disabilities Research Reviews, 10*(4), 234-47. https://doi.org/10.1002/mrdd.20038

Semple, Randye & Reid, Elizabeth & Miller, Lisa. (2005). Treating anxiety with mindfulness: An open trial of mindfulness training for anxious children. *Journal of Cognitive Psychotherapy. 19.* 379-392. 10.1891/088983905780907702.

Serpell, L., Treasure, J., Teasdale, J., & Sullivan, V. (1999). Anorexia nervosa: Friend or foe? *International Journal of Eating Disorders, 25*(2), 177-86. https://doi.org/10.1002/(SICI)1098-108X(199903)25:2<177::AID-EAT7>3.0.CO;2-D

Shaffer, D., Fisher, P., Lucas, C. P., Dulcan, M. K., & Schwab-Stone, M. E. (2000). NIMH Diagnostic Interview Schedule for Children Version IV (NIMH DISC-IV): Description, differences from previous versions, and reliability of some common diagnoses. *Journal of the American Academy of Child & Adolescent Psychiatry, 39*(1), 28-38. https://doi.org/10.1097/00004583-200001000-00014

Shakespeare-Finch, J., & Lurie-Beck, J. (2014). A meta-analytic clarification of the relationship between posttraumatic growth and symptoms of posttraumatic distress disorder. *Journal of Anxiety Disorders, 28*(2), 223–229. https://doi.org/10.1016/j.janxdis.2013.10.005

Shang, C. Y., Lin, H. Y., Tseng, W. Y., & Gau, S. S. (2018). A haplotype of the dopamine transporter gene modulates regional homogeneity, gray matter volume, and visual memory in children with attention-deficit/hyperactivity disorder. *Psychological Medicine, 48*(15), 2530-40. https://doi.org/10.1017/S0033291718000144

Shao, D., Gao, Q., Li, J., Xue, J., Guo, W., Long, Z., & Cao, F. (2015). Test of the stress sensitization model in adolescents following the pipeline explosion. *Comprehensive Psychiatry, 62,* 178-86. https://doi.org/10.1016/j.comppsych.2015.07.017

Sharma-Patel, K., & Brown, E. J. (2016). Emotion regulation and self blame as mediators and moderators of trauma-specific treatment. *Psychology of Violence, 6*(3), 400-409. https://doi.org/10.1037/vio0000044

Shaw, K.A., Maenner, M.J., Baio, J., Washington, A., Christensen, D.L., Wiggins, L.D., Pettygrove, S., Andrews, J. G., White, T., Rosenberg, C. R., Constantino, J. N., Fitzgerald, R. T., Zahorodny, W., Shenouda, J., Daniels, J. L., Salinas, A., Durkin, M. S., & Dietz, P. M. (2020). Early identification of autism spectrum disorder among children aged 4 years—Early Autism and Developmental Disabilities Monitoring

Network, Six Sites, United States, 2016. *MMWR Surveillance Summaries, 69*(3), 1-11. https://doi.org/10.15585/mmwr.ss6903a1

Sheeber, L., Hops, H., Alpert, A., Davis, B., & Andrews, J. (1997). Family support and conflict: Prospective relations to adolescent depression. *Journal of Abnormal Child Psychology, 25*(4), 333-44.

Shelleby, E. C., & Kolko, D. J. (2015). Predictors, moderators, and treatment parameters of community and clinic-based treatment for child disruptive behavior disorders. *Journal of Child and Family Studies, 24*(3), 734-48. https://doi.org/10.1007/s10826-013-9884-1

Shields, A., & Cicchetti, D. (1998). Reactive aggression among maltreated children: The contributions of attention and emotion dysregulation. *Journal of Clinical Child Psychology, 27*(4), 381-95.

Shiffman, M., VanderLaan, D. P., Wood, H., Hughes, S. K., Owen-Anderson, A., Lumley, M. M., Lollis, S. P., & Zucker, K. J. (2016). Behavioral and emotional problems as a function of peer relationships in adolescents with gender dysphoria: A comparison with clinical and nonclinical controls. *Psychology of Sexual Orientation and Gender Diversity, 3*(1), 27-36. https://doi.org/10.1037/sgd0000152

Shortt, A. L., Barrett, P. M., & Fox, T. L. (2001). Evaluating the FRIENDS program: A cognitive-behavioral group treatment for anxious children and their parents. *Journal of Clinical Child Psychology, 30*(4), 525-35.

Shumway, S., & Wetherby, A. M. (2009). Communicative acts of children with autism spectrum disorders in the second year of life. *Journal of Speech, Language, and Hearing Research, 52,* 1139-56. https://doi.org/10.1044/1092-4388(2009/07-0280)

Sibley, M. H., Altszuler, A. R., Morrow, A. S., & Merrill, B. M. (2014). Mapping the academic problem behaviors of adolescents with ADHD.

School Psychology Quarterly, 29*(4), 422-37. https://doi.org/10.1037/spq0000071

Sicile-Kira, J. (2017). About the artist. Retrieved from https://www.jeremysvision.com/about-the-artist

Silberman, S. (2016). *Neurotribes: The legacy of autism and the future of neurodiversity.* Avery.

Silk, J. S., Steinberg, L., & Morris, A. S. (2003). Adolescents' emotion regulation in daily life: Links to depressive symptoms and problem behavior. *Child Development, 74*(6), 1869-80.

Siller, M., Hutman, T., & Sigman, M. (2013). A parent-mediated intervention to increase responsive parental behaviors and child communication in children with ASD: A randomized clinical trial. *Journal of Autism and Developmental Disorders, 43*(3), 540-55. https://doi.org/10.1007/s10803-012-1584-y

Siller, M., Swanson, M., Gerber, A., Hutman, T., & Sigman, M. (2014). A parent-mediated intervention that targets responsive parental behaviors increases attachment behaviors in children with ASD: Results from a randomized clinical trial. *Journal of Autism and Developmental Disorders, 44*(7), 1720-32. https://doi.org/10.1007/s10803-014-2049-2

Silverman, W. K., & Alfano, A. M. (1996a). *Anxiety Disorder Interview Schedule for DSM-IV—Child Version: Child interview schedule.* Oxford University Press.

Silverman, W. K., & Alfano, A. M. (1996b). *Anxiety Disorder Interview Schedule for DSM-IV—Child Version: Parent interview schedule.* Oxford University Press.

Silverman, W.K., & Hinshaw, S.P. (2008). The second special issue on evidence-based psychosocial treatments for children and adolescents: A 10-year update. *Journal of Clinical Child and Adolescent Psychology 37*(1), 1-7. https://doi.org/15374410701817725

Silverman, W. K., & Ollendick, T. H. (2005). Evidence-based assessment of anxiety and its disorders in children and adolescents. *Journal of Clinical Child and Adolescent Psychology, 34*(3), 380-411.

Silverman, W. K., Ortiz, C. D., Viswesvaran, C., Burns, B. J., Kolko, D. J., Putnam, F. W., & Amaya-Jackson, L. (2008). Evidence-based psychosocial treatments for child and adolescent exposed to traumatic events: A review and meta-analysis. *Journal of Clinical Child & Adolescent Psychology, 37*(1), 156-83.

Simoneau, T. L., Miklowitz, D. J., Richards, J. A., Saleem, R., & George, E. L. (1999). Bipolar disorder and family communication: Effects of a psychoeducational treatment program. *Journal of Abnormal Psychology, 108*(4), 588-97.

Simonoff, E., Pickles, A., Charman, T., Chandler, S., Loucas, T., & Baird, G. (2008). Psychiatric disorders in children with autism spectrum disorders: Prevalence, comorbidity, and associated factors in a population-derived sample. *Journal of the American Academy of Child & Adolescent Psychiatry, 47*(8), 921-29. https://doi.org/10.1097/CHI.0b013e318179964f

Singh, M., Kelley, R., Chang, K., & Gotlib, I. (2015). Intrinsic amygdala functional connectivity in youth with bipolar I disorder. *Journal of the American Academy of Child and Adolescent Psychiatry, 54*(9), 763-70.

Siqueland, L., Kendall, P. C., & Steinberg, L. (1996). Anxiety in children: Perceived family environments and observed family interaction. *Journal of Clinical Child Psychology, 25*(2), 225-37.

Skagerberg, E., Di Ceglie, D., & Carmichael, P. (2015). Brief report: Autistic features in children and adolescents with gender dysphoria. *Journal of Autism and Developmental Disorders, 45*(8), 2628-32. https://doi.org/10.1007/s10803-015-2413-x

Skogan, A. H., Zeiner, P., Egeland, J., Rohrer-Baumgartner, N., Urnes, A. G., Reichborn-Kjennerud, T., & Aase, H. (2014). Inhibition and working memory in young preschool children with symptoms of ADHD and/or oppositional-defiant disorder. *Child Neuropsychology, 20*(5), 607–624. https://doi.org/10.1080/09297049.2013.838213

Skoglund, C., Chen, Q., D'Onofrio, B. M., Lichtenstein, P., & Larsson, H. (2014). Familial confounding of the association between maternal smoking during pregnancy and ADHD in offspring. *Journal of Child Psychology and Psychiatry, and Allied Disciplines, 55*(1), 61–68. https://doi.org/10.1111/jcpp.12124

Slof-Op 't Landt, M. C., Meulenbelt, I., Bartels, M., Suchiman, E., Middeldorp, C. M., Houwing-Duistermaat, J. J., van Trier, J., Onkenhout, E. J., Vink, J. M., van Beijsterveldt, C. E., Brandys, M. K., Sanders, N., Zipfel, S., Herzog, W., Herpertz-Dahlmann, B., Klampfl, K., Fleischhaker, C., Zeeck, A., de Zwaan, M., Herpertz, S., ... Slagboom, P. E. (2011). Association study in eating disorders: TPH2 associates with anorexia nervosa and self-induced vomiting. *Genes, Brain, and Behavior, 10*(2), 236–243. https://doi.org/10.1111/j.1601-183X.2010.00660.x

Smid, G. E., van der Velden, P. G., Lensvelt-Mulders, G. M., Knipscheer, J. W., Gersons, B. R., & Kleber, R. J. (2012). Stress sensitization following a disaster: A prospective study. *Psychological Medicine, 42*(8), 1675-86. https://doi.org/10.1017/S0033291711002765

Smink, F. E., van Hoeken, D., Oldehinkel, A. J., & Hoek, H. W. (2014). Prevalence and severity of DSM-5 eating disorders in a community cohort of adolescents. *International Journal of Eating Disorders, 47*(6), 610-19. https://doi.org/10.1002/eat.22316

Smith, B. H., Barkley, R. A., & Shapiro, C. J. (2007). Attention-deficit/hyperactivity disorder. In E. J. Mash & R. A. Barkley (Eds.), *Assessment of childhood disorders., 4th ed.* (pp. 53–131). The Guilford Press.

Smith, P., Perrin, S., Yule, W., & Rabe-Hesketh, S. (2001). War exposure and maternal reactions in the psychological adjustment of children from Bosnia-Hercegovina. *Journal of Child Psychology and Psychiatry, 42*(3), 395-404. https://doi.org/10.1111/1469-7610.00732

Smith, P., Yule, W., Perrin, S., Tranah, T., Dalgleish, T., & Clark, D. M. (2007). Cognitive-behavioral therapy for PTSD in children and adolescents: A preliminary randomized controlled trial. *Journal of the American Academy of Child & Adolescent Psychiatry, 46*(8), 1051-61. https://doi.org/10.1097/CHI.0b013e318067e288

Smith, T. (2001). Discrete trial training in the treatment of autism. *Focus on Autism and Other Developmental Disabilities, 16*(2), 86-92. https://doi.org/10.1177/108835760101600204

Smith, T. (2010). Early and intensive behavioral intervention in autism. In J. R. Weisz & A. E. Kazdin (Eds.), *Evidence-based psychotherapies for children and adolescents* (2nd ed., pp. 312-26). Guilford.

Smith, T., Eikeseth, S., Klevstrand, M., & Lovaas, O. I. (1997). Intensive behavioral treatment for preschoolers with severe mental retardations and pervasive developmental disorder. *American Journal on Mental Retardation, 102*(3), 238-49. https://doi.org/10.1352/0895-8017(1997)102<0238:IBTFPW>2.0.CO;2

Smith, T., Groen, A. D., & Wynn, J. W. (2000). Randomized trial of intensive early intervention for children with pervasive developmental disorder. *American Journal on Mental Retardation, 105*(4), 269-85. https://doi.org/10.1352/0895-8017(2000)105<0269:RTOIEI>2.0.CO;2

Smith, T., & Iadarola, S. (2015). Evidence base update for autism spectrum disorder. *Journal of Clinical Child and Adolescent Psychology, 44*(6), 897-922. https://doi.org/10.1080/15374416.2015.1077448

Smith, Y. S., Van Goozen, S. M., & Cohen-Kettenis, P. T. (2001). Adolescents with gender identity disorder who were accepted or rejected for sex reassignment surgery: A prospective follow-up study. *Journal of the American Academy of Child and Adolescent Psychiatry, 40*(4), 472-81.

Smith, Y. S., Van Goozen, S. M., Kuiper, A. J., & Cohen-Kettenis, P. T. (2005). Sex reassignment: Outcomes and predictors of treatment for adolescent and adult transsexuals. *Psychological Medicine, 35*(1), 89-99. https://doi.org/10.1017/S0033291704002776

Smith-Boydston, J. M., Holtzman, R. J., & Roberts, M. C. (2014). Transportability of multisystemic therapy to community settings: Can a program sustain outcomes without MST services oversight? *Child & Youth Care Forum, 43*(5), 593-605. https://doi.org/10.1007/s10566-014-9255-0

Smith Slep, A. M., & O'Leary, S. G. (1998). The effects of maternal attributions on parenting: An experimental analysis. *Journal of Family Psychology, 12*, 234-43.

Smoller, J. W., & Finn, C. T. (2003). Family, twin, and adoption studies of bipolar disorder. *American Journal of Medical Genetics Part C: Seminars in Medical Genetics, 1*, 48-58.

Snoek, H. M., van Strien, T., Janssens, J. M., & Engels, R. E. (2009). Longitudinal relationships between fathers', mothers', and adolescents' restrained eating. *Appetite, 52*(2), 461-68. https://doi.org/10.1016/j.appet.2008.12.009

Snyder, J., Schrepferman, L., Oeser, J., Patterson, G., Stoolmiller, M., Johnson, K., & Snyder, A. (2005). Deviancy training and association with deviant peers in young children: Occurrence and contribution to early-onset conduct problems. *Development and Psychopathology, 17*(2), 397-413.

Solleveld, M. M., Schrantee, A., Baek, H. K., Bottelier, M. A., Tamminga, H. G. H., Bouziane, C., Stoffelsen, R., Lucassen, P. J., Van Someren, E. J. W., Rijsman, R. M., & Reneman, L. (2020).

Effects of 16 weeks of methylphenidate treatment on actigraph-assessed sleep measures in medication-naive children with ADHD. *Frontiers in Psychiatry*, *11*, 82. https://doi.org/10.3389/fpsyt.2020.00082

Sollie, H., & Larsson, B. (2016). Parent-reported symptoms, impairment, helpfulness of treatment, and unmet service needs in a follow-up of outpatient children with attention-deficit/hyperactivity disorder. *Nordic Journal of Psychiatry*, *70*(8), 582-90. https://doi.org/10.1080/08039488.2016.1187204

Sollie, H., Mørch, W., & Larsson, B. (2016). Parent and family characteristics and their associates in a follow-up of outpatient children with ADHD. *Journal of Child and Family Studies*, *25*(8), 2571-84. https://doi.org/10.1007/s10826-016-0411-z

Sonuga-Barke, E. S., Thompson, M., Abikoff, H., Klein, R., & Brotman, L. M. (2006). Nonpharmacological interventions for preschoolers with ADHD: The case for specialized parent training. *Infants & Young Children*, *19*(2), 142-153. doi:10.1097/00001163-200604000-00007

Sorensen, L., Dodge, K., & Conduct Problems Prevention Research Group. (2016). How does the Fast Track intervention prevent adverse outcomes in young adulthood? *Child Development*, *87*(2), 429-45. http://doi.org/10.1111/cdev.12467

Southammakosane, C., & Schmitz, K. (2015). Pediatric psychopharmacology for treatment of ADHD, depression, and anxiety. *Pediatrics*, *136*(2), 352-59.

Southern Baptist Convention. (2014). On transgender identity. Retrieved from http://sbc.net/resolutions/2250/on-transgender-identity

Sowerby, P., & Tripp, G. (2009). Evidence-based assessment of attention-deficit hyperactivity disorder (ADHD). In J. L. Matson, F. Andrasik, & M. L. Matson (Eds.), *Assessing childhood psychopathology and developmental disabilities* (pp. 209–239). Springer. https://doi.org/10.1007/978-0-387-09528-8_8

Sparks, B. F., Friedman, S. D., Shaw, D. W., Aylward, E. H., Echelard, D., Artru, A. A., Maravilla, K. R., Giedd, J. N., Munson, J., Dawson, G., & Dager, S. R. (2002). Brain structural abnormalities in young children with autism spectrum disorder. *Neurology*, *59*(2), 184-92. https://doi.org/10.1212/wnl.59.2.184

Sparrow, S. S., Cicchetti, D. V., & Balla, D. A. (2005). *Vineland adaptive behavior scales, Second edition (Vineland II), survey interview form/caregiver rating form*. Pearson Assessments.

Spencer, R., Devilbiss, D., & Berridge, C. (2015). The cognition-enhancing effects of psychostimulants involve direct action in the prefrontal cortex. *Biological Psychiatry*, *77*(11), 940-50. https://doi.org/10.1016/j.biopsych.2014.09.013

Spikol, A., McAteer, D., & Murphy, J. (2019). Recognising autism: A latent transition analysis of parental reports of child autistic spectrum disorder 'red flag' traits before and after age 3. *Social Psychiatry and Psychiatric Epidemiology: The International Journal for Research in Social and Genetic Epidemiology and Mental Health Services*, *54*, 703-13. https://doi.org/10.1007/s00127-019-01664-3

Spivey, L., & Edwards-Leeper, L. (2019). Future directions in affirmative psychological interventions with transgender children and adolescents. *Journal of Clinical Child and Adolescent Psychology*, *48*(2), 343-56. https://doi.org/10.1080/15374416.2018.1534207

Sroufe, L. A. (1995). *Emotional development: The organization of emotional life in the early years*. Cambridge University Press.

Sroufe, L. A. (1997). Psychopathology as an outcome of development. *Development and Psychopathology*, *9*(2), 251-68.

Sroufe, L. A., & Rutter, M. (1984). The domain of developmental psychopathology. *Child Development*, *55*(1), 17.

Stark, K. D., Reynolds, W. M., & Kaslow, N. J. (1987). A comparison of the relative efficacy of self-control therapy and a behavioral problem-solving therapy for depression in children. *Journal of Abnormal Child Psychology, 15*, 91-113.

Stark, K. D., Sander, J., Hauser, M., Simpson, J., Schnoebelen, S., Glenn, R., & Molnar, J. (2006). Depressive disorders during childhood and adolescence. In E. J. Mash & R. A. Barkely (Eds.), *Treatment of childhood disorders* (3rd ed., pp. 336-407). Guilford.

Stark, K. D., Streusand, W., Krumholz, L. S., & Patel, P. (2010). Cognitive-behavioral therapy for depression: The ACTION treatment program for girls. In J. R. Weisz & A. E. Kazdin (Eds.), *Evidence-based psychotherapies for children and adolescents* (2nd ed., pp. 93-109). Guilford.

Steensma, T. D., Biemond, R., de Boer, F., & Cohen-Kettenis, P. T. (2010). Desisting and persisting gender dysphoria after childhood: A qualitative follow-up study. *Clinical Child Psychology and Psychiatry, 16*(4), 499-516. https://doi.org/10.1177/1359104510378303

Steensma, T. D., & Cohen-Kettenis, P. T. (2015). More than two developmental pathways in children with gender dysphoria? *Journal of the American Academy of Child and Adolescent Psychiatry, 54*(2), 147-48.

Steensma, T., & Cohen-Kettenis, P. (2018). A critical commentary on "a critical commentary on follow-up studies and "desistence" theories about transgender and gender nonconforming children." *International Journal of Transgenderism, 19*(2), 225-30. https://doi.org/10.1080/15532739.2018.1468292

Steensma, T. D., Kreukels, B. P., de Vries, A. L., & Cohen-Kettenis, P. T. (2013). Gender identity development in adolescence. *Hormones and Behavior, 64*(2), 288-97.

Steensma, T. D., McGuire, J. K., Kreukels, B. C., Beekman, A. J., & Cohen-Kettenis, P. T. (2013). Factors associated with desistence and persis-tence of childhood gender dysphoria: A quantitative follow-up study. *Journal of the American Academy of Child & Adolescent Psychiatry, 52*(6), 582-90. https://doi.org/10.1016/j.jaac.2013.03.016

Stein, B. D., Jaycox, L. H., Kataoka, S. H., Wong, M., Tu, W., Elliott, M. N., & Fink, A. (2003). A mental health intervention for schoolchildren exposed to violence: A randomized controlled trial. *JAMA: Journal of the American Medical Association, 290*(5), 603-11. https://doi.org/10.1001/jama.290.5.603

Stein, M. B., Jang, K. L., Taylor, S., Vernon, P. A., & Livesley, W. J. (2002). Genetic and environmental influences on trauma exposure and posttraumatic stress disorder symptoms: A twin study. *The American Journal of Psychiatry, 159*(10), 1675-81. https://doi.org/10.1176/appi.ajp.159.10.1675

Steinberg, A. M., Brymer, M. J., Kim, S., Briggs, E. C., Ippen, C. G., Ostrowski, S. A., Gully, K. J., & Pynoos, R. S. (2013). Psychometric properties of the UCLA PTSD reaction index: Part I. *Journal of Traumatic Stress, 26*(1), 1-9. http://dx.doi.org/10.1002/jts.21780

Steinberg, L. D., & Silk, J. S. (2002). Parenting adolescents. In M. Bornstein (Ed.), *Handbook of parenting* (2nd ed., Vol. 3, pp. 103-33). Erlbaum.

Steinhausen, H. (2002). The outcome of anorexia nervosa in the 20th century. *The American Journal of Psychiatry, 159*(8), 1284-93. https://doi.org/10.1176/appi.ajp.159.8.1284

Stenseng, F., Belsky, J., Skalicka, V., & Wichstrøm, L. (2016). Peer rejection and attention deficit hyperactivity disorder symptoms: Reciprocal relations through ages 4, 6, and 8. *Child Development, 87*(2), 365-73. https://doi.org/10.1111/cdev.12471

Stice, E., Marti, C. N., & Rohde, P. (2013). Prevalence, incidence, impairment, and course of the proposed DSM-5 eating disorder diagnoses in an 8-year prospective community study of young women. *Journal of Abnormal Psychology, 122*(2), 445-57. https://doi.org/10.1037/a0030679

Stice, E., & Peterson, C. B. (2007). Eating disorders. In E. J. Mash & R. A. Barkley (Eds.), *Assessment of childhood disorders* (4th ed., pp. 751-80). Guilford.

Stigler, K. A., McDonald, B. C., Anand, A., Saykin, A. J., & McDougle, C. J. (2011). Structural and functional magnetic resonance imaging of autism spectrum disorders. *Brain Research, 1380,* 146–161. https://doi.org/10.1016/j.brainres.2010.11.076

Stillman, W. (2006). *Autism and the God connection.* Sourcebooks, Inc.

Striegel-Moore, R. H., Fairburn, C. G., Wilfley, D. E., Pike, K. M., Dohm, F., & Kraemer, H. C. (2005). Toward an understanding of risk factors for binge-eating disorder in black and white women: A community-based case-control study. *Psychological Medicine, 35*(6), 907-17. https://doi.org/10.1017/S0033291704003435

Stone, W., Ousley, O., Yoder, P., Hogan, K., & Hepburn, S. (1997). Nonverbal communication in two- and three-year-old children with autism. *Journal of Autism and Developmental Disorders, 27*(6), 677-96. https://doi.org/10.1023/A:1025854816091

Stonehouse, C. (1998). *Joining children on the spiritual journey: Nurturing a life of faith.* Baker Academic.

Storebø, O. J., Simonsen, E., & Gluud, C. (2016). Methylphenidate for attention-deficit/hyperactivity disorder in children and adolescents. *JAMA: Journal of the American Medical Association, 315*(18), 2009-10. https://doi.org/10.1001/jama.2016.3611

Strakowski, S. M., Adler, C. M., Almeida, J., Altshuler, L. L., Blumberg, H. P., Chang, K. D., DelBello, M. P., Frangou, S., McIntosh, A., Phillips, M. L., Sussman, J., & Townsend, J. D. (2012). The functional neuroanatomy of bipolar disorder: A consensus model. *Bipolar Disorders, 14*(4), 313-25.

Sucksdorff, M., Lehtonen, L., Chudal, R., Suominen, A., Joelsson, P., Gissler, M., & Sourander, A. (2015). Preterm birth and poor fetal growth as risk factors of attention-deficit/hyperactivity disorder. *Pediatrics, 136*(3), e599–e608. https://doi.org/10.1542/peds.2015-1043

Sue, D. W., & Sue, D. (2013). *Counseling the culturally diverse: Theory and practice.* Wiley.

Sullivan, A. E., & Miklowitz, D. J. (2010). Family functioning among adolescents with bipolar disorder. *Journal of Family Psychology, 24*(1), 60-67. https://doi.org/10.1037/a0018183

Sullivan, E. L., Holton, K. F., Nousen, E. K., Barling, A. N., Sullivan, C. A., Propper, C. B., & Nigg, J. T. (2015). Early identification of ADHD risk via infant temperament and emotion regulation: A pilot study. *Journal of Child Psychology and Psychiatry, 56*(9), 949-57. https://doi.org/10.1111/jcpp.12426

Sullivan, M., Finelli, J., Marvin, A., Garrett-Mayer, E., Bauman, M., & Landa, R. (2007). Response to joint attention in toddlers at risk for autism spectrum disorder: A prospective study. *Journal of Autism and Developmental Disorders, 37*(1), 37-48. https://doi.org/10.1007/s10803-006-0335-3

Sullivan, P. F., Neale, M. C., & Kendler, K. S. (2000). Genetic epidemiology of major depression: Review and meta-analysis. *American Journal of Psychiatry, 157,* 1552-62.

Sullivan, S. A., Thompson, A., Kounali, D., Lewis, G., & Zammit, S. (2017). The longitudinal association between external locus of control, social cognition and adolescent psychopathology. *Social Psychiatry and Psychiatric Epidemiology, 52*(6), 643-55. https://doi.org/10.1007/s00127-017-1359-z

Sundberg, M. L. (2008) *Verbal behavior milestones assessment and placement program: The VB-MAPP.* AVB Press.

Sundermann, J. M., & DePrince, A. P. (2015). Maltreatment characteristics and emotion regulation (ER) difficulties as predictors of mental health symptoms: Results from a community-recruited sample of female adolescents. *Journal of Family Violence, 30*(3), 329-38. https://doi.org/10.1007/s10896-014-9656-8

Susman, E. J., Dockray, S., Schiefelbein, V. L., Herwehe, S., Heaton, J. A., & Dorn, L. D. (2007). Morningness/eveningness, morning-to-afternoon cortisol ratio, and antisocial behavior problems during puberty. *Developmental Psychology, 43*(4), 811-22.

Sutandar-Pinnock, K., Woodside, D. B., Carter, J. C., Olmsted, M. P., & Kaplan, A. S. (2003). Perfectionism in anorexia nervosa: A 6–24-month follow-up study. *International Journal of Eating Disorders, 33*(2), 225-29. https://doi.org/10.1002/eat.10127

Suveg, C., Sood, E., Barmish, A., Tiwari, S., Hudson, J. L., & Kendall, P. C. (2008). "I'd rather not talk about it": Emotion parenting in families of children with an anxiety disorder. *Journal of Family Psychology, 22*, 875-84.

Suveg, C., & Zeman, J. (2004). Emotion regulation in children with anxiety disorders. *Journal of Clinical Child and Adolescent Psychology, 33*(4), 750-59.

Suzuki, L. A., Lee, E., & Short, E. L. (2017). Psychological assessment. In J. M. Casas, L. A. Suzuki, C. M. Alexander, & M. A. Jackson (Eds.), *Handbook of multicultural counseling* (4th ed., pp. 259-68). Sage.

Swanson, S. (2010). Experiential religion: A faith formation process for children with autism. *Journal of Religion, Disability, and Health, 14*, 238-55.

Swanson, S. A., Crow, S. J., Le Grange, D., Swendsen, J., & Merikangas, K. R. (2011). Prevalence and correlates of eating disorders in adolescents: Results from the national comorbidity survey replication adolescent supplement. *Archives of General Psychiatry, 68*(7), 714-23. https://doi.org/10.1001/archgenpsychiatry.2011.22

Syed-Abdul, S., Fernandez-Luque, L., Jian, W., Li, Y., Crain, S., Hsu, M., Wang, Y., Khandregzen, D., Chuluunbaatar, E., Nguyen, P. A., & Liou, D. (2013). Misleading health-related information promoted through video-based social media: Anorexia on YouTube. *Journal of Medical Internet Research, 15*(2), 137-49. https://doi.org/10.2196/jmir.2237

Sylva, K., Barreau, S., Melhuish, E., Sammons, P., Siraj-Blatchford, I., & Taggart, B. (2007). *The effect of the home learning environments on children's development and outcomes at age 7: EPPE results*. London: DfES/Institute of Education, University of London.

Sylva, K., Melhuish, E., Sammons, P., Siraj-Blatchford, I., & Taggart, B. (2008). *Final report from the primary phase: pre-school, school, and family influences on children's development during key stage 2 (age 7–11)*. Nottingham: Department for Children, Schools and Families.

Tan, P. Z., Forbes, E. E., Dahl, R. E., Ryan, N. D., Siegle, G. J., Ladouceur, C. D., & Silk, J. S. (2012). Emotional reactivity and regulation in anxious and nonanxious youth: a cell-phone ecological momentary assessment study. *Journal of Child Psychology and Psychiatry, and Allied Disciplines, 53*(2), 197–206. https://doi.org/10.1111/j.1469-7610.2011.02469.x

Tan, S. Y. (1987). Cognitive-behavior therapy: A biblical approach and critique. *Journal of Psychology and Theology, 15*(2), 103-12.

Tan, S. Y. (2007). Use of prayer and Scripture in cognitive-behavioral therapy. *Journal of Psychology and Christianity, 26*(2), 101-11.

Tandon, M., & Pergjika, A. (2017). Attention deficit hyperactivity disorder in preschool-age children. *Child and Adolescent Psychiatric Clinics of North America, 26*(3), 523-38. https://doi.org/10.1016/j.chc.2017.02.007

Tanner, K. (2010). *Christ the key*. Cambridge University Press.

Tannous, J., Amaral-Silva, H., Cao, B., Wu, M.-J., Zunta-Soares, G. B., Kazimi, I., Zeni, C., Mwangi, B., & Soares, J. C. (2018). Hippocampal subfield volumes in children and adolescents with mood disorders. *Journal of Psychiatric Research, 101*, 57-62. https://doi.org/10.1016/j.jpsychires.2018.03.003

Tanofsky-Kraff, M., Yanovski, S. Z., & Yanovski, J. A. (2005). Comparison of child interview and parent reports of children's eating disordered behaviors. *Eating Behaviors, 6*(1), 95-99. https://doi.org/10.1016/j.eatbeh.2004.03.001

Tarbox, J., La Cava, S., & Hoang, K. (2016). Types of assessment. In J. L. Matson (Ed.), *Handbook of assessment and diagnosis of autism spectrum disorder* (pp. 11-26). Springer International Publishing. https://doi.org/10.1007/978-3-319-27171-2

Taylor, J., Iacono, W. G., & Mc Gue, M. (2000). Evidence for a genetic etiology of early-onset delinquency. *Journal of Abnormal Psychology, 109*(4), 634-643. https://doi.org/10.1037/0021-843X.109.4.634

Taylor, J. H., Lebowitz, E. R., Jakubovski, E., Coughlin, C. G., Silverman, W. K., & Bloch, M. H. (2018). Monotherapy insufficient in severe anxiety? Predictors and moderators in the Child/Adolescent Anxiety Multimodal Study. *Journal of Clinical Child and Adolescent Psychology, 47*(2), 266-81. https://doi.org/10.1080/15374416.2017.1371028

Taylor, J. L., & Seltzer, M. M. (2010). Changes in the autism behavioral phenotype during the transition to adulthood. *Journal of Autism and Developmental Disorders, 40*(12), 1431-46. https://doi.org/10.1007/s10803-010-1005-z

Taylor, J. L., & Seltzer, M. M. (2011). Employment and post-secondary educational activities for young adults with autism spectrum disorders during the transition to adulthood. *Journal of Autism and Developmental Disorders, 41*(5), 566-74. https://doi.org/10.1007/s10803-010-1070-3

Taylor, L. K., & Weems, C. F. (2009). What do youth report as a traumatic event? Toward a developmentally informed classification of traumatic stressors. Psychological Trauma: Theory, Research, Practice, and Policy, 1(2), 91–106. https://doi.org/10.1037/a0016012

Tedeschi, R. G., & Calhoun, L. G. (1995). *Trauma & transformation: Growing in the aftermath of suffering*. Sage. https://doi.org/10.4135/9781483326931

Tedeschi, R. G., & Calhoun, L. G. (1996). The Posttraumatic Growth Inventory: Measuring the positive legacy of trauma. *Journal of Traumatic Stress, 9*(3), 455-72. https://doi.org/10.1002/jts.2490090305

Tedeschi, R. G., Cann, A., Taku, K., Senol-Durak, E., & Calhoun, L. G. (2017). The posttraumatic growth inventory: A revision integrating existential and spiritual change. *Journal of Traumatic Stress, 30*(1), 11-18. https://doi.org/10.1002/jts.22155

Telfer, M. M., Tollit, M. A., Pace, C. C., & Pang, K. C. (2020). *Australian standards of care and treatment guidelines for trans and gender diverse children and adolescents* (version 1.2). The Royal Children's Hospital.

Temple Newhook, J., Pyne, J., Winters, K., Feder, S., Holmes, C., Tosh, J., Sinnott, M., Jamieson, A., & Pickett, S. (2018). A critical commentary on follow-up studies and "desistance" theories about transgender and gender-nonconforming children. *International Journal of Transgenderism, 19*(2), 212-24. https://doi.org/10.1080/15532739.2018.1456390

Theule, J., Wiener, J., Tannock, R., & Jenkins, J. M. (2013). Parenting stress in families of children with ADHD: A meta-analysis. *Journal of Emotional and Behavioral Disorders, 21*(1), 3-17.

Thompson, M. J., Davies, P. T., Hentges, R. F., Sturge-Apple, M. L., & Parry, L. Q. (2020). Understanding how and why effortful control moderates children's vulnerability to interparental conflict. *Developmental Psychology, 56*(5), 937-50. https://doi.org/10.1037/dev0000909

Thornback, K., & Muller, R. T. (2015). Relationships among emotion regulation and symptoms during trauma-focused CBT for school-aged children. *Child Abuse & Neglect,* 50, 182-92.

Thurm, A., Lord, C., Lee, L.-C., & Newschaffer, C. (2007). Predictors of language acquisition in pre-school children with autism spectrum disorders. *Journal of Autism and Developmental Disorders, 37,* 1721-34. https://doi.org/10.1007/s10803-006-0300-1

Thurm, A., Manwaring, S. S., Luckenbaugh, D. A., Lord, C., & Swedo, S. E. (2014). Patterns of skill attainment and loss in young children with autism. *Development and Psychopathology, 26*(1), 203-14. https://doi.org/10.1017/S0954579413000874

Tick, B., Bolton, P., Happé, F., Rutter, M., & Rijsdijk, F. (2016). Heritability of autism spectrum disorders: a meta-analysis of twin studies. *Journal of Child Psychology and Psychiatry and Allied Disciplines, 57*(5), 585–595. https://doi.org/10.1111/jcpp.12499

Tiemeier, H., Velders, F. P., Szekely, E., Roza, S. J., Dieleman, G., Jaddoe, V. W. V., Uitterlinden, A. G., White, T. J. H., Bakermans-Kranenburg, M. J., Hofman, A., Van Ijzendoorn, M. H., Hudziak, J. J., & Verhulst, F. C. (2012). The Generation R Study: A review of design, findings to date, and a study of the 5-HTTLPR by environmental interaction from fetal life onward. *Journal of the American Academy of Child & Adolescent Psychiatry, 51*(11), 1119-35.

Timbremont, B., & Braet, C. (2004). Cognitive vulnerability in remitted depressed children and adolescents. *Behaviour Research and Therapy, 42*(4), 423-37.

Tishelman, A. C., Kaufman, R., Edwards-Leeper, L., Mandel, F. H., Shumer, D. E., & Spack, N. P. (2015). Serving transgender youth: Challenges, dilemmas, and clinical examples. *Professional Psychology: Research and Practice, 46*(1), 37-45. https://doi.org/10.1037/a0037490

Tobin, J. (2004). Introduction. In J. Tobin (Ed.), *Pikachu's Global Adventure: The Rise and Fall of Pokémon* (pp. 3-11). Duke University Press.

Tomanik, S. S., Pearson, D. A., Loveland, K. A., Lane, D. M., & Shaw, J. B. (2007). Improving the reliability of autism diagnoses: Examining the utility of adaptive behavior. *Journal of Autism and Developmental Disorders, 37,* 921-28. https://doi.org/10.1007/s10803-006-0227-6

Topham, G. L., Hubbs-Tait, L., Rutledge, J. M., Page, M. C., Kennedy, T. S., Shriver, L. H., & Harrist, A. W. (2011). Parenting styles, parental response to child emotion, and family emotional responsiveness are related to child emotional eating. *Appetite, 56*(2), 261-64. https://doi.org/10.1016/j.appet.2011.01.007

Toth, K., Munson, J., Meltzoff, A. N., & Dawson, G. (2006). Early predictors of communication development in young children with autism spectrum disorder: Joint attention, imitation, and toy play. *Journal of Autism and Developmental Disorders, 36,* 993-1005. https://doi.org/10.1007/s10803-006-0137-7

Toupin, J., Déry, M., Pauzé, R., Mercier, H., & Fortin, L. (2000). Cognitive and familial contributions to conduct disorder in children. *Journal of Child Psychology and Psychiatry, 41*(3), 333-44.

Tourian, L., LeBoeuf, A., Breton, J., Cohen, D., Gignac, M., Labelle, R., Guile, J.-M., & Renaud, J. (2015). Treatment options for the cardinal symptoms of disruptive mood dysregulation disorder. *Journal of the Canadian Academy of Child and Adolescent Psychiatry, 24*(1), 41-54.

Towner, W. S. (2008). Children and the image of God. In M. J. Bunge (Ed.), *The child in the Bible* (pp. 307-23). Eerdmans.

Trace, S. E., Thornton, L. M., Baker, J. H., Root, T. L., Janson, L. E., Lichtenstein, P., Pedersen, N. L., & Bulik, C. M. (2013). A behavioral-genetic investigation of bulimia nervosa and its relationship with alcohol use disorder. *Psychiatry Research*, *208*(3), 232-37. https://doi.org/10.1016/j.psychres.2013.04.030

Treadwell, K. R., & Kendall, P. C. (1996). Self-talk in youth with anxiety disorders: States of mind, content specificity, and treatment outcome. *Journal of Consulting and Clinical Psychology*, *64*(5), 941-50.

Treatment for Adolescents with Depression Study (TADS). (2000). *Protocol*. Retrieved from http://tads.dcri.org/wp-content/uploads/2015/11/TADS_Protocol.pdf

Treatment for Adolescents with Depression Study (TADS). (2004). Fluoxetine, cognitive-behavioral therapy, and their combination for adolescents with depression: Treatment for Adolescents with Depression Study (TADS) randomized controlled trial. *JAMA: Journal of the American Medical Association*, *292*(7), 807-20.

Treatment for Adolescents with Depression Study (TADS). (2005). *Cognitive behavior therapy manual*. Retrieved from http://tads.dcri.org/wp-content/uploads/2015/11/TADS_CBT.pdf

Treatment for Adolescents with Depression Study (TADS). (2009). The Treatment for Adolescents with Depression Study (TADS): Outcomes over 1 year of naturalistic follow-up. *American Journal of Psychiatry*, *166*, 1141-49.

Trentacosta, C. J., & Shaw, D. S. (2009). Emotional self-regulation, peer rejection, and antisocial behavior: Developmental associations from early childhood to early adolescence. *Journal of Applied Developmental Psychology*, *30*(3), 356-65.

Trickey, D., Siddaway, A. P., Meiser-Stedman, R., Serpell, L., & Field, A. P. (2012). A meta-analysis of risk factors for post-traumatic stress disorder in children and adolescents. *Clinical Psychology Review*, *32*(2), 122-38. https://doi.org/10.1016/j.cpr.2011.12.001

Tripp, T. (1995). *Shepherding a child's heart*. Shepherd Press.

Troop-Gordon, W., Rudolph, K. D., Sugimura, N., & Little, T. D. (2015). Peer victimization in middle childhood impedes adaptive responses to stress: A pathway to depressive symptoms. *Journal of Clinical Child & Adolescent Psychology*, *44*(3), 432-45.

True, W. R., Rice, J., Eisen, S. A., Heath, A. C., Goldberg, J., Lyons, M. J., & Nowak, J. (1993). A twin study of genetic and environmental contributions to liability for posttraumatic stress symptoms. *Archives of General Psychiatry*, *50*(4), 257–264. https://doi.org/10.1001/archpsyc.1993.01820160019002

Tung, I., Brammer, W. A., Li, J. J., & Lee, S. S. (2015). Parenting behavior mediates the intergenerational association of parent and child offspring ADHD symptoms. *Journal of Clinical Child and Adolescent Psychology*, *44*(5), 787–799. https://doi.org/10.1080/15374416.2014.913250

Turner, S. M., Beidel, D. C., & Costello, A. (1987). Psychopathology in the offspring of anxiety disorders patients. *Journal of Consulting and Clinical Psychology*, *55*(2), 229-35.

Turpyn, C. C., Chaplin, T. M., Cook, E. C., & Martelli, A. M. (2015). A person-centered approach to adolescent emotion regulation: Associations with psychopathology and parenting. *Journal of Experimental Child Psychology*, *136*, 1-16.

Twenge, J. M., & Nolen-Hoeksema, S. (2002). Age, gender, race, socioeconomic status, and birth cohort differences on the Children's Depression Inventory: A meta-analysis. *Journal of Abnormal Psychology*, *111*, 578-88.

Udwin, O., Boyle, S., Yule, W., Bolton, D., & O'Ryan, D. (2000). Risk factors for long-term psychological effects of a disaster experienced in adolescence: predictors of post traumatic stress disorder. *Journal of Child Psychology and Psychiatry and Allied Disciplines, 41*(8), 969–979.

Ugueto, A. M., Santucci, L. C., Krumholz, L. S., & Weisz, J. (2014). Problem-solving skills training. In E. S. Sburlati, H. J. Lyneham, C. A. Schniering, & R. M. Rapee (Eds.), *Evidence-based CBT for anxiety and depression in children and adolescents: A competencies-based approach* (pp. 247-59). John Wiley & Sons.

Umbarger, G. T., III. (2017). Advances in neurobiological and medical research. In D. Zager, D. F. Cihak, & A. Stone-MacDonald (Eds.), *Autism spectrum disorders: Identification, education, and treatment., 4th ed.* (pp. 66–95). Routledge/Taylor & Francis Group.

US Department of Health and Human Services, Administration for Children and Families, Administration on Children, Youth and Families, Children's Bureau. (2013). *Child maltreatment 2012.* Government Printing Office. Available from https://www.acf.hhs.gov/sites/default/files/cb/cm2012.pdf

Usami, M., Iwadare, Y., Watanabe, K., Kodaira, M., Ushijima, H., Tanaka, T., Harada, M., Tanaka, H., Sasaki, Y., & Saito, K. (2014). Decrease in the traumatic symptoms observed in child survivors within three years of the 2011 Japan earthquake and tsunami. *PLOS ONE, 9*(10), e110898.

van Beijsterveldt, C. E., Hudziak, J. J., & Boomsma, D. I. (2006). Genetic and environmental influences on cross-gender behavior and relation to behavior problems: a study of Dutch twins at ages 7 and 10 years. *Archives of Sexual Behavior, 35*(6), 647-58.

Van Beveren, B., Mezulis, A., Wante, L., & Braet, C. (2019). Joint contributions of negative emotionality, positive emotionality, and effortful control on depressive symptoms in youth. *Journal of Clinical Child and Adolescent Psychology, 48*(1), 131-42. https://doi.org/10.1080/15374416.2016.1233499

van Brakel, A. L., Muris, P., Bögels, S. M., & Thomassen, C. (2006). A multifactorial model for the etiology of anxiety in non-clinical adolescents: Main and interactive effects of behavioral inhibition, attachment and parental rearing. *Journal of Child & Family Studies, 15*(5), 568-78.

van den Bulk, B. G., Somerville, L. H., van Hoof, M., van Lang, N. J., van der Wee, N. A., Crone, E. A., & Vermeiren, R. M. (2016). Amygdala habituation to emotional faces in adolescents with internalizing disorders, adolescents with childhood sexual abuse related PTSD and healthy adolescents. *Developmental Cognitive Neuroscience, 21,* 15-25. https://doi.org/10.1016/j.dcn.2016.08.002

Vanderburgh, R. (2009). Appropriate therapeutic care for families with pre-pubescent transgender/gender-dissonant children. *Child & Adolescent Social Work Journal, 26*(2), 135-54. https://doi.org/10.1007/s10560-008-0158-5

van der Kolk, B. A. (2005). Developmental Trauma Disorder: Toward a rational diagnosis for children with complex trauma histories. *Psychiatric Annals, 35*(5), 401-8.

VanderLaan, D. P., Leef, J. H., Wood, H., Hughes, S. K., & Zucker, K. J. (2015). Autism spectrum disorder risk factors and autistic traits in gender dysphoric children. *Journal of Autism and Developmental Disorders, 45*(6), 1742-50. https://doi.org/10.1007/s10803-014-2331-3

van der Meer, D., Hartman, C. A., van Rooij, D., Franke, B., Heslenfeld, D. J., Oosterlaan, J., Faraone, S. V., Buitelaar, J. K., & Hoekstra, P. J. (2017). Effects of dopaminergic genes, prenatal adversities, and their interaction on attention-deficit/hyperactivity disorder and neural correlates of response inhibition. *Journal of Psychiatry & Neuroscience, 42*(2), 113–121. https://doi.org/10.1503/jpn.150350

van der Meer, D., Hoekstra, P. J., Bralten, J., van Donkelaar, M., Heslenfeld, D. J., Oosterlaan, J., Faraone, S. V., Franke, B., Buitelaar, J. K., & Hartman, C. A. (2016). Interplay between stress response genes associated with attention-deficit hyperactivity disorder and brain volume. *Genes, Brain, and Behavior, 15*(7), 627–636. https://doi.org/10.1111/gbb.12307

van der Meer, D., Hoekstra, P. J., Zwiers, M., Mennes, M., Schweren, L. J., Franke, B., Heslenfeld, D. J., Oosterlaan, J., Faraone, S. V., Buitelaar, J. K., & Hartman, C. A. (2015). Brain correlates of the interaction between 5-HTTLPR and psychosocial stress mediating attention deficit hyperactivity disorder severity. *The American Journal of Psychiatry, 172*(8), 768-75. https://doi.org/10.1176/appi.ajp.2015.14081035

Van der Oord, S., Prins, P. M., Oosterlaan, J., & Emmelkamp, P. G. (2008). Efficacy of methylphenidate, psychosocial treatments and their combination in school-aged children with ADHD: A meta-analysis. *Clinical Psychology Review, 28*(5), 783-800. https://doi.org/10.1016/j.cpr.2007.10.007

van Lieshout, M., Luman, M., Twisk, J. R., Faraone, S. V., Heslenfeld, D. J., Hartman, C. A., Hoekstra, P. J., Franke, B., Buitelaar, J. K., Rommelse, N. N. J., & Oosterlaan, J. (2017). Neurocognitive predictors of ADHD outcome: A 6-year follow-up study. *Journal of Abnormal Child Psychology, 45*(2), 261-72. https://doi.org/10.1007/s10802-016-0175-3

Van Oort, F. A., Greaves-Lord, K., Verhulst, F. C., Ormel, J., & Huizink, A. C. (2009). The developmental course of anxiety symptoms during adolescence: The TRIALS study. *Journal of Child Psychology and Psychiatry, 50*, 1209-17.

van Steensel, F. J., Bogels, S. M., & Perrin, S. (2011). Anxiety disorders in children and adolescents with autistic spectrum disorders: A meta-analysis. *Clinical Child and Family Psychology Review, 14*(3), 302-17. https://doi.org/10.1007/s10567-011-0097-0

Vasey, M. W., El-Hag, N., & Daleiden, E. L. (1996). Anxiety and the processing of emotionally threatening stimuli: Distinctive patterns of selective attention among high- and low-test-anxious children. *Child Development, 67*(3), 1173-85.

Vera, J., Granero, R., & Ezpeleta, L. (2012). Father's and mother's perceptions of parenting styles as mediators of the effects of parental psychopathology on antisocial behavior in outpatient children and adolescents. *Child Psychiatry and Human Development, 43*(3), 376-92. https://doi.org/10.1007/s10578-011-0272-z

Verduijn, N. C., Vincken, M. B., Meesters, C. G., & Engelhard, I. M. (2015). Emotional reasoning in acutely traumatized children and adolescents: An exploratory study. *Journal of Child and Family Studies, 24*(10), 2966-74. https://doi.org/10.1007/s10826-014-0100-8

Verduin, T. L., & Kendall, P. C. (2003). Differential occurrence of comorbidity within childhood anxiety disorders. *Journal of Clinical Child and Adolescent Psychology, 32*(2), 290-95.

Vernberg, E. M., La Greca, A. M., Silverman, W. K., & Prinstein, M. J. (1996). Prediction of posttraumatic stress symptoms in children after Hurricane Andrew. *Journal of Abnormal Psychology, 105*(2), 237-48. https://doi.org/10.1037/0021-843X.105.2.237

Vetter, N. C., Backhausen, L. L., Buse, J., Roessner, V., & Smolka, M. N. (2020). Altered brain morphology in boys with attention deficit hyperactivity disorder with and without comorbid conduct disorder/oppositional defiant disorder. *Human Brain Mapping, 41*(4), 973-83. https://doi.org/10.1002/hbm.24853

Vidal, S., Steeger, C. M., Caron, C., Lasher, L., & Connell, C. M. (2017). Placement and delinquency outcomes among system-involved youth referred to multisystemic therapy: A propensity score matching analysis. *Administration and Policy in Mental Health and Mental Health Services Research, 44*(6), 853-66. https://doi.org/10.1007/s10488-017-0797-y

Viktorin, A., Uher, R., Reichenberg, A., Levine, S. Z., & Sandin, S. (2017). Autism risk following antidepressant medication during pregnancy. *Psychological Medicine,* 47(16), 2787-96. https://doi.org/10.1017/S0033291717001301

Virués-Ortega, J. (2010). Applied behavior analytic intervention for autism in early childhood: Meta-analysis, meta-regression and dose–response meta-analysis of multiple outcomes. *Clinical Psychology Review, 30*(4), 387-99. https://doi.org/10.1016/j.cpr.2010.01.008

Vitiello, B. (2013). How effective are the current treatments for children diagnosed with manic/mixed bipolar disorder? *CNS Drugs, 27*(5), 331-33.

Vitiello, B., Rohde, P., Silva, S., Wells, K., Casat, C., Waslick, B., Simons, A., Reinecke, M., Weller, E., Kratochvil, C., Walkup, J., Pathak, S., Robins, M., March, J., & TADS Team (2006). Functioning and quality of life in the Treatment for Adolescents with Depression Study (TADS). *Journal of the American Academy of Child and Adolescent Psychiatry,* 45(12), 1419–1426. https://doi.org/10.1097/01.chi.0000242229.52646.6e

Vivanti, G., Paynter, J., Duncan, E., Fothergill, H., Dissanayake, C., & Rogers, S. J. (2014). Effectiveness and feasibility of the Early Start Denver Model implemented in a group-based community childcare setting. *Journal of Autism and Developmental Disorders, 44*(12), 3140-53. https://doi.org/10.1007/s10803-014-2168-9

Wachholtz, A. B., & Pargament, K. I. (2005). Is spirituality a critical ingredient of meditation? Comparing the effects of spiritual meditation, secular meditation, and relaxation on spiritual, psychological, cardiac, and pain outcomes. *Journal of Behavioral Medicine, 28*(4), 369-84.

Wade, T. D., Bulik, C. M., Neale, M., & Kendler, K. S. (2000). Anorexia nervosa and major depression: Shared genetic and environmental risk factors. *The American Journal of Psychiatry,* 157(3), 469-71. https://doi.org/10.1176/appi.ajp.157.3.469

Wade, T. D., Gordon, S., Medland, S., Bulik, C. M., Heath, A. C., Montgomery, G. W., & Martin, N. G. (2013). Genetic variants associated with disordered eating. *International Journal of Eating Disorders, 46*(6), 594-608. https://doi.org/10.1002/eat.22133

Wagner, D. V., Borduin, C. M., Sawyer, A. M., & Dopp, A. R. (2014). Long-term prevention of criminality in siblings of serious and violent juvenile offenders: A 25-year follow-up to a randomized clinical trial of multisystemic therapy. *Journal of Consulting and Clinical Psychology,* 82, 492–499. https://doi.org/10.1037/a0035624

Walker, D. F., Ahmed, S., Milevsky, A., Quagliana, H. L., & Bagasra, A. (2013). Sacred texts. In D. F. Walker & W. L. Hathaway (Eds.), *Spiritual interventions in child and adolescent psychotherapy* (pp. 155-80). American Psychological Association.

Walker, D. F., Doverspike, W., Ahmed, S., Milevsky, A., & Woolley, J. D. (2013). Prayer. In D. F. Walker & W. L. Hathaway (Eds.), *Spiritual interventions in child and adolescent psychotherapy* (pp. 181-207). American Psychological Association.

Walker, D. F., Partridge, K. J., Whitesell, A., Montes, B., & Hall, S. E. (2014). Cognitive-behavioral approaches to treatment. In K. S. Flanagan & S. E. Hall (Eds.), *Christianity and developmental psychopathology: Theory and application for working with youth* (pp. 319-86). InterVarsity Press.

Walker, D. F., Quagliana, H. L., Wilkinson, M., & Frederick, D. (2013). Christian-accommodative trauma-focused cognitive-behavioral therapy for children and adolescents. In E. L. Worthington, E. L. Johnson, J. N. Hook, & J. D. Aten (Eds.), *Evidence-based practices for Christian counseling and psychotherapy* (pp. 101-21). InterVarsity Press.

Walker, D. F., Reese, J. B., Hughes, J. P., & Troskie, M. J. (2010). Addressing religious and spiritual issues in trauma-focused cognitive behavior therapy with children and adolescents. *Professional Psychology: Research and Practice, 41*(2), 174-80.

Walkup, J. T., Albano, A. M., Piacentini, J., Birmaher, B., Compton, S. N., Sherrill, J. T., Ginsburg, G., Rynn, M., McCracken, J., Waslick, B., Iyengar, S., March, J., & Kendall, P. C. (2008). Cognitive behavioral therapy, sertraline, or a combination in childhood anxiety. *New England Journal of Medicine, 359*, 2753-66.

Waller, R., Hyde, L. W., Klump, K. L., & Burt, S. A. (2018). Parenting is an environmental predictor of callous-unemotional traits and aggression: A monozygotic twin differences study. *Journal of the American Academy of Child & Adolescent Psychiatry, 57*(12), 955-63. https://doi.org/10.1016/j.jaac.2018.07.882

Wallien, M. S., & Cohen-Kettenis, P. T. (2008). Psychosexual outcome of gender-dysphoric children. *Journal of the American Academy of Child and Adolescent Psychiatry, 47*(12), 1413-23.

Walsh, M. (2016). Autism, culture, church: From disruption to hope. *Journal of Disability & Religion, 20*(4), 343-51. https://doi.org/10.1080/23312521.2016.1239916

Wampold, B. (2015). How important are the common factors in psychotherapy? An update. *World Psychiatry, 14*(3), 270-77. https://doi.org/10.1002/wps.20238

Wamser-Nanney, R., & Vandenberg, B. R. (2013). Empirical support for the definition of a complex trauma event in children and adolescents. *Journal of Traumatic Stress, 26*(6), 671-78. https://doi.org/10.1002/jts.21857

Wang, C., Chan, C. W., & Ho, R. H. (2013). Prevalence and trajectory of psychopathology among child and adolescent survivors of disasters: A systematic review of epidemiological studies across 1987–2011. *Social Psychiatry and Psychiatric Epidemiology, 48*(11), 1697-1720. https://doi.org/10.1007/s00127-013-0731-x

Wang, D. C., Aten, J. D., Boan, D., Jean-Charles, W., Griff, K. P., Valcin, V. C., Davis, E. B., Hook, J. N., Davis, D. E., Van Tongeren, D. R., Abouezzeddine, T., Sklar, Q., & Wang, A. (2016). Culturally adapted spiritually oriented trauma-focused cognitive–behavioral therapy for child survivors of restavek. *Spirituality in Clinical Practice, 3*(4), 224-36. https://doi.org/10.1037/scp0000101

Wang, M., Tian, X., & Zhang, W. (2020). Interactions between the combined genotypes of 5-HTTLPR and BDNF Val66Met polymorphisms and parenting on adolescent depressive symptoms: A three-year longitudinal study. *Journal of Affective Disorders, 265*(15), 104-11. https://doi.org/10.1016/j.jad.2020.01.064

Wang, Y., Tian, L., Guo, L., & Huebner, E. S. (2020). Family dysfunction and adolescents' anxiety and depression: A multiple mediation model. *Journal of Applied Developmental Psychology, 66.* https://doi.org/10.1016/j.appdev.2019.101090

Waszczuk, M. A., Zavos, H. S., Gregory, A. M., & Eley, T. C. (2014). The phenotypic and genetic structure of depression and anxiety disorder symptoms in childhood, adolescence, and young adulthood. *JAMA Psychiatry, 71*, 905-16.

Watson, J. R. (2002). *An annotated anthology of hymns.* Oxford University Press.

Way, B. M., & Taylor, S. E. (2010). Social influences on health: is serotonin a critical mediator? *Psychosomatic Medicine, 72*(2), 107-12.

Weathers, J., Lippard, E. T. C., Spencer, L., Pittman, B., Wang, F., & Blumberg, H. P. (2018). Longitudinal diffusion tensor imaging study of adolescents and young adults with bipolar disorder. *Journal of the American Academy of Child & Adolescent Psychiatry, 57*(2), 111-17. https://doi.org/10.1016/j.jaac.2017.11.014

Webb, C., Hayes, A. M., Grasso, D., Laurenceau, J., & Deblinger, E. (2014). Trauma-focused cognitive behavioral therapy for youth: Effectiveness in a community setting. *Psychological Trauma: Theory, Research, Practice, and Policy, 6*(5), 555-62. https://doi.org/10.1037/a0037364

Webb, M. (2012). Toward a theology of mental illness. *Journal of Religion, Disability & Health, 16*(1), 49-73. https://doi.org/10.1080/15228967.2012.645608

Webster-Stratton, C. (1994). Advancing videotape parent training: A comparison study. *Journal of Consulting and Clinical Psychology, 62*(3), 585-93.

Webster-Stratton, C., & Hammond, M. (1998). Conduct problems and levels of social competence in Head Start children: Prevalence, pervasiveness, and associated risk factors. *Clinical Child Psychology and Family Psychology Review, 1,* 101-24.

Webster-Stratton, C., & Reid, M. J. (2010). The Incredible Years Parents, Teachers, and Children Training Series: A multifaceted treatment approach for young children with conduct disorders. In J. R. Weisz & A. E. Kazdin (Eds.), *Evidence-based psychotherapies for children and adolescents* (2nd ed., pp. 194-210). Guilford.

Webster-Stratton, C., Reid, M. J., & Hammond, M. (2004). Treating children with early-onset conduct problems: Intervention outcomes for parent, child, and teacher training. *Journal of Clinical Child and Adolescent Psychology, 33*(1), 105-24.

Wechsler, D. (2008). *Wechsler Adult Intelligence Scale—Fourth Edition.* Pearson Clinical.

Wechsler, D. (2012). *Wechsler Preschool and Primary Scale of Intelligence—Fourth Edition.* Pearson Clinical.

Wechsler, D. (2014). *Wechsler Intelligence Scale for Children—Fifth Edition.* Pearson Clinical.

Weems, C. (2008). Developmental trajectories of childhood anxiety: Identifying continuity and change in anxious emotion. *Developmental Review, 28*(4), 488–502. https://doi.org/10.1016/j.dr.2008.01.001

Weems, C. F., & Carrión, V. G. (2008). Brief report: Diurnal salivary cortisol in youth—clarifying the nature of posttraumatic stress dysregulation. *Journal of Pediatric Psychology, 34*(4), 389-95. https://doi.org/10.1093/jpepsy/jsn087

Weems, C. F., Klabunde, M., Russell, J. D., Reiss, A. L., & Carrión, V. G. (2015). Post-traumatic stress and age variation in amygdala volumes among youth exposed to trauma. *Social Cognitive and Affective Neuroscience, 10*(12), 1661-67. https://doi.org/10.1093/scan/nsv053

Weems, C. F., Silverman, W., Rapee, R., & Pina, A. (2003). The role of control in childhood anxiety disorders. *Cognitive Therapy and Research, 27*(5), 557-68. https://doi.org/10.1023/A:1026307121386

Weersing, V., Jeffreys, M., Do, M., Schwartz, K., & Bolano, C. (2017). Evidence base update of psychosocial treatments for child and adolescent depression. *Journal of Clinical Child and Adolescent Psychology, 46*(1), 11-43. https://doi.org/10.1080/15374416.2016.1220310

Wei, C., Cummings, C. M., Villabø, M. A., & Kendall, P. C. (2014). Parenting behaviors and anxious self-talk in youth and parents. *Journal of Family Psychology, 28*(3), 299-307.

Wei, Y., Wang, L., Wang, R., Cao, C., Shi, Z., & Zhang, J. (2013). Prevalence and predictors of posttraumatic stress disorder among Chinese youths after an earthquake. *Social Behavior and Personality*, *41*(10), 1613-24. https://doi.org/10.2224/sbp.2013.41.10.1613

Weinstein, S. M., Henry, D. B., Katz, A. C., Peters, A. T., & West, A. E. (2015). Treatment moderators of child- and family-focused cognitive-behavioral therapy for pediatric bipolar disorder. *Journal of the American Academy of Child & Adolescent Psychiatry*, *54*(2), 116-25.

Weiss, B., & Garber, J. (2003). Developmental differences in the phenomenology of depression. *Development and Psychopathology*, *15*(2), 403-30.

Weissman, M. M., Markowitz, J. C., & Klerman, G. L. (2000). *A comprehensive guide to interpersonal therapy*. Basic Books.

Weisz, J. R., Donenberg, G. R., Han, S. S., & Weiss, B. (1995). Bridging the gap between laboratory and clinic in child and adolescent psychotherapy. *Journal of Consulting and Clinical Psychology*, *63*(5), 688-701. https://doi.org/10.1037/0022-006X.63.5.688

Weisz, J. R., McCarty, C. A., Eastman, K. L., Chaiyasit, W., & Suwanlert, S. (1997). Developmental psychopathology and culture: Ten lessons from Thailand. In S. S. Luthar, J. A. Burack, D. Cicchetti, & J. R. Weisz (Eds.), *Developmental psychopathology: Perspectives on adjustment, risk, and disorder* (pp. 568-92). Cambridge University Press.

Werling, D. M., & Geschwind, D. H. (2015). Recurrence rates provide evidence for sex-differential, familial genetic liability for autism spectrum disorders in multiplex families and twins. *Molecular Autism*, *6*, 27. https://doi.org/10.1186/s13229-015-0004-5

Werner, E., Dawson, G., Munson, J., & Osterling, J. (2005). Variation in early developmental course in autism and its relation with behavioral outcome at 3-4 years of age. *Journal of Autism and Developmental Disorders*, *35*(3), 337-50. https://doi.org/10.1007/s10803-005-3301-6

Werner, E. E., & Smith, R. S. (1992). *Overcoming the odds: High risk children from birth to adulthood*. Cornell University Press.

West, A. E., Jacobs, R. H., Westerholm, R., Lee, A., Carbray, J., Heidenreich, J., & Pavuluri, M. N. (2009). Child and family-focused cognitive-behavioral therapy for pediatric bipolar disorder: pilot study of group treatment format. *Journal of the Canadian Academy of Child and Adolescent Psychiatry*, *18*(3), 239-46.

West, A. E., & Pavuluri, M. N. (2009). Psychosocial treatments for childhood and adolescent bipolar disorder. *Child and Adolescent Psychiatric Clinics of North America*, *18*(2), 471-82.

West, A. E., Weinstein, S. M., Peters, A. T., Katz, A. C., Henry, D. B., Cruz, R. A., & Pavuluri, M. N. (2014). Child- and family-focused cognitive-behavioral therapy for pediatric bipolar disorder: A randomized clinical trial. *Journal of the American Academy of Child and Adolescent Psychiatry*, *53*(11), 1168-78.

Westerberg-Jacobson, J., Edlund, B., & Ghaderi, A. (2010a). A 5-year longitudinal study of the relationship between the wish to be thinner, lifestyle behaviours and disturbed eating in 9–20-year old girls. *European Eating Disorders Review*, *18*(3), 207-19. https://doi.org/10.1002/erv.983

Westerberg-Jacobson, J., Edlund, B., & Ghaderi, A. (2010b). Risk and protective factors for disturbed eating: A 7-year longitudinal study of eating attitudes and psychological factors in adolescent girls and their parents. *Eating and Weight Disorders*, *15*(4), e208-e218. https://doi.org/10.1007/BF03325302

White, F. W., Brislin, S., Sinclair, S., Fowler, K. A., Pope, K., & Blair, R. J. R. (2013). The relationship between large cavum septum pellucidum and antisocial behavior, callous-unemotional traits, and psychopathy and adolescents. *Journal of Child Psychology and Psychiatry*, *54*(5), 575-81.

White, J., Shelton, K. H., & Elgar, F. J. (2014). Prospective associations between the family environment, family cohesion, and psychiatric symptoms among adolescent girls. *Child Psychiatry and Human Development, 45*(5), 544-54.

Whitehead, A. L. (2018). Religion and disability: Variation in religious service attendance rates for children with chronic health conditions. *Journal for the Scientific Study of Religion, 57*(2), 377-95.

Wichstrøm, L., & von Soest, T. (2016). Reciprocal relations between body satisfaction and self-esteem: A large 13-year prospective study of adolescents. *Journal of Adolescence, 47*, 16-27. https://doi.org/10.1016/j.adolescence.2015.12.003

Widstrom, A. M., Ransjo-Arvidson, A. B., & Christensson, K. (1987). Gastric suction in healthy newborn infants: Effects on circulation and developing feeding behaviour. *Acta Paediatrica Scandinavica, 76*(4), 566-72.

Wierenga, C., Bischoff-Grethe, A., Melrose, A., Torres, L., Irvine, L., & Bailer, U. F. (2014). Hunger does not motivate reward in women remitted from anorexia nervosa. *Biological Psychiatry, 77*(7), 642-52. https://doi.org/10.1016/j.biopsych.2014.09.024

Wierenga, C. E., Ely, A., Bischoff-Grethe, A., Bailer, U. F., Simmons, A. N., & Kaye, W. H. (2014). Are extremes of consumption in eating disorders related to an altered balance between reward and inhibition? *Frontiers in Behavioral Neuroscience, 8*, 410.

Wigal, T., Greenhill, L., Chuang, S., McGough, J., Vitiello, B., Skrobala, A., Swanson, J., Wigal, S., Abikoff, H., Kollins, S., McCracken, J., Riddle, M., Posner, K., Ghuman, J., Davies, M., Thorp, B., & Stehli, A. (2006). Safety and tolerability of methylphenidate in preschool children with ADHD. *Journal of the American Academy of Child & Adolescent Psychiatry, 45*(11), 1294-1303. https://doi.org/10.1097/01.chi.0000235082.63156.27

Wiggs, K., Elmore, A. L., Nigg, J. T., & Nikolas, M. A. (2016). Pre- and perinatal risk for attention-deficit hyperactivity disorder: Does neuropsychological weakness explain the link? *Journal of Abnormal Child Psychology, 44*(8), 1473-85. https://doi.org/10.1007/s10802-016-0142-z

Wilens, T., Martelon, M., Joshi, G., Bateman, C., Fried, R., Petty, C., & Biederman, J. (2011). Does ADHD predict substance-use disorders? A 10-year follow-up study of young adults with ADHD. *Journal of the American Academy of Child & Adolescent Psychiatry, 50*(6), 543-53. https://doi.org/10.1016/j.jaac.2011.01.021

Wilens, T. E., Robertson, B., Sikirica, V., Harper, L., Young, J. L., Bloomfield, R., Lyne, A., Rynkowski, G., & Cutler, A. J. (2015). A randomized, placebo-controlled trial of guanfacine extended release in adolescents with attention-deficit/hyperactivity disorder. *Journal of the American Academy of Child & Adolescent Psychiatry, 54*(11), 916-25. https://doi.org/10.1016/j.jaac.2015.08.016

Willcutt, E. G. (2012). The prevalence of DSM-IV attention deficit/hyperactivity disorder: A meta-analytic review. *Neurotherapeutics, 9*(3), 490-99.

Willcutt, E. G., Doyle, A. E., Nigg, J. T., Faraone, S. V., & Pennington, B. F. (2005). Validity of the executive function theory of attention-deficit/hyperactivity disorder: A meta-analytic review. *Biological Psychiatry, 57*(11), 1336-46. https://doi.org/10.1016/j.biopsych.2005.02.006

Williams, G., Chamove, A. S., & Millar, H. R. (1990). Eating disorders, perceived control, assertiveness and hostility. *British Journal of Clinical Psychology, 29*(3), 327-35. https://doi.org/10.1111/j.2044-8260.1990.tb00889.x

Williams, N. M., Franke, B., Mick, E., Anney, R. L., Freitag, C. M., Gill, M., Thapar, A., O'Donovan, M., Owen, M., Holmans, P., Kent, L., Middleton, F., Zhang-James, Y., Liu, L., Meyer, J., Nguyen, T. T., Romanos, J., Romanos, M., Seitz, C., . . . Faraone, S. V. (2012). Genome-wide analysis of copy number variants in attention deficit hyperactivity disorder: The role of rare variants and duplications at 15q13.3. *The American Journal of Psychiatry, 169*(2), 195-204. https://doi.org/10.1176/appi.ajp.2011.11060822

Winje, D., & Ulvik, A. (1998). Long-term outcome of trauma in children: The psychological consequences of a bus accident. *Journal of Child Psychology and Psychiatry, 39*(5), 635-42.

Winters, K., Temple Newhook, J., Pyne, J., Feder, S., Jamieson, A., Holmes, C., Sinnott, M., Pickett, S., & Tosh, J. (2018). Learning to listen to trans and gender diverse children: A response to Zucker (2018) and Steensma and Cohen-Kettenis (2018). *International Journal of Transgenderism, 19*(2), 246-50. https://doi.org/10.1080/15532739.2018.1471767

Wolford, S. N., Cooper, A. N., & McWey, L. M. (2019). Maternal depression, maltreatment history, and child outcomes: The role of harsh parenting. *American Journal of Orthopsychiatry, 89*(2), 181-91. https://doi.org/10.1037/ort0000365

Wolke, D., Rizzo, P., & Woods, S. (2002). Persistent infant crying and hyperactivity problems in middle childhood. *Pediatrics, 109*(6), 1054-60.

Wolmer, L., Hamiel, D., Versano-Eisman, T., Slone, M., Margalit, N., & Laor, N. (2015). Preschool Israeli children exposed to rocket attacks: Assessment, risk, and resilience. *Journal of Traumatic Stress, 28*(5), 441-47. https://doi.org/10.1002/jts.22040

Wolpe, J. (1990). *The practice of behavior therapy* (4th ed.). Pergamon.

Wolraich, M. L., McKeown, R. E., Visser, S. N., Bard, D., Cuffe, S., Neas, B., Geryk, L. L., Doffing, M., Bottai, M., Abramowitz, A. J., Beck, L., Holbrook, J. R., & Danielson, M. (2014). The prevalence of ADHD: Its diagnosis and treatment in four school districts across two states. *Journal of Attention Disorders, 18*(7), 563-75. https://doi.org/10.1177/1087054712453169

Woltering, S., Lishak, V., Hodgson, N., Ganic, N., & Zelazo, P. D. (2016). Executive function in children with externalizing and comorbid internalizing behavior problems. *Journal of Child Psychology and Psychiatry, 57*(1), 30-38.

Wong, H. M., & Goh, E. L. (2014). Dynamics of ADHD in familial contexts: Perspectives from children and parents and implications for practitioners. *Social Work in Health Care, 53*(7), 601-16. https://doi.org/10.1080/00981389.2014.924462

Wood, A. G., Nadebaum, C., Anderson, V., Reutens, D., Barton, S., O'Brien, T. J., & Vajda, F. (2015). Prospective assessment of autism traits in children exposed to antiepileptic drugs during pregnancy. *Epilepsia, 56*(7), 1047-55. https://doi.org/10.1111/epi.13007

Woolfenden, S., Sarkozy, V., Ridley, G., & Williams, K. (2012). A systematic review of the diagnostic stability of autism spectrum disorder. *Research in Autism Spectrum Disorders, 6*(1), 345-54. https://doi.org/10.1016/j.rasd.2011.06.008

World Health Organization. (1995). *Environmental Health Criteria 165: Inorganic Lead.* International Programme on Chemical Safety.

World Professional Association for Transgender Health. (2012). Standards of care for the health of transsexual, transgender, and gender nonconforming people. Retrieved from https://wpath.org/publications/soc

Wozniak, J., Biederman, J., Kiely, K., Stuart, A. J., Faraone, S. V., Mundy, E., & Mennin, D. (1995). Mania-like symptoms suggestive of childhood-onset bipolar disorder in clinically referred children. *Journal of the American Academy of Child and Adolescent Psychiatry, 34*(7), 867-76.

Wu, M., Hartmann, M., Skunde, M., Herzog, W., & Friederich, H. (2013). Inhibitory control in bulimic-type eating disorders: A systematic review and meta-analysis. *PLOS ONE 8*(12): e83412. https://doi.org/10.1371/journal.pone.0083412

Wyciszkiewicz, A., Pawlak, M. A., & Krawiec, K. (2017). Cerebellar volume in children with attention-deficit hyperactivity disorder (ADHD): Replication study. *Journal of Child Neurology, 32*(2), 215-21. https://doi.org/10.1177/0883073816678550

Wymbs, B. T., Wymbs, F. A., & Dawson, A. E. (2015). Child ADHD and ODD behavior interacts with parent ADHD symptoms to worsen parenting and interparental communication. *Journal of Abnormal Child Psychology, 43*(1), 107-19. https://doi.org/10.1007/s10802-014-9887-4

Xie, P., Kranzler, H. R., Poling, J., Stein, M. B., Anton, R. F., Brady, K., Weiss, R. D., Farrer, L., & Gelernter, J. (2009). Interactive effect of stressful life events and the serotonin transporter 5-HTTLPR genotype on posttraumatic stress disorder diagnosis in 2 independent populations. *Archives of General Psychiatry, 66*(11), 1201-9. https://doi.org/10.1001/archgenpsychiatry.2009.153

Xu, J., Zwaigenbaum, L., Szatmari, P., & Scherer, S. W. (2004). Molecular cytogenetics of autism. *Current Genomics, 5*(4), 347-64. https://doi.org/10.2174/1389202043349246

Xu, K., & Yuan, P. (2014). Effects of three sources of social support on survivors' posttraumatic stress after the Wenchuan earthquake. *Journal of Loss and Trauma, 19*(3), 229-43. https://doi.org/10.1080/15325024.2013.791516

Xu, M., Jiang, W., Du, Y., Li, Y., & Fan, J. (2017). Executive function features in drug-naive children with oppositional defiant disorder. *Shanghai Archives of Psychiatry, 29*(4), 228-36.

Yamazaki, Y., & Omori, M. (2016). The relationship between mothers' thin-ideal and children's drive for thinness: A survey of Japanese early adolescents and their mothers. *Journal of Health Psychology, 21*(1), 100-111. https://doi.org/10.1177/1359105314522676

Yap, M. H., Allen, N. B., & Sheeber, L. (2007). Using an emotion regulation framework to understand the role of temperament and family processes in risk for adolescent depressive disorders. *Clinical Child and Family Psychology Review, 10*(2), 180-96.

Yap, M. H., Schwartz, O. S., Byrne, M. L., Simmons, J. G., & Allen, N. B. (2010). Maternal positive and negative interaction behaviors and early adolescents' depressive symptoms: Adolescent emotion regulation as a mediator. *Journal of Research on Adolescence, 20*(4), 1014-43.

Yarhouse, M. A. (2015). *Understanding gender dysphoria: Navigating transgender issues in a changing culture.* InterVarsity Press.

Yarhouse, M. A., & Carr, T. L. (2012). MTF transgender Christians' experiences: A qualitative study. *Journal of LGBT Issues in Counseling, 6*(1), 18-33.

Yeung, N. C. Y., Lau, J. T. F., Yu, N. X., Zhang, J., Xu, Z., Choi, K. C., Zhang, Q., Mak, W. W. S., & Lui, W. W. S. (2018). Media exposure related to the 2008 Sichuan Earthquake predicted probable PTSD among Chinese adolescents in Kunming, China: A longitudinal study. *Psychological Trauma: Theory, Research, Practice, and Policy, 10*(2), 253-62. https://doi.org/10.1037/tra0000121

Ying, L., Wu, X., Lin, C., & Jiang, L. (2014). Traumatic severity and trait resilience as predictors of posttraumatic stress disorder and depressive symptoms among adolescent survivors of the Wenchuan earthquake. *PLOS ONE, 9*(2), e89401. https://doi.org/10.1371/journal.pone.0089401

Yoder, P. J., & McDuffie, A. S. (2006). Treatment of responding to and initiating joint attention. In T. Charman & W. Stone (Eds.), *Social & communication development in autism spectrum disorders: Early identification, diagnosis, & intervention* (pp. 117-42). Guilford.

Yoo, H. (2015). Genetics of autism spectrum disorder: Current status and possible clinical applications. *Experimental Neurobiology, 24*, 257-72.

Youngstrom, E. A., & Algorta, G. P. (2014). Pediatric bipolar disorder. In E. J. Mash & R. A. Barkley (Eds.), *Child psychopathology* (3rd ed., pp. 264-316). Guilford.

Youngstrom, E. A., Findling, R. L., Danielson, C. K., & Calabrese, J. R. (2001). Discriminative validity of parent report of hypomanic and depressive symptoms on the General Behavior Inventory. *Psychological Assessment, 13*(2), 267-76.

Youngstrom, E. A., Findling, R. L., Youngstrom, J. K., & Calabrese, J. R. (2005). Toward an evidence-based assessment of pediatric bipolar disorder. *Journal of Clinical Child and Adolescent Psychology, 34*(3), 433-48.

Yuen, R. K., Thiruvahindrapuram, B., Merico, D., Walker, S., Tammimies, K., Hoang, N., Chrysler, C., Nalpathamkalam, T., Pellecchia, G., Liu, Y., Gazzellone, M. J., D'Abate, L., Deneault, E., Howe, J. L., Liu, R. S., Thompson, A., Zarrei, M., Uddin, M., Marshall, C. R., Ring, R. H., … Scherer, S. W. (2015). Whole-genome sequencing of quartet families with autism spectrum disorder. *Nature Medicine, 21*(2), 185–191. https://doi.org/10.1038/nm.3792

Yule, W., Bolton, D., Udwin, O., Boyle, S., O'Ryan, D., & Nurrish, J. (2000). The long-term psychological effects of a disaster experienced in adolescence: I: The incidence and course of PTSD. *Journal of Child Psychology and Psychiatry, 41*(4), 503-11. https://doi.org/10.1111/1469-7610.00635

Zarychta, K., Mullan, B., Kruk, M., & Luszczynska, A. (2017). A vicious cycle among cognitions and behaviors enhancing risk for eating disorders. *BMC Psychiatry, 17*, 154.

Zastrow, A., Kaiser, S., Stippich, C., Walther, S., Herzog, W., Tchanturia, K., Belger, A., Weisbrod, M., Treasure, J., & Friederich, H. C. (2009). Neural correlates of impaired cognitive-behavioral flexibility in anorexia nervosa. *American Journal of Psychiatry, 166*(5), 608–616. https://doi.org/10.1176/appi.ajp.2008.08050775

Zastrow, B., Martel, M., & Widiger, T. (2018). Preschool oppositional defiant disorder: A disorder of negative affect, surgency, and disagreeableness. *Journal of Clinical Child & Adolescent Psychology, 47*(6), 967-77. https://doi.org/10.1080/15374416.2016.1225504

Zendarski, N., Sciberras, E., Mensah, F., & Hiscock, H. (2017). Academic achievement and risk factors for adolescents with attention-deficit hyperactivity disorder in middle school and early high school. *Journal of Developmental and Behavioral Pediatrics, 38*(6), 358-68. https://doi.org/10.1097/DBP.0000000000000460

Zhang, J., Zhu, S., Du, C., & Zhang, Y. (2015). Post-traumatic stress disorder and somatic symptoms among child and adolescent survivors following the Lushan earthquake in China: A six-month longitudinal study. *Journal of Psychosomatic Research, 79*(2), 100-106. https://doi.org/10.1016/j.jpsychores.2015.06.001

Zhang, W., Jiang, X., Ho, K., & Wu, D. (2011). The presence of post-traumatic stress disorder symptoms in adolescents three months after an 8·0 magnitude earthquake in southwest China. *Journal of Clinical Nursing, 20*(21-22), 3057-69. https://doi.org/10.1111/j.1365-2702.2011.03825.x

Zhang, W., Liu, H., Jiang, X., Wu, D., & Tian, Y. (2014). A longitudinal study of posttraumatic stress disorder symptoms and its relationship with coping skill and locus of control in adolescents after an earthquake in China. *PLOS ONE, 9*(2), e88263. https://doi.org/10.1371/journal.pone.0088263.

Zhang, Y., Zhang, J., Zhu, S., Du, C., & Zhang, W. (2015). Prevalence and predictors of somatic symptoms among child and adolescents with probable posttraumatic stress disorder: A cross-sectional study conducted in 21 primary and secondary schools after an earthquake. *PLOS ONE, 10*(9), e0137101.

Zhou, X., Wu, X., Fu, F., & An, Y. (2015). Core belief challenge and rumination as predictors of PTSD and PTG among adolescent survivors of the Wenchuan earthquake. *Psychological Trauma: Theory, Research, Practice, and Policy*, *7*(4), 391-97. https://doi.org/10.1037/tra0000031

Zhu, J. L., Olsen, J., Liew, Z., Li, J., Niclasen, J., & Obel, C. (2014). Parental smoking during pregnancy and ADHD in children: The Danish National Birth Cohort. *Pediatrics*, *134*(2), e382-e388. https://doi.org/10.1542/peds.2014-0213

Zimmer-Gembeck, M. J., Nesdale, D., Webb, H. J., Khatibi, M., & Downey, G. (2016). A longitudinal rejection sensitivity model of depression and aggression: Unique roles of anxiety, anger, blame, withdrawal and retribution. *Journal of Abnormal Child Psychology*, *44*, 1291-1307. https://doi.org/10.1007/s10802-016-0127-y

Ziobrowski, H. N., Sonneville, K. R., Eddy, K. T., Crosby, R. D., Micali, N., Horton, N. J., & Field, A. E. (2019). Maternal eating disorders and eating disorder treatment among girls in the Growing Up Today Study. *Journal of Adolescent Health*, *65*(4), 469-75. https://doi.org/10.1016/j.jadohealth.2019.04.031

Zisser, A., & Eyberg, S. M. (2010). Parent-Child Interaction Therapy and the treatment of disruptive behavior disorders. In J. R. Weisz & A. E. Kazdin (Eds.), *Evidence-based psychotherapies for children and adolescents* (2nd ed., pp. 179-93). Guilford.

Zisser-Nathenson, A. R., Herschell, A. D., & Eyberg, S. M. (2018). Parent-child interaction therapy and the treatment of disruptive behavior disorders. In J. R. Weisz & A. E. Kazdin (Eds.), *Evidence-based psychotherapies for children and adolescents* (3rd ed., pp. 103-21). Guilford Press.

Ziv, Y. (2012). Exposure to violence, social information processing, and problem behavior in preschool children. *Aggressive Behavior, 38*(6), 429-41.

Zucker, K. (2018). The myth of persistence: Response to "A critical commentary on follow-up studies and 'desistance' theories about transgender and gender non-conforming children" by Temple Newhook et al. (2018). *International Journal of Transgenderism, 19*(2), 231-45. https://doi.org/10.1080/15532739.2018.1468293

Zucker, K. J., & Bradley, S. J. (1995). *Gender identity disorder and psychosexual problems in children and adolescents*. Guilford Press.

Zucker, K. J., Wood, H., Singh, D., & Bradley, S. J. (2012). A developmental, biopsychosocial model for the treatment of children with gender identity disorder. *Journal of Homosexuality, 59*(3), 369-97. https://doi.org/10.1080/00918369.2012.653309

Zucker, K. J., Wood, H., & VanderLaan, D. P. (2014). Models of psychopathology in children and adolescents with gender dysphoria. In B. P. C. Kreukels, T. D. Steensma, & A. L. C. de Vries (Eds.), *Gender dysphoria and disorders of sex development: Progress in care and knowledge* (pp. 171-92). Springer.

Zwaigenbaum, L., Bauman, M. L., Fein, D., Pierce, K., Buie, T., Davis, P. A., Newschaffer, C., Robins, D. L., Wetherby, A., Choueiri, R., Kasari, C., Stone, W. L., Yirmiya, N., Estes, A., Hansen, R., McPartland, J. C., Natowicz, M. R., Carter, A., Granpeesheh, D., . . . Wagner, S. (2015). Early screening of autism spectrum disorder: Recommendations for practice and research. *Pediatrics, 136*(Suppl 1), S41-S59. https://doi.org/10.1542/peds.2014-3667D

Zwaigenbaum, L., Bryson, S., Rogers, T., Roberts, W., Brian, J., & Szatmari, P. (2005). Behavioral manifestations of autism in the first year of life. *International Journal of Developmental Neuroscience, 23*(2-3), 143-52. https://doi.org/10.1016/j.ijdevneu.2004.05.001

Subject Index

Scripture Index

Also Available

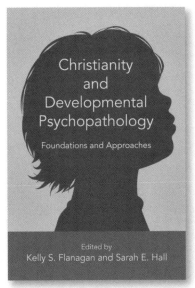

***Christianity and Developmental
Psychopathology***
978-0-8308-2855-5

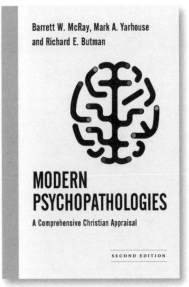

Modern Psychopathologies
978-0-8308-2850-0

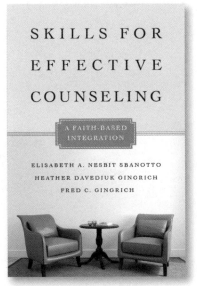

Skills for Effective Counseling
978-0-8308-2860-9

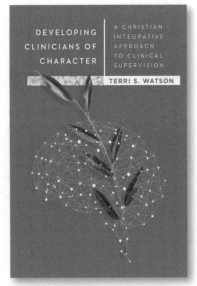

***Developing Clinicians
of Character***
978-0-8308-2863-0

Finding the Textbook You Need

The IVP Academic Textbook Selector
is an online tool for instantly finding the IVP books
suitable for over 250 courses across 24 disciplines.

---

ivpacademic.com